STRESS

STRESS
Neurobiology and Neuroendocrinology

Edited by

MARVIN R. BROWN

University of California, San Diego
San Diego, California

GEORGE F. KOOB

Research Institute of the Scripps Clinic
La Jolla, California

University of California, San Diego
San Diego, California

CATHERINE RIVIER

The Salk Institute
La Jolla, California

MARCEL DEKKER, INC.   New York · Basel · Hong Kong

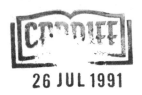

Library of Congress Cataloging-in-Publication Data

Stress: neurobiology and neuroendocrinology / edited by Marvin R. Brown,
George Koob, Catherine Rivier.
  p. cm.
Includes bibliographical references.
Includes index.
ISBN 0-8247-8325-5 (alk. paper)
1. Stress (Physiology) 2. Stress (Psychology) 3. Homeostasis. 4. Neuroendo-
crinology. 5. Medicine, Psychosomatic. 6. Neurophysiology. I. Brown, Marvin
R. II. Koob, George F. III. Rivier, Catherine.
  [DNLM: 1. Disease—etiology. 2. Homeostasis—physiology. 3. Neuroimmuno-
modulation. 5. Stress, Psychological—physiopathology. WM 172 S91546]
QP82.2.S8S883   1990
616.9'8—dc20
DNLM/DLC
for Library of Congress   90-14098
                                                                            CIP

This book is printed on acid-free paper

MARCEL DEKKER, INC.
270 Madison Avenue, New York, New York 10016

Current printing (last digit):
10 9 8 7 6 5 4 3 2 1

PRINTED IN THE UNITED STATES OF AMERICA

PREFACE

In recent years it has become evident that the stress response plays an important role in the development of a variety of human diseases. In contrast to other types of pathologies, stress-related diseases often represent a complication or side effect of the actions of the body's regulatory systems. A complex array of regulatory mechanisms work to ensure the smooth functioning and maintenance of the organism's physiological systems when facing physical or psychological challenges. Indeed, an animal's ability to successfully respond to short- or long-term threats to its homeostasis represents a hallmark of successful adaptation.

In attempting to maintain homeostasis, regulatory systems can go awry, sometimes compromising the organism's survival. The etiology of many human diseases involves regulatory components which are working to maintain "milieu interieur" stability in response to stressors.

It is unlikely that a single genetic defect can explain the role of the stress response in the development of human disease. It is more likely that complex interactions between the systems involved in homeostasis and the organism's particular genetic and pathologic makeup determine the emergence of stressor-associated disease processes.

The principal purpose of this book is to assemble the research and opinions of selected investigators who have explored and characterized the mechanisms of stressor-induced diseases. The four broad areas of discussion include historical perspectives on the study of stress, the regulation and integration of homeostatic processes, the role of the regulatory processes in the development of stressor-induced pathophysiology, and a description of stress management. The goal of this text is to encapsulate scientific information pertinent to stress processes and stressor-induced diseases, and to serve as a catalyst for the development of innovative methods and approaches for further studies in stress biology.

Marvin R. Brown
George F. Koob
Catherine Rivier

CONTENTS

ROLE OF HOMEOSTATIC PROCESSES IN THE DEVELOPMENT OF
PATHOPHYSIOLOGY FOLLOWING STRESS

CONTRIBUTORS

Byron J. Allen, M.D. Department of Medicine, University of California School of Medicine, Irvine Medical Center, Orange, California

Nathan M. Appel, Ph.D. Neuropeptide Unit, Neuroscience Branch, Addiction Research Center, National Institute on Drug Abuse, National Institutes of Health, Bethesda, Maryland

J.A. Barbosa, M.D. Department of Medicine, University of California and Veterans Administration Medical Center, San Diego, California

Michael A. Brodsky, M.D. Department of Medicine, University of California School of Medicine, Irvine Medical Center, Orange, California

Marvin R. Brown, M.D. Professor, Departments of Medicine and Surgery, University of California, San Diego, San Diego, California

Thomas F. Burks, Ph.D. Professor and Head, Department of Pharmacology, University of Arizona College of Medicine, Tucson, Arizona

J.H. Cervenka, M.D. Department of Medicine, University of California and Veterans Administration Medical Center, San Diego, California

Y.M. Chang, M.D. Department of Medicine, University of California and Veterans Administration Medical Center, San Diego, California

Helen M. Chao, M.D. Laboratory of Neuroendocrinology, Rockefeller University, New York, New York

Ronald H. Cox, Ph.D. Associate Professor, Department of Physical Education, Health, and Sport Studies and Center for Health Enhancement, Miami University, Oxford, Ohio

Mary F. Dallman, Ph.D. Professor, Department of Physiology, University of California School of Medicine, San Francisco, California

Errol B. DeSouza, Ph.D. Chief, Neuropeptide Unit, Neuroscience Branch, Addiction Research Center, National Institute on Drug Abuse, National Institutes of Health, Bethesda, Maryland

Laurel A. Fisher, Ph.D. Assistant Professor, Department of Pharmacology, University of Arizona College of Medicine, Tucson, Arizona

Maureen N. Gannon, M.D. Laboratory of Neuroendocrinology, Rockefeller University, New York, New York

John S. Gottdiener, M.D. University of Maryland School of Medicine, Baltimore, Maryland

Thackery S. Gray, Ph.D. Assistant Professor, Department of Anatomy, Loyola Stritch School of Medicine, Maywood, Illinois

Ashley B. Grossman, M.D. Senior Lecturer, Department of Endocrinology and Honorary Consultant Physician, St. Bartholomew's Hospital, London, England

R.J. Hsiao, M.D. Department of Medicine, University of California, and Veterans Administration Medical Center, San Diego, California

Michael Irwin, Ph.D. Associate Director, Clinical Center on Alcoholism, Veterans Administration Medical Center; Assistant Professor, Department of Psychiatry, University of California School of Medicine, San Diego, California

Ned H. Kalin, Ph.D. Department of Psychiatry, William S. Middleton Memorial VA Hospital, Madison, Wisconsin

Jacob Klein, M.D. Division of Cardiology, Cedars-Sinai Medical Center, University of California School of Medicine, Los Angeles, California

George F. Koob, M.D. Division of Preclinical Neuroscience and Endocrinology, Department of Basic and Clinical Research, Research Institute of the Scripps Clinic, La Jolla, California

David S. Krantz, Ph.D. Uniformed Services University of the Health Sciences, Bethesda, Maryland

Seymour Levine, Ph.D. Department of Psychiatry and Behavioral Sciences, Stanford University School of Medicine, Stanford, California

Bruce S. McEwen, Ph.D. Professor, Laboratory of Neuroendocrinology, Rockefeller University, New York, New York

Klaus A. Miczek, Ph.D. Professor, Department of Psychology, Tufts University, Medford, Massachusetts

Charles B. Nemeroff, M.D., Ph.D. Associate Professor of Psychiatry and Pharmacology; Director, Laboratory of Psychoneuroendocrinology, Duke University Medical Center, Durham, North Carolina

Daniel O'Connor, M.D. Associate Professor, Department of Medicine, University of California, and Veterans Administration Medical Center, San Diego, California

R.J. Parmer, M.D. Department of Medicine, University of California and Veterans Administration Medical Center, San Diego, California

Paul M. Plotsky, M.D. The Clayton Foundation Laboratories for Peptide Biology, The Salk Institute, La Jolla, California

Daniel Porte, Jr., M.D. Professor, Department of Medicine, Veterans Administration Medical Center; University of Washington, Seattle, Washington

James C. Pryor, M.D. Instructor, Department of Psychiatry, Vanderbilt University School of Medicine, Nashville, Tennessee

Catherine Rivier, M.D. The Clayton Foundation Laboratories for Peptide Biology, The Salk Institute, La Jolla, California

Alan Rozanski, M.D. Division of Cardiology, Cedars-Sinai Medical Center, University of California School of Medicine, Los Angeles, California

Robert M. Sapolsky, M.D. Department of Biological Science, Stanford University School of Medicine, Stanford, California

Paul E. Sawchenko, Ph.D. Associate Professor, Developmental Neurobiology Laboratory, The Clayton Foundation Laboratories for Peptide Biology, The Salk Institute, La Jolla, California

David Shannahoff-Khalsa, M.D. The Khalsa Foundation for Medical Science, Del Mar, California

Robert L. Spencer, M.D. Laboratory of Neuroendocrinology, Rockefeller University, New York, New York

Susan L. Stoddard, Ph.D. Associate Professor, Department of Neuroscience, Indiana University School of Medicine, Fort Wayne, Indiana

Gerald J. Taborsky, Jr., M.D. Professor, Department of Medicine, Veterans Administration Medical Center, University of Washington, Seattle, Washington

Yvette Taché, Ph.D. Center for Ulcer Research and Education, Veterans Administration Medical Center; Professor, Department of Medicine, Brain Research Institute, University of California School of Medicine, Los Angeles, California

M.A. Takiyyuddin, M.D. Department of Medicine, University of California and Veterans Administration Medical Center, San Diego, California

Michael L. Thompson, Ph.D. Department of Psychology, Tufts University, Medford, Massachusetts

Walter Tornatzky, Ph.D. Research Associate, Department of Psychology, Tufts University, Medford , Massachusetts

Holger Ursin Institute of Psychology, University of Bergen, Bergen, Norway

Richard C. Veith, M.D. Director, Geriatric Research Education, and Clinical Center, Seattle/American Lake Veterans Administration Medical Center; Associate Professor, Department of Psychiatry and Behavioral Sciences, University of Washington School of Medicine, Seattle, Washington

Richard L. Verrier, Ph.D. Professor, Department of Pharmacology, Georgetown University Medical Center, Washington, D.C.

Herbert Weiner, M.D. Department of Psychiatry and Biobehavioral Sciences, University of California, Los Angeles, California

Perspectives on Stress

1

WHAT IS STRESS?

Seymour Levine
Stanford University School of Medicine, Stanford, California
Holger Ursin
University of Bergen, Bergen, Norway

TERMINOLOGY

Both of the authors have repeatedly attempted to eliminate the term stress, but without any success. We admit defeat and will try to accept that the term stress is with us to stay. The concept has very high face validity. Every human subject we have tested seems to have his or her own understanding of the term; it has even become integrated into the vocabulary of young children. There seems to be no language barrier, at least within the Western world, regarding this term. In our personal experience, in both the United States and Scandinavia, we have never encountered difficulties in communicating to research subjects, students, or colleagues from other continents and cultures what area of human experience we are addressing. Difficulties arise only when we try to provide a concise and stringent definition that all stress researchers will agree upon. It is even difficult to find a definition that a plurality of researchers will accept.

This state of affairs must be accepted. The scientific use of any terminology must go beyond common sense usage. There are an abundance of authors who complain about the diversity of definitions of stress and the lack of consensus. Quite frequently, the conclusion is that the term is meaningless (1). However, this should not be used as an argument against the concept or against the existence of the problem area. A commonly used approach is to put forward an operational definition based on one preferred questionnaire or physiological indicator. This is perfectly valid, but this state of affairs will not result in any agreement on what is the proper definition.

The major problem with the concept of stress is that we are faced with a composite, multidimensional concept. All existing definitions include some components. We can identify three main subclasses, and will deal with them separately. These three main subclasses are the input (stress stimuli); the processing systems, including the subjective experience of stress; and the output (stress responses). One basic difficulty is that these subclasses interact. The essential picture we want to convey is one of a complex system with feedback and control loops, no less but no more complicated than any other of the body's self-regulated systems. This system affects many other biological processes and may function as a common alarm and drive system, whenever there is a real or apparent challenge to the self-regulating systems of the organism.

INPUT: THE STIMULI

There are no common physical characteristics of the stimuli classified as stressful by human subjects or that function as stress stimuli in experiments with humans or animals. All sensory modalities may be used and any amplitude, duration, type of energy, and level of complexity may constitute stress as long as it is above the sensory threshold.

The list of potential stressful stimuli for an airline pilot consists of such events as aircraft failure, information workload, weather conditions, fatigue, and recent life events at home. Job stress questionnaires deal with problems with the boss (as well as colleagues), the information flow in the organization, salary conditions, stability of the employment situation, and to what extent the work interferes with social relations (2). Questionnaires on stressful life events are the primary tool utilized in behavioral epidemiology research on stress. A wide range of life events, from weddings to funerals, are included (3). In animal research, stress stimuli range from physical stimuli (e.g., electric shock, hemorrhage, etc.) to psychosocial disruptions (e.g., separation of mother and offspring). Our first consensus conclusion is that if there is anything common to the stimuli that produce the state of stress and the stress responses, it is not a function of their physical characteristics.

The alternative hypothesis is that stress stimuli may be classified and defined psychologically. If we accept that only the perceiver of the stimuli can translate it, this may lead to the conclusion that all stress stimuli are psychological (4). However, this definition would not represent consensus.

There are, for example, many clinical situations where it appears necessary to deal with all input stimuli as "stress." Thus a patient, because of increased vulnerability, should be protected from all types of stimuli (i.e., noise, cold, heat, etc.) that may affect the final outcome. This notion is in part embedded in Selye's (5) concept of the nonspecificity of the stress stimuli.

An additional source of confusion is that Selye used the terms stress and strain differently from their use in Hooke's (1635-1703) equation for the relationship between stress and strain in an elastic body. Instead of strain being produced by stress, Selye did not use the term *strain*, and assumed that stress was produced by stimuli he referred to as *stressors*, a term that has since been used by many of the writers in this field.

Specifically for analyses of stress in the workplace, it is often useful to classify all input as "loads" rather than as potential stress or stressors. Inputs that have to be dealt with by one or several of the effector systems of the individual represent a load for that system. In the literature that deals with work tasks and human performance (6), one discriminates between physical loads on the organism (e.g., physical work, muscle load, physical factors such as heat, light, etc.), and psychological loads. The latter may be differentiated into mental workload (e.g., task characteristics, degree of difficulty, amount of information to be handled) and emotional loads (e.g., threats, ambition, fear of failure). With the help of this nomenclature, it should be possible to reach a second consensus conclusion: Psychological emotional "loads" are the most frequently reported stress stimuli, and are given as reasons for most stress responses for most individuals in most situations. They are also a major component of commonly used stimuli in animal research and must be taken into account even when investigators assume that they are dealing with a strictly physical load.

Since the emotional aspect is so important and depends on psychological factors of the perceiver, there is no reason to expect to find a "Hooke"-type linear relationship between what is imposed and what occurs in the organism. Even if we disregard the emotional aspect, there is still little reason to expect a linear relationship. This would presume that the brain functions as a reflex automaton, with inborn and stereotypic reflex pathways from stimulus to response. The brain is a complex network of self-regulating systems. We have no a priori reason to expect to be able to predict the effects of a given stimulus on the organism without knowledge of how the brain of any individual is going to process a specific stimulus in a particular situation. This depends on the information stored in this specific brain for this stimulus situation. In other words, this depends on previous experience, or learning. In the next section, we will discuss the processing systems that determine the fate of the stimuli. We will attempt to treat this in expectancy terms, and will try to show how this should be acceptable whether one considers the brain from a cognitive or a learning theory point of view.

PROCESSING VARIABLES: THE CENTRAL STAGE

Input Filters

An evaluation of stimulus inputs by each individual, therefore, is crucial in determining whether a stimulus is to be considered as "stress" or not. This evaluation of the stimulus, rather than the stimulus itself, is a central theme in most contemporary writings on stress. The third consensus conclusion is that the main reason for the lack of linearity between the input and what occurs within the organism is that the input is being evaluated or filtered before it gains access to any response system.

These filters should perhaps be regarded as gates, but they do not appear as digital (all-or-none) logical units. The fate of the input is determined by central factors or the state of the central data processor, the brain. In most cases, some form of comparison is the basic principle for the stimulus treatment. This is true even for a simple response such as the orienting reflex (7). Novelty can only be detected by signal evaluation taking place within the central nervous system (CNS). The same is true for uncertainty, ambiguity, and threats. The information has access to parts of the brain, where the information is compared with what has been stored previously. In our opinion, these comparisons may be regarded most simply as expectations.

Thus, purely psychological events, such as the failure to meet expectations or the absence of previously expected positive reinforcement, appear to be critical elements that elicit a stress response. Another way of eliciting the stress response is the imposition of more apparent physical stimuli, such as cold or events producing tissue damage. However, the expectation of such stimuli, or failure to meet previously established expectations of being able to avoid such stimuli, are also capable of eliciting stress responses. We will deal with the best known stress-related "filters" within this framework of expectancies.

Filter 1: Defense and Stimulus Expectancies

The first filtering mechanism has only been demonstrated in humans and many researchers would claim that it is specific to this species, since it seems to depend on rather complex cognitive functions. When humans perceive a threat signal, they may distort and deny the true or probable consequences of that signal. Since Freud this has been referred to as "defense." In its most primitive forms, defense may block threat signals from producing stress responses. The price for this may be a failure to behave appropriately in dangerous situations (8,9).

We do not know whether animals have similar defense mechanisms. However, if we define this property as a mechanism affecting stimulus expectancies, this phylogenetic difference may not be as dramatic. Stimulus expectancy (10) refers to the storing of information that one stimulus precedes another (i.e., classic conditioning). When an aversive event is expected (i.e., signaled by other stimuli), the stress response occurs. When this relationship is misperceived by the individual through mechanisms distorting the true relationship, the individual is said to use "cognitive defense." Denial, for instance, is defined as a distortion of true relationships between stimuli resulting in the refusal to accept a threat as a real threat. Although these have not been identified, there is no a priori reason why animals could not have mechanisms that distort stimulus expectancies.

Filter 2: Response Outcome Expectancies

The second type of expectancy results from learning about the consequences of acts. This type of expectancy is referred to as response outcome expectancy (10) and is related to instrumental conditioning. In principle, three classes of such expectancies are important in determining whether the individual will or will not show stress responses: coping, helplessness, and hopelessness.

Coping is used in two different ways. One way in which coping is commonly used refers to the coping strategies used to face a challenge or threat. These strategies may be executed both under high and low levels of stress. Therefore, there is no relationship between this meaning of coping and the physiological state of the individual. A second meaning, which will be used in this chapter, refers to established positive response outcome expectancies. Coping, by our definition, is the result of a learning process. An individual expects a positive affective outcome with a high degree of probability. This definition of coping predicts reduced stress in the individual. This has been demonstrated both in animals (11) and humans (12).

The development of a positive response outcome expectancy is dependent upon whether the individual can *control* or perceive control in a specific situation or experimental paradigm. This, again, depends on the capacity to make active responses in the presence of aversive stimuli, and to register the consequences of such acts. If the responses result in a positive outcome, such as by either escaping or avoiding a noxious event, or by being able to obtain positive reinforcement, the brain will then store these relationships as positive outcome expectancies. This type of learning requires not only that such positive events occur, but the brain must also be able to record these results. This is often referred to as *feedback*. Rapid and clear feedback is necessary for control and, therefore, coping to occur.

The inability to cope is due primarily to the failure to utilize appropriate coping mechanisms (i.e., control) and results in high levels of stress (13). Stress responses may be reduced when an individual is exposed to signals that a particular need is to be satisfied. Establishment of a positive outcome expectancy reduces physiological activation both in humans (12) and in animals (11). The presence of positive reinforcers or signals representing positive reinforcers reduces stress responses, and this reduction depends on the probability of reinforcement rather than its density (14,15).

It is perhaps more surprising that absence of positive reinforcers, and clear signals that such reinforcement will not occur, also reduces the stress response. This latter phenomenon is less well known, but seems to be a very important mechanism for survival. A hungry rat does not run around after food in an environment where there obviously is no food present. Only when signals occur that may indicate food do we observe the increased activity (16,17).

Helplessness refers to psychological situations in which the individual cannot determine any relationship between the responses available and the probable outcomes. In our opinion, this definition is reasonably close to the original definition offered by Overmier and Seligman (18). Within our theoretical framework, helplessness exists when the subject has learned that there is a very low probability that responses will lead to any consequences at all. This state has been established mainly in experimental situations involving stimuli that are highly negative (aversive), but it may exist also in situations with positive affective values. The effect on the internal state under the latter circumstances have not been measured. The state under the threat of highly negative outcomes, unless rectified by the individual, is high arousal.

Hopelessness means that the individual has acquired a perceived probability that the available responses will lead to aversive or negative events, such as punishment. Whatever the subject does, something, or most things, goes wrong. This state is more related to the guilt-ridden depression often typical of human depressive states. Helplessness has often been used as a theoretical model for depression (19); however, in our opinion, hopelessness may be a better model (20).

The interactional or "transactional" model of stress of Lazarus (21) is also based on expectancies and appraisals. The subject first evaluates whether the stimulus situation is a threat or not (primary appraisal), and then considers whether this threat can be met with the resources he or she has (secondary appraisal). Stress occurs when the subject believes that these resources are insufficient. There are considerable points of agreement between this position and ours. Major differences are due to Lazarus' use of *coping* as a term for the strategies used to handle stress and his lack of distinction between *defense* and *coping*. In our opinion, this definition of coping offers little or no possibility to predict physiological consequences of the stimuli. We disagree with Lazarus and Folkman (22) in their critique of defining stress stimuli based only on the response they elicit. In principal, they do this themselves since they rely primarily on verbal reports from their subjects as to whether they find a particular situation stressful or not. To us one of the essential elements in the definition of stress must be that we deal with stimuli that have particular physiological and/or overt behavioral effects. This is the validation of the concept. However, the stress response is also a very complex set of phenomena, and not all responses are valid indicators of the central state being evaluated.

Individual Differences

Insofar as one of the crucial factors in our current attempt to define stress is the processing variable, it is important to elaborate that there are factors that can permanently alter the state of the CNS so that what appear to be identical inputs frequently result in markedly different outputs, both behaviorally and physiologically. Although it is not possible to identify all of the factors that constitute individual differences, some developmental experiences have been shown to alter what we have called *processing*. Thus, stimulation in infancy has been shown to affect many of the outcome variables. It has been demonstrated that behavioral, endocrinologic, neurochemical, and immunologic outcomes in response to identical stimulus inputs are very different when infant rodents are exposed to stimulation either in the form of handling or exposure to mild electric shocks during critical periods in development (23). Although exceptions have been reported (24), in general, the effect appears to be an overall diminution of the output variables. The central state of the processor can also be altered for long durations, if not permanently, by experiences in adulthood. Exposure to inescapable and unpredictable shock appears to result in an organism that is, in general, hyperreactive to input stimuli and shows exaggerated outcome responses (25,26). These exaggerated responses do not appear to be task dependent and seem to be generalized to numerous input stimuli, as was discussed above in reference to response outcome expectancies referred to as helplessness and hopelessness.

Although the evidence presented above represents the best documented demonstration of experientially induced individual differences, there is evidence that other ontogenetic variables also permanently alter these processing systems. Factors such as prenatal stress (27), differential mother–infant interactions (28,29), nutritional factors (30), and altered hormonal states during development (31) have all been implicated.

Finally, although the evidence is not yet compelling, a growing body of information suggests a strong genetic component as a determinant of individual differences (32). This evidence suggests that both in animals and in humans the individual differences observed in many of our cherished outcome variables may indeed be genetically determined.

In humans, there are also social factors that produce individual differences. It seems well established that the presence of social support increases tolerance to stressful life events and has a general beneficiary effect on health (33). Similar stress-reducing effects of the social interaction may be seen also in animals that have complex social structures (34).

STRESS RESPONSES: THE OUTCOME VARIABLES

The stress responses are overt behavioral and physiological changes. From a physiological, medical, and biological point of view, the final validation of the concept and its measurements is that there are physiological changes. Our theoretical framework has this as an essential component. If there are discrepancies between the various response indicators of the assumed central state, we will defer to the biological indicators. This has made it possible to arrive at theoretical explanations of why there are sometimes such discrepancies. On the other hand, we admit that the subjective report of stress and discomfort from a human being must be accepted as meaningful and valid data.

Reports of Stress Experience

Subjective verbal reports on what aspects of the work situation are stressful seem reasonably consistent, and give reproducible results. Questionnaires yield valid results from a wide range of occupations (2), in the United States, Great Britain, and Scandinavia. Results have been found to correlate with other subjective statements on, for instance, anxiety, depression, and health problems such as muscle pain (35), and objective measures of health variables believed to be influenced by stress such as blood pressure (36) and immunoglobulins (37,38).

The experience of stress is, as is the case with anxiety, often based on an experience of one or several of the many peripheral components of the stress response. Indeed, we have previously admitted that in our first extensive discussions of stress and coping one of us defined coping (the inverse of stress) as the state when the stomach did not hurt (39). This might be read as a simplified version of the more formal statement that even if the behavior is inappropriate, the absence of physiological responses or related symptoms indicates that coping has occurred. Conversely, the existence of such phenomena indicates that stress is present, regardless of the behavioral response. In general, the subjective reports seem to follow the physiological state. However, as with all verbal statements from human subjects, there are reasons to question if they are always truthful, or if we hear what the subjects for some reason want us to hear. Verbal reports may be regarded as one aspect of the total number of responses available to a subject. The relationship between the internal state and overt behavior is not as simple as one might believe, even in animals.

Behavior and Physiological Relationships

If one exposes a feral-born squirrel monkey living by itself (individually housed) to a snake housed in a Plexiglas box above the cage, several behaviors are observed. The monkey will emit numerous alarm calls, display increased activity, and will avoid the snake by maintaining maximal distance. All of these behaviors can be defined as stress related. An analysis of endocrine changes also indicates marked elevations of cortisol in this situation. If the snake is presented in the same way to squirrel monkeys living in a social group (group-housed), all of the behaviors emitted remain much the same. However, under the group-housed condition, the squirrel monkey fails to show any change in the activity of the pituitary-adrenal system (40).

When the behavioral and physiological indices of stress are concordant there is little problem in interpreting the outcome. The problem arises when there is discordance or dissociation between these two or more of the traditionally used outcome variables. Discordance may occur in any number of ways. The response of the group-housed squirrel monkey exposed to a snake is one example in which all the behavioral indices would indicate stress, but this is not substantiated by the physiological parameter (plasma cortisol) measured. Another example of discordance is seen in a series of experiments on primate mother-infant separations. Traditionally stress and/or distress has been inferred in infant mammals primarily on the basis of one important behavior, namely vocalization. An increase in infant vocalization following environmental disturbances that include separation from the mother has been linearly equated with stress. However, we have demonstrated in infant primates (both squirrel and Rhesus) (41) that under many circumstances there exists an inverse relationship between vocalization and some physiological indices of stress. Under certain conditions of separation (i.e., when the mother is visually present), the infant emits significantly more vocalizations but the levels of plasma cortisol and cerebrospinal fluid (CSF) 3-methoxy-4-hydroxyphenylethylene glycol (MHPG) are significantly reduced in comparison to when the infant is totally isolated from its mother and other conspecifics (42). It has been hypothesized that under these circumstances, vocalization is an instrumental act that serves as a coping response to reduce levels of arousal.

Whereas discordance implies that two variables change in different directions but are assumed to be causally related, dissociation implies that neither variable is related. There may be instances in which dissociation between the behavioral and physiological responses may occur. Nonhuman primate infants subjected to repeated separations from the mother display a significant reduction in vocalization emitted by the third separation and by the sixth hardly vocalize at all (43). However, some physiological indications (plasma cortisol levels) remain elevated even following the sixth separation, long after most of the initial behavioral response caused by the separation has ceased to occur. In rodents, when an infant separated from its mother is placed in a novel environment there is an increase in ultrasonic vocalization as well as elevated plasma corticosterone levels. The elevation of corticosterone remains even when the presence of a sibling in the novel environment causes vocalizations to cease (44).

There are theoretical grounds on which to differentiate between behavioral and physiological arousal indices. Groves and Thompson (45) have drawn a distinction between stimulus-response (S-R) or motor symptoms, with direct neural pathways, and state or arousal systems, with diffuse CNS connections. When a motor system is evoked, both the S-R and arousal systems are activated. However, the two systems appear to be independent. When a motor response is elicited repeatedly, the amplitude of the response may decrease (habituation) or increase (sensitization). Habituation is primarily phasic and believed to occur in the S-R system. Sensitization is tonic and regulated by the arousal system. Since S-R and arousal systems appear to be subject to different stimulation parameters (i.e., frequency has strong effects on habituation, intensity is directly related to sensitization), dissociation between the two systems is likely, particularly in the case of repeated stimulation.

Another interesting issue is raised when there is discordance between the various physiological indicators. One example occurred in a study on the psychobiology of stress in men undergoing parachute training (12). Prior to and following the initial jump all behavioral (fear rating) and physiological (hormone and autonomic) indices were elevated. However, following repeated jumps from the training tower, the behavioral and most of the hormonal elevations no longer were present. However, increases in testosterone levels, urinary epinephrine levels, and heart rate were present throughout the training. Other instances of directional differences between endocrine and autonomic systems have been demonstrated in humans (46) and in animals (47). One might conclude that these different physiological systems reflecting arousal are responding to different psychological parameters, or are differentially regulated by the CNS.

The ultimate task facing the researcher in this field is somehow to resolve these apparent paradoxes. When behavior can be presumed to be functioning as an instrumental or coping response, there are few problems since the behavior can be seen as functional and adaptive. However, since we are assuming that behavior (motor systems) and arousal are regulated differentially by the CNS, some physiological output controlled by the arousal system must be altered for us to infer that the stimulus input is being processed as stress. To discuss this further, we must briefly review arousal or activation theory, and add some elements to account for the data discussed above.

Physiological Responses

The general response to the type of stimuli we have called stressful or stress-eliciting is referred to as the *stress response*. We have chosen to explain this within the framework of arousal or activation theory, as it is known in neurophysiology (48-50). In the present context, we assume that arousal or activation is a process in the CNS that increases the activity in the brain from one level to a higher level, and that may maintain this level. The emphasis of this concept is on changes in these levels, and maintenance of them.

The strong correlations between the subjective feeling of wakefulness versus drowsiness and the corresponding changes in the electroencephalogram (EEG)

(51) were the basis for the original classification of the EEG by Berger (52). This was also the foundation for the neurophysiological arousal or activation concept as we know it today. The essential aspect for the use in the present context is the relationship between this central state and vegetative (53), endocrine (54), and immunological processes (55). The changes produced in these subsystems are to be regarded as parts of the total activation or arousal response. The various subsystems are contributing parts, but none of them are essential elements. Surgical or chemical manipulation of one or several of these systems may dampen activation, but such procedures do not seem to eliminate activation.

In our opinion, there is no particular reason to pick one specific marker of the general response as the one and only "stress marker." A good stress marker is the one that works for a particular laboratory. It must be reliable, quantifiable, and sensitive. However, no particular physiological response that meets these specifications is more valid than any other.

Since the presence of activation may be regarded as the driving force behind the solution of problems, stress responses are not to be accepted as something that should be avoided at all costs. Activation may be regarded not only as an alarm system but also as the driving force that makes an animal or a human act to reduce needs. Therefore, activation is in this context an essential element in the total adaptive system of the organism (56). Feelings of stress, or related states such as anxiety, are not necessarily evils to be dampened by psychopharmacological interventions, even if they may appear to be unpleasant. They may be adequate responses to stimuli requiring full attention and integrated action for solution, and subsequent reduction of the source of the stress response. The purpose of the response is to eliminate not only itself but also the source of the state.

This alarm system or driving force will remain activated until there is an agreement between the set value and the actual value, or until the brain gives lower priority to the set value. It is of particular interest that activation also seems to depend on the probability (or the expectancy) of solution to a particular discrepancy.

There is consensus that no matter what the response is to be called, it affects most other physiological systems. It is a general, nonspecific, and strong response system. All endocrine systems, the autonomic system, and the immune system, have been shown to be "sensitive" to environmental changes via these mechanisms. This has also been shown for the biochemical activity in the brain. There is reasonable agreement that the system is activated whenever there is a discrepancy between what the organism is set for regarding an important variable and what really exists (actual value of the same variable). This is only a reformulation of homeostatic theory. There is also agreement that in situations with homeostatic imbalance, and whenever expectancies are not met, two types of responses occur. The first is the general alarm or stress response. This is in principle a nonspecific, general response. The second type or class of responses is specific to the situation and the experience of this particular individual.

There is no consensus as to what extent there really is a general activation system dependent on the reticular formation. It is generally agreed that the specific ascending systems from the brain stem are involved, but these specific subsystems have not been incorporated into a larger systematic theory that replaces general activation theory. However, there is some evidence of specificity between particular behavioral strategies or response systems and particular hormones.

Specific Activation Systems

The first differentiation to be made is between the types of responses seen in coping versus noncoping subjects, or in the early versus late stages of the parachutist training mentioned above. When coping has been established, there is still a short-lasting activation that has been referred to as "phasic" activation, in contrast to the general, and longer-lasting, activation seen in the noncoping subject (57). The phasic activation in the coping individual is characterized by epinephrine release (not norepinephrine) (58), pulse rate increases (59), and a modest but significant rise in plasma levels of testosterone (60). Arnetz (61) produced this type of activation in elderly subjects as a response to an intervention program, and pointed out the desirable anabolic aspects of this type of activation.

The second differentiation is more complex. Pribram and McGuiness (62) identified three separate but interacting neural systems for the control of attention. The immediate behavioral and physiological responses to a novel stimulus, the orienting response, they referred to as "arousal," the more tonic readiness necessary for solving a problem they called "activation," and the coordination between these two they referred to as "effort." They suggested that the effort mechanism was dependent on amygdala and the arousal mechanism on hippocampus. The long-lasting tonic activation we have identified as the possible pathogenic factor in the stress response, is related to the "activation" concept of Pribram and McGuiness, and the shortlasting, phasic or anabolic response in coping subjects relates to their "arousal" concept. The effort invested in any given task represents a combination of these two, as suggested by Pribram and McGuiness. When the evaluation of the expected outcome takes the effort to be invested into account for one particular task in one particular situation, Bandura (63) refers to this as *efficacy*.

Response expectancies such as helplessness and hopelessness are assumed to be rather general. When these occur in a situation that persists, the long-lasting, tonic activation occurs that is believed to be the pathogenic part of the stress response. There is no a priori reason to attach pathogenic effects to the short-lasting phasic and anabolic activation referred to as arousal by Pribram and

McGuiness, even if it may be experienced as uncomfortable. Task-oriented, planned, and directed allocation of resources in a person who believes him- or herself able to handle a situation, therefore, is probably no health risk. If this is referred to as stress, it should be clear that in this case stress may be adaptive and result in training rather than straining.

Henry and Meehan (64) have suggested that there is endocrine specificity to these activation mechanisms. They believe that the amygdala effort mechanism may be tied to catecholamines and the hippocampus arousal mechanism to corti- sol. Bohus (47) has reported experimental animal data to support these notions. In humans, factor analyses of endocrine responses have consistently turned up at least three reasonably stable factors: a catecholamine, a cortisol, and a testos- terone factor (59,65,66). Further statistical analyses have revealed stable rela- tionships between these factors and psychological traits. It is generally accepted that the tendency to react with sympathetic activation and catecholamines (the catecholamine factor) is reliably related to the behavioral pattern commonly identified as type A behavior, which is believed to be coronary-prone, at least when it occurs with hostility and lack of coping (59,67,68). There are also rather consistent data on relations between the tendency to react with cortisol (the cortisol factor) and the psychological defense mechanisms we have described as filter 1 (69). There seems to be a surprisingly constant relationship between the cortisol factor and psychological defense, on the one hand, and plasma levels of immunoglobulins on the other (55).

CONCLUSIONS

We have defined stress as consisting of three major components that include stimuli input, the evaluation or processing system, and the outcome or response. We believe that all existing definitions of stress include one or another compo- nent. Thus, in order for us to define any event as stress all components of this definition must be present, but the investigator does not have to deal with all the aspects. We do not believe that any one aspect of our definition is more important than any other, in principle, but accept that different research tradi- tions differ in what they choose to study and measure.

Stress, as we have defined it, is an integral part of an adaptive biological system. Both the behavioral and physiological response to stress are required for both humans and animals to function within the confines of a dynamic and fre- quently challenging environment. It should not be viewed as an atavistic mecha- nism no longer suited for civilized humans (70,71). Some of the perceived sensations from the stress response may be described as uncomfortable, but this is not a signal that the process is necessarily pathogenic.

The responses elicited by stress appear to have multiple functions, one of these may be to drive the organism to express behaviors that may eliminate the source of stress-inducing stimuli. One of the recurrent themes in many of the chapters in this volume is that biological responses are part of a homeostatic mechanism. The psychological processes we have discussed must also be regarded as part of the general principle of homeostasis. Thus, the behavioral mechanisms we have described are fundamental to the organism's adaptation to the environment, and as such must be considered within the context of adaptive mechanisms regulated by the brain.

The initial phase of the response may function as a positive feedback mechanism. Increased muscle tension plus the vegetative components of the response give rise to sensations that are essential elements in the sensation of stress. This tends to facilitate further development of the stress state. The process is described in the original James–Lange theory of emotions that emphasized the experience of the peripheral components of emotion as essential for the emotional experience (the "real" emotion).

At the peak of the response physiological resources are mobilized and result in enhanced function; there is also improved performance from a psychological point of view in many tasks (48). In complex tasks, the limit for performance may be surpassed; in such cases high stress levels may be incompatible with peak performance. The general effect of the response is to improve the chances of dealing with the stressful situation and eliminate the source of stress. The uncomfortable aspect of the sensation is not pathogenic, but should drive the subject to proper behaviors. Only when the situation becomes chronic may the stress response be inadequate and pathological in response to a crisis.

However, the later stages of the acute stress response are characterized by the release of slower-reacting hormones such as cortisol. Munck and colleagues (72) have hypothesized that this aspect of the total stress response functions as a suppressive mechanism to dampen some of the acute reactions. This "tail" of the acute reaction may again be regarded as a homeostatic device to reestablish physiological balance. The possible pathological results appear to be associated with prolonged, sustained states in which the homeostatic mechanisms are taxed.

The contemporary view of stress can be characterized as an imposition model. In one sense it represents the misuse of the load concept, which has been discussed previously. This view is fostered by the voluminous number of studies, originating with Selye, in which severely traumatic stimuli were used to elicit the stress response. The perspective we have taken suggests a very different approach. In so far as many of the responses to such diverse stimuli such as maternal loss, frustration, electric shock, and surgical trauma appear to be the same, one can assume that there must be elements common to these inputs. Our hypothesis is that all stress-inducing stimuli have the property of representing the absence of critical features in the environment. By this we mean that there is a lack of information (uncertainty or unpredictability) concerning the obtaining of positive outcomes or avoidance of negative outcomes. Thus, stress stimuli, or signals representing these stimuli, indicate that something is missing or about to disappear and that this something is highly relevant and desirable to the organism. Therefore stress is presumed to be the state that is created whenever the processor (brain) registers this informational discrepancy.

Both in animals and humans there has been a consistent finding that uncertainty, lack of information, and the absence or loss of control all produce alarm states. Conversely, the presence of information (in the form of clear and salient safety signals), behaviors that lead to positive outcomes, and behaviors that result in control, reduce or eliminate the alarm states, with the concomitant reduction of the physiological responses associated with this state.

We have attempted to provide what we feel is a broader and more comprehensive definition of "what is stress." In the process our views have departed from many of the more traditional approaches to the problem area. We arrive at our *final consensus* conclusion: The concept of stress is not unlike many other life events; it is difficult to live with but impossible to live without.

ACKNOWLEDGMENTS

S. Levine was supported by grants HD-02881 from NIMH & HD and MH-19936 from NIMH. H. Ursin was supported by the Norwegian Research Council for Science and Industrial Research, and Statoil. We wish to thank Sandra Wiener for her advice.

REFERENCES

1. Engel B T. Stress is a noun! No, a verb! No, an adjective. In: Field TM, McCabe PM, Schneiderman N, eds. Stress and coping. Hillsdale, NJ: Lawrence Erlbaum Assoc, 1985: 3-12.
2. Cooper C L. The stress check. New York: Prentice Hall, 1981.
3. Lundberg U, Theorell T. Scaling of life changes: differences between three diagnostic groups and between recently experienced and nonexperienced events. J Hum Stress 1976; 2:7-17.
4. Mason J W. Motivational factors in psychosocial development. In: Arnold WJ, Page MM, eds. Nebraska symposium on motivation. 1970, vol. 18. 1971: 35-67.
5. Selye H. A syndrome produced by diverse nocuous agents. Nature 1936; 138: 32.
6. Moray N. Mental workload. New York: Plenum Press, 1979.
7. Sokolov E N. Neuronal models and the orienting reflex. In: Brazier MAB, ed. The central nervous system and behavior. Hillsdale, NJ: Lawrence Erlbaum Assoc, 1960; 187-276.
8. Kragh U. The defense mechanism test: a new method for diagnosis and personnel selection. J Appl Psychol 1960; 44: 303-309.

9. Varnes R. The defense mechanism test predicts inadequate performance under stress. Scand J Psychol 1982; 23: 37–43.
10. Bolles R C. Reinforcement, expectancy and learning. Psychol Rev 1972; 79: 394–409.
11. Coover G D, Ursin H, Levine S. Plasma corticosterone levels during active-avoidance learning in rats. J Comp Physiol Psychol 1973; 82: 170–174.
12. Ursin H, Baade E, Levine S, eds. Psychobiology of stress. New York: Academic Press, 1978.
13. Ursin H, Murison R, eds. Biological and psychological basis of psychosomatic disease. Oxford: Pergamon Press, 1983.
14. Goldman L, Coover G D, Levine S. Bidirectional effects of reinforcement shifts on pituitary–adrenal activity. Physiol Behav 1973; 10: 209–214.
15. Levine S, Coover G D. Environmental control of suppression of the pituitary–adrenal system. Physiol Behav 1976; 17: 35–37.
16. Coover G D, Murison R, Sundberg H, Jellestad F, Ursin H. Plasma corticosterone and meal expectancy in rats: effects of low probability cues. Physiol Behav 1984; 179–184.
17. Davis H, Levine S. Predictabiity, control, and the pituitary–adrenal response in rats. J Comp Physiol Psychol 1982; 96: 393–404.
18. Overmier J B, Seligman M E P. Effect of inescapable shock upon subsequent escape and avoidance responding. J Comp Physiol Psychol 1967; 63: 28–33.
19. Seligman M E P. Helplessness: on depression, development and death. San Francisco: WH Freeman 1975.
20. Prociuk T J, Breen L, Lussier R J. Hopelessness, internal–external locus of control and depression. J Clin Psychol 1976; 32: 299–300.
21. Lazarus R S. Psychological stress and the coping process. New York: McGraw-Hill, 1966.
22. Lazarus R S, Folkman S. Stress, appraisal, and coping. New York: Springer, 1984.
23. Levine S. An endocrine theory of infantile stimulation. In: Ambrose A, ed. Stimulation in early infancy. London: Academic Press, 1969; 45–63.
24. Levine S. Plasma-free corticosteroid response to electric shock in rats stimulated in infancy. Science 135: 1962; 795–796.
25. Brett L P, Patterson J, Levine S. Adjunctive drinking and the pituitary–adrenal response: effects of prior aversive stimulation (preshock). Physiol Behav 1982; 219–223.
26. Weinberg J, Erskine M, Levine S. Shock-induced fighting attenuates the effects of prior shock experience in rats. Physiol Behav 1980; 25: 9–16.
27. Fride E, Dan Y, Feldon J, Halevy G, Weinstock M. Effects of prenatal stress on vulnerability to stress in prepubertal and adult rats. Physiol Behav 1986; 37: 681–687.
28. Hennessy M B, Vogt J, Levine S. Strain of foster mother determines long-term effects of early handling: evidence for maternal mediation. Physiol Psychol 1982; 10: 153–157.

29. Treiman D M, Fulker D W, Levine S. Interaction of genotype and environment as determinants of corticosteroid response to stress. Dev Psychobiol 1970; 3(2): 131-140.
30. Wiener S G, Levine S. Perinatal malnutrition and early handling: interactive effects on the development of the pituitary-adrenal system. Dev Psychobiol 1978; 11(4): 335-352.
31. Bohn M C. Glucocorticoid induced teratologies of the nervous system. In: Yanai J, ed. Neurobehavioral teratology. Amsterdam: Elsevier Science Publ., 1984: 365-387.
32. Suomi S J. Genetic and maternal contributions to individual differences in Rhesus monkey biobehavioral development. In: Krasnegor N A, Blass E M, Hofer M A, Smotherman W P, eds. Perinatal development—a psychobiological perspective. Orlando: Academic Press, 1987; 397-419.
33. Isacsson S O, Janzon L, eds. Social support—health and disease. Stockholm: Almqvist and Wiksell, 1986: 193.
34. Stanton M E, Patterson J M, Levine S. Social influences on conditioned cortisol secretion in the squirrel monkey. Psychoneuroendocrinology 1985; 10: 125-134.
35. Ursin H, Endresen I, Ursin G. Psychological factors and self-reports of muscle pain. Eur J Appl Physiol 1985; 57: 282-290.
36. Knox S, Theorell T, Svensson J, Waller D. The relation of social support and working environment to medical variables associated with elevated blood pressure in young men: a structural model. Soc Sci Med 1985; 21: 526-531.
37. Ursin H, Mykletun R, Tonder O, Vaernes R, Relling G, Isaksen E, Murison R. Psychological stress-factors and concentrations of immunoglobulins and complement components in humans. Scand J Psychol 1984; 25: 340-347.
38. Vaernes R, Knardahl S, Roemsing J, Aakvaag A, Toender O, Walther B, Ursin H. Relations between environmental problems, psychology and health among shift-workers in the Norwegian process industry. Work Stress 1988; 2: 7-15.
39. Levine S, Weinberg J, Ursin H. Definition of the coping process and statement of the problem. In: Ursin H, Baade E, Levine S, eds. Psychobiology of stress: a study of coping men. New York: Academic Press, 1978: 3-21.
40. Vogt J L, Coe C L, Levine S. Behavioral and adrenocorticoid responsiveness of squirrel monkeys to a live snake: is flight necessarily stressful? Behav Neural Biol 1981; 32: 391-405.
41. Levine S. Psychobiologic consequences of disruption in mother—infant relationships. In: Krasnegor N A, Blass E M, Hofer M A, Smotherman P W, eds. Perinatal development: a psychobiological perspective. New York: Academic Press, 1987: 359-376.
42. Wiener S G, Coe C L, Levine S. Endocrine and neurochemical sequelae of primate vocalizations. In: Newman J, ed. The physiological control of mammalian vocalizations. New York: Plenum Press, 1988: 367-394.

43. Coe C L, Glass J C, Wiener S G, Levine S. Behavioral, but not physiological, adaptation to repeated separation in mother and infant primates. Psychoneuroendocrinology 1983; 8: 401-409.

44. Levine S, Gutierrez Y R, Stanton M E. Maternal separation and the ontogeny of pituitary-adrenal activity. In: Chrousos GP, Loriaux DL, Gold PW, eds. Physical and emotional stress: mechanisms and clinical implications. New York: Plenum Press.

45. Groves P M, Thompson R F. Habituation: a dual process theory. Psychol Rev 1970; 77: 419-450.

46. Frankehaeuser M, Lundberg U. Sympathetic-adrenal and pituitary-adrenal response to challenge. In: Pichot P, Berner P, Wolf R, Thau K, eds. Psychiatry, vol. 2. London: Plenum Press, 1985: 699-704.

47. Bohus B. Limbic-midbrain mechanisms and behavioral physiology of interactions with CRF, ACTH, and adrenal hormones. In: Hellhammer D, Florin I, Weiner H, eds. Neurobiological approaches to human disease. Toronto: H. Huber, 1988: 267-285.

48. Moruzzi G, Magoun H W. Brain stem reticular formation and activation of the EEG. Electroencephalogr Clin Neurophysiol 1949; 1: 455-473.

49. Lindsley D B. Emotion. In Stevens S, ed. Handbook of experimental psychology. New York: Wiley, 1951.

50. Vanderwolf C H, Robinson T E. Reticulo-cortical activity and behavior. A critique of the arousal theory and a new synthesis. Brain Behav Sci 1981; 4: 459-514.

51. Jones B E. Understanding the physiological correlates of a behavioral state as a constellation of events. Brain Behav Sci 1981; 4: 482-483.

52. Berger H. Ueber das Elektroenkephalogramm des Menschen. II. J Physiol Neurol 1930; 40: 60-179.

53. Malmo R B. Studies of anxiety. Some clinical origins of the activation concept. In: Spielberger C D, ed. Anxiety and behavior. New York: Academic Press, 1966; 157-177.

54. Hennessy J W, Levine S. Stress, arousal and the pituitary-adrenal system: A psychoendocrine model. In: Sprague JM, Epstein AN, eds. Progress in psychobiology and physiological psychology, vol. 8. New York: Academic Press, 1979: 133-178.

55. Ursin H, Mykletun R, Tonder O, Vaernes R, Relling G, Isaksen E, Murison R. Psychological stress-factors and concentrations of immunoglobulins and complement components in humans. Scand J Psychol 1984; 25: 340-347.

56. Ursin H. Expectancy and activation: an attempt to systematize stress theory. In: Hellhammer D, Florin I, Weiner H, eds. Neurobiological approaches to human disease. Toronto: H. Huber, 1988.

57. Ursin H. Personality, activation, and somatic health. A new psychosomatic theory. In Levine S, Ursin H, eds. Coping and health. New York: Plenum Press, 1980: 259-279.

58. Hansen J R, Stoa K F, Blix A S, Ursin H. Urinary levels of epinephrine and norepinephrine in parachutist trainees. In: Ursin H, Baade E, Levine S, eds. Psychobiology of stress. A study of coping men. New York: Academic Press, 1978: 63-74.

59. Stromme S B, Wikeby P C, Blix A S, Ursin H. Additional heart rate. In: Ursin H, Baade E, Levine S, eds. Psychobiology of stress. A study of coping men. New York: Academic Press, 1978: 83–89.
60. Davidson J, Smith E R, Levine S. Testosterone. In: Ursin H, Baade E, Levine S, eds. Psychobiology of stress. A study of coping men. New York: Academic Press, 1978; 57–62.
61. Arnetz B. The potential role of psychosocial stress on levels of hemoglobin Alc (HbAlC) and fasting plasma glucose in elderly people. J Gerontol 1984; 39: 424–429.
62. Pribram K, McGuiness D. Arousal, activation and effort in the control of attention. Psychol Rev 1975; 82 116–149.
63. Bandura A. Self-efficacy mechanisms in physiological activation and health-promoting behavior. In: Madden JIV, Mathysee S, Barchas J, eds. Adaptation, learning and affect. New York: Raven Press, 1986.
64. Henry J P, Meehan J P. Psychosocial stimuli physiological specificity, and cardiovascular disease. In: Weiner H, Hofer MA, Stunkard A J, eds. Brain, behaviour and bodily disease. New York: Raven Press, 1981.
65. Rose R M, Poe R O, Mason J W. Observations on the relationship between psychological state, 17-OHCS excretion, and epinephrine, norepinephrine, insulin, BEI, estrogen and androgen levels during basic training. Psychosom Med 1967; 29: 544.
66. Ellertsen B, Johnsen T B, Ursin H. Relationship between the hormonal responses to activation and coping. In: Ursin H, Baade E, Levine S, eds. Psychobiology of stress. A study of coping men. New York: Academic Press, 1978; 105–122.
67. Jenkins C D. Psychosocial risk factors for coronary heart disease. Acta Med Scand 1982; 660 (suppl.): 123–136.
68. Glass D C. Stress, behavior patterns, and coronary disease. Am Scientist 1977; 65: 177–187.
69. Vaernes R, Ursin H, Darragh A, Lambe R. Endocrine response patterns and psychological correlates. J Psychosom Res 1982; 26: 123–131.
70. Levi L. Stress and distress in response to psychosocial stimuli. Stockholm: Almquist and Wiksell, 1972.
71. Charvat J, Dell P, Folkow B. Mental factors and cardiovascular disorders. Cardiologia 1964; 44: 124–141.
72. Munck A, Guyre P M, Holbrook N J. Physiological functions of glucocorticoids in stress and their relation to pharmacological actions. Endocr Rev 1984; 5: 25–44.

2

BEHAVIORAL BIOLOGY OF STRESS AND PSYCHOSOMATIC MEDICINE

Herbert Weiner

University of California, Los Angeles, California

WHAT IS STRESS?

No agreed-upon definition of "stress" exists. As recently as 1970, Hans Selye (1) defined it as ". . . the non-specific response of the body to any demand made upon it." Missing from this definition was the observation that stressors also have behavioral and psychological as well as physical consequences. For example, different animals have a variety of behavioral strategies for survival in dealing with the threat of predators; these behavioral responses must be appropriate to the threat or challenge if they are to succeed; were they random or indiscriminate (nonspecific), survival would not be assured. When the threat to survival is an infection, the appropriate response is immunological. If the threat to reproductive success is competition among males for mates, the appropriate response is to fight the rival, submit to him, or flee from him to find another mating partner.

Despite the fact that the credit for the concept of stress is customarily accorded to Claude Bernard, Walter B. Cannon, and Hans Selye, the principles briefly enunciated in the previous paragraph were first laid down by Sir Charles Darwin. It is to him that we owe a complete reassessment of the relationship of the organism to its environment, incorporated in the concept of natural selection. In his view the environment was in constant change (seasonal, climatic, chemical, geological, etc.), or it was continually being altered by its inhabitants. In the organism's struggle for existence, the environment is potentially threatening or dangerous due to the withdrawal of resources, the disruption of health by infection, starvation, heat, or cold, and the threat of predators and competitors. By virtue of our own activities—the promotion of war and torture; the pollution of the atmosphere, water and ground; and the invention of dangerous technologies—we add to nature's threats and dangers.

In Darwin's formulation, the environment was challenging, dangerous, "stressfull," and full of potential or actual obstacles. Only the fittest survived. Thus the question arose: How does the organism deal with these challenges and stresses, avoid danger, and overcome obstacles to survive and reproduce?

Yet the environment also contains resources, cooperative conspecifics, and shelter. It is a source of information for the reception and processing of which peripheral receptors and the brain have evolved. This information is analyzed, classified, stored, checked against past stores, and synthesized by the brain, and it leads to specific and appropriate actions. These actions include selection of environments by the organism to bring it into more favorable conditions than mere random movements would. Animals determine which aspects of the environment are relevant and which can be ignored; they sense and respond to environmental changes with coordinated physiological and behavioral patterns (2).

Thus biologists study changing response patterns to some aspect of the environment or other organisms in it (e.g., the shadow of a predator hawk; the odor, sight, or sound of a sexually mature or dominant male). Behavioral responses (and their physiological correlates) are usually indicators of food, sexual partners, or danger; they are often short-term but are subject to intense selection because they may fail. One reason for their failure is that both individuals and species vary in their capacities to respond to a given environmental challenge: they are differently adapted.

The environmental challenges and threats to the organism that elicit response patterns may be called stresses or stressors. Although the physiological responses to stressors are, with some exception, similar (3) in different species and genera, what differs between similar species is the interpretation of the challenging or threatening signal. As Levins and Lewontin (2, p. 43) have pointed out, "the most advantageous response to a signal does not depend on . . . [its] . . . physical form but on its value as a predictor or correlate." Different environments or contexts "require different responses." Conversely, different environments may require the same behavioral response as long as it is likely to guarantee survival. In addition, the very system (the brain) that interprets the environment and upon which the organism depends for survival must (or should) be protected from being disrupted by external or internal forces.

The concept of stress is therefore by no means new (in fact, it goes back to Aristotle). Furthermore, the stressors that Selye (4) employed in his first study overwhelmed his animals: They were rendered incapable of, or were prevented from mounting a patterned response. However, even under the most dire challenge, animals capable of making an avoidant response suffered less organ damage than those who were prevented from doing so (5).

Furthermore, stress research has been biased by a tradition of controlled experiments in biologically irrelevant (e.g., electric shock), inappropriate (e.g., injections of croton oil), or impoverished contexts (e.g., social animals isolated in cages). Stress has been equated with anesthesia (e.g., ether stress). In other studies it was administered to highly trained animals made to perform stereotyped, biologically, irrelevant tasks, except the avoidance of pain. From such unnatural experimental conditions and the effects they produced (gastric erosions, adrenal hyperplasia, and hemorrhagic damage to the organs of the immune system) conclusions were drawn about how animals behave in nature, how the brain "works," and how disease (organ damage) is produced.

A DEFINITION OF STRESS

The concept of stress flows naturally from Darwin's formulation of natural selection. Stresses are selective pressures that derive from the physical and social environment. They are challenging or threatening to the survival, integrity, and reproductive success of individuals and of groups. In animals, they are particularly intense at certain times during the life cycle, for example, during breeding. Breeding requires a chain of favorable or optimal environmental conditions that ensure food supplies, housing of offspring, the correct temperature conditions, and relative protection from predators (6).

Organisms vary in their capacity to respond to, meet, deal with, overcome, or escape from challenges and threats; those who cannot or do not fail to survive or fall ill. Therefore, it should not be surprising that individual differences in response to stress occur, which is a principle we also owe to Darwin.

Thus stress can be conceived of as a threat or challenge to the integrity and survival of the organism. Based on this idea and in the case of humans, it may be possible to provide an initial and crude taxonomy of stress (7) in the following manner:

1. Natural disasters: Earthquakes, floods, volcanic eruptions, fire, tornadoes, avalanches, mud slides, pestilence, infections, toxins, drought, and famine
2. Manmade disasters: War, technological inventions, economic disasters, vehicular accidents, hostage-taking, torture, rape, genocide, incarceration, child abuse
3. Personal experiences: Disruption of human relationships by bereavement, separation, or divorce; marital and family discord; migration; forced unemployment; poverty; occupational change; "paced" work; surgery, injury, illness, and disease; examinations

Each of these several categories may have both general and individual consequences. Each person interprets such experiences in his or her own manner; they
have personal meanings and a different impact on each person. Some find challenges or danger exciting, others shrink or flee from them. Some welcome death;
others will go to any length to survive. Therefore, it is not the event or experience per se that is stressful, but how it is perceived by, and what it means to, its
beholder that initiates a process that may end in its being considered stressful.
Each stressor is associated with attempts to deal with it; these, in turn, may be
appropriate or not. A critical variable in the process is a person's sense of control
over the experience, and over his or her actions in dealing with it. Loss of control is experienced as helplessness (or "giving-up"), for example, and is regularly
associated with corticosteroid secretion in humans and animals (8).

Stress cannot only be defined in physiological terms as it often has in the
past. As Darwin had pointed out, behavior and physiology are inseparable.
Together they constitute an integrated, organismic response to challenge, threat,
or danger. These patterned responses (including anticipatory ones) are highly
discriminated and appropriate to the specific experience. What generates behavioral (action) and physiological patterns?: They are presumed to be due to
complex neural and hormonal pattern generators and motor programs involving
oscillatory processes.

STRESS AND HOMEOSTASIS

Since Selye's time, quite another definition of stress has been put forward: It is
"any threat to, or disturbance of homeostasis" (9–11). This definition of stress is
again restricted to physiological responses to stress and it is as problematic as
Selye's previously cited definition for some of the same reasons. Stress research
in recent years has taught us that "threats" or "disturbances" are not equivalent.
The patterned and coordinated changes in behavior and physiology in response
to a stress are exquisitely attuned to each other: A patterned "disturbance" in
the circulation produced by orthostasis differs from that produced by exercise,
or by a threatening fight between animals. (It also seems to be stretching the
meaning of the concept to include orthostasis or exercise in any classification of
stress.)

The concept of homeostasis has outlived its usefulness. The basis of this
idea (owed to Bernard and Cannon) was that every physiological variable
maintains a steady-state equilibrium; when that is perturbed, physiological
reactions occurred to restore the steady state. In the past two or three decades,
biologists and physiologists have realized every critical variable goes through
oscillations: no steady state exists. The body's fundamental operating modes are
oscillatory: respiration; body temperature; blood pressure; the pulse of the
heart; sleep stages; chewing; food intake; menstruation; the levels of hormones,

neurotransmitters, immunocytes, membrane receptors, and enzyme activity; and the cell cycle all go through regular oscillations on a number of time scales (second by second, hourly, circadian, monthly, seasonal, etc.) (12–14).

One reason for the existence of oscillations is that most, if not all, subsystems and systems of the body are arranged in and regulated by negative feedback loops: For example, the subsystem controlling ovarian secretion begins with the hypothalamic luteinizing hormone-releasing hormone (LHRH), which stimulates oscillatory (pulsatile) secretion of luteinizing hormone (LH) by the anterior pituitary gland, which in turn causes estradiol (E_2) to be produced and secreted by the ovary. Estradiol usually inhibits LHRH secretion (15,16). If this inhibition is sufficiently steep, the overall system will oscillate. The steepness of the inhibition may increase to critical levels at puberty because the hypothalamic (preoptic and arcuate) neurons become more "sensitive" to E_2. As a result, oscillation in the system begins (a bifurcation has occurred) and menarche is reached. Of course, the system is more complexly regulated: throughout the menstrual cycle E_2 and progesterone levels change, to account in part for intermittence in the menstrual cycle. In addition, hypothalamic, catecholaminergic, and peptidergic neurons regulate the secretion of LHRH and its (gonadotrophin) associated peptide.

The nonlinear concept of bifurcation entails a qualitative change from one (stable) oscillatory mode to another. An example of such a transition is the midcycle LH pulse that ends with ovulation. This intermittent process cannot be accounted for by any single-loop, oscillatory system. To complicate the matter even further, a single variable may oscillate within two separate time frames: Five to six oscillations (with a mean duration of 28 min) in serum cortisol occur in humans during any 24 h period. These are in turn superimposed on a circadian oscillation (also about 24 h in length) whose nadir occurs in the first hours of the night. Of equal importance is that the adrenocorticotropic hormone (ACTH) shows a similar circadian oscillation. Yet, and despite its close link to episodic corticosteroid secretion, it also oscillates 10 times in a 24 h period with a duration of each oscillation of about 140 min. In addition, oscillatory systems may appear to be closely coupled: sleep and the circadian oscillation of cortisol secretion. We know, however, that these systems may be uncoupled (e.g., by sleep reversal).

Abnormal functioning (illness or disease), according to this view, occurs when a system loses the stability of its usual operating mode (engineers calls this a "failure mode"). Each form of abnormal functioning can be conceived of as a bifurcation to a mode that "models the dynamical patterns of the pathology" (14). The mode may either revert to an earlier one or it may take the form of an oscillatory instability: tetanic contractions, arrhythmias and dysrhythmias, and various other altered temporal patterns. In other idioms, discontrol or disregulation has occurred.

One may, therefore, reconceptualize the effects of a stressor. The perturbations of a system produced by it do not alter the homeostatic steady state, but they induce bifurcations, forcing a system into oscillatory instability, or producing a reversion to an earlier functioning mode.

On the other hand, a subsystem that had previously oscillated by virtue of its participation in a negative feedback loop may be taken out of the loop (e.g., by ectopic tumors that produce peptides—pancreatic gastrinomas, lung tumors secreting ACTH, etc.—or when receptors are preempted by an autoantibody (e.g., in Graves' disease) that continually stimulates unregulated thyroid hormone secretion (17). Yet we do not know how stressors interact with such nonoscillating systems, if they do at all.

STRESS, ILLNESS, AND DISEASE
Concepts of Disease

The oldest pathogenetic concept of disease in western medicine is that its cause(s) is (are) exogenous; it is visited upon a helpless victim by supernatural agents: angry gods, spirits, demons, witches, and so on. This view was reinforced in parallel with a gradually developing taxonomy of specific diseases (initially suggested by Sydenham). When Morgagni and Bichat developed first an organ and later a tissue pathology, they correlated changes in structure with symptoms. The material basis for defining disease was thus established in terms of gross organ and histological changes in dead tissue. The specific anatomical changes were both the cause of the disease(s) and the basis for their classification. Virchow extended pathology to the level of cells. He proclaimed that the nosology of disease must be based on the causes of the cellular pathology. The discovery of bacteria by Pasteur was not only a significant advance in our understanding of the cause of (infectious) diseases but also reinforced the concept of their exogenous causation. This linear concept established (and overstated) the causes and pathogenesis of disease: An external agent attacks a healthy but passive organism to produce material changes in it that *are* the disease (18).

Koch, by his experiments with *M. tuberculosis*, reinforced this grossly oversimplified view of the pathogenesis of tuberculosis by overwhelming his animals with massive doses of the mycobacterium. Selye, as already mentioned, did the same to his animals by other means (restraint, injury, injection of toxins) to produce disease. The relationship of stress to disease was conceptualized as another exogenous source of anatomical damage; it was as linear a concept as the infections theory of disease.

However, many factors in addition to exposure to *M. tuberculosis* determine its expression as a disease. Among these factors are the age of the host at the time of exposure to and infection with the organism; the host's nutritional and immunological status; and his or her ethnicity, economic status, and genetic origin. In addition, the anatomical lesions of sarcoidosis very closely resemble those produced by the tubercle bacillus, and yet they are not due to infection by it. Thus the specific histological validity of tuberculosis is also suspect.

These examples, among many others, suggest that an endogenous concept of disease is closer to reality. According to this second view, external causes interact with responses of the host to produce symptoms of disease. The responses of the host to the inciting external cause may be limited or are altered. Among the factors that limit or alter the person's capacity to response are genetic ones. However, the same genetic defect may have different outcomes: The X-linked form of agammaglobulinemia places the person at high risk for repeated infection in childhood and rheumatoid arthritis and malignant disease in later life. In patients with phenylketonuria, the absence of the enzyme phenylalanine hydroxylase results in an inability to metabolize phenylalanine, and is associated for unknown reasons with mental deficiency. It limits the learning ability of the child with phenylketonuria; living in a complex society, such a limitation impairs the acquisition of adaptive "tools." In some environments, a genetic defect (the hemoglobin S trait) endows its heterozygous owner with increased resistance to infection with the malaria parasite. In other geographic environments, in which no malaria exists, we see only the effects of sickle-cell disease in heterozygotes, with which this trait is also associated.

The interaction of the host with the environment is not only a product of his or her capacity to mount a response to infection. There are many other classes of interaction. The capacity of the organism to maintain response to challenge or threat is also determined by genes and by intrauterine, perinatal, and early postnatal experience; by nutritional, educational, intellectual, familial, and cultural factors; and by aging. These limit or enhance the adaptive capacity of the organism in its interaction with the environment.

Whereas the traditional exogenous theory of disease is linear, deterministic, and unifactorial, the endogenous theory is nonlinear, multifactorial, and probabilistic. This second theory resembles in part the modern theory of psychosomatic medicine (19,20) and it accords more closely with darwinian principles than does the traditional biomedical model.

Selye's Diseases of Adaptation

The intimate association between stress and disease was already apparent in Selye's initial paper. In the next 10 years he placed the burden on the glucocorticoids as the main incitors of the anatomical effects he had produced. As many have pointed out, most recently Munck et al. (11), Selye seemed to have forgotten earlier observations that adrenalectomy markedly enhances the sensitivity of animals to injury, infection, and so on. But at that time, 40 years ago, it was quite unclear whether in the normal animal the permissive role of the corticosteroids in endowing the animal with some resistance to stress was due to the mineralo- or the glucocorticosteroids. Nonetheless, Selye believed that many diseases (hypertension, peptic ulcer, allergic, rheumatic, and collagen diseases) were the product of excessive or "adaptive" reactions in which the corticosteroids played a pathogenetic role. He demonstrated, for example, that a high-salt diet and treatment with deoxycorticosterone acetate in a nephrectomized animal produced high blood pressure (BP). He called these heterogeneous group of illnesses diseases of adaptation, thus implying that disease was the product of "abnormal" or excessive responses to stress.

There is, however, no evidence that the most common forms of hypertension are the product of excessive levels of mineralocorticoids (the role of salt in this disease remains enigmatic to this date). But the coup de grace to his theory of disease was given by the demonstration that ACTH and the corticosteroids actually suppress the manifestations of allergic, rheumatic, and collagen diseases (21).

WHAT IS PSYCHOSOMATIC MEDICINE?

The idea that there is a special category of psychosomatic disease or illness is wrong. Equally outdated is the concept that psychosomatic medicine is limited to the study of the role of the emotions in clinical medicine (22).

What is psychosomatic medicine? It is an alternative to the traditional and predominant Western biomedical, disease-oriented model. Psychosomatic medicine is a patient-oriented medicine. It seeks to render a comprehensive account of a person's predisposition to, the precipitation and perpetuation of, illness and disease (23) as well as the patient's responses to them and to treatment. Therefore, its purview goes beyond a more limited concern with the proximate mechanisms of disease, which are the central focus of the traditional medical model. Because its ambitious program is so comprehensive it remains incomplete. We know, for example, a great deal about the social contributions to averting and inciting many diseases, that is, how many diseases are unequally distributed in populations. Much information has also been collected about the many onset conditions of a variety of illnesses and diseases. Genetic factors are also known to contribute to the variation in the causes of disease. Because of its historical concerns, medicine has acquired much knowledge of the pathophysiology and anatomical pathology of disease that are integrated into the foregoing. What is often missing is a true understanding of pathogenesis and the specific link between the antecedent causative factors of a disease and its development. Many gaps remain to be filled in before a full account of any disease can be rendered.

Psychosomatic medicine attempts to describe comprehensively the cause of disease, with an emphasis on the factors that limit the host's capacity to resist

challenges and threats. This, as noted above, is the product of genetic endow-
ment and a variety of experiences in the environment during maturation and
development. Psychosomatic medicine is based on the axiom that many factors
in combination enhance or impede persons' adaptive capacities, respectively, to
promote health in some, or to place others at risk for illness and disease on meeting threats, challenges, infection, or disaster.

At the same time, it incorporates into its concepts the observation that a
person's conduct may also place him or her at risk for a number of serious
diseases. Certain sexual practices or intravenous drug abuse antecede infection
with the human immunodeficiency virus. The smoking and chewing of tobacco
products are hazards that contribute to atherosclerosis, pulmonary emphysema
and carcinoma, and cancer of the mouth and larynx. Pregnant mothers who
smoke tobacco or abuse drugs and alcohol deliver babies of low birth weight
who may be addicted to drugs and suffer from the fetal alcohol syndrome. While
alcohol abuse may eventuate in disease in virtually every organ of the body, it is
also strongly associated with trauma, disability, or death due to automobile
accidents and with physical assault on, and sexual abuse of, other persons.

Traditional medicine studies the biochemical pharmacology and toxicology
of alcohol, nicotine, and other drugs. It waits to correct the damage wrought by
them after it has occurred, rather than preventing their social, familial, economic, and other antecedents. The abuse of alcohol and tobacco, for example,
increases sharply in male workers who are forcibly unemployed (24).

Psychosomatic medicine asks why persons fall ill at a particular time in their
lives, and with one disease and not another. The answers to such questions can
only be found by determining the context in which illness and disease begins,
and by an inquiry into the array of predispositions to a particular disease. The
context in which disease begins is presumed to be perceived as stressful and not
controllable; therefore, the experience of the stress is often unpleasant and distressing to its beholder. Specific emotions are aroused that signal danger and
adversity (i.e., fear or anger); if the situation is averted or overcome, relief is
generated; if the outcome is uncertain, hope is experienced; if the challenge or
threat is uncontrollable and the person is defeated by it, hopelessness and helplessness are felt: The person gives up (25). Controllability means the capacity of
a person to mount the appropriate response to challenge or threat; in part, this
ability is a function of knowledge as to how to go about doing so; in part, it is a
function of regulating the cognitive-emotional responses to such a threat. Many
of the stresses that have been correlated with illness and disease onset are
dramatic and sudden. However, a chronic background of distress, irritation,
and frustration is also conducive to demoralization, a chronically depressed
mood, and a variety of diseases (26,27).

Coping with challenge and threat mediates the impact of such stresses. Age
and maturity are critical variables in the ability to cope with them (i.e., control

them). Coping entails the realistic appraisal of the stressful situation, the requisite information for handling it, and a program of action designed to overcome it (28). At times other strategies are used to regulate the meaning and emotional impact of the event. Of crucial importance in coping with stress is the help, support, and advice of other people; in medicine these are often the physician or nurse. In fact, social cohesion, close personal relationship, and a slow rate of sociocultural change buffer the effects of high-fat diets and obesity that are some of the risk factors for coronary atherosclerosis and thus sudden death or myocardial infarction (29,30).

Bereavement (A Specific Stressful Onset Condition) and the Role of Human Relationships in Disease and Illness

In the past 25 years there has been a discernible shift in psychosomatic medicine from concerns about the personal characteristics of patients with specific diseases to the role of bereavement or separation as a general and frequent onset condition of disease and illness, and in determining their prognosis (including recovery from disease and surgery). These observations, together with research on the behavioral and physiological effects of separating young animals from their mothers, has led to a reconceptualization of the critical role of personal relationships in health, illness, and disease (31-35).

The usual and personal response of human beings to bereavement or separation is grief. A decline in health occurs within the first year following bereavement and a sharp increase in the incidence of depression, the risk of suicide, and mortality are observed. Bereaved persons smoke more tobacco, experience sleeplessness, drink more alcohol, and increase their use of "tranquilizers" (36,37). Bereaved persons not only change their habits but also are at risk for a wide variety of diseases or the exacerbation of previous disease (35, pp. 311-312). It is clear that bereavement does not specify one disease; other interactive factors do so.

Our knowledge of the psychobiology of bereavement in humans is also in a rudimentary state: in some persons, but not all, corticosteroid excretion levels are elevated. Older subjects of both sexes facing bereavement, or who have been widowed, have higher urinary levels of norepinephrine or epinephrine; when they are anxious or depressed, their serum prolactin and growth hormone levels are elevated (38). A depressed mood mediates the effects of bereavement in both men and women, and is associated with decreased responses of peripheral lymphocytes to mitogen stimulation (39,40) and natural killer cell cytotoxicity (41). However, it is not yet known how such immunological changes affect health outcomes.

In contrast to our dearth of knowledge of the human psychobiology of bereavement, much is known about the effects of separating young animals from their mothers. Such an experience has both immediate and long-term psychobiological effects. The latter include a predisposition to high BP (when the animal is subsequently returned to the colony); later persistent elevations of basal heart rate; disturbances in growth and of sleep and body temperature regulation; persistent immunosuppression and a predisposition to opportunistic infection; a marked increase in the incidence of gastric erosions (when rats are later challenged); disturbances in the regulation of polyamine synthesis; and a lowering of the catecholamine and nucleoprotein content of the brain (35, pp. 317-319).

Based on an extensive series of his and other investigators' studies that systematically examined the short-term effects of separation on the behavior and physiology of infant rats (and monkeys) while separate aspects of the mother-infant interaction were varied, Hofer (32) has concluded that the mother regulates her offspring's behavior and physiology until the time of weaning. For instance, her milk regulates the infant's heart rate, her body heat maintains its body temperature, her licking its neck sustains the infant's growth hormone levels, a pheromone secreted by the areolae produces attachment to her nipple, and her touch controls its activity. The vital role of these interactions is attested to by the profound consequences of a 48 h separation at 14 days of age that places the young animal at risk for later disease. One may conclude that prior to weaning the mother acts as an external regulator of the behavior of its infant and the normal maturation of its brain and bodily systems, even to the point of influencing gene expression.

There is also an abundant literature from human subjects which suggests that children and adults who are personally immature (especially reliant on others) are at morbid risk (42). Among other factors, immaturity makes them particularly sensitive to bereavement and separation, and less capable (without the intervention of others) of regulating their own behavior and bodily function.

How Do Stresses Incite Disease?

What is far less clear is how acute or chronic stress and distress, and the failure to cope with them, contribute to the onset of one disease or illness and not another. Despite decades of research in autonomic psychophysiology, psychoneuroendocrinology, and now psychoneuroimmunology (43), progress in answering this question has proceeded slowly. It is one thing to demonstrate that in nature or in the laboratory stressors produce physiological changes in every bodily system, but it is quite another to demonstrate that such acute changes do or do not lead to disease. Thus it may very well be true that the normotensive children of a hypertensive parent have larger and more persistent BP responses (44), but it is quite another matter to demonstrate that this BP "hyperreactivity" eventuates in hypertension (45). In fact, the evidence mounts quite to the contrary.

In part, the failure to solve the problem of how stressful experience is transduced into physiological change is blamed on our inability to "solve" the "mind–brain–body" problem. This age-old conundrum reappears in theories about the relationship of stress to disease in the guise of the postulate that emotions engendered by stress linearly "produced" physiological change. The failure to solve this particular puzzle came about because the theory did not take into account that behavior (including the emotions) and physiology are inseparable. One does not cause the other; they are part of an integrated, organismic response to stress, and are specifically attuned to the threat or challenge. (The cat about to fight another shows specific behaviors and cardiovascular changes that differ from those observed during the fight, and from those that obtain upon victory or defeat [46]. Furthermore, these physiological changes are patterned ones: each pattern differs during the various phases of the fight).

Therefore, one major scientific task is to discover the way in which physiology and behavior are coordinated. An approach to the eventual solution to this question is to determine the common principles that guide their functioning (17).

Acute organismic changes are imposed on long-standing social arrangements. Social animals establish hierarchies. Each member of the hierarchy has his or her "place" in it. Each "place" has its own psychobiology. In stable primate societies, the background levels or patterns of a neurotransmitter (serotonin), or of LH and progesterone, depend on the animal's status in the social hierarchy. They differ markedly in the dominant and subordinate male and female, respectively. The subordinate female marmoset monkey does not ovulate. Subordinate females are harassed by the dominant and excluded from food resources and male partners; their mean levels of LH and progesterone are low. When they are removed from the colony, oscillatory LH patterns in the subordinate resume and mean levels of LH and progesterone rise. A preovulatory LH surge occurs. When the animals are returned to the colony, the situation is reversed. Yet when LHRH (1 μg every 2 h) is infused into subordinates living in the colony, LH pulses, a preovulatory LH surge, and raised progesterone levels are seen (47). In the subordinate female living with a dominant one, LH secretion is under tonic inhibitory control, possibly by beta-endorphin, which is in turn released by the corticotropin-releasing factor (CRF).

These observations provide new insights into the relationship of social arrangements to physiology. They lead to new questions: How does the submissive female monkey, already altered physiologically, respond to another challenge? Her baseline "psychobiology" differs from that of the dominant female. Also, her lack of menstrual cycling and ovulation cannot really be considered a disease. Yet in a woman it might be considered as such.

Role of the Neuropeptides in Stress

The discovery of the neuropeptides ushered in a new era in our understanding of how stress generates patterns of physiological change (48), and of how behavior and physiology are integrated (49). They have provided us with surprising new insights into how stress antecedes and induces disease. At least in rats, some of the peptides seem to play a role in the induction and prevention of gastric erosions by (cold-restraint) stress. Both thyrotropin-releasing hormone (TRH) and CRF are released by cooling animals (50,51). However, these two peptides, which are centrally administered and vagally mediated, have opposite actions on gastric acid secretion, contractions, and erosion formation. The TRH provokes them, CRF inhibits them, and also counteracts the effects of TRH when both are instilled into the cisterna magna of rats (52-54).

These observations begin to link stress, mediated by the brain, to disease outcome, yet the relevance of these observations on rats to the pathogenesis of human gastric or duodenal ulceration remains questionable. Among the reasons for questioning their applicability is the fact that every disease is heterogeneous and the pathogenesis of each subform may differ. Thus the matter becomes even more complex.

Heterogeneity of Disease

The likelihood that each disease, defined by some common anatomical configuration, is not uniform further complicates our understanding: The lesion is but the final outcome of different pathogenetic (or combinations thereof) processes. Thus the question of the role of stress in pathogenesis is raised to another level of complexity.

Variation characterizes each disease. Diabetes mellitus occurs in at least two forms (types I and II). Patients with duodenal ulcer may have elevated (inherited as an autosomal dominant trait) or normal serum levels of the pepsinogen (PG) I isoenzyme; other patients have elevated or normal PG-II isoenzyme levels (55). Several different forms of altered regulation of gastric acid secretion occur in duodenal ulcer (56). Heterogeneity occurs in hypertension (e.g., defined in terms of the distribution of serum renin levels), bronchial asthma, rheumatoid arthritis, systemic lupus erythematosus, and other diseases. At least 100 forms of "cancer" are known. Correlated with the different forms of one disease, psychological heterogeneity also exists (57-59). Their psychological heterogeneity further suggests that patients prone to each of the subforms of a disease differ in their special sensitivity to one stressor and not another. This hypothesis, although testable, remains to be further proven.

How psychobiological variation interacts with patterned physiological change induced by stress is not understood. For example, the question of how bereavement interacts with the various regulatory disturbances that have been identified in peptic duodenal ulcer is not known. In fact, there is some beginning evidence from investigations in rats that the pathogenesis (the proximate mechanisms) of gastric erosions is not uniform either. Various combinations of increased gastric contractions and acid secretion with diminished bicarbonate, somatostatin, mucus, and serotonin secretion may all play a role.

Many pathways have been identified that lead to the development of bronchial asthma: infection, allergic reactions to an array of antigens, the mediation of immunoglobulin E, and the secretion of the mediators of the immediate forms of hypersensitivity, exercise, excitement, and excessive interpersonal closeness (or distance). But the asthmatic attack will not occur unless bronchial hyperreactivity is already present. The tendency to bronchoconstriction is mediated by the vagus and excessive muscarinic cholinergic receptor activity on bronchial smooth muscle.

New Concepts of the Nature of Disease

These two examples, among many others, illustrate a new concept of disease. No longer defined in terms of an anatomical change as the final end-product, disease is conceptualized as a disturbance in the communication between cells and organs, leading to disturbances in their regulation (17,20,60-62). The organism is an intricate communication system of information exchange that regulates behavior and physiology. Cells communicate with one another by coded messenger signals: electrical impulses, ions, neurotransmitters, amino acids, peptides, proteins, carbohydrates, and fatty acids; they influence each other locally and at a distance. The signals they emit are carefully regulated by numerous influences (17). The signal is emitted intermittently. It operates in an oscillatory mode (see above) because the subsystems of communication signals are arranged in a series of negative feedback loops. Disease occurs when the mode in which the system usually operates goes through a bifurcation.

The organism is also integrated into a larger system of information exchange. It receives signals from the physical and social environment, and emits coded signals (sounds, gestures, postures, smells, words, etc.) into it. The received signals are transduced and digitized at peripheral receptors. The signal is processed in parallel by the brain of the organism and is capable of selecting and analyzing it. The organism may respond to one aspect or to all of the signal, or may choose not to, depending in part on the contextual framework in which it occurs.

Until recently we have not known how the transduced signal is communicated to those integrating areas of the brain that produce patterned changes in hormones: the autonomic and immune system. Only recently have some of the communication channels (pathways) been mapped. For example, neural pathways from peripheral receptors are now known to release CRF (63); they occur in parallel with those that end in cortical receptive fields. Parallel pathways of this kind form the basis of integrated behavioral and physiological responses.

STRESS AND DISEASE: ISCHEMIC HEART DISEASE

What is the evidence for these (psychosomatic) assertions? A very limited number of examples will be used to support them, including coronary artery disease (CAD) and its consequences. Its incidence and prevalence are low in stable communities and societies. In other societies, its point prevalence is inversely correlated with social class (64), being highest in those least educated and lowest on the social scale. Obesity is also more prevalent in American women in the lower social classes (65). Obesity is a risk factor for CAD, as it is for sleep apnea and type II diabetes mellitus, both of which in turn predispose to CAD.

It is claimed that CAD is a disease of well-nourished people who exercise little and ingest excess calories and saturated fats. Yet the relationship of low levels of exercise and excessive food intake is usually associated with obesity only in women (66). However, men are more prone to CAD.

Saturated fats raise low-density lipoprotein (LDL) levels. A low ratio of high-density lipoprotein (HDL) to LDL levels is a metabolic risk factor for CAD. In familial (genetic) hypercholesterolemia, LDL levels are high and CAD occurs at an early age (67). Thus genetic factors play a crucial role in one form of CAD. On the other hand, the HDL/LDL ratio falls in unemployed male workers without their having this genetic trait (68).

Another frequent antecedent of CAD is hypertension, which in turn may be exacerbated by obesity and excess calories. In addition, hypertension is conducive to myocardial hypertrophy and relative myocardial insufficiency and failure, especially in the presence of CAD.

Additional risk factors play a role in CAD: the use of tobacco, and possibly the type A behavior pattern (TABP). However, the evidence of the role of this behavior pattern in predisposing to CAD and myocardial infarction (MI) is by no means persuasive, except in the group of subjects first described by Friedman and Rosenman (69). In fact, recent evidence suggests that TABP contributes mainly to sudden death in patients with CAD who have recovered from an MI, but not to angina pectoris or MI itself (70).

A number of risk factors for CAD have been described, but none so far except low socioeconomic status can be classified as potential stresses culminating in CAD, MI, or sudden death. To make the matter even more problematic, there is evidence that coronary atherosclerosis develops early in the life of young men and evolves over many years (71), which suggests that whatever the causative role of stress, it is more likely to be "permissive" and interactive rather than directly causal.

What are these "stresses?" How do they manifest themselves? Blue collar workers who do heavy manual labor or shift work and are exposed to excessive noise are especially prone to MI (72). A chronic work overload, especially that over which the worker has no control (e.g., paced work), is also conducive to MI. Siegrist et al. (73) have prospectively studied 416 blue collar workers exposed to working conditions over which they exerted little control. Some of them responded by attempts to enhance their control and to increase their commitment to work, which, under the circumstances, lead to frustration and irritation but a refusal to quit. These workers were initially free of any discernable signs of CAD. When compared to matched workers not exposed to "forced" work, those who responded with the psychological reactions just described had higher BP levels ($r^2 = 0.35$) than those who did not ($r^2 = 0.09$), and higher LDL and lower HDL levels. In 365 of these blue collar workers evaluated for 3 years, the incidence of MI was 19.2% (compared to an incidence of 6.0% in a normal, matched, male control population). Of particular interest was that 50% of such workers who responded to their work with frustration and irritation also experienced sleep disturbances (20% in controls). Forty percent of those with sleep disturbances suffered from sleep apnea, which was associated with cardiac arrhythmias. Those who did not have sleep disturbances maintained high heart rates throughout the night, or showed greater heart rate variability during sleep.

These studies are both unique and need to be repeated. Equally interesting is that both sudden death and MI occur with excess frequency in the morning hours when the person is alert and active.

Some further understanding of the role of alertness and activity in CAD has been obtained in studying the phenomenon of silent myocardial ischemia, which is a product of coronary vasospasm and is not necessarily associated with ST segment changes on the electrocardiogram (EKG)- and/or with angina pectoris.

Coronary blood flow may be reduced by narrowing or occlusion of a coronary artery, which leads to pain and ischemia when the myocardial oxygen requirement increases, for example, with exercise. However, it is now well known that vasospasm occurs in arteries compromised by atherosclerosis and/or thrombosis even during acute MI (74). Yet vasospasm can occur with or without coronary atherosclerosis, and in any phase of ischemic heart disease. During vasospasm myocardial perfusion is diminished and left ventricular wall motion abnormalities may occur ("silent" ischemia). When anginal pain is present and cardiac perfusion deficits are seen, the EKG may show no abnormalities. On the other hand, elevations or depression of the ST segment of the EKG (as a criterion of myocardial ischemia at rest) were only accompanied by pain in 32% of 6009 episodes in 33 patients (75). These EKG changes may occur without any or consistent increases in heart rate or BP.

The question is: how and under what conditions does silent ischemia occur? It is recognized that in patients with such a condition a variety of pharmacological agents (ergonovine, histamine, norepinephrine, and neuropeptide Y) (76) can produce vasospasm. However, of greater interest to those investigating the role of stressors in the inception of silent ischemic episodes with ST segment changes is the work of Deanfield et al. (77). They showed that in 16 patients with angina pectoris, episodes of transient myocardial ischemia occurred in the absence of physical exertion. During the performance of serial subtraction (100 minus 7, etc.), 12 of the 16 had abnormalities of regional myocardial perfusion measured by positron emission tomography with rubidium 82. While subtracting numbers, only 6 of the 12 showed ST segment depression, and 4 complained of angina. Exercise produced perfusion abnormalities and ST-segment depression in all 16, and angina pectoris in 15. In addition to simple subtraction, the act of public speaking may induce a fall in ejection fraction in about one-third of patients with CAD. Regional wall motion abnormalities occur while reading a book, during the Stroop test, or while performing mental arithmetic in 59% of 23 of these patients. Public speaking and exercise were equivalent in producing cardiac dysfunction (78).

It is now quite clear that the incidence of anginal pain is a severe underestimate of the true prevalence of myocardial ischemia (as adjudged by ST segment changes or perfusion deficits). The EKG changes in turn do not reflect faithfully myocardial perfusion deficits that result from coronary vasospasm induced by everyday tasks and events. Despite this obvious source of error, it is now more certain that myocardial ischemia occurs during everyday physical and mental activities in patients with CAD and less frequently while they are asleep (79). (The ischemia is, however, potentially damaging to the myocardium.)

Patients with CAD may either die suddenly or develop an MI when excited, during arguments or exercise, or while they urinate or defecate. The question, of course, is whether all of these routine activities should be considered stresses. Clearly they are not.

Additional factors play an antecedent role in sudden death and MI. In several studies, the unemployed seeking work had increased mortality ratios (1.3:1.0), accounted for by sudden death and MI when contrasted to employed workers; or they were at increased risk for ischemic heart disease (24). An interaction between bereavement, age, and death (predominatly from heart disease) has been reported. Recent widowers (231 of 4486), 55 years and older, died within the first 6 months after the death of their wives: an increase of 40% above that expected for married men of the same age (80,81). In a somewhat older group of 361 elderly widowed men and women, an excess mortality occurred especially in the men. The best independent predictors of mortality were unhappiness, anxiety and depression, and minimal social contacts (82). Furthermore, the prognosis at every point during a period of 10 years following myocardial infarction in 140 married and unmarried men and women was considerably worse in both unmarried groups (83).

The traditional biomedical approach is concerned with the biochemical and molecular processes in coronary atherogenesis (84). The psychosomatic approach is to chart all the avenues that lead to CAD and its outcomes. It is apparent from this review that there is no one pathway. Furthermore, a number of distal and proximate factors interact with CAD to place persons at risk for serious and often fatal disease. Even routine and trivial perturbations may throw a person with CAD into the oscillatory instability known as ventricular tachycardia or fibrillation (85), and death. One may conclude that the role of stress in CAD and its complications is subtle. It is most evident that it may play an important role over time in workers whose jobs are of low status, demanding, and over which they have little or no control; in those with few human contacts; the unemployed who want to work; those with major financial worries; and in divorced or widowed men (86).

A number of proximate events may antecede or surround the occurrence of sudden death or MI in middle-aged men, including the death of a spouse.

STRESS AND ILL HEALTH

Both traditional medicine and, until recently, psychosomatic medicine have preoccupied themselves with disease defined by alterations in the material structure of organs and cells. When no such changes occur but a patient is ill (in ill health), he or she is either neglected or subjected to unnecessary diagnostic or surgical procedures designed to search out the nonexistent lesion.

To put it another way, medical traditionalists consider that structural change is the only cause of illness and their only concern. Yet a patient may have a disease and be in good health, or be ill. The patient may also be ill without a disease, but he or she cannot both be in ill and good health at the same time.

Most patients who seek medical care (other than at major medical centers) do not have diseases but are in ill health. Ill health constitutes a major burden to patients, their families, and society. Those in chronic ill health spend 7 days a month in bed (normal amount, ½ day). Their annual medical care costs exceed by a factor of 9 the annual expenditure of the average U.S. citizen (87).

Persons in ill-health are symptomatic and disabled. Ill health has clearly been related to stress, for example, the threat of or an actual job loss is associated with a 70% increase in episodes of illness, 150% increase in medical consultations, and 200% increase in attendance at OPD. (88).

The graver and the more frequent life events, other than job loss, are adjudged to be by patients, the longer they are likely to be symptomatic, absent from work, prone to disrupt their daily routine, and visit physicians (89). The reasons for consultation are a large variety of symptoms referable to the cardiorespiratory, neuromuscular, and gastrointestinal systems and associated with anxiety and depression, which are often misdiagnosed (90).

These symptoms cluster into groups in an unsystematic manner, for instance, patients with a functional or an irritable bowel syndrome hyperventilate. Hyperventilators in turn complain of neuromuscular symptoms. In fact, these patients express personal distress in terms of bodily symptoms.

A more precise analysis of the symptoms leads to the conclusion that they represent physiological changes in vital biological functions: in respiratory and cardiac rhythms, food intake, digestion, elimination, reproduction, sleep rhythms, pain modulation, and others. Most of these functions are oscillatory; they are disturbed when their usual oscillatory mode is changed.

These vital biological functions can be disrupted by stress; in fact such a disruption is the more usual outcome of stress than is disease. Stress, as one of the many possible factors involved in the pathogenesis of disease, actually has a low probability of inciting it: even in a high risk population the probability is 0.14 (91). The accumulated observational evidence is that stress experienced as distress manifests itself as a gamut of bodily symptoms that express disrupted biological functions. These assertions will be supported by two of the many "functional" syndromes of ill health.

Hyperventilation

In this syndrome, the ventilatory effort exceeds the body's need for oxygen, with the result that the partial pressure of carbon dioxide ($PaCO_2$) in arterial blood falls and respiratory alkalosis ensues. The chronic hyperventilator shows irregular (oscillatory) patterns of breathing, characterized by upper thoracic excursions interspersed with deep (often irregularly occurring) inspirations. Chronic hyperventilators may trigger a new attack by a single inspiration (92). About two-thirds of all chronic hyperventilators have persistently low $PaCO_2$ levels, to which the respiratory center has adapted. They are, however, no longer alkalotic.

Changes in inspiratory depth occur with sighing, gasping, exercise, excitement, and fear. Grief-stricken patients sigh; pain can produce a gasp. Each of these changes in rhythmic respirations may set off the symptoms and complex metabolic changes of the syndrome (93) (Table 1).

Acute attacks of hyperventilation may produce cardiovascular changes. In association with a reduced $PaCO_2$ level and alkalosis, an initial arterial vasodilation occurs, mean BP falls, and cardiac output and heart rate increase. A few minutes later arterial vasoconstriction (including the coronary arteries) occurs (94), and the changes in BP, cardiac output, and heart rate disappear.

Hyperventilating patients may manifest sinus tachycardia and arrhythmias at rest, ST segment elevations or depressions (95), and supraventricular and

TABLE 1   Signs and Symptoms of Hyperventilation Syndrome (HVS)

General
  Chronic and easy fatigability, weakness, sleep disturbances, headache, excessive sweating, sensation of feeling cold, poor concentration and performance of tasks
Neurologic
  Numbness and tingling especially of distal extremities, giddiness, syncope, blurring or tunneling of vision, and impaired thinking
Respiratory
  Sensation of breathlessness or inability to take a deep enough breath with sighing, yawning, and excessive use of upper chest and accessory muscles of respiration, nocturnal dyspnea superficially mimicking paroxysmal nocturnal dyspnea of cardiovascular origin, and nonproductive cough with frequent clearing of throat
Cardiovascular
  Chest pains often mimicking angina, palpitations, and tachycardia
Gastrointestinal
  Aerophagia resulting in full/bloated sensation, belching, flatus, esophageal reflux and heartburn, sharp lower chest pain, dry mouth, and sensation of lump in throat
Musculoskeletal
  Myalgias, increased muscle tone with muscle tightness (stiffness), cramps, with occasional carpopedal spasms and, rarely, a more generalized tetany
Psychiatric
  Anxious, irritable, and tense although may superficially appear calm (suppression of emotional release), depersonalization or a feeling of being far away, phobias, and panic attacks
Metabolic
  Hypocapnia ($PaCO_2$), alkalosis (in acute not chronic HVS), left shift of O_2 dissociation curve, hypophosphatemia (due to intracellular shift), deionization of Ca^{2+}
Renal
  Increased excretion of HCO_3^-, increased formation and excretion of ammonium ion and titratable acid, increase in Na l and K^+
Neural
  Resetting of respiratory center to low $PaCO_2$, beta-adrenergic discharge, ? release of histamine
Cardiac
  Vasodilation followed by constriction (i.e., first fall in mean BP, peripheral resistance, increase in HR and CO, then return to baseline), ST-segment depression or elevation, coronary vasoconstriction, sinus arrhythmia or tachycardia, PVCs
Cerebrovascular
  Vasoconstriction, decreased flow, EEG: high-voltage delta activity

Source: Ref. 93.

ventricular premature beats. Hypocapnic alkalosis reduces coronary arterial blood flow (96) and produces coronary vasospasm in patients with and without Prinzmetal's variant angina (97), and coronary atherosclerosis. In fact, hyperventilation in some patients may eventuate in MI, probably by producing coronary vasospasm and silent ischemia.

These observations, taken together with those described above, may explain why patients with anxiety and panic disorders have a shortened lifespan (98,99). At least 50% of all patients diagnosed as having these disorders actually hyperventilate. Thus it seems likely that a functional syndrome—one of ill-health—can eventuate in ischemic heart disease and its fatal sequelae (100).

Functional Bowel Disorders

It is of some historical interest that the same physician, DaCosta, who described "soldier's heart" (i.e., the hyperventilation syndrome) also described membranous enteritis: the functional (irritable) bowel disorder (FBD) in 1871. This topic is still fraught with confusion and the syndrome goes by a multitude of descriptive names. It has only recently been realized, however, that the putative local variants of FBD ("mucous" or "spastic" colitis) are only a part of a more general functional disturbance of the entire gut with symptoms (101,102). The prevalence of other associated symptoms (headache, backache, muscular aches, chest pain, hyperventilation, anxiety, and depression, in 78%) do not point to the gut as the sole source of origin of the FBD. The entire, distressed person is afflicted. It is also a common disorder: Its lifetime prevalence in a population may be 50-75% (103).

Among the more distressing forms of FBD is gastroesopheageal reflux (GER), which may result in esophagitis and esophageal strictures. In GER, gastric acid is cleared less often or forcefully from the esophagus by reflex peristaltic waves. At the same time the lower esophageal sphincter tone is reduced. Because refluxing occurs most frequently at night, sleep recordings have demonstrated that patients with GER awaken too transiently, and do not clear their esophagus or constrict the sphincter. It is thus basically a sleep disorder (104).

Related to GER is diffuse esophageal spasm that may be expressed as chest pain and is, therefore, often mistaken for ischemic heart disease. In this form of FBD, nonperistaltic tetanic waves occur in the esophagus and the lower sphincter does not open. A bifurcation (phase transition) in the usual rhythmic, sequential patterns of esophageal contractions on swallowing has therefore occurred. In other forms of spasm, spontaneous or interrupted contractile rhythms occur. The esophagus can be thrown into tetanic spasm experimentally by stresses (105). Patients with this disorder are also frequently and diagnosably depressed, anxious, or alcohol abusers.

Rhythmic disturbances occur in the stomach in FBD. The usual rhythmic three to four cycle/min gastric pacemaker potential may be irregular, tetanic, or intermittent at either increased or decreased frequencies (106,107). In other patients jejunal motility and migratory motor complexes (MMC) are irregular or absent. In fact, the MMC is extraordinarily sensitive to any environmental change, including noise and cold. (Motility disturbances occur in animals when stressed: They consist of an inhibition of small bowel contractions and reduced colonic transit time [108], which may be due to the release of CRF by the stressor).

The predominantly colonic form of FBD is associated with psychological distress in 80% of all patients. The sources of distress are marital discord, work, and concern about children in persons who are chronic worriers, or are always fearful (109). The distress they experience often takes the form of a depressed mood or a somatization disorder and is present in at least 80% of such patients (110,111).

Some of these patients are also unusually sensitive to the pain of abdominal distention (112). They also respond to distention or to the eating of a meal not by a single contraction but by tetanic oscillations of the colon (113). The electrical activity in the colonic form of FBD in some patients is marked by an increase in the proportion of slow myoelectric activity (114). These slow potentials also persist much longer after a meal.

Our knowledge of the psychophysiology of the FBD is far from complete. The FBD is clearly not a physiological disorder of the gut alone but of the whole distressed person. The sources of his or her distress are not fully worked out, and it is obviously not one disorder because different distrubances of colonic function have been recorded (115).

CONCLUSION

We have attempted to redefine stress, according to Sir Charles Darwin's ideas, and guided by the principles of evolutionary and organismic biology. In so dong, it becomes apparent that stresses are selective pressures with which all creatures must contend. It is not surprising that some of these pressures occur because animals are social beings: competition and predation are part of life. We add to these selective pressures, which are in part occasioned by conflict with our fellows. Animals are alerted to danger by internal signals, and respond to victory, defeat, discovery, and other emotional states. The responses to selective pressures must be specific and discriminated in order to succeed. The entire organism participates in them. However, injury, defeat, infection, and malnutrition may be followed by disease.

Because the organism is one and indivisible, any part definition of stress "responses" must necessarily fail. Therefore, they cannot be defined only by the physiological response, or by an outdated concept such as disturbed homeostasis. Every function of the organism is oscillatory; no functional (homeostatic) steady state exists. New concepts are needed to understand how stresses and oscillatory modes of functioning interact.

Because stresses are selective pressures that challenge or threaten whole organisms, one can only study them in intact creatures. Such a line of approach is not traditional in medicine, because of its historical concern with material alterations in organs and cells and with the proximate mechanisms of disease. Therefore, a medicine of whole organisms arose, poorly named psychosomatic medicine. The aim of this newer conceptual approach was to study the factors that aided persons in, or prevented them from, meeting or overcoming selective pressures. When they were incapable of doing so, with or without the help of others, profound changes in behavior and physiology occurred. The failure to overcome stresses is experienced by persons as defeat or inability to control the situation and to regulate their behavior and physiology. The specific mediators of this state of being and the development of disease remain known. Thus the pathogenetic puzzle about disease production remains with us. Persons are also "programmed" to develop specific diseases; each program, to add to the complexity of this issue, is not uniform. Thus a comprehensive understanding of the role of stress in disease remains unattained.

However, most persons seen by physicians do not have diseases but are in ill health. The links between stress and the various syndromes of ill health are more tightly forged. These syndromes are characterized by bifurcations (phase transitions) in the usual oscillatory operating modes of basic and vital biological functions.

REFERENCES

1. Selye H. The evolution of the stress concept. Am Scietist 1970; 61:692–699.
2. Levins R, Lewontin R. The dialectical biologist. Cambridge: Harvard University Press, 1985.
3. Gibbs D M. Vasopressin and oxytocin: hypothalamic modulators of the stress response. Psychoneuroendocrinology 1986; 11:131–140.
4. Selye H. A syndrome produced by diverse nocuous agents. Nature 1936; 148:84–85.
5. Weiss J M. Effects of coping behavior with and without a feedback signal on stress pathology in rats. J Comp Physiol Psychol 1971; 77:22–30.
6. Crews D, Moore M D. Evolution of mechanisms controlling mating behavior. Science 1986; 231:121–125.
7. Weiner H. The concept of stress in the light of studies on disasters, unemployment, and loss: a critical analysis. In: Zales M R, ed. Stress in health and disease. New York: Brunner/Mazel, 1985; 24–94.
8. Sapolsky R M. Lessons of the Sergenti: why some of us are more susceptible to stress. Sciences 1988; May/June: 38–42.
9. Hinkle L E Jr. Stress and disease: the concept after 50 years. Soc Sci Med 1987; 25:561–566.

10. Kopin I. Adrenergic responses following recognition of stress. In Zinder O, Bresnitz S, ed. Molecular biology of stress. UCLA symposia on molecular and cellular biology, new series, vol. 97. New York: Alan R. Liss, 1988.

11. Munck A, Guyre P M, Holbrook N. Physiological functions of glucocorticoids in stress and their relation to pharmacological actions. Endocr Rev 1984; 5:25-44.

12. Rapp P E, Mees A I, Sparrow C T. Frequency encoded biochemical regulation is more accurate than amplitude dependent control. J Theor Biol 1981; 90:531-544.

13. Yates F E. Outline of a physical theory of physiological systems. Can J Physiol Pharmacol 1982; 60:217-248.

14. Garfinkel A. A mathematics for physiology. Am J Physiol 1983; 245: R455-R466.

15. Smith W. Hypothalamic regulation of pituitary secretion of luteinizing hormone. II. Feedback control of gonadotropin secretion. Bull Math Biol 1980; 42:57-78.

16. Abraham R. Dynamical models for physiology. Am J Physiol 1983; 245: R467-R472.

17. Weiner H, Mayer E. The organism in health and disease: towards an integrated biomedical model. Submitted for publication.

18. Copeland D D. Concepts of disease and diagnosis. Perspect Biol Med 1977; 20:528-538.

19. Engel G L. The need for a new medical model: a challenge for biomedicine. Science 1977; 196:129-136.

20. Weiner H. Psychobiology and human disease. New York: Elsevier, 1977.

21. Hench P S, Kendall E C, Slocumb C N, Polley H F. The effect of a hormone of the adrenal cortex (17-hydroxy-11-dehydrocorticosterone: compound E) and of pituitary adrenocorticotropic hormone on rheumatoid arthritis. Proc Staff Mtgs Mayo Clin 1949; 24:181-197.

22. Weiner H. Die Geschichte der psychosomatischen Medizin und das Leib-Seele-Problem in der Medizin. Psychother Med Psychol 1986; 36:361-391.

23. Mirsky I A. Physiologic, psychologic, and social determinants in the etiology of duodenal ulcer. Am J Dig Dis 1958; 3:285-314.

24. Farrow S C. Unemployment and health: a review of methodology. In: Cullen J, Siegrist J, eds. Breakdown in human adaptation to stress, vol. 1. Boston: Martinus Nijhoff, 1984; 149-158.

25. Engel G L. A life setting conducive to illness: the giving-up, given-up complex. Arch Intern Med 1968; 69:293-300.

26. Hinkle L E Jr. The effect of exposure to culture change, social change and changes in interpersonal relationships on health. In: Dohrenwend BS, Dohrenwend BP, eds. Stressful life events: their nature and effects. New York: Wiley, 1974:9-44.

27. Brown G W, Harris T. Social origins of depression. London: Tavistock Press, 1978.

28. Lazarus R S. Psychological stress and the coping process. New York: McGraw-Hill, 1966.

29. Bruhn J G, Chandler B, Miller M C, Wolf J, Lynn T N. Social aspects of coronary heart disease in two adjacent, ethnically different communities. Am J Public Health 1966; 56:1493–1506.
30. Marmot M G, Syme S L. Acculturation and coronary heart disease in Japanese-Americans. Am J Epidemiol 1976; 104:225–247.
31. Hofer M A. On the relationship between attachment and separation processes in infancy. In: Plutchick R, ed. Emotion, theory, research, and experience: emotions in early development-2. New York: Academic Press, 1982.
32. Hofer M A. Relationships as regulators. Psychosom Med 1984; 46:183–187.
33. Taylor G J. Psychosomatic medicine and contemporary psychoanalysis. Madison, CT: International Universities Press, 1987.
34. Weiner H. The prospects for psychosomatic medicine: selected topics. Psychosom Med 1982; 44:488–517.
35. Weiner H. Human relationships in health, illness, and disease. In: Magnusson D, Ohman A, eds. Psychopathology: an interactional perspective. Orlando, FL: Academic Press, 1987:305–323.
36. Parkes C M, Brown R J. Health after bereavement. Psychosom Med 1972; 34:449–461.
37. Jacobs S, Ostfeld A. An epidemiological review of the mortality of bereavement. Psychosom Med 1977; 39:344–357.
38. Jacobs S C. Psychoendocrine aspects of bereavement. In: Zisook S, ed. Biopsychosocial aspects of bereavement. Washington, DC: American Psychiatric Press, 1987:141–155.
39. Bartrop R W, Luckhurst E, Lazarus L, Kiloh L G, Perry R. Depressed lymphocyte function after bereavement. Lancet 1977; 1:834–836.
40. Schleifer S J, Keller S E, Camarino M, Thornton J C, Stein M. Suppression of lymphocyte stimulation following bereavement. JAMA 1983; 250:374–377.
41. Irwin M, Daniels M, Bloom E T, Smith T L, Weiner H. Life events, depressive symptoms, and immune function. Am J Psychiatry 1987; 144:437–441.
42. Ruesch J. The infantile personality: the core problem of psychosomatic medicine. Psychosom Med 1948; 10:133–144.
43. Ader R. Psychoneuroimmunology. New York: Academic Press, 1981.
44. Light K, Obrist P. Cardiovascular reactivity to behavioral stress in young males with and without marginally elevated casual systolic pressures: comparison of clinic, home and laboratory measure. Hypertension 1980; 2:802–808.
45. Weder A B, Julius S. Editorial: behavior, blood pressure variability and hypertension. Psychom Med 1985; 47:406–414.
46. Zanchetti A, Baccelli G, Mancia G. Fighting, emotion and exercise: cardiovascular effects in the cat. In: Onesti G, Fernandez M, Kim K E. eds. Regulation of blood pressure by the central nervous system. New York: Grune & Stratton, 1976.

47. Abbott D H. Behaviourally mediated suppression of reproduction in female primates. J Zool 1987; 213:1–16.

48. Brown M, Fisher L. Corticotropin-releasing factor: effects on the autonomic nervous system and visceral systems. Fed Proc FASEB 1985; 44: 243–248.

49. Weiner H. Overview of the symposium. In: Weiner H, Hellhammer D, Florin I, Murison RC, eds. Neuronal control of bodily function: basic and clinical aspects: vol. IV, frontiers in stress research. Toronto: Hans Huber, 1989.

50. Arancibia S, Tapia-Arancibia L, Assenmacher I, Astier H. Direct evidence of short-term cold-induced TRH release in the median eminence of unanesthesized rats. Neuroendocrinology 1983; 37:225–228.

51. Chappell P B, Smith M A, Kilts C D, Bissette G, Ritchie J, Anderson C, Nemeroff C B. Alterations in corticotropin-releasing factor-like immunoreactivity in discrete rat brain regions after acute and chronic stress. J Neurosci 1986; 6:2908–2914.

52. Taché Y. Role of brain neuropeptides in the regulation of gastric secretion. In: Weiner H, ed. Specialty conference: neurobiologic and psychobiologic mechanisms in gastric function and ulceration. West J Med 1985; 143:215–218.

53. Garrick T, Veiseh A, Sierra A, Weiner H, Taché Y. Corticotropin-releasing factor acts centrally to suppress stimulated gastric contractility in the rat. Regul Pept 1988; 21:173–181.

54. Stephens R L, Ishikawa T, Weiner H, Novin D, Taché Y. TRH analogue, RX 77368, injected into dorsal vagal complex stimulates gastric secretion in rats. Am J Physiol 1988; 254:G639–G634.

55. Rotter J I, Rimoin D L. Peptic ulcer disease—a heterogeneous group of disorders? Gastroenterology 1977; 73:604–607.

56. Grossman M I. Abnormalities of acid secretion in patients with duodenal ulcer. Gastroenterology 1978; 75:524–526.

57. Julius S, Esler M D. Autonomic nervous cardiovascular regulation in borderline hypertension. Am J Cardiol 1975; 36:685–672.

58. Thailer S A, Friedman R, Harshfield G A, Pickering T G. Psychologic differences between high-, normal-, low-renin hypertensives. Psychosom Med 1985; 47:294–297.

59. Vollhardt B R, Ackerman S H, Grayzel A I, Barland P. Psychologically distinguishable groups of rheumatoid arthritis patients: a controlled, single blind study. Psychosom Med 1982; 44:353–362.

60. Weiner H. Are psychosomatic diseases, diseases of regulation? Psychosom Med 1975; 37:289–291.

61. Melnechuk T. Cell receptor disorders. LaJolla, CA: Western Behavioral Sciences Institute, 1978.

62. Rubenstein E. Diseases caused by impaired communication among cells. Sci Am 1980; 242:102–121.

63. Feldman S. Neural pathways mediating adrenocortical responses. Fed Proc FASEB 1985; 44:169–175.

64. Marmot M G, Rose G, Shipley M, Hamilton P J S. Employment grade and coronary heart disease in British civil servants. J Epidemiol Commun Health 1978; 32:244–249.

65. Goldblatt P B, Moore M E, Strunkard A J. Social factors in obesity. JAMA 1965; 192:1039–1044.

66. Stunkard A J. From explanation to action in psychosomatic medicine: the case of obesity. Psychosom Med 1975; 37:195–236.

67. Brown M S, Goldstein J L. A receptor mediated pathway for cholesterol homeostasis. Science 1986; 232:34–47.

68. Saxena K. Physiological effects of job loss. Paper presented at the Annual Meeting of the International Society for the Prevention of Stress, 1980.

69. Friedman M, Rosenman R H. Association of a specific overt behavior pattern with blood and cardiovascular findings. JAMA 1959; 169:1286–1295.

70. Brackett C D, Powell L H. Psychosocial and physiological predictors of sudden cardiac death after healing of acute myocardial infarction. Am J Cardiol 1988; 61:979–983.

71. Enos W F, Holmes R H, Beyer J. Coronary heart disease among United States soldiers killed in action in Korea. JAMA 1953; 152:1090–1093.

72. Siegrist J. Interaction between short- and long-term stress in cardiovascular disease. In: L'Abbate A, ed. Breakdown in human adaptation to 'stress.' Part 5, vol. II. Boston: Martinus Nijhoff, 1984:892–899.

73. Siegrist J, Matschinger H, Siegrist K. Socio-emotional inputs to central neuronal regulation of the cardiovascular system. In Hellhammer D, Florin I, Weiner H, eds. Neuronal control of bodily function: basic and clinical aspects. Neurobiological approaches to human disease, vol. III. Toronto: Hans Huber, 1988:174–190.

74. Hackett D, Davies G, Chierchia S, Maseri A. Intermittent coronary occlusion in acute myocardial infarction: value of combined thrombolytic and vasodilator therapy. N Engl J Med 1987; 317:1055–1059.

75. Maseri A, Severi S, DeNes M, et al. "Variant" angina: one aspect of a continuous spectrum of vasospastic myocardial ischemia. Am J Cardiol 1978; 42:1019–1035.

76. Gu J, Polak J M, Adrian T E, Allen J M, Tatemoto K, Bloom S R. Neuropeptide tyrosine (NPY)—a major cardiac neuropeptide. Lancet 1983; 1:1008–1010.

77. Deanfield J E, Shea M, Kensett M, et al. Silent myocardial ischaemia due to mental stress. Lancet 1984; 2:1001–1005.

78. Rozanski A, Bairey C N, Krantz D S, et al. Mental stress and the induction of silent myocardial ischemia in patients with coronary artery disease. N Engl J Med 1988; 318:1005–1012.

79. Barry J, Selwyn A P, Nabel E G, et al. Frequency of ST-segment depression produced by mental stress in stable angina pectoris from coronary artery disease. Am J Cardiol 1988; 61:989–993.

80. Young M, Benjamin B, Wallis C. The mortality of widowers. Lancet 1963; 2:454–456.
81. Helsing K J, Szklo M, Comstock G W. Factors associated with mortality after widowhood. Am J Public Health 1981; 71:802–809.
82. Bowling A, Charlton J. Risk factors for mortality after bereavement: a logistic regression analysis. J R Coll Gen Pract 1987; 37:551–554.
83. Chandra V, Szklo M, Goldberg R, Tonascia J. The impact of marital status on survival after an acute myocardial infarction: a population-based study. Am J Epidemiol 1983; 117:320–325.
84. Ross R. The pathogenesis of atherosclerosis—an update. N Engl J Med 1986; 314:488–500.
85. Glass L, Mackey M C. Pathological conditions resulting from instabilities in physiological control systems. Ann NY Acad Sci 1979; 316:214–235.
86. Ruberman W, Weinblatt E, Goldberg J D, Chaudhary B S. Psychosocial influences on mortality after myocardial infarction. N Engl J Med 1984; 311:552–559.
87. Smith G R Jr, Monson R A, Ray D C. Patients with multiple unexplained symptoms: their characteristics, functional health and health care utilization. Arch Intern Med 1986; 146:69–72.
88. Beale N, Nethercott S. Job-loss and health—the influence of age and previous morbidity. J R Coll Gen Pract 1986; 36:261–264.
89. Norman G R, McFarlane A H, Streiner D L. Patterns of illness among individuals reporting high and low stress. Can J Psychiatry 1985; 30:400–405.
90. Smith G R Jr, Monson R A, Ray D C. Psychiatric consultation in somatization disorder: a randomized controlled study. N Engl J Med 1986; 314:1407–1413.
91. Weiner H, Thaler M, Reiser M F, Mirsky I A. Etiology of duodenal ulcer. I. Relation of specific psychological characteristics to rate of gastric secretion. Psychosom Med 1957; 19:1–10.
92. Lum L C. The syndrome of chronic habitual hyperventilation. In: Hill O W, ed. Modern trends in psychosomatic medicine. London: Butterworth, 1976; 196–230.
93. Magarian G J. Hyperventilation syndromes: infrequently recognized common expressions of anxiety and stress. Medicine 1982; 61:219–236.
94. Kontos H A, Richardson D W, Raper A J, Zubair-Ulhassen, Patterson J L. Mechanisms of action of hypocapnic alkalosis on limb blood vessels in man and dog. Am J Physiol 1972; 223:1296–1307.
95. Tzivoni D, Stein A, Keren A, Stern S. Electrocardiographic characteristics of neurocirculatory asthenia during everyday activities. Br Heart J 1980; 44:426–432.
96. Neill W A, Hattenhauer M. Impairment of myocardial supply due to hyperventilation. Circulation 1975; 52:854–858.
97. Mortensen S A, Vilhelmson R, Sande E. Prinzmetal's variant angina (PVA). Circadian variation in response to hyperventilation. Acta Med Scand Suppl 1981; 644:38–41.

98. Coryell W, Noyes R, Clarcy J. Excess mortality in panic disorder: a comparison with primary unipolar depression. Arch Gen Psychiatry 1982; 39:701-703.
99. Coryell W, Noyes R, House J D. Mortality among outpatients with anxiety disorders. Am J Psychiatry 1986; 143:508-510.
100. Haines A P, Imeson J D, Meade T W. Phobic anxiety and ischaemic heart disease. Br Med J 1987; 295:297-299.
101. Dotevall G J, Svedlund J, Sjodin I. Symptoms in irritable bowel disease. Scand J Gastroenterol (Suppl) 1982; 79:16-19.
102. Lennard-Jones J E. Functional gastrointestinal disorders. N Engl J Med 1983; 308:431-435.
103. Texter E C Jr, Butler R C. The irritable bowel syndrome. Am Fam Physician 1975; 11:169-173.
104. Dent J, Dodds W J, Friedman R H, et al. Mechanism of gastroesophageal reflux in recumbent asymptomatic human subjects. J Clin Invest 1980; 65:226-267.
105. Schuster M M. Disorders of the esophagus: application of pscyhophysiological methods to treatment. In: Holzl R, Whitehead WE, eds. Psychophysiology of the gastrointestinal tract. New York: Plenum Press, 1983; 33-42.
106. You C H, Lee K T, Chey W H, Menguy R. Electrogastrographic study of patients with unexplained nausea, bloating and vomiting. Gastroenterology 1980; 79:311-314.
107. You, C H, Chey, W H, Lee K T, Menguy R, Bortoff A. Gastric and small intestinal myoelectric dysrhythmia associated with chronic intractable nausea and vomiting. Ann Intern Med 1981; 95:449-451.
108. Williams C L, Villar R G, Peterson J M, Burks T F. Stress-induced changes in intestinal transit in the rat: a model for irritable bowel syndrome. Gastroenterology 1988; 94:611-621.
109. Chaudhary N A, Truelove S C. The irritable colon syndrome: a study of the clinical features, predisposing causes and prognosis in 130 cases. Q J Med 1962; 31:307-323.
110. Hislop I G. Psychological significance of the irritable colon syndrome. Gut 1971; 12:452-457.
111. Alpers D H. Functional gastrointestinal disorders. Hosp Pract 1983; 18: 139-153.
112. Whitehead W E, Engel B T, Schuster M M. Irritable bowel syndrome: physiological and psychological differences between diarrhea-predominant and constipation-predominant patients. Dig Dis Sci 1980; 25:404-413.
113. Connell A M, Jones F A, Rowlands E N. Motility of the pelvic colon. IV: Abdominal pain associated with colonic hypermotility after meals. Gut 1965; 6:105-112.
114. Snape W J, Cohen S. How colonic motility differs in normal subjects and patients with IBS. Pract Gastroenterol 1979; 3:21-25.
115. Weiner H. The functional bowel disorders. In: Weiner H, Baum A, eds. Perspectives in behavioral medicine: eating regulation and discontrol. Hillsdale, NJ: Lawrence Erlbaum, 1988:137-161.

Regulation and Integration of Homeostatic Responses

3

THE FINAL COMMON PATH

Issues Concerning the Organization of Central Mechanisms Controlling Corticotropin Secretion

Paul E. Sawchenko

The Salk Institute, La Jolla, California

The isolation and characterization of a 41-residue peptide now acknowledged to be the principal corticotropin-releasing factor (CRF) of the hypothalamus (1) was the crucial event that permitted access to central pathways that govern pituitary-adrenal responses to stress. Even at our currently crude level of understanding, these have proven to be quite complex, involving a host of interconnected pathways, many of which express multiple transmitter/modulator agents and appear capable of situation-specific plastic adaptations. In keeping with the spirit of this volume, the present chapter will endeavor less to provide a recantation of what is known about central stress-related circuitry than to use a sketch of current understanding as a means to frame lingering questions and raise organizational possibilities.

ORIGINS

Based on results gleaned from a variety of approaches, many have surmised that a tightly clustered group of cells in a discrete (dorsal medial) part of the parvocellular division of the paraventricular nucleus of the hypothalamus (PVH) comprises the principal source for the delivery of CRF to the hypophyseal portal vasculature (Fig. 1). This has now been supported using a combined retrograde transport–immunohistochemical approach in adrenalectomized rats (2); the failure to use colchicine pretreatment in these experiments, due to technical constraints, leaves open to question whether minor contributions to

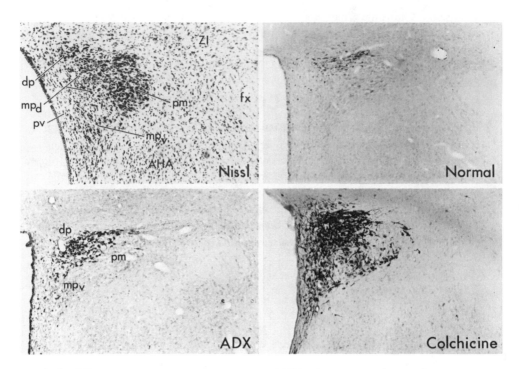

FIGURE 1 CRF immunostaining in the PVH of untreated (normal), adrenal-ectomized (ADX), and colchicine-treated rats; a section through a similar level stained for Nissl material is shown for reference. In the untreated rat, a relatively small number of cells, centered in a discrete subdivision (mpd), are stained weakly for CRF. After ADX, the number and staining intensity of cells display-ing CRF–IR are augmented, but their distribution is similar; these correspond to hypophysiotropic neurons. Colchicine treatment enhances immunostaining for CRF not only in PVHmpd but also in autonomic-related (dp, mpv), other parvo-cellular neurosecretory (pv) and magnocellular neurosecretory (pm) regions (all micrographs X80; reprinted with permission from ref. 12).

the hypophysiotropic projection may arise from CRF-immunoreactive (CRF–IR) neurons in the preoptic area and other hypothalamic regions, as has been suggested on the basis of lesion studies (3).

The more pressing question concerning the central triggering of the stress response has to do with the role that may be played by *magnocellular* neurosecretory neurons (Fig. 2). Both oxytocin (OT) and vasopressin (AVP) are present, and differentially regulated in hypophyseal portal plasma (4,5) and both interact with CRF to promote ACTH secretion. As discussed below, adrenal steroid-dependent expression of AVP in parvocellular neurosecretory CRF neurons has been established, but OT has not been localized in more than a handful of cells in regions that project prominently to the median eminence (6; see Fig. 3). Magnocellular neurons are currently the only viable candidate sources for such an influence (Fig. 2). Moreover, calcium-dependent, potassium-stimulated release of AVP from magnocellular axons has been demonstrated in vitro (7) and

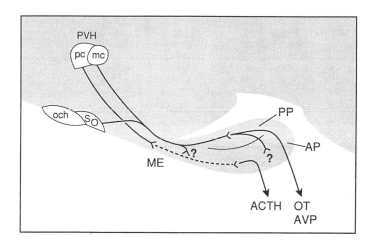

FIGURE 2 Schematic sagittal view of the basal diencephalon and pituitary shows the organization of magnocellular (mc) and parvocellular (pc) neurosecretory components of the PVH, and potential sites at which secretions of magnocellular neurons may interact with the parvocellular system. CRF contained in axonal projections from the parvocellular division of the PVH to the external zone of the median eminence (ME) is transported to the anterior pituitary (AP) via the portal vasculature (dashed line). Projections of magnocellular neurosecretory neurons from the PVH and the supraoptic nucleus (SO) pass through the internal lamina of the median eminence en route to the posterior lobe (PP), where oxytocin (OT) and vasopressin (AVP) are released into the systemic circulation. Magnocellular secretions may gain access to the portal vasculature via exocytotic release at the level of the median eminence or via vascular links between the posterior and anterior lobes (question marks).

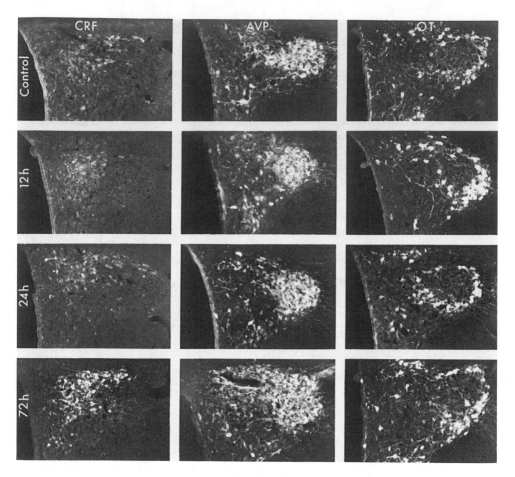

FIGURE 3 Organization and response to steroid withdrawal of CRF, oxytocin (OT), and vasopressin (AVP) neurons in the PVH. Micrographs show peptide staining patterns in control animals and in those subjected to pharmacological inhibition of steroid synthesis for 12, 24, or 72 h. CRF-IR neurons are concentrated in the parvocellular division of the nucleus and show a graded enhancement to steroid withdrawal. OT- and AVP-IR cells are normally seen in topographically distinctive parts of the magnocellular division of the nucleus. After 72 h of steroid inhibition, expression of AVP-IR in the hypophysiotropic zone is apparent. OT-IR, by contrast, is not influenced at any time. Magnocellular neurons constitute the only currently viable candidates for the delivery of OT to the portal vasculature, while AVP may arise from parvocellular and magnocellular elements (all micrographs X 80; reprinted with permission from ref. 63).

exocytotic release of neurosecretory granules has been seen ultrastructurally from magnocellular "axons-of-passage" coursing through the internal lamina (8). In addition, vascular links permitting blood flow from the neural to the anterior lobes have been described (9). It is clear that magnocellular neurons appear capable of releasing secretory products at loci with access to the portal plexus and/or to corticotropes directly. The conditions under which they might do so, and how such release might be integrated with the mechanisms that regulate nonapeptide biosynthesis in the magnocellular nuclei, and secretion from the neurohypophysis, are important and daunting questions yet to be explored systematically. There exists strong physiological evidence that CRF serves primarily to set the stimulatory tone on corticotropes, with the situational response determined largely by the relative abundance of cosecretagogues (10). At a most basic level, therefore, we still do not know whether, or under what circumstances, magno- versus parvocellular neurosecretory elements comprise the dominant impetus in driving corticotropin secretion.

CHEMICAL MAKEUP

It has been established that variously sized subsets of the parvocellular neurosecretory CRF–IR neuron are capable of expressing one or more of at least seven additional biologically active peptides (see 11,12). These include some molecules (AVP, angiotensin II, cholecystokinin, vasoactive intestinal polypeptide, PHI) that exhibit activity, alone and/or in synergy with CRF, in stimulating ACTH secretion (13), and others (enkephalin, neurotensin) that are ostensibly inert with respect to direct actions on corticotropes. Like CRF, at least some of the former (AVP, angiotensin II, cholecystokinin) are down-regulated by glucocorticoids (14-16; Fig. 3), while the latter appear not to be (14). A number of the agents that have been localized in "precorticotropes" have been shown to be active at physiologically reasonable concentrations in influencing the secretions of other adenohypophyseal cell types (e.g., 17,18). Insofar as current methods can resolve, it would seem unlikely that all hypophysiotropic CRF neurons express all seven additional peptides, or even that neurons capable of expressing a common complement necessarily respond similarly to regulatory influences. For example, Whitnall has marshalled evidence to suggest that cells in which CRF and AVP coexist may be partitioned into topographically distinctive steroid-responsive and nonresponsive pools (e.g., 19). These kind of data raise the possibility that micropopulations of parvocellular neurosecretory neurons may be defined on the basis of colocalization patterns and/or responsivity to extrinsic influences. Such an organization is, at first blush, perplexing, in view of the fact that, in the end, the contents of such elaborately specified subpopulations would be unceremoniously dumped together into portal plasma. If, however, such micropopulations prove to be differentiated entities subject to uniquely specified or weighted patterns of neural and hormonal influences, we may be catching a glimpse of an organization that can provide the subtle moment-to-moment adjustments in integrated pituitary output that allow the adaptational gymnastics of which the neuroendocrine system seems fully capable. We tend to regard phylogenetically ancient neurosecretory neurons as being primitive, and their capacity for multiple peptide expression as a manifestation of a relatively undifferentiated status. One is led at least to entertain the possibility that perhaps nothing could be further from the truth.

AFFERENT CONTROL

When considered relative to immediately adjoining populations of magnocellular neurosecretory and autonomic-related projection neuron pools in the PVH, the CRF-rich hypophysiotropic zone is distinguished by its great number and diversity of afferents [20]. This may be construed teleologically as being consistent with the multiplicity of sensory modalities and specific stimuli capable of eliciting or modifying stress responses. For didactic purposes, anatomically defined afferents may be grouped into five categories: visceral, somatic/special sensory, hypothalamic, circumventricular, and limbi (Fig. 4). Only a few features will be highlighted briefly here.

Pathways for the tramsission of visceral, or interoceptive, information are the most fully characterized set of inputs to the CRF neuron and are likely to comprise the arena in which a detailed anatomy of substrates underlying modality-specific influences on the CRF neuron will first be achieved (Fig. 5). This circuitry revolves about the nucleus of the solitary tract (NTS), the principal recipient of primary vagal and glossopharyngeal afferents. Three distinct territories of the NTS, which carry adrenergic, noradrenergic, and multiple peptidergic signatures, project to the CRF-rich zone of the PVH, as do at least two major projection fields of the NTS, the C1 adrenergic cell group and the lateral parabrachial nucleus (21–26). Lesions that involve various components of these pathways can disrupt pituitary-adrenal responses to such diverse challenges as ether stress, hemorrhage, and circadian cues (27-29). The obvious and pressing need is to determine how specific kinds of interoceptive information are gated across these parallel, yet differentiated, conduction lines, and what implications such organization might have for our understanding of the behavior of the system.

Real or perceived perturbations in the external environment can also activate the HPA axis, although the routes by which pertinent somatic and special sensory information may reach the hypothalamus have remained obscure. Some insight has been suggested in a recent study of mesencephalic and pontine projections to the PVH (26; Fig. 4). These included inputs from pontine cholinergic cell groups, which receive somatosensory inputs via the lemniscal and spinothalamic systems (see 30); the intergeniculate leaflet, a thalamic cell group that

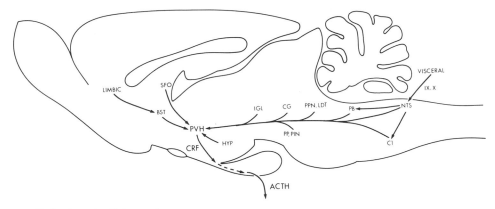

FIGURE 4 Schematic summary in a sagittal view of the rat brain of some afferent inputs to the CRF-rich region of the PVH. Visceral sensory inputs may reach the nucleus via direct projections from the nucleus of the solitary tract (NTS), which receives primary vagal (X) and glossopharyngeal (IX) afferents, or via projections relayed through the C1 adrenergic cell group or the parabrachial nucleus (PB). Other ascending sensory modalities may gain access to the CRF neuron via relays in the midbrain and pons; these include the pedunculopontine (PPN) and laterodorsal tegmental (LDT) nuclei (somatic sensory), the central gray (nociception and other modalities), the peripeduncular (PP) and posterior intralaminar (PIN) nuclei (auditory), and the intergeniculate leaflet (IGL; visual). Nearly all recognized hypothalamic (HYP) cell groups project to the PVH. Prominent inputs also arise from the subfornical organ (SFO), a circumventricular structure specialized for transducing influences of circulating angiotensin II. The bed nucleus of the stria terminals (BST) provides a potential conduit for acknowledged influences of several limbic system cell groups, which themselves do not project directly to the PVH.

receives a direct visual input (31); the central gray, which is involved in processing information from a number of sensory modalities, including nociception (e.g., 32); and several mesencephalic cell groups that are interconnected with auditory relay nuclei (33). The latter are particularly intriguing, since they, via connections with the hypothalamus and amygdala, have been implicated by LeDoux and colleagues (34) as mediating behavioral and cardiovascular components of emotional responses conditioned to an auditory stimulus.

Manipulation of principal components of the limbic region of the telencephalon (including the hippocampal formation and the septal and amygdaloid nuclear complexes) clearly affect HPA axis output, and, as discussed below, these limbic system structures have often been implicated as potential targets for corticosteroid feedback (e.g., 35). Problematic is the fact that with the sole exception of a moderate input from the central nucleus of the amygdala (36), none of

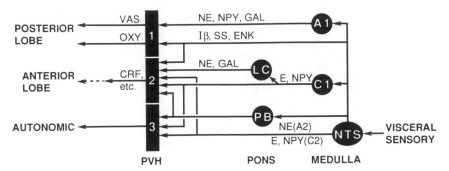

FIGURE 5 Schematic diagram of the organization and chemical coding of some visceral sensory inputs to the PVH. Three major classes of PVH output neurons are numbered, and their principal targets and chemical makeup indicated. The distribution and coding of some major direct and second-order pathways from the NTS to the PVH are also shown. Note the target specificity of each anatomically defined projection, upon which are superimposed complex and partly overlapping biochemical specificities. PB, parabrachial nucleus; LC, locus ceruleus; NE, norepinephrine; E, epinephrine, NPY, neuropeptide Y; GAL, galanin; Iβ; inhibinβ; ENK, enkephalin; SS, somatostatin; VAS, vasopressin; OXY, oxytocin.

these structures projects at all prominently to the PVH, especially to the "CRF zone" (37,38). Most do, however, project to or through regions immediately adjacent to the PVH, in which are found gamma-aminobutyric (GABA)ergic neurons that project, in turn, into the nucleus (unpublished observations, 1989). Local GABA cells thus appear worthy of consideration as potentially providing an avenue by which inputs to the perinuclear zone, such as those from several limbic system structures, may come to influence PVH mechanisms. As an alternative, components of the septum, hippocampus, and amygdala are each prominently interconnected with the bed nucleus of the stria terminalis (e.g., 39), a discrete (caudolateral) part of which projects strongly to the PVH (37). The bed nucleus remains a viable candidate site for integrating limbic system influences on the CRF neuron, although this has yet to be explored.

Immunohistochemically defined afferents to the PVH are almost invariably distributed across a number of the functional domains (of which the CRF-rich zone is but one) that have been defined on the basis of cellular architecture, connections, and/or neurochemical markers (40). Such distributions then ostensibly define potential substrates for invoking in tandem (i.e., integrating) various combinations of parvocellular neurosecretory, magnocellular neurosecretory, and autonomic-related outputs of the nucleus. In most of those few instances in which the origins and distributions of the individual cells groups contributing to any given chemically specified afferent have been scrutinized closely, a clear anatomically based dissociability has been evident. Thus, the three cell groups that contribute to the broadly distributed noradrenergic projection individually provide topographically distinctive, and largely nonoverlapping, inputs, only one of which (from the A2 cell group of the caudal nucleus of the solitary tract) is distributed prominently to the "CRF zone" of the PVH (21). Similar, although less pronounced, dissections seem to apply to the neuropeptide Y- and galanin-IR inputs (41,42). The adrenergic projections are exceptional, in that the input from each of the contributing (C1, C2, and C3) cell groups appears to mirror the distribution of the adrenergic input as a whole (22).

As with their hypothalamic targets, many of the principal afferents to the CRF neuron display multiple neurochemical markers. The patterns of coexpression are varied, ranging from a near-complete identity to coexistence within small subsets, and appear generally not to be fully in register with the anatomical organization. For example, NPY-IR is present within the vast majority of brainstem adrenergic neurons that project primarily to the parvocellular division of the PVH, in a subset of A1 noradrenergic neurons that project to the magnocellular division (41), and in nonaminergic neurons in the arcuate nucleus of the hypothalamus whose projections to the PVH have not been rigorously defined (43). The imprecise superimposition of biochemical phenotypes on a near point-to-point manner of anatomical organization would seem to broaden the potential for close regulation of afferent control of the system, if, for example, relevant neuroactive substances expressed in subsets of various groups of projection neurons are subject to regulation as a class, as well as individually by their own unique sets of neural and humoral influences.

CORTICOSTEROID REGULATION

Adrenal steroids exert potent inhibitory effects on the proximal limbs of the HPA axis (44). The array of target molecules and the site(s) and mechanisms by which such effects may be brought to bear remain to be fully clarified. Delivery of the synthetic glucocorticoid dexamethasone to the PVH can inhibit adrenalectomy-induced increases in CRF and AVP immunoreactivity and mRNA (45–47). Corticosterone, which is the principal native glucocorticoid in the rat, is inert in similar paradigms but does attenuate the corticotropin response to steroid withdrawal when delivered to various other brain regions (35; see below). The existence of distinct high-affinity, low-capacity (type I) and low-affinity, high-capacity (type II) glucocorticoid receptors has been demonstrated and show partly overlapping distributions, particularly in several limbic system cell groups (48, 49). In the PVH, by contrast, CRF-IR neurons express the type II receptor (50) but apparently not the type I (49). The challenge here is to determine the degree of inhibition that may be effected by local versus distant steroid-receptive elements under various conditions.

OTHER REGULATORY INFLUENCES

Neuronal

Pertinent to the identity of the site(s) at which negative feedback effects on the CRF neuron may be exerted is a consideration of the role that neural inputs might play in modifying peptide expression in the CRF neuron, apart from, or concomitant with, their roles in conventional synaptic transmission. Differential transsynaptic effects on the synthesis, as well as the release, of coexisting effector agents in target neuron pools has been shown in other systems (e.g., 51), and several lines of evidence support the view that some form(s) or fraction of corticosteroid feedback effects on the HPA axis may be mediated via neural inputs to the CRF neuron (see 44). Two classes of inputs have been implicated prominently in this context.

Catecholaminergic projections arising from the brainstem are in a position to relay interoceptive stimuli to the CRF neuron (52). In addition, evidence exists to suggest that the integrity of these pathways may be required for corticosteroid feedback influences to be exerted in at least some models (53-55). This, coupled with the fact that the cells of origin of these projections express the type II glucocorticoid receptor (56,57), raised the possibility that some form or fraction of feedback may be mediated remotely, via the aminergic projections. Transections of these pathways in intact and steroid-manipulated rats, however, resulted in effects on CRF and AVP immunostaining that were opposite in sign and independent from those that resulted from manipulations in steroid titers (58,49; see Fig. 6). Moreover, these lesions fail to exert effects on CRF or AVP mRNA levels (59), which are known to be regulated by glucocorticoids. Thus, while the aminergic pathways appear capable of modifying peptide dynamics in the CRF neuron, the effect appears to be exerted posttranscriptionally. The mechanism(s) through which such effects may be exerted, and how they might be integrated with the synaptic signaling properties of these pathways, remain to be clarified.

A second class of projections that have been implicated as targets for corticosteroid feedback are those in the limbic region of the telencephalon, including the hippocampal formation, the septal nuclei, and the amygdala. Neurons at these sites harbor the types I and II glucocorticoid receptors in abundance (48, 49), and physiological evidence supports a role for these sites in mediating feedback effects. This is perplexing from an anatomical perspective, since, with the possible exception of the amygdala (36), these limbic structures provide at most meager projections to the PVH, particularly to its parvocellular division (37,38). Nonetheless, delivery of corticosterone, the principal native glucocorticoid in the rat, to several limbic regions can significantly attenuate the corticotropin response to adrenalectomy (35). Di- and polysynaptic routes by which limbic system inputs may reach the PVH are easily envisaged (see above), but questions

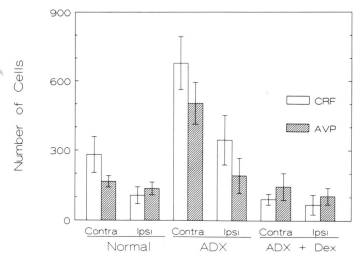

FIGURE 6 Effects of unilateral catecholamine deafferentation on CRF- and AVP-IR in the parvocellular division of the PVH in normal rats and in adrenalectomized (ADX) rats treated with vehicle or dexamethasone (Dex). Cell counts (mean ± SEM) from the sides of the brain ipsilateral (ipsi) and contralateral (contra) to the lesion are given. Note that the overall tendency on the lesioned side is to reduce the number of cells stained for either peptide, but that the essential direction of the response to manipulation of steroid status remains intact (data replotted from ref. 58).

remain as to how the integrity of feedback-related information, per se, can be maintained in the flow of information across synapses. That is, how might the CRF cell "know" that any second or third order limbic system input is related to feedback, when that information would likely be diluted by its convergence with presumably non-feedback-related afferent influences on "interneurons" in the circuit? Moreover, and as the catecholamine data summarized above attest (58,60), not all synaptic inputs appear to have access to the transcriptional control mechanisms at which the influence of glucocorticoids is exerted.

Hormonal

Although there is no dispute as to the preeminence of glucocorticoids as hormonal modulators of peptide expression in the parvocellular neurosecretory CRF neuron, we have recently obtained evidence for additional bloodborne influences. It has long been suspected that "short-loop" negative feedback effects of ACTH may be exerted on the production and/or release of hypothalamic CRF(s) (61). The observation that hypophysectomy (HYPOX) results in more profound enhancements of CRF and AVP immunostaining in the PVH-median eminence projection system than ADX (14) prompted an evaluation of the effect of ACTH replacement on peptide staining in this system in HYPOX–ADX rats. The results (unpublished observations, 1989) indicated that systemic ACTH exerted surprisingly potent effects in mitigating the expected enhancement of AVP-IR, while CRF-staining was less profoundly affected (Fig. 7). These observations raise intriguing questions as to the site(s) and mechanisms by which the effects of ACTH may be exerted. If central (e.g., PVH) sites of action are involved, how does the peptide cross the blood–brain barrier, and how might such signals be integrated with neuronal ACTH-containing inputs to the CRF neuron (62)? Perhaps more importantly, the results suggest that additional bloodborne factors may play significant roles in regulating the hypophysiotropic "CRF neuron," and that such effects may be exerted differentially on colocalized secretagogues for corticotropin. Broadly construed, this would be in keeping with the idea that the peptides coexpressed with CRF and that are capable of influencing several adenohypophyseal cell types should be subject to at least some differential regulatory influences.

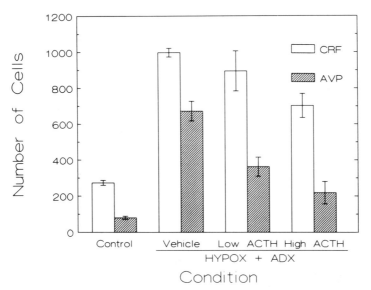

FIGURE 7 Effects of systemic ACTH on the number (mean ± SEM) of CRF- and AVP-IR cells in the PVH of hypophysectomized (HYPOX) and adrenalectomized (ADX) rats. Data from normal (control) and vehicle-treated HYPOX–ADX animals are given for comparison. ACTH significantly attenuates the HYPOX–ADX-induced enhancement in AVP-IR, while CRF-IR cells are less prominently affected. N = four to seven rats per group.

CONCLUSIONS

It seems clear that the chain-link view of the central limb of the HPA axis as comprising merely a homogeneous pool of CRF neurons, regulated by glucocorticoids and played upon by the sensorium via an array of neural pathways, is restrictive and no longer tenable. The "CRF neuron" is a multiply determined class of cell types that has the potential at times to function as prethyrotropes and prelactotropes, as well as precorticotropes. Moreover, other cell types with access to the portal vasculature almost certainly contribute significantly to the situation-specific drive on corticotropin secretion. Glucocorticoids are principal, but not exclusive, bloodborne regulators of hypothalamic CRFs. A highly differentiated set of afferents may function, in addition to conventional information-bearing capacities, to regulate pertinent peptide expression at transcriptional and/or posttranscriptional levels. A more expansive approach to the system should foster insight into substrates underlying the integrated hypothalamic response to particular challenges, as well as those pertinent to the control of corticotropin secretion, per se.

ACKNOWLEDGMENTS

Work from the author's laboratory summarized here was supported by NIH grants (NS-21182 and HL-35137, and was conducted in part by the Clayton Foundation for Research, California Division. P.E.S. is a Clayton Foundation Investigator. I am grateful to Drs. E. T. Cunningham Jr. and M. C. Levin for allowing me to cite some of their unpublished data.

REFERENCES

1. Vale W, Speiss J, Rivier C, Rivier J. Characterization of a 41-residue ovine hypothalamic peptide that stimulates the secretions of corticotropin and β-endorphin. Science 1983; 213:1394–1397.
2. Kawano H, Daikoku S, Shibasaki T. CRF-containing neuron systems in the rat hypothalamus: retrograde tracing and immunohistochemical studies. J Comp Neurol 1988; 272:260–268.
3. Merchenthaler I, Hynes, M A, Vigh S, Schally A V, Petrusz P. Corticotropin releasing factor (CRF): origin and course of afferent pathways to the median eminence (ME) of the rat hypothalamus. Neuroendocrinology 1984; 39: 296–306.
4. Gibbs D M. Measurement of hypothalamic corticotropin-releasing factors in hypophyseal portal blood. Fed Proc 1985; 44:203–206.
5. Plotsky P M. Hypophyseotropic regulation fo adenohypophyseal adrenocorticotropin secretion. Fed Proc 1985; 44:207–213.

6. Sawchenko P E, Swanson L W, Vale W W. Corticotropin-releasing factor: co-expression within distinct subsets of oxytocin-, vasopressin- and neurotensin-immunoreactive neurons in the hypothalamus of the male rat. J Neurosci 1984; 4:1118-1129.

7. Holmes M C, Antoni F A, Aguilera G, Catt K J. Magnocellular axons in passage through the median eminence release vasopressin. Nature 1986; 391:326-329.

8. Buma P and Nieuwenhuys R. Ultrastructural demonstration of oxytocin and vasopressin release sites in the neural lobe and median eminence of the rat by tannic acid and immunogold methods. Neurosci Lett 1987; 74:151-157.

9. Page R B. The pituitary portal system. In: Ganten D, Pfaff D, eds. Current topics in neuroendocrinology, Vol. 7. Morphology of the hypothalamus and its connections. Berlin: Springer-Verlag, 1986:1-47.

10. Plotsky P M, Bruhn T O, Vale W. Hypophysiotropic regulation of adrenocorticotropin secretion in response to insulin-induced hypoglycemia. Endocrinology 1985; 117:323-329.

11. Swanson L W, Sawchenko P E, Lind R Wm Rho J-H. The CRH motoneuron: differential peptide regulation in neurons with possible synaptic, paracrine, and endocrine outputs. Ann NY Acad Sci 1987; 512:12-23.

12. Sawchenko P E, Swanson L W. Organization of CRF immunoreactive cells and fibers in the rat brain: immunohistochemical studies. In: DeSouza, E B, Nemeroff C B. Boca Raton, FL: CRC Uniscience, 1989; 29-51.

13. Antoni F A. Hypothalamic control of adrenocorticotropin-releasing factor. Endocr Rev 1986; 7:351-378.

14. Sawchenko P E. Adrenalectomy-induced enhancement of CRF and vasopressin immunoreactivity in parvocellular neurosecretory neurons: anatomic peptide and steroid specificity. J Neurosci 1987; 7:1093-1106.

15. Lind R W, Swanson L W, Sawchenko P E. Anatomical evidence that neural circuits related to the subfornical organ contain angiotensin II. Brain Res Bull 1985; 15:79-82.

16. Mezey E, Reseine T D, Skirboll L, Beinfeld M, Kis J Z. Role of cholecystokinin in corticotropin release: coexistence with vasopressin and corticotropin-releasing factor in cells of the rat hypothalamic paraventricular nucleus. Proc Natl Acad Sci USA 1986; 83:3510-3513.

17. Lumpkin M D, Samson W K, & McCann S M. Arginine vasopressin as a thyrotropin-releasing hormone. Science 1987; 235:1070-1073.

18. Schramme C, Denef C. Stimulation of spontaneous and dopamine-inhibited prolactin release from anterior pituitary reaggregate cell cultures by angiotensin peptides. Life Sci 1984; 34:1651-1658.

19. Whitnall M H. Distributions of pro-vasopressin expressing and provasopressin deficient CRH neurons in the paraventricular hypothalamic nucleus of colchicine-treated normal and adrenalectomized rats. J Comp Neurol 1988; 275:13-28.

20. Sawchenko P E, Cunningham E T Jr, Levin M C, Bittencourt J C, Roberts V J. Chemical neuroanatomy of the paraventricular nucleus. J Neuroendocrinol 1990; in press.

21. Cunningham E T Jr, Sawchenko P E. Anatomical specificity of noradrenergic inputs to the paraventricular and supraoptic nuclei of the rat hypothalamus. J Comp Neurol 1988; 274:60–76.
22. Cunningham E T Jr, Bohn M C, Sawchenko P E. The organization of adrenergic projections to the paraventricular and supraoptic nuclei of the rat hypothalamus. J Comp Neurol 1990; in press.
23. Sawchenko P E, Benoit R, Brown M R. Somatostatin 28-immunoreactive inputs to the paraventricular nucleus: origin from nonaminergic neurons in the nucleus of the solitary tract. J Chem Neuroanat 1988; 1:81–94.
24. Sawchenko P E, Plotsky P M, Cunningham E T Jr, et al. Inhibin β-immunoreactivity in a visceral sensory system controlling oxytocin secretion in the rat brain. Nature 1988; 344:315–317.
25. Saper C B, Loewy A D. Efferent connections of the parabrachial nucleus in the rat. Brain Res 1980; 197:291–317.
26. Levin M C, Cunningham E T Jr, Sawchenko P E. The organization of mesencephalic and pontine afferents to the paraventricular and supraoptic nuclei in the rat. Soc Neurosci Abstr 1987; 13:1166.
27. Carlson D E, Gann D S. Responses of adrenocorticotropin and vasopressin to hemorrhage after lesions of the caudal ventrolateral medulla in rats. Brain Res 1987; 406:385–389.
28. Darlington D N, Shinsako J, Dallman M F. Medullay lesions eliminate ACTH responses to hypotensive hemorrhage. Am J Physiol 1986; 251: R106–R115.
29. Szafarczyk A, Alonso G, Ixart G, Malaval F, Assenmacher I. Diurnal-stimulated and stress-induced ACTH release is mediated by ventral noradrenergic bundle. Am J Physiol 1985; 249:E219–E226.
30. Rye D B, Saper C B, Lee H J, Wainer B H. Pedunculopontine tegmental nucleus of the rat: cytoarchitecture, cytochemistry and some extrapyramidal connections of the mesopontine tegmentum. J Comp Neurol 1987; 259:483–528.
31. Pickard G E. Bifurcating axons of retinal ganglion cells terminate in the hypothalamic suprachiasmatic nucleus and the intergeniculate leaflet of the thalamus. Neurosci Lett 1985; 55:211–217.
32. Mayer D J, Price D D. Central nervous system mechanisms of analgesia. Pain 1976; 2:379–404.
33. LeDoux J E, Ruggiero D A, Reis D J. Projections to the subcortical forebrain from anatomically defined regions of the medial geniculate body in the rat. J Comp Neurol 1985; 242:182–213.
34. LeDoux J E, Sakaguchi A, Reis D J. Subcortical efferent projections of the medial geniculate nucleus mediate emotional responses conditioned to acoustic stimuli. J Neurosci 1984; 4:683–698.
35. Kovacs K J, Makara G B. Corticosterone and dexamethasone act at different brain sites to inhibit adrenalectomy-induced adrenocorticotropin hypersecretion. Brain Res 1988; 474:205–210.
36. Gray T S, Carney M E, Magnuson D J. Direct projections from the central amygdaloid nucleus to the hypothalamic paraventricular nucleus: possible role in stress induced ACTH release. Neuroendocrinology 1990; in press.

37. Sawchenko P E, Swanson L W. The organization of forebrain afferents to the paraventricular and supraoptic nuclei of the rat. J Comp Neurol 1983; 218:121–144.

38. Oldfield B J, Hou-Yu A, Silverman A J. A combined electron microscopic HRP and immunocytochemical study of the limbic projections to rat hypothalamic nuclei containing vasopressin and oxytocin neurons. J Comp Neurol 1985; 231:221–231.

39. Swanson L W, Cowan W M. The connections of the septal region in the rat. J Comp Neurol 1979; 186:621–656.

40. Swanson L W, Sawchenko P E. Hypothalamic integration: organization of the paraventricular and supraoptic nuclei. Annu Rev Neurosci 1983; 6: 269–324.

41. Sawchenko P E, Swanson L W, Grzanna R, et al. Colocalization of neuropeptide Y immunoreactivity in brainstem catecholaminergic neurons that project to the paraventricular and supraoptic nuclei in the rat. J Comp Neurol 1985; 241:138–153.

42. Levin M C, Sawchenko P E, Howe P R C, Bloom S R, Polak J M. The organization of galanin-immunoreactive inputs to the paraventricular nucleus with special reference to their relationship to catecholaminergic afferents. J Comp Neurol 1987; 261:562–582.

43. Bai F L, Yamano M, Shiotani Y, et al. An arcuato-paraventricular and dorsomedial hypothalamic neuropeptide Y-containing system which lacks norepinephrine in the rat. Brain Res 1985; 331:172–175.

44. Keller-Wood M E, Dallman M F. Corticosteroid inhibition of ACTH secretion. Endocr Rev. 1984; 5:1–24.

45. Kovacs K , Kiss J Z, Makara G. Glucocorticoid implants around the hypothalamic paraventricular nucleus prevent the increase of corticotropin-releasing factor and arginine vasopressin immunostaining induced by adrenalectomy. Neuroendocrinology 1986; 44:229–234.

46. Sawchenko P E. Evidence for a local site of action for glucocorticoids in inhibiting CRF and vasopressin in the paraventricular nucleus. Brain Res 1987; 403:213–226.

47. Kovacs K, Mezey E. Dexamethasone inhibits corticotropin releasing factor gene expression in the paraventricular nucleus of the rat. Neuroendocrinology 1987; 46:365–368.

48. Fuxe K, Cintra A, Harfstrand A, et al. Central glucocorticoid receptor immunoreactive neurons: new insights into the endocrine regulation of the brain. Ann NY Acad Sci 1987; 512:362–393.

49. Arriza J L, Simerly R B, Swanson L W, Evans R M. The neuronal mineralocorticoid receptor as a mediator of glucorticoid response. Neuron 1988; 1: 887-900.

50. Agnati L F, Fuxe K, Yu Z-Y, et al. Morphometrical analysis of the distribution of corticotropin-releasing factor, glucocorticoid receptor and phenylethanolamine-N-methyltransferase immunoreactive structures in the paraventricular hypothalamic nucleus of the rat. Neurosci Lett 1986; 54:147–152.

51. Black I B, Adler J E, LaGamma E F. Impulse activity differentially regulates co-localized transmitters by altering messenger RNA levels. Prog Brain Res 1986; 68:121–127.

52. Sawchenko P E, Swanson L W. The organization of noradrenergic pathways from the brainstem to the paraventricular and supraoptic nuclei. Brain Res Rev 1982; 4:275–325.

53. Feldman S, Siegel R A, Wiedenfeld J, Conforti N, Melamed E. Role of medial forebrain bundle catecholaminergic fibers in the modulation of glucocorticoid negative feedback effects. Brain Res 1983; 260:297–300.

54. Kaneko M, Hiroshige T. Site of fast, rate-sensitive feedback inhibition of adrenocorticotropin secretion during stress. Am J Physiol 1978; 234: R46–R51.

55. Smythe G A, Bradshaw J E, Vining R F. Hypothalamic monoamine control of stress-induced adrenocorticotropin release in the rat. Endocrinology 1983; 113:1062–1071.

56. Harfstrand A, Fuxe K, Cintra A, et al. Glucocorticoid receptor immunoreactivity in monoaminergic neurons of rat brain. Proc Natl Acad Sci USA 1986; 83:9779–9783.

57. Sawchenko P E, Bohn M C. Glucocorticoid receptor immunoreactivity in C1, C2 and C3 adrenergic neurons that project to the hypothalamus or to the spinal cord in the rat. J Comp Neurol 1989; 285:107–116.

58. Sawchenko P E. The effects of catecholamine-depleting medullary knife cuts on CRF- and vasopressin-immunoreactivity in the hypothalamus of normal and steroid-manipulated rats. Neuroendocrinology 1988; 48:459–470.

59. Alonso G, Szafarczyk A, Balmefrezol M, Assenmacher I. Immunocytochemical evidence for stimulatory control by the ventral noradrenergic bundle of the paraventricular nucleus secreting corticotropin releasing factor and vasopressin in rats. Brain Res 1986; 397:297–307.

60. Swanson L W, Simmons D M. Differential steroid hormone and neural influences on peptide mRNA levels in CRH cells of the paraventricular nucleus: a hybridization histochemical study in the rat. J Comp Neurol 1989; 285:413–435.

61. Seiden G, Brodish A. Physiological evidence for "short-loop" feedback effects of ACTH on hypothalamic CRF. Neuroendocrinology 1971; 8:154–164.

62. Liposits Z S, Sievers L, Paull W K. Neuropeptide-Y and ACTH-immunoreactive innervation of corticotropin releasing factor (CRF)-synthesizing neurons in the hypothalamus of the rat. Histochemistry 1988; 88:227–234.

63. Plotsky P M, Sawchenko P E. Hypophysial–portal plasma levels, median eminence content and immunohistochemical straining of corticotropin-releasing factor, arginine vasopressin and oxytocin following pharmacological adrenalectomy. Endocrinology 1987; 120:1361–1369.

4

LIMBIC PATHWAYS AND NEUROTRANSMITTERS AS MEDIATORS OF AUTONOMIC AND NEUROENDOCRINE RESPONSES TO STRESS

The Amygdala

Thackery S. Gray
Loyola Stritch School of Medicine, Maywood, Illinois

Anxiety or expressed fear associated with real or imagined threat constitutes psychological stress. One set of biological changes that occur during stress includes a profile of responses that have been classically described as the "flight or fight" defense response. Normally this cluster of biological responses helps to increase the readiness and execution of behaviors that will ultimately increase the probability of survival of the organism. These include appropriate changes in the cardiovascular, respiratory, and other visceral systems. The importance of providing an accurate account of how stress affects the integrity of biological systems is apparent. Chronic fear and anxiety can harm the body organs physically and contribute to the development of cardiovascular, gastrointestinal, and other visceral pathological conditions as well as maladaptive behaviors. Prevention and treatment of stress-related disorders are predicated on an increased understanding of the biological substrates that mediate visceral changes associated with both acutely and chronically threatening conditions.

The regions of the central nervous system responsible for mediating the perception and expression of fear and anxiety are currently the subjects of intense study. The limbic system is considered one of the pivotal systems in this regard. The limbic system is composed primarily of diencephalic and telencephalic structures that provide an interface between the neocortex and regions within the brainstem and spinal cord that control somatomotor, visceromotor, and neuroendocrine systems.

The amygdala, located within the temporal lobe of the brain, is one such region. The amygdala is unique among limbic structures in that it has direct anatomical connections with neocortex, hypothalamic neuroendocrine cells, and preganglionic autonomic regions of the brainstem. Stimulation of the amygdala in humans produces acute perceptions of anxiety or fear that are strikingly realistic (1,2). Activation of the amygdala in humans and animals also can produce somatomotor and visceral-autonomic changes that typically accompany defense responses (1-8). Destruction of the amygdala markedly affects various measures of fear/anxiety and blunts learned visceral/somatomotor responses to fear-provoking stimuli (3,9-11). The amygdala contains a high density of benzodiazepine receptors, which suggests that it is an important site for anxiolytic drug actions (12). The amygdala has also been implicated in animal models of stress-related pathological conditions including hypertension (6,13,14) and gastric ulcers (15).

This chapter will review how the amygdala might integrate or participate in the expression of autonomic, neuroendocrine, and somatomotor response to stress-evoking (i.e., threatening) stimuli. This chapter is not intended to be comprehensive in terms of the overall functions and pathways of the amygdala. The emphasis will instead be on the possible neurotransmitters and anatomical pathways that mediate autonomic and neuroendocrine responses to stress. In doing so, recent data in the literature and from the author's laboratory will be discussed. In this regard the emphasis will be on the amygdaloid central nucleus because this part of the amygdala is more directly involved in the central visceral neuroanatomic circuitry (16-19). For a more complete review of the amygdala the reader is encouraged to consult several recent papers (18-20).

AMYGDALA AND NEUROPEPTIDES

An area of intense interest within the last two decades has been the relationship between the relatively newly described peptide-containing neurons of the central nervous system and their possible role in biological integration of stress. The significance of adrenocorticotropic hormone (ACTH) and other peptide hormones in stress responses is discussed in other chapters of this book. However, there is good reason to believe that neuropeptides may also act as neurotransmitters and/or neuromodulators within the central nervous system to affect parameters of stress (See also Brown chapter in this book). The amygdala, especially the central nucleus, contains a high concentration and abundance of many different neuropeptides. These peptides are located in extrinsically projecting neurons, intrinsic neurons, and extra-amygdaloid afferents. It is important to determine whether the anatomical circuitry of the amygdala can be coded in terms of peptide specific pathways. Studies using combined immunocytochemistry and lesions or retrograde tracing techniques have provided some data on the source and destination of amygdaloid efferents and afferents (21-28,cf. 29).

Figure 1 summarizes the peptides identified to date within cells that project out of the amygdala of rat. In terms of the output neurons, corticotropin-releasing factor (CRF), neurotensin, somatostatin, substance P, and galanin producing cells are the primary output neurons to the brainstem. The enkephalin-containing cells of the amygdala appear to be intrinsic neurons and reciprocally connect the amygdala to homologous regions of the bed nucleus of the stria terminalis. The enkephalin cells also contain gamma amino butyric acid. Most other peptide cell types studied so far also participate in the bidirectional pathway between the central amygdala and bed nucleus of the stria terminalis. The peptidergic output neurons of the amygdala-brainstem pathway show little target specificity,

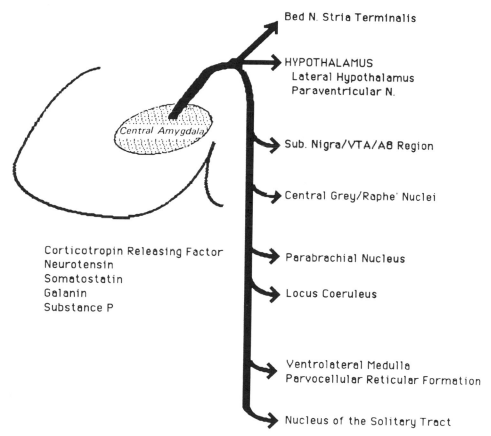

FIGURE 1   Peptides identified within cells that project out of rat amygdala.

although further amygdaloid termination regions need to be examined (e.g., lateral hypothalamus, substantia nigra, ventrolateral medulla). All five peptide-containing cell types contribute axons to the central grey, parabrachial region, and the vagal complex. A recent study has suggested a somatostatin input from the amygdala to the A8 dopaminergic cell groups; however, the possibility that other peptides innervate this region was not tested (25). The parabrachial nucleus receives the strongest input from amygdaloid peptidergic neurons. For example, over 60% of the CRF containing cells in the central amygdaloid nucleus project to the parabrachial nucleus compared to slightly over 30% to the central grey and 15% to the dorsal vagal complex. Thus, the amygdaloid neurons may release the same peptides at multiple sites within the brainstem. These peptides may have a similar effect upon their target regions to promote the stress response, dependent on the individual properties of each peptide. For example, neurotensin has an excitatory effect upon neurons within the central grey and bed nucleus of the stria terminalis (30,31). Or, alternatively, peptides may act differentially due to target specific differences in distributions of receptors and/ or the cells of the particular area innervated. Somatostatin reduces excitability of neurons of the nucleus of the solitary tract, although enhancement of excit-ability has been observed in other regions of the brain (32).

The differential effects of these peptides could form the substrates for differ-ential activation of components of the defense response. There is evidence that different target regions of the amygdala mediate different components of re-sponses to aversive stimuli. For example, lesions of the midbrain central grey will abolish freezing response to a tone that signals electric shock in rats (33,34). The same lesion, however, will not affect the cardiovascular response to the tone (34). Destruction of cells within the lateral hypothalamus will affect the cardiovascu-lar response to the tone but not the freezing response. This suggests that there is some degree of segregation in terms of the components of the stress response integrated by target regions of amygdaloid neurons. However, it should be noted that integrated defense responses have been elicited by stimulation of amygda-loid pathways from the amygdala through the hypothalamus and into the central grey (4). The inputs of the central amygdala are far more complex. Compared to the efferent cells, there are more afferents and many more types of peptides within the terminals of the central amygdaloid nucleus. Figure 2 summarizes the sources and types of peptide terminals within the central amygdaloid nucleus. The source of thyrotropin-releasing factor (TRF), bombesin, angiotensin II, and atrial natriuretic peptide-containing terminals is unknown. Some peptide-con-taining afferents arise from multiple sources. For example, enkephalin and neurotensin arise from cells within the parabrachial nucleus and nucleus of the solitary tract. Peptide afferents from multiple sources may convey the general activity of the neural circuitry associated with the amygdala or a subset of that circuitry that serves a common function. Some peptide afferents show clear

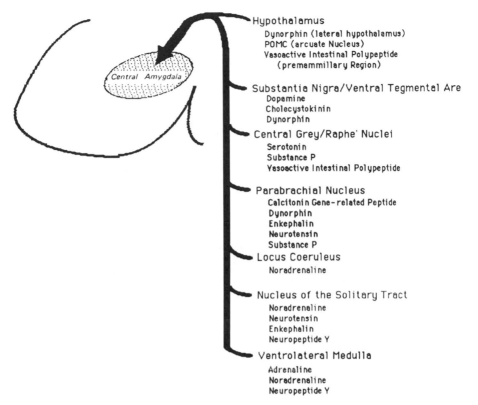

FIGURE 2 Sources and types of peptide terminals within the central amygdaloid nucleus.

single-source selectivity. The most interesting example is calcitonin gene-related peptide (CGRP), which comes exclusively from the parabrachial nucleus. The parabrachial nucleus has been associated with cardiovascular, respiratory, and special visceral afferent functions (for review see 35). Information of this nature may be transmitted via CGRP release. Some peptide inputs coexist with catecholamines. Many amygdaloid terminals probably contain both cholecystokinin and dopamine that arise from the same neurons within the substantia nigra (36). Thus, modulation of the amygdaloid functions by other brain regions can be coded to some degree according to the type of peptide-containing terminal and its source and whether it coexists with another putative neurotransmitter.

As noted above, activation of the amygdala in awake, behaving animals produces autonomic changes that resemble responses to "psychological" stressors. Based on immunocytochemical studies, there are over 15 different peptides contained within terminals of the amygdala. It is reasonable to hypothesize that release of one or several of these peptides may be at least partly responsible for some of the cardiovascular or other measurable autonomic changes that occur during activation of amygdaloid neurons. One approach that has been taken is to inject peptides into the amygdala of awake rats and measure changes in heart rate, blood pressure, and plasma catecholamine levels. Of the 16 peptides studied to date, only CGRP and TRF caused increases in both heart rate and blood pressure (37.38). Injections of either TRF or CGRP into the amygdala increased plasma levels of norepinephrine (38). Thyrotropin-releasing factor, but not CGRP, increased plasma epinephrine levels (38). Thus, TRF and CGRP can stimulate amygdaloid neurons to increase cardiovascular activity ultimately through decreased vagal activity and increased activity of the sympathetic nervous system.

AMYGDALA AND CATECHOLAMINES

The relationship between stress and central release of catecholamines has been the subject of numerous investigations (e.g., 39-42). It is not yet clear what specific roles the different catecholaminergic systems play in affecting the biological response to stress. However, there is considerable evidence that noradrenergic, adrenergic, and dopaminergic brain cells are involved in responses to stress. The question we asked was whether descending amygdaloid neurons innervated specific subsets of brainstem catecholaminergic neurons. If so, perhaps amygdaloid activation of selective catecholaminergic pathways may be a mechanism contributing to the expression of components of the stress response. To accomplish this, the highly specific anatomical tracer *Phaseolus vulgaris* leukoagglutinin lectin was injected into the amygdala of rats (43). This tracer fills the cell bodies at the injection site and is transported into their axons and terminals. The neurons that contain the tracer can then be localized by standard immunohistochemical techniques. The cell bodies, axons, and terminals of the neurons that contain the anatomical tracer will appear brown. The same tissue can then be processed using antibodies to catecholamine enzymes (i.e., tyrosine hydroxylase, dopamine beta hydroxylase, and phenylethanolamine N-methyltransferase) using a different color reaction (44). The distribution of amygdaloid terminals was examined within the well-described dopaminergic, noradrenergic, and adrenergic cell groups of the brainstem (45).

The results of a recent set of experiments in our laboratory are summarized in Figure 3 (46,47). Amygdaloid neurons heavily innervated a continuum of dopaminergic cells that extended from lateral substantia nigra (A9) into the retrorubral field (A8). In the pons and amygdaloid, terminals were found on noradrenergic cells within rostral portions of the locus coeruleus (A6). In the medulla, adrenergic cells within the nucleus of the solitary tract and ventrolateral medulla

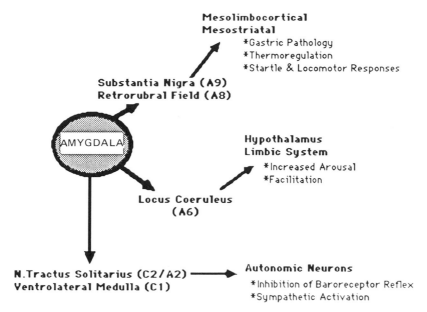

FIGURE 3 Possible functions of amygdala catecholamine pathways.

were associated with amygdaloid terminals. Noradrenergic cells with the nucleus of the solitary tract were also innervated by the amygdala. Areas that were not heavily innervated by the amygdala included dopaminergic cells of the ventral tegmental area (A10) and more ventral parts of the substantia nigra, the main body of the locus coeruleus, the subcoeruleus, and Kolliker-Fuse nucleus. Also amygdaloid terminals were not distributed heavily within the A5 catecholamine group and the noradrenergic cells of the caudal ventrolateral medulla.

Thus, the results of this study favor the hypothesis that the amygdala can selectively affect the activity of specific dopaminergic cells of the midbrain, the rostral locus coeruleus and noradrenergic/adrenergic cells of the medulla. The possible functions of these pathways are summarized in Figure 3. The lateral portion of A9 and the A8 cells contribute dopaminergic fibers to the mesostriatal pathway and the mesolimbocortical pathway (26,48). Both the mesostriatal and mesolimbocortical systems have possible roles during stress. The mesolimbocortical pathway, which projects back to the amygdala, is involved in the maintenance of gastric mucosal integrity in the presence of stressors (49). The protective effect could be related to the amygdaloid dopamine neuronal processing of reward-related behaviors (50). Recent studies suggest that there is an important interaction in terms of stress-induced gastric pathological conditions and TRH, neurotensin, and dopamine within the amygdala (51).

However, there are other possible functions of amygdala pathway to dopaminergic brainstem neurons. Dopamine levels are increased in the prefrontal cortex in response to various types of stressors, presumably through activation of the mesolimbocortical dopaminergic system (52). The amygdala could be partly responsible for cortical release of dopamine. The mesostriatal pathway is involved in the central control of thermoregulation by its action upon heat-dissipation mechanisms (53). This could be related to temperature changes observed during stress.

The amygdala innervated rostral portions of the locus coeruleus noradrenergic cell group. Intermittent (over 3-4 h) electrical stimulation of the amygdala in cats will produce the defense response and will also reduce overall levels of cerebral norepinephrine (54). The region of the locus coeruleus innervated by the amygdala projects back upon the hypothalamus and limbic system. As noted above, stimulation of the amygdala also results in increases in plasma norepinephrine. These findings would explain the close temporal relationship between the release of norepinephrine within the amygdala and plasma increases of norepinephrine (55). The function of this pathway could be to facilitate or inhibit limbic system activity further. For example, injections of alpha-2 receptor agonists into the central amygdala of rats prevents air stress from increasing renal nerve activity. This did not, however, block increases of blood pressure normally observed in response to noise stress (56). Administration of beta-adrenoreceptor antagonists into the amygdala had no effect on renal nerve activity or blood pressure increases. However, injection of beta-adrenoreceptor antagonists into the amygdala does impair learned cardiovascular responses to aversive stimuli in rabbits (57). This suggests a possible separation of cardiovascular and sympathetic modulation, depending on differential receptor activation within the amygdala. This may occur through differential activation of peptidergic neurons within the amygdala. The exact mechanisms by which this could occur are unclear. However, disruption of the noradrenergic input to the amygdala reduces neurotensin immunoreactivity with the cell bodies of the amygdaloid central nucleus (58). This may occur through differential receptor activation of amygdaloid peptide containing neurons (e.g., in this case neurotensin cells).

Amygdaloid terminals frequently contacted cells of the adrenergic C2 and noradrenergic A2 cell groups of the nucleus of the solitary tract (NTS). Stimulation of the Ce attenuates the baroreceptor reflex (5) and injections of epinephrine or, to a lesser degree, norepinephrine within the NTS decrease the activity of neurons that participate in the baroreceptor reflex (59,60). Thus it is possible that Ce neurons could excite adrenergic and/or noradrenergic neurons within the NTS, causing their release, which may in turn have an inhibitory action on the baroreceptive modulating neurons. This postulated amygdala-mediated baroreceptor reflex inhibition could contribute to the hypertensive cardiovascular response observed when the amygdala is activated.

AMYGDALA AND ACTH RELEASE

A number of studies have implicated the amygdala as an important part of the neural circuitry that mediates ACTH and corticosterone responses (61-64). Changes in plasma corticosterone or ACTH levels have been observed after electrical stimulation of the amygdala in awake rats and cats (64-67). Both increases and decreases in the corticosterone response have been observed; however, stimulation of the corticomedial amygdala usually elicited increases in awake animals (64,66). Destruction of the amygdala inhibits adrenocortical responses to stress-inducing olfactory and somatosensory stimuli (68). Bilateral lesions of the amygdala also attenuate hypersecretion of ACTH that is usually observed after adrenalectomy (61). More specific lesion studies of the amygdala have emphasized the importance of the central amygdaloid nucleus in the mediation of ACTH release. Lesions of the central amygdaloid nucleus dramatically attenuated ACTH responses to immobilization stress (62). Baseline secretion of ACTH is not altered after ablation of the central amygdala. Destruction of the central amygdaloid nucleus increases the serotonergic activity of many of the regions within the hypothalamus and the amygdala (63). The serotonergic system is considered important in the delayed negative feedback actions of glucocorticoid feedback to the ACTH stimulating parts of the hypothalamus (cf. 63). Destruction of the Ce and its subsequent effect upon the serotonergic neurons may be at least partly responsible for blocking of ACTH hypersecretion observed after adrenalectomy (61).

The specific pathway or pathways by which the amygdala can activate corticotropin-releasing cells (i.e., cells that effect pituitary release of ACTH) of the hypothalamus have not been defined. Amygdaloid neurons could be connected to the pituitary activating regions of the paraventricular nucleus of the hypothalamus (PVN) via monosynaptic and/or multisynaptic pathways. The central amygdaloid nucleus neurons were only sparsely labeled after injections of retrograde tracer into the PVN (69,70), although medial amygdaloid nucleus neurons were consistently retrogradely labeled. Other anatomical studies suggest that Ce projections to the PVN are mediated via an indirect pathway from the Ce to the bed nucleus of the stria terminalis, which in turn projects heavily upon the PVN (71). As an alternative, the Ce projects upon brainstem regions that have direct connections with PVN (17,19).

The cells that affect the release of ACTH from the pituitary are located within the parvocellular parts of the PVN. Certainly CRF-containing neurons are among the most important neurons in this regard. However, other peptide containing neurons such vasopressin and oxytocin cells are important modulators of the release of ACTH and other opiomelanocortins (see Rivier chapter). The question we asked was whether the central amygdaloid nucleus and/or the bed nucleus of the stria terminalis (BST) directly projected upon the parvocellular PVN, and if so what types of neurons within the PVN are innervated. To answer this question *Phaseolus vulgaris* leukoagglutinin lectin tracer injections were used to label amygdaloid and BST terminals (see above) within the hypothalamus and immunocytochemical reactions to vasopressin, oxytocin and CRF were investigated (72,73, unpublished data).

The results of this study are summarized in Figure 4. Central amygdaloid and BST terminals were found on all three types of parvocellular PVN neurons (i.e., CRF, vasopressin, and oxytocin). The projection from the BST to the parvocellular PVN was much heavier compared to the amygdala. In addition, the BST neurons appeared to innervate directly magnocellular vasopressin and oxytocin cells of the PVN and supraoptic nucleus. Thus, the central amygdala can both directly and indirectly (probably disynaptically) activate CRF, vasopressin, and oxytocin cells within the parvocellular PVN. In addition, the projections to the BST could be the anatomical pathways through which it modulates the release of vasopressin, and possibly oxytocin, from magnocellular hypothalamic neurons (74).

SUMMARY AND CONCLUSIONS

A clear picture of the relationship and function of the amygdala to its pathways and possible neurotransmitters has yet to emerge. However, based on the more

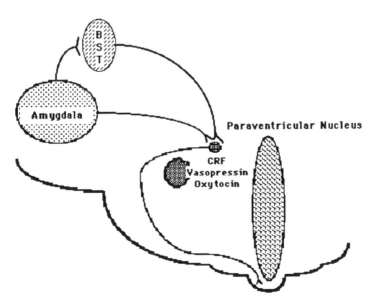

FIGURE 4   Central amydaloid and BST terminals in the paraventricular nucleus.

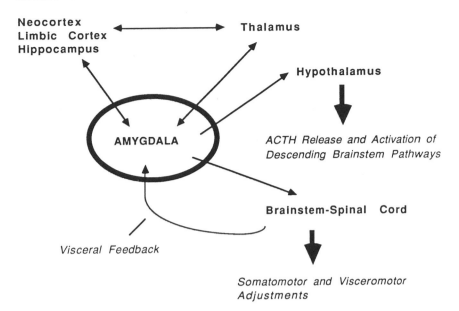

FIGURE 5 Model of sensory processing and recognition.

recent data, an extension of a model proposed by Gloor (75) can be discussed. This model is illustrated in part by Figure 5. Cortical and thalamic inputs to the amygdala probably convey information regarding the complex sensory properties of a threatening or nonthreatening stimulus. The significance of the stimulus may be coded via interactions through associated neural circuitry (e.g., cortex and hippocampus) and/or within amygdala itself. The amygdala then may transmit the appropriate output to the hypothalamus, other limbic regions and the brainstem. This may be mediated via the release of peptides and yet to be identified amygdaloid neurotransmitters. The function of catecholamines may be generally to facilitate and coordinate neuroendocrine, autonomic, and somatomotor output, depending on the particular cell group affected.

Brainstem projections upon the amygdala could be carrying visceral sensory feedback and information regarding input received by the forebrain. In general, this input could function to reduce or increase amygdaloid activity. In more specific terms, the visceral feedback could augment or attenuate the emotional perception of the threatening circumstances, depending on the function of the particular neural circuitry and the psychological or physiological state of the animal. Changes in autonomic functions are perceived at the conscious and unconscious levels. At the conscious level this visceral feedback allows us to define the seriousness of the threat or stressor that confronts us. Probably at the unconscious level, the visceral feedback contributes to the formation of an "emotional or affective" significance to the threatening stimulus (i.e., learning). For example, CGRP terminals within the amygdala (as noted above) originate from the parabrachial nucleus. One of the proposed functions of the parabrachial nucleus is to relay visceral input from the NTS to the amygdala (35). Thus, one could speculate that CGRP inputs to the amygdala may produce the same visceral sensation in the animal that occurs when stress-evoking stimuli are present. Also at the unconscious level are reflexes that attempt to maintain autonomic homeostasis. A clear example is the baroreceptor reflex, which serves to maintain heart rate and blood pressure at a relatively steady state. Activation of the amygdala normally overrides this reflex, but as amygdaloid activity is reduced it may serve to return amygdaloid activity further to normal basal levels.

REFERENCES

1. Chapman W P, Schroeder H R, Geyer G, et al. Physiological evidence concerning importance of the amygdaloid nuclear region in the integration of circulatory function in man. Science 1954; 120: 949-950.
2. Gloor P. Role of the human limbic system in perception, memory, and affect: lessons from temporal lobe epilepsy. In Doan BK, Livingston KE, eds. The limbic system: functional organization and clinical disorders. New York: Raven Press, 1986: 159-169.
3. Kaada B R. Stimulation and regional ablation of the amygdaloid complex with reference to functional representations. In Eleftheriou BE, ed. The neurobiology of the amygdala. New York: Plenum Press, 1972: 205-281.
4. Hilton S B, Zbrozyna A W. Amygdaloid region for defense reaction and its efferents pathway to the brain stem. J Physiol 1963; 165: 106-184.
5. Stock G, Rupprecht U, Stumpf H, Schlor K H. Cardiovascular changes during arousal elicited by stimulation of amygdala, hypothalamus and locus coeruleus. J Autonom Nerv Syste 1981; 3: 503-510
6. Galeno T M, Brody M J. Hemodynamic responses to amygdaloid stimulation in spontaneously hypertensive rats. Am J Physiol 1983; 245: R281-R286.
7. Iwata J, Chida K, LeDoux J E. Cardiovascular responses elicited by stimulation of neurons in the central nucleus of amygdala in awake, but not anesthesized rats, resemble conditioned emotional responses. Brain Res 1987; 418: 183-188
8. Harper R M, Frysinger R C, Trelease R B, Marks J D. State dependent alteration of respiratory cycle timing by stimulation of the central nucleus of amygdala. Brain Res 1984; 306: 1-8
9. Kapp B S, Pascoe J P, Bixler M A. The amygdala: a neuroanatomical systems approach to its contribution to aversive conditioning. In: Butters N, Squire L, eds. The neuropsychology of memory. New York: Guilford Press, 1985; 473-488.

10. Iwata J, LeDoux J, Meeley M P, et al. Intrinsic neurons in the amygdaloid field projected to by the medial geniculate body mediate emotional responses conditioned to acoustic stimuli. Brain Res 1986; 383: 195–214.

11. Vanderwolf C H, Kelly M E, Kraemer P, Streather A. Are emotion and motivation localized in the limbic system and nucleus accumbens? Behav Brain Res 1986; 27: 45–58.

12. Niehoff D L, Kuhar M J. Benzodiazepine receptors: localization in rat amygdala. J Neurosci 1983; 3: 2091–2097.

13. Folkow B, Hallback-Norlander M, Martner J, Nordborg C. Influence of amygdala lesions on cardiovascular responses to alerting stimuli, on behaviour and on blood pressure development in spontaneously hypertensive rats. Acta Physiol Scand 1982; 116: 133–139.

14. Galeno T M, Van Hoesen B W, Maixner W, Johnson A K, Brody M J. Contribution of the amygdala to the development of spontaneous hypertension. Brain Res 1982; 246: 1–6.

15. Henke P G. Recent studies of the central nucleus of the amygdala and stress ulcers. Neurosci Biobehav Rev 1988; 12: 143–150.

16. Loewy A D, McKellar S. The neuroanatomical basis of central cardiovascular control. Fed Proc 1980; 39: 2495–2503.

17. Van Der Kooy D, Koda L Y, McGinty J R, Gerfen C R, Bloom F E. The organization of projections from the cortex, amygdala, and hypothalamus to the nucleus of the solitary tract in rat. J Comp Neurol 1984; 224: 1–24.

18. LeDoux J E. Emotion. In: Plum F, ed. Handbook of physiology—the nervous system V. Baltimore: Waverly, 1984: 419–459.

19. Price J L, Russchen F T, Amaral D G. The limbic region. II: The amygdaloid complex. In Emson PC, ed. Handbook of chemical neuroanatomy. Vol. 5: Integrated systems of the CNS, Part I. New York: Raven Press, 1987: 279–388.

20. Sarter M, Markowitsch H J. Involvement of the amygdala in learning and memory: a critical review with emphasis on anatomical relations. Behav Neurosci 1985; 99: 342–380.

21. Yamano M, Hillyard C J, Girgis S, et al. Presence of a substance P-like immunoreactive neurone system from the parabrachial area to the central amygdaloid nucleus of the rat with reference to coexistence with calcitonin gene-related peptide. Brain Res 1988; 451: 179–188.

22. Schwaber J S, Sternini C, Brecha N C, Rogers W T, Card J P. Neurons containing calcitonin gene-related peptide in the parabrachial nucleus project to the central nucleus of the amygdala. J Comp Neurol 1988; 270: 416–426.

23. Shiosaka S, Sakanaka M, Inagaki S, et al. Putative neurotransmitters in the amygdaloid complex with special reference to peptidergic pathways. In: Emson PC, ed. Chemical neuroanatomy. New York: Raven Press, 1983; 359–388.

24. Zardetto-Smith A M, Gray T S. Catecholaminergic cells of the ventrolateral medulla and nucleus of the solitary tract innervate the central nucleus of the amygdala in the rat. Soc Neurosci Abstr 1988; 14: 1318.

25. Deutch A Y, Bean A J, Roth R H. Regulation of A8 dopamine neurons by somatostatin. Eur J Pharmacol 1988; 147: 317-320.

26. Loughlin S E, Fallon J H. Dopaminergic projections to amygdala from substantia nigra and ventral tegmental area. Brain Res 1983; 262: 334-338.

27. Fallon J H. Histochemical characterization of dopaminergic, noradrenergic and serotonergic projections to the amygdala. In: Ben-Ari Y, ed. The amygdaloid complex. New York: Elsevier, 1981; 175-184.

28. McDonald A J. Somatostatinergic projections from the amygdala to the bed nucleus of the stria terminalis and medial preoptic-hypothalamic region. Neurosci Lett 1987; 75: 271-277.

29. Gray T S. Autonomic neuropeptide connections of the amygdala. In Tache Y, Morley JE, Brown MR, Neuropeptides and stress: Hans Selye symposium on neuronedocrinology and stress. New York: Springer-Verlag, 1988; 92-106.

30. Behbehani M M, Shipley M T, McLean J H. Effect of neurotensin on neurons in the periaqueductal gray: an in vitro study. J Neurosci 1987; 7: 2035-2040.

31. Sawada S, Takada S, Yamomoto C. Electrical activity recorded from thin sections of bed nucleus of the stria terminalis and effects of neurotensin. Brain Res 1980; 188: 578-581.

32. Jacquin T, Champagnat J, Madamba S, Denavit-Suabie M, Siggins G R. Somatostatin depresses excitability in neurons of the solitary tract complex through hyperpolarization and augmentation of IM, a noninactivating voltage-dependent outward current blocked by muscarinic agonists. Proc Natl Acad Sci 1988; 85: 948-952.

33. Liebman J, Mayer D J, Liebsekin J C. Mesencephalic central grey lesions and fear-motivated behavior in rats. Brain Res 1970; 23: 353-370.

34. LeDoux J E, Iwata J, Cicchetti P, Ries D J. Different behavioral correlates of conditioned fear. J Neurosci 1988; 8: 2517-2529.

35. Fulwiler C E, Saper C B. Subnuclear organization of the efferent connections of the parabrachial nucleus in the rat. Brain Res Rev 1984; 7: 229-259.

36. Hokfelt T, Skirboll L, Rehfeld J F, Goldstein M, Markey K, Dann O. A subpopulation of mesencephalic dopamine neurons projecting to limbic areas contains a cholecystokinin-like peptide: evidence from immunohistochemistry combined with retrograde tracing. Neuroscience 1980; 5: 2093-2124.

37. Nguyen K Q, Sills M A, Jacobowitz D M. Cardiovascular effects produced by microinjections of calcitonin gene-related peptide in the rat central amygdaloid nucleus. Peptides 1986; 7: 337-339.

38. Brown M R, Gray T S. Peptide injections into the amygdala of conscious rats: effects on blood pressure, heart rate and plasma catecholamines. Regul Pept 1988; 21: 95-10.

39. Irwin J, Ahluwalia P, Zacharko R M, Anisman H. Central norepinephrine and plasma corticosterone following acute and chronic stressors: influence of social isolation and handling. Pharm Biochem Behav 1986; 24: 1151–1154.

40. Svenson T H. Peripheral, autonomic regulation of locus coeruleus noradrenergic neurons in brain: putative implications of psychiatry and psychopharmacology. Psychopharmacology 1987; 92: 1–7.

41. Tilders F J H, Berkenbosch F. CRF and catecholamines; their place in central and peripheral regulation of the stress response. Acta Endocrinol 1986; 276: 63–75.

42. Loewy A D, Neil J J. The role of descending monoaminergic systems in central control of blood pressure. Fed Proc 1981; 40: 2778–2785.

43. Gerfen C R, Sawchenko P E. An anterograde neuroanatomical tracing method that shows the detailed morphology of neurons, their axons and terminals: immunohistochemical localization of an axonally transported lectin. Brain Res 1984; 290: 219–238.

44. Piekut D T. Interactions of immunostained ACTH1-39 fibers and CRF neurons in the paraventricular nucleus of rat hypothalamus: application of avidin–glucose oxidase to dual immunostaining procedures. J Histochem Cytochem 1987; 35: 261–265.

45. Hökfelt T, Martensson R, Bjorklund A, Kleinau S, Goldstein M. Distributional maps of tyrosine–hydroxylase-immunoreactive neurons in the rat brain, In: Bjorklund A, Hokfelt T, eds. Handbook of chemical neuroanatomy. Vol. 2: Classical transmitters in the CNS. Part I. New York: Elsevier Press, 1984; 277–379.

46. Wallace D M, Magnuson D J, Gray T S. The amygdalo-brainstem pathway: selective innervation of dopaminergic, noradrenergic and adrenergic cells in the rat. Neurosci Lett 1989; 97: 252–258.

47. Cassell M D, Gray T S. The amygdala directly innervates adrenergic (C1) neurons in the ventrolateral medulla in the rat. Neurosci Lett 1989; 97: 163–168.

48. Deutch A, Goldstein M, Baldino F B Jr, Roth R. Telencephalic projections of the A8 dopamine cell group. Ann NY Acad Sci 1989;

49. Ray A, Henke P G, Sullivan R M. Central dopamine systems and gastric stress pathology in rats. Physiol Behav 1988; 42: 359–364.

50. Nakano Y, Lenard L, Oomura Y, Nishino H, Aou S, Yamamoto T. Functional involvement of catecholamines in reward-related neuronal activity of the monkey amygdala. J Neurophysiol 1987; 57: 72–91.

51. Henke P G, Sullivan R M, Ray A. Interactions of thyrotropin-releasing hormone (TRH) with neurotensin and dopamine in the central nucleus of the amygdala during stress ulcer formation in rats. Neurosci Lett 1988; 91: 95–100.

52. Dunn A J, Kramarcy M R. Neurochemical responses during stress: relationships between the hypothalamic-pituitary-adrenal and catecholamine systems, In: Iversen L I, Iversen S D, Snyder S H, eds. Handbook of psychopharmacology. vol. 18. New York: Plenum Press, 1984: 455–515.

53. Lee T F, Mora F, Myers R D. Dopamine and thermoregulation: an evalua-
     tion with special reference to dopaminergic pathways. Neurosci Biobehav
     Rev 1985; 9: 589-598.
54. Reis D J, Gunne L-M. Brain catecholamines: relation to the defense reac-
     tion evoked by brain stimulation in the cat. Science 1965; 156: 1768-
     1770.
55. Dietl H. Temporal relationship between noradrenaline rlease in the central
     amygdala and plasma noradrenaline secretion in rats and tree shrews.
     Neurosci Lett 1985; 55: 41-46.
56. Koepke J P, Jones S, DiBona G F. a_2-Adrenoreceptors in amygdala control
     renal sympathetic nerve activity and renal function in conscious sponta-
     neously hypertensive rat. Brain Res 1987; 404: 80-88.
57. Gallagher M, Kapp B S. Influence of amygdala opiate-sensitive mechanisms,
     fear motivated responses and memory processes for aversive experiences.
     In: Martinez JL, Jensen RA, Messing RB, Regter H, McGaugh, JL, eds
     Endogenous peptides and learning and memory processes. New York: Aca-
     demic Press, 1981; 445-461.
58. Kawakami F, Fukui K, Okamura H, et al. Influence of ascending noradren-
     ergic fibers on the neurotensin-like immunoreactive perikarya and evidence
     of direct projection of ascending neurotensin-like immunoreactive fibers in
     the rat. Neurosci Lett 1984; 51: 231-234.
59. Felman P D, Moises H C. Adrenergic responses of baroreceptor cells in the
     nucleus tractus solitarii of the rat: a microiontophoretic study. Brain Res
     1987; 420: 351-361.
60. Saavedra J M, Fernandez-Pardal J, Torda T, Reis D, Ross C. Dissociation
     between rat hypothalamic and brainstem PNMT after stress and between
     hypothalamic catecholamines and PNMT after midbrain hemitransections.
     In: Usdin E, Kvetnansky E, Axelrod J, eds. Stress: the role of catechol-
     amines and other neurotransmitters. vol. 1. New York: Gordon and Breach,
     1983; 137-146.
61. Allen J P, Allen C F. Role of amygdaloid complexes in the stress-induced
     release of ACTH in the rat. Neuroendocrinology 1974; 15: 220-230
62. Beaulieu S, Di Paolo T, Cote J, Barden N. Participation of the central
     amygdaloid nucleus in the response of adrenocorticotropin (ACTH) secre-
     tion to immobilization stress: opposing roles of the noradrenergic and
     dopaminergic systems. Neuroendocrinology 1987; 45: 37-46.
63. Beaulieu S, Di Paolo T, Barden N. Control of ACTH secretion by the
     central nucleus of the amygdala: implication of the serotonergic system and
     its relevance to the glucocorticoid delayed feedback mechanism. Neuro-
     endocrinology 1986; 44: 247-254.
64. Redgate E S, Fahringer E E. A comparison of the pituitary-adrenal activity
     elicited by electrical stimulation of preoptic, amygdaloid and hypothalamic
     sites in the rat brain. Neuroendocrinology 1973; 12: 334-343.
65. Dunn J D, Whitener J. Plasma corticosterone responses to electrical stimula-
     tion of the amygdaloid complex: cytoarchitectural specificity. Neuro-
     endocrinology 1986; 42: 211-217.

66. Matheson B K, Branch B J, Taylor A N. Effects of amygdaloid stimulation on pituitary-adrenal activity in conscious cats. Brain Res 1971; 32: 151–167.
67. Zolovick A J. Effects of lesions and electrical stimulation of the amygdala on hypothalamic-hypophyseal regulation. In: Eleftheriou BE, ed. The neurobiology of the amygdala. New York: Plenum Press 1972: 643–685.
68. Feldman S, Conforti N. Amygdalectomy inhibits adrenocorticotropin responses to somatosensory and olfactory stimulation. Neuroendocrinology 1981; 5: 1323–1329.
69. Silverman A J, Hoffman D L, Zimmerman E A. The descending afferent connections of the paraventricular nucleus of the hypothalamus (PVN). Brain Res Bull 1981; 6: 47–61.
70. Tribollet E, Dreifuss J J. Localization of neurones projecting to the hypothalamic paraventricular nucleus of the rat: a horseradish peroxidase study. Neuroscience 1981; 7: 1215–1328.
71. Swanson L W. The Hypothalamus. In; Bjorklund A, Hokfelt T, Swanson LW, eds. Handbook of chemical neuroanatomy. Integrated systems of the CNS. Part I. Hypothalamus, hippocampus, amygdala and retina. Amsterdam: Elsevier/North-Holland Biomedical Press. 1987.
72. Magnuson D J, Gray T S. Amygdala directly innervates parvocellular paraventricular hypothalamic CRF, vasopressin and oxytocin containing cells. Soc Neurosci Abstr 1988; 14: 1288.
73. Gray T S, Carney M E, Magnuson D J. Direct projections from the central amygdaloid nucleus to the hypothalamic paraventricular nucleus: possible role in stress-induced ACTH release. Neuroendocrinology, 1989; 50: 433–446.
74. Hayward J N. The amygdaloid nuclear complex and mechanisms of release of vasopressin from the neurohypophysis. In: Eleftheriou BE, ed. The neurobiology of the amygdala. New York: Plenum Press, 1972; 685–740.
75. Gloor P. Inputs and outputs of the amygdala: what the amygdala is trying to tell the rest of the brain. In: Livingston KE, Hornykiewicz O, eds. Limbic mechanisms. The continuing evolution of the limbic system concept. New York: Plenum Press, 1978: 189–209.

5

DISTRIBUTION OF BRAIN AND PITUITARY RECEPTORS INVOLVED IN MEDIATING STRESS RESPONSES

Errol B. De Souza and Nathan M. Appel

National Institute on Drug Abuse, National Institutes of Health
Bethesda, Maryland

The mammalian response to stress is characterized by a wide variety of endocrine, autonomic, and behavioral sequelae that are representative of Selye's "general adaptation syndrome" (1). The principal endocrine response to stress involves stimulation of the hypothalamic–pituitary–adrenocortical axis, which results in coordinated secretion of corticotropin-releasing factor (CRF), adrenocorticotropic hormone (ACTH), and glucocorticoid, respectively. A major component of the autonomic response to stress is activation of sympathetic outflow, resulting in release of epinephrine from the adrenal medulla and norepinephrine from sympathetic nerve endings. These hormones (glucocorticoids, epinephrine, and norepinephrine) subserve homeostasis by altering a variety of cardiovascular, metabolic, and immune parameters.

Pharmacological studies have demonstrated that a variety of brain transmitters produce effects on endocrine, autonomic, behavioral, and/or immune parameters that are reminiscent of stress responses. However, their physiological role in mediating stress responses is less well defined. Three of the better-characterized brain neurotransmitter systems involved in coordinating endocrine, autonomic, behavioral, and immune responses to stress are the catecholamines, CRF, and opioid peptides. A detailed comparison of the relative density and precise distribution of these "stress neurotransmitter" receptors in the central nervous system (CNS) is necessary for us to define better some of the neuroanatomical substrates mediating the various effects of these neurotransmitters to coordinate the organism's response to stress. This chapter will focus on the distribution of catecholamine, CRF, and opioid receptors in brain nuclei that play important roles in coordinating the autonomic and endocrine responses to stress. In addition, since altered anterior pituitary hormone secretion is a major component of the neuroendocrine stress response, the role of pituitary receptors in modulating this aspect of the mammalian response to stress will also be addressed.

DISTRIBUTION OF ANTERIOR PITUITARY AND HYPOTHALAMIC RECEPTORS MEDIATING ENDOCRINE RESPONSE TO STRESS

The mammalian endocrine response to stress is characterized by altered secretion of a variety of anterior pituitary hormones. These include the proopiomelano-cortin (POMC)-derived peptides ACTH and β-endorphin/β-lipotropin, prolactin, thyroid-stimulating hormone, growth hormone, and the gonadotropins: luteiniz-ing hormone and follicle-stimulating hormone. The best characterized endocrine responses to stress are increased ACTH and prolactin secretion. On the other hand, thyrotropin, gonadotropin, and growth hormone responses to stress are not stereotypic and may vary subject to the nature, frequency, and/or duration of the stressor as well as the species under investigation. Since substantial evi-dence suggests that the brain in general, and the hypothalamus in particular, exerts the primary influence on anterior lobe hormone secretion, the distribu-tion in these areas of the primary neurohormone membrane receptors involved in modulating secretion of prolactin and POMC-derived peptides from the anterior pituitary will be described.

Dopamine Receptors

Considerable evidence supports a seminal role for dopamine as an inhibitor of prolactin secretion from the anterior pituitary (2,3). Dopamine, released from hypothalamic tuberoinfundibular neurons (originating in the arcuate nucleus and projecting to median eminence), inhibits prolactin secretion by acting at specific high-affinity receptors in the plasma membrane of mammotrophs (4). Radioligand binding studies have identified D_2 dopamine receptors in membrane preparations of anterior pituitary (see 5). In addition, receptor autoradiographic studies in rat (6) and human (7) pituitary glands have identified D_2 dopamine receptors in the anterior lobe. In rat, there is uniform distribution of D_2 dopa-mine receptors in the anterior lobe (6), which suggests a more generalized role for D_2 dopamine receptors in regulating anterior pituitary hormone secretion. In contrast, human anterior pituitary displays clusters of D_2 dopamine receptors corresponding to the clustering of mammotrophs, which suggests a primary role for these receptors in modulating prolactin secretion in humans (7).

CRF Receptors

Stress-induced secretion of POMC-derived peptides from the anterior pituitary is regulated primarily by CRF, which is derived from neurons whose cell bodies reside in the parvocellular portion of the paraventricular nucleus of the hypothalamus and project axons to the median eminence. The CRF acts on specific high-affinity binding sites in the anterior pituitary whose distribution in both rat and human anterior pituitary closely resembles the clustering of corticotrophs (8,9) (see Fig. 1). Although low densities of CRF-binding sites have been localized in hypothalamus (10), their role in mediating feedback effects of the peptide on its own release is at present undefined.

Adrenergic Receptors

A role for central noradrenergic and adrenergic neurons in regulating POMC-derived peptide secretion is well established; however, their role in modulating prolactin secretion is less well defined (11,12). Alpha- and β-adrenergic agents have been shown to alter ACTH secretion both in vivo and in pituitary cells in vitro (see 13, 14). Norepinephrine and, in particular, epinephrine may affect pituitary POMC-derived hormone release via the systemic circulation or may influence anterior pituitary function via the hypothalamohypophyseal portal system. The concentration of epinephrine in the hypophyseal portal blood reaching the anterior lobe cells under basal conditions, and the higher peripheral levels of circulating epinephrine and norepinephrine present in stressed states, are sufficient to activate adrenergic receptors in the pituitary gland (see 13, 15).

The direct actions of catecholamines to stimulate ACTH secretion at the pituitary level appear to be mediated primarily by β-adrenergic receptors (see 13). Radioligand binding studies have identified β-adrenergic receptors in anterior pituitary homogenates and have further demonstrated that these binding sites are predominantly of the β_2 subtype (see 13, 16). Receptor autoradiographic studies have revealed a uniform distribution of β_2-adrenergic receptors in bovine, rat, and human pituitary glands (16). The evidence supporting a physiological role for β_2-adrenergic receptors in the anterior pituitary in modulating ACTH responses to stress is based on studies demonstrating that insulin and stress-induced release of ACTH were blocked by the β-adrenergic antagonist propranolol (see 13, 17). The upregulation of β_2-adrenergic receptors in anterior pituitary following removal of circulating epinephrine is further support for a physiological role of these receptors in modulating anterior pituitary function (17).

Direct a_1-mediated adrenergic stimulation of POMC-derived peptide secretion has been demonstrated in primary cultures of anterior pituitary (see 14) and putative a_1-adrenergic receptors have been identified and characterized in rat

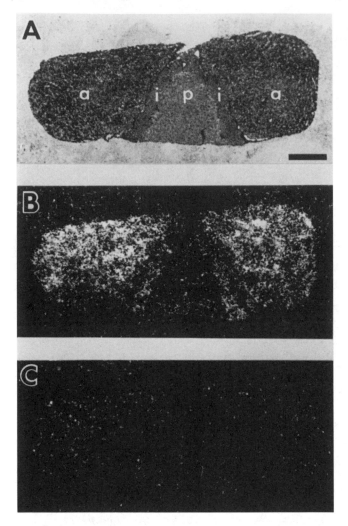

FIGURE 1 Autoradiographic localization of corticotropin-releasing factor (CRF)-binding sites in rat pituitary labeled with Nle^{21}, $[^{125}I]\,Tyr^{32}$–ovine CRF. A. Brightfield photomicrograph of a section of rat pituitary (horizontal plane) B. Darkfield photomicrograph shows the autoradiographic grain distribution in the same section. In darkfield illumination, the high densities of binding sites show up as the bright areas. Note the clustering of CRF binding sites in the anterior lobe (a) and the relatively uniform pattern of distribution in the intermediate lobe (i); no specific binding sites are present in the posterior lobe (p). C. Darkfield photomicrograph illustrates the absence of specific receptor binding in an adjacent serial section when 1 μM unlabeled ovine CRF was included in the incubation buffer. Bar = 500 μm (reproduced with permission from ref. 8).

anterior pituitary cells in culture (18). However, the role of these receptors in mediating in vivo effects of catecholamines remains controversial. Autoradiographic studies have demonstrated an absence of α_1-adrenergic receptors in anterior pituitary (15). Moreover, recent data suggest that the α_1-adrenergic control of ACTH secretion in anterior pituitary cultures may, in fact, be an acquired response due to culture conditions (19).

While the effect of catecholamines to stimulate ACTH secretion at the pituitary level appears to be mediated primarily through action at β_2-adrenergic receptors, their effects in brain to alter stress-induced POMC-derived peptide secretion, through effects on CRF, appear less well defined. The precise role of the noradrenergic/adrenergic system either to facilitate or inhibit stress-induced CRF and POMC-derived peptide secretion remains unresolved (11,20,21). It is, however, clear from the literature that the actions of catecholamines are mediated through α- and/or β-adrenergic receptors in hypothalamus. Low to moderate densities of β-adrenergic receptors displaying a relatively uniform distribution have been localized in hypothalamus (22). In addition, these hypothalamic β-adrenergic receptors appear to be equally divided into the β_1 and β_2 subtypes (22).

Alpha$_1$-adrenergic receptors are, for the most part, fairly uniformly distributed throughout hypothalamus and are of low to moderate density within this brain region (23, 24). However, within the paraventricular nucleus, the density of α_1-adrenergic receptors associated with the medial parvocellular CRF-containing region is greater than that associated with the lateral magnocellular portion of this nucleus (25). Furthermore, recent data demonstrating decreases in the density of α_1-adrenergic receptors in the medial portion of the paraventricular nucleus in response to the stress of dehydration support the importance of these binding sites in mediating stress responses (25). In contrast to the relatively uniform distribution of α_1- and β-adrenergic receptors receptors in hypothalamus, there is a striking regional distribution of α_2-adrenergic receptors in this brain region (26). The highest densities of α_2-adrenergic receptors in hypothalamus are associated with both the magnocellular and parvocellular portions of the paraventricular and periventricular nuclei, the arcuate nucleus, and the median eminence (26) (see Fig. 2).

Serotonin Receptors

Serotonin has been shown to regulate pituitary hormone secretions both through effects in brain and directly at the level of the pituitary gland (11,12). Serotonin receptors in brain have been classified into several subtypes including 5-HT$_1$ and 5-HT$_2$ receptors. Furthermore, several subclassifications of the 5-HT$_1$ serotonin receptor subtype have been described (27). Direct in vitro effects of serotonin have been reported on ACTH (28) and prolactin (29) secretion, and these effects

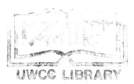

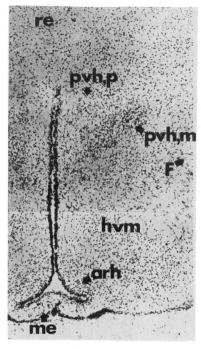

A

FIGURE 2 The distribution of [³H]para-aminoclonidine ([³H]PAC) -labeled
α_2-adrenergic receptors in rat medial hypothalamus. A. Histologic appearance of
a toluidine-blue-stained section. B. Autoradiographic distribution of [³H]PAC.
The darkfield autoradiogram shows the distribution of [³H]PAC binding sites.
Bright regions represent areas of high receptor density. C. Darkfield autoradiogram of a section adjacent to that shown in B labeled with [³H]PAC in the
presence of 10⁻⁵ M phentolamine is shown to demonstrate nonspecific binding.
Bar = 300 μm. arh, arcuate nucleus; F, fornix; hvm, ventromedial hypothalamus;
me, median eminence; pvh-m, paraventricular nucleus of the hypothalamus,
magnocellular part; pvh-p, paraventricular nucleus of the hypothalamus, parvocellular part; re, nucleus reuniens (courtesy of Drs. J.R. Unnerstall and M.J.
Kuhar; reproduced with permission from ref. 26).

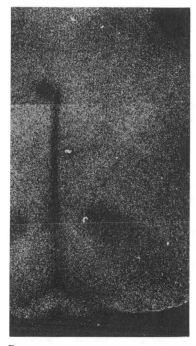

B

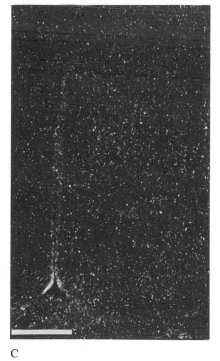

C

appear to be mediated through 5-HT$_2$ serotonin receptors. Autoradiographic studies have revealed low densities of 5-HT$_2$ serotonin receptors in rat anterior pituitary (6).

Early studies using fairly nonselective ligands suggested that serotonin may act in hypothalamus to stimulate ACTH and prolactin secretion through mechanisms involving primarily 5-HT$_2$ serotonin receptors. However, more recent evidence using more selective ligands also suggests the involvement of 5-HT$_1$ receptors in modulating ACTH and prolactin secretion (30). Within hypothalamus, high densities of 5-HT$_1$ serotonin receptors are present in the ventromedial nucleus, significantly lower densities are present in the remainder of the hypothalamus and these 5-HT$_1$ receptors appear to belong to the 5-HT$_{1B}$ subclass (31). The distribution of 5-HT$_2$ serotonin receptors in hypothalamus is less striking; low densities of receptors are evident throughout hypothalamus, with the exception of the mammillary nucleus, which contains a high concentration of 5-HT$_2$ serotonin receptors (32).

Opioid Receptors

Opioid peptides and their receptors have been widely implicated in the endocrine responses to stress. For example, opioids have been demonstrated to mediate the release of a variety of pituitary hormones including ACTH, luteinizing hormone, thyrotropin, and prolactin (33,34). Opioid receptors have been classified into at least three major categories: mu, delta, and kappa. Recent evidence suggests that the diverse endocrine effects of opioids may be mediated through specific opioid receptor subtypes (34). Hypothalamic kappa and mu opioid receptors appear to mediate the ACTH release, while opioid-induced prolactin secretion appears to be mediated primarily at mu binding sites (35-37). Hypothalamus contains moderate to high densities of both mu and kappa opioid receptors, while there is a notable absence of delta receptors (38-41) (see Fig. 3). The localization of kappa opioid receptors in the area of the paraventricular nucleus of hypothalamus may provide a substrate for the effects of opioids to stimulate ACTH secretion through effects mediated by CRF. In addition, there are high densities of mu opioid receptors in the ventromedial and dorsomedial nuclei and, in particular, the arcuate nucleus. The effects of opioids on prolactin secretion may involve both serotonergic and dopaminergic mechanisms (see 33). Opioids have been demonstrated to decrease the release of newly synthesized dopamine, thereby providing a mechanism for opioid-induced prolactin secretion (42). Given the high densities of mu opioid receptors in the region of the arcuate nucleus, this hypothalamic region may provide a site of action for opioids to alter dopamine release.

An interesting aspect of the effects of opioids on hypothalamic–pituitary–adrenocortical secretion is that it is very species dependent. In rats, opioids

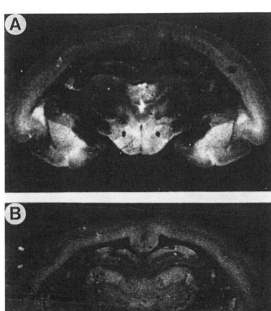

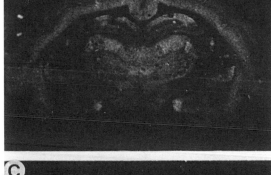

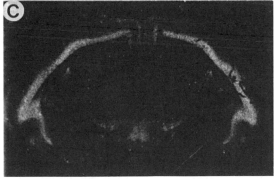

FIGURE 3   Distribution of mu (A), delta (B), and kappa (C) opioid receptors in guinea pig brain. The photomicrographs show the distribution of autoradiographic grains in coronal sections of guinea pig brain at the level of diencephalon. Bright areas correspond to high densities of binding sites. Mu, delta, and kappa opioid receptors were selectively labeled using previously described conditions (38). Mu, 1.8 nM [^{3}H]-dihydromorphine; delta, 4 nM [^{3}H]-D-ala^2-D-leu^5-enkephalin + 30 nM morphine; kappa, 1.6 nM [^{3}H]-(-)-ethylketocyclazocine + 30 nM morphine + 100 nM D-ala^2-D-leu^5-enkephalin.

primarily stimulate the axis, while in humans the effects of opioids involve inhibition of ACTH and cortisol secretion (see 33). These differential effects of opioids may relate, in part, to the differential distribution of mu, delta, and kappa receptors in the CNS of different species. For example, receptor-binding studies in homogenates reveal that brain membranes from pig, guinea pig, and human are comprised of approximately 35–50% kappa-, 30–40% mu-, and 20–30% delta-binding sites, whereas kappa sites represent a much smaller proportion (10% kappa, 60% mu, and 25% delta) in rat (see 38). Thus, the relatively higher concentration of kappa opioid receptors in human hypothalamus compared to that of rat may help to explain the opposing effects of some opioids on ACTH secretion in these species.

Benzodiazepine/Gamma Aminobutyric Acid Receptors

Benzodiazepine receptor agonists such as diazepam not only alleviate anxiety associated with stress but also inhibit stress-induced increases in anterior pituitary hormone secretion (see 43, 44). A variety of data obtained in clinical and laboratory settings have demonstrated that β-carbolines, a class of active benzodiazepine receptor "inverse agonists," elicit behavioral and neuroendocrine changes reminiscent of anxiety and stress (see 43). In other studies, effects of stress-induced activation of the hypothalamus–pituitary–adrenocortical axis and prolactin secretion have been reported (see 45, 46). GABAergic effects in brain are mediated by two distinct recognition sites classified as the $GABA_A$ and $GABA_B$ receptors (47). Moreover, the benzodiazepine receptors in brain are part of a complex consisting of $GABA_A$ receptors and an associated chloride ionophore with multiple allosteric binding sites (48).

GABA may alter pituitary hormone secretion through direct effects at the pituitary level; GABA receptors have been identified in anterior pituitary (see 45, 49). The literature also suggests involvement of both $GABA_A$ and $GABA_B$ receptors in hypothalamus to mediate the suppressive effects of GABA on CRF secretion (see 50). There is good evidence to suggest that $GABA_B$ binding sites in hypothalamus are involved in mediating the effects of stress to stimulate prolactin secretion (51). However, the demonstration that benzodiazepines (which act to potentiate the effects of GABA at $GABA_A$ receptors) are potent inhibitors of stress-induced ACTH and prolactin secretion (see 43, 44) provide evidence that $GABA_A$ binding sites also play important roles in modulating stress-induced anterior pituitary hormone secretion. Both $GABA_A$ and $GABA_B$ receptors have been identified in hypothalamus by autoradiography; however, their density is relatively low in comparison with other brain regions (52). On the other hand, moderate to high concentrations of central-type benzodiazepine receptors have been identified in this brain region (see 53, 54).

Cholinergic Receptors

Central cholinergic mechanisms have been postulated to participate in regulating ACTH and prolactin responses to stress (see 55). In addition, direct hypothalamic effects of acetylcholine to stimulate CRF secretion through mechanisms that involve both muscarinic and nicotinic cholinergic receptors have been demonstrated. The presence of nicotinic cholinergic receptors in rat hypothalamus is controversial. Early studies reported high densities of [^{125}I]-bungarotoxin binding sites in hypothalamus, while more recent studies using [^{3}H] nicotine or [^{3}H] methylcarbamylcholine suggest the presence of low to negligible densities of nicotinic binding sites in this brain region (56-58). A recent study examining the distribution of nicotinic binding sites with respect to CRF-immunoreactive perikarya in rat hypothalamus demonstrated higher densities of [^{3}H] nicotine binding sites within the neurophil surrounding the paraventricular and supraoptic nuclei than in other hypothalamic nuclei (59). Low to moderate densities of muscarinic cholinergic binding sites have also been localized in hypothalamus; both M_1 and M_2 muscarinic binding sites are present in this brain region (60).

Vasoactive Intestinal Peptide Receptors

Vasoactive intestinal peptide (VIP) has been implicated in modulating endocrine responses to stress. Immunoneutralization studies have shown that an antiserum directed against VIP attenuates or blocks stress-induced prolactin secretion (61). VIP receptors are found in very high densities in a variety of hypothalamic nuclei, with a particularly discrete localization in the magnocellular paraventricular nucleus (62-64) (see Fig. 4). The paraventricular nucleus has recently been implicated in mediating the prolactin secretory responses to restraint stress, ether stress, and serotonergic agents in rat (65). High densities of VIP receptors have also been visualized in the arcuate nucleus of the hypothalamus (62-64), providing a substrate for VIP to alter prolactin secretion through indirect effects on dopamine release.

Neuropeptide Y Receptors

Neuropeptide Y (NPY) has been demonstrated to modulate stress responses. Recent studies report that NPY is released in response to stress (66) and that direct administration of NPY in hypothalamic areas such as the paraventricular nucleus results in increased ACTH and suppressed prolactin secretion (see 67). The demonstration of NPY receptors in the paraventricular nucleus of the hypothalamus (67) provides a site of action for NPY to modulate stress-induced pituitary hormone secretion.

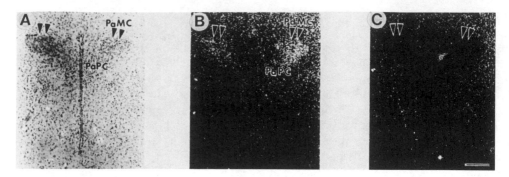

FIGURE 4 Distribution of VIP receptors in the paraventricular nucleus of the hypothalamus. A, Brightfield photomicrograph shows a high-power view of the paraventricular nucleus of the hypothalamus. B, Darkfield photomicrograph shows the total [^{125}I] VIP binding sites distribution on emulsion-coated coverslips over an area identical to that corresponding to A. In B, note the higher concentration of grains in the magnocellular portion (PaMC) than in the parvocellular region (PaPC) of this nucleus. C, Darkfield photomicrograph of a serial section adjacent to B shows the absence of specific receptor binding sites when 10^{-7} M unlabeled VIP is included in the incubation buffer. Bar = 100 μm.

Interleukin-1 Receptors

The cytokine interleukin-1 (IL-1) is one of the key mediators of the immune response to stress, infection, or antigenic challenge (see 68). IL-1 has recently been reported to stimulate hypothalamic–pituitary–adrenocortical hormone secretion (see 69). Interleukin-1 has been reported to stimulate ACTH and to inhibit prolactin secretion by pituitary cells in culture and to stimulate CRF secretion into the hypophyseal portal circulation, thus providing evidence that both brain and pituitary sites of action may be involved in the effects of IL-1 on stress-induced hormone secretion (see 69). In keeping with a role for both brain and pituitary in modulating the effects of IL-1, high densities of IL-1 binding sites have been identified in anterior pituitary and lower concentrations are present in brain (70).

DISTRIBUTION OF BRAIN AND SPINAL CORD RECEPTORS MODULATING AUTONOMIC RESPONSES TO STRESS

Many CNS nuclei have been implicated in regulating autonomic responses to stress. The CNS pathways involved in autonomic regulation have been described in great detail in previous chapters (see Chapters by Sawchenko, Gray and Loewy). In this section, we will address the relevance of various neuro-transmitter receptors that modulate autonomic responses to stress in the context of their distribution within these nuclei.

In mammals, cell bodies of the preganglionic neurons, which represent the final common pathway through which activation of sympathetically innervated targets is accomplished, are located mainly in the intermediolateral nucleus (IML) of the thoracic and upper lumbar spinal cord (see 71). In turn, IML perikarya receive descending inputs from numerous supraspinal centers that include, but are not limited to, the paraventricular nucleus of hypothalamus, the Kolliker-Füse nucleus, various catecholaminergic cell groups, nucleus of the solitary tract, rostral ventrolateral medulla, and caudal raphe nuclei. Other brain nuclei further influence sympathetic outflow through afferent and efferent connections with the nuclei described above. They include the parabrachial nucleus, central nucleus of the amygdala, and bed nucleus of the stria terminalis. A summary of the relative distribution of select receptors that may modulate sympathetic outflow via these nuclei is given in Table 1. In the following sections we will describe, in more detail, the relevant CNS sites of action and receptor subtypes through which catecholamine, opioid peptides, and CRF appear to produce their effects on autonomic responses to stress.

Alpha$_2$-Adrenergic Receptors

Norepinephrine and epinephrine are critical neurotransmitters that modulate adaptive responses to stress through their actions at various parts of the neuronal circuitry involved in regulating autonomic function. Although these catecholamines can act at both α- and β-adrenergic receptors, a great deal of evidence suggests that norepinephrine and epinephrine act primarily at α_2-adrenergic receptors in CNS to regulate autonomic activity. Much of this evidence is based on effects of the α_2-adrenergic receptor agonist clonidine to alter cardiovascular responses to stress (see 26). Unnerstall et al. (26) carried out a detailed study examining the distribution of α_2 agonist binding sites in rat and human CNS and discussed their relevance in regulating both sympathetic and parasympathetic outflow. The following represents a summary of their findings (for review, see 26). The presence of moderate to high densities of α_2-adrenergic receptors in nuclei of the medullary baroreceptor reflex arc provides an excellent example of the role of α_2-adrenergic receptors to subserve autonomic function. Some of the highest densities of α_2-adrenergic receptors in CNS are found in the nucleus tractus solitarius, nucleus commissuralis, and the dorsal motor nucleus of the vagus, which together make up the dorsal motor complex of the medulla (see Fig. 5). Thus, α_2-adrenergic receptors in this brain area could mediate baroreceptor and stretch receptor afferent input, which is transmitted via cranial nerves IX and X and integrated within the nucleus tractus solitarius. These receptors can

TABLE 1   Relative distribution of α_2-Adrenergic, CRF, and Opioid Receptors in Major Rat CNS Nuclei Mediating Autonomic Responses to Stress

Region	α_2-Adrenergic[a]	CRF[a]	Opioid[b]		
			μ	δ	κ
Spinal cord		++	+	+	
IML	+++				
Nucleus tractus solitarius	+++	++	+	+	
Dorsal motor nucleus of vagus	+++	+			
Nucleus commissuralis	+++				
Nucleus ambiguus	+		+	+	
Rostral ventrolateral medulla		+/++	-	-	-/+
C1	++				
A5	++				
Nucleus parabrachialis	++	++			
Kolliker-Füse nucleus	+				
Locus ceruleus	+++	+	+	-	+
Raphe nuclei			+	-	+
Dorsalis	++	+	+	-	+
Magnus	+				
Amygdala	+++	+/++	+	-/+	-/+
Hippocampus	+++	+	+	-/+	+
Bed nucleus of stria terminalis	+++	+	-/+	-/+	+
Hypothalamus		+	+		
Anterior	++	+	-	-	+
Paraventricular	+++	++	-	-	+
Medial preoptic	++				
Septum	+++	+/++	-/+	-/+	-/+
Cingulate cortex	++	++	+	+	-/+
Insular cortex	+++	++/+++	-	+	+

[a]The distributions of α_2-adrenergic and CRF receptors are adapted from refs. 26 and 10, respectively. For α_2-adrenergic and CRF receptors: +++, high; ++, medium; +, low density of binding sites.
[b]The distributions of opioid receptors are adapted from refs. 39–41. Since there is disagreement regarding the distribution of opioid receptor subtypes, they are listed as either present (+) or absent (-).

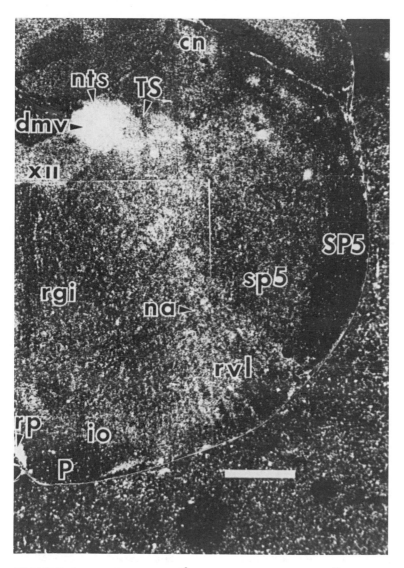

FIGURE 5 Distribution of [³H] para-aminoclonidine ([³H]PAC)-labeled α_2-adrenergic receptors in the medulla oblongata of the rat. Bar = 800 μm. cn, cuneate nucleus; dmv, dorsal motor nucleus of the vagus; io, inferior olivary nucleus; na, nucleus ambiguus; nts, nucleus of the solitary tract; P, pyramidal tract; rp, raphe pallidus; rvl, ventrolateral medulla, rostral part; sp5, nucleus of the trigeminal; SP5, spinal tract of the trigeminal; TS, solitary tract; XII, hypoglossal nucleus (courtesy of Drs. J.R. Unnerstall and M.J. Kuhar; reproduced with permission from ref. 26).

subsequently mediate effects on parasympathetic outflow through connections between nucleus tractus solitarius and the dorsal motor nucleus of the vagus and the ventrolateral medulla, which sites also contain moderate densities of a_2 receptors (see Fig. 5). Alpha$_2$-adrenergic agonists can inhibit sympathetic activity through actions at receptors in the ventrolateral medulla, which projects to the preganglionic sympathetic neurons in the IML of spinal cord. Sympathetic outflow could be specifically affected by the presence of moderate densities of a_2-adrenergic receptors in the vicinity of C1 epinephrine and A5 norepinephrine nuclei. As an alternative, since there is enrichment of a_2-adrenergic receptors over preganglionic sympathoadrenal neurons within IML, this site may represent a more direct locus of action for a_2 agonists to inhibit sympathetic activity (72).

The autoradiographic demonstration of a_2-adrenergic receptors in supramedullary brain areas involved in autonomic regulation further supports the importance of these binding sites in mediating autonomic effects of catecholamines. These brain regions, which include locus ceruleus, several hypothalamic nuclei (the paraventricular nucleus in particular) (see Fig. 2), bed nucleus of the stria terminalis, central nucleus of the amygdala, septum, hippocampus, and cingulate and insular cortices, all contain varying densities of a_2-adrenergic receptors (see Table 1). These receptors may function to integrate ascending visceral information relayed from medulla to forebrain areas regulating autonomic function, either through direct connections from the medulla to forebrain regions or through pontine relay centers such as locus ceruleus, parabrachial nucleus, and dorsal raphe nucleus; these latter brain regions have moderate to high densities of a_2-adrenergic receptors. Reciprocal connections between some forebrain regions, such as the paraventricular nucleus and medulla, suggest that receptors at these sites may also play important roles in integrating autonomic and endocrine responses to stress.

Opioid Receptors

Although there is substantial evidence in the literature demonstrating effects of opioids on a variety of autonomic parameters, the role of endogenous opioids in modulating stress-induced autonomic function is less well defined. This confusion relates, in part, to the multiplicity of endogenous opioids and their respective receptors (34). Interpretation of experimental data is further confounded by route of drug administration, species under investigation, and use of anesthesia (73,74). For the most part, in conscious animals, opioid receptor agonists administered into CNS (either into the ventricular space or directly into brain) affect a variety of autonomic parameters including heart rate and blood pressure through mechanisms involving a balance between stimulation of sympathetic and parasympathetic outflows. Microinjection studies into discrete brain nuclei using more selective mu, delta, and kappa opioid receptor agonists and antagonists have implicated both hypothalamic and brainstem sites of action. Possible hypothalamic sites mediating the effects of opioids on autonomic outflow include the paraventricular, anterior hypothalamic, and medial preoptic nuclei (75-78). In addition, a number of investigators have examined the role of the three opioid receptor subtypes in the nucleus ambiguus and nucleus tractus solitarius in mediating autonomic effects of opioids (73,74,77,79). For the most part, there is general agreement on a role for mu receptors in mediating the effects of opioid peptides on cardiovascular parameters through actions at these sites. As a specific example, pressor and tachycardic responses to selective mu opioid receptor agonists have been reported following injection of these compounds into the ambiguus and solitary nuclei, as well as into the anterior, paraventricular, and medial preoptic hypothalamic nuclei (74). The importance of mu opioid receptors in modulating stress-induced autonomic responses is further supported by studies demonstrating that microinjections of a mu opioid receptor agonist blunted restraint stress-induced tachycardia, apparently by vagal mechanisms, since this effect was blocked by atropine methylnitrate (78).

The role of delta opioid receptors in modulating autonomic function is less well defined. Delta receptor agonists have been reported to alter a variety of autonomic parameters; however, microinjection studies have demonstrated that higher doses of delta receptor agonists are required to produce effects comparable to those seen with mu receptor agonists (74,75). This discrepancy may relate, in part, to the overall paucity of delta receptors in rat hypothalamus (see Fig. 5) and brainstem (38-41) (see Table 1). On the other hand, there are low to moderate concentrations of mu and kappa receptors in both rat brain regions. Within hypothalamus, significantly higher densities of kappa than mu receptors are present, while in brainstem nuclei there is a higher density of mu than kappa opioid receptors (38). Microinjection of various kappa opioid receptor agonists into discrete hypothalamic areas, including paraventricular and medial preoptic nuclei, and into brainstem regions including nucleus ambiguus and nucleus tractus solitarius, decreases blood pressure and heart rate in anesthesized rats (74,79). These data clearly implicate kappa receptors in mediating some of the cardiovascular effects of opioids, but it is unclear whether these effects of kappa agonists are indeed opposite to those of mu opioid receptor agonists or whether these differences simply relate to the presence of anesthetic. Other studies have reported opposite blood pressure responses to injections of enkephalin analogues in anterior hypothalamus of anesthetized versus conscious rats (74-76).

The presence of opioid receptors in other brainstem and forebrain nuclei involved in autonomic regulation provide additional potential sites of action for opioids in modulating autonomic function. For example, high densities of opioid receptors are found in brain regions such as locus ceruleus, dorsal motor nucleus of the vagus, raphe magnus, ventrolateral medulla, bed nucleus of the stria terminalis, and amygdala (38-41). The predominant receptor types in these brain regions are mu and kappa, with significantly lower densities of delta receptors. However, since many of the studies examining the effects of opioids on autonomic outflow have been carried out in rat, and given the different proportions of mu, delta, and kappa opioid receptors across species (see above), caution must be exercised in extrapolating these findings to humans.

Opioid receptors have been visualized by autoradiography in spinal cord, but there appears to be no enrichment of opioid receptors in IML compared to adjacent regions (38,72). Nevertheless, opioid receptors in spinal cord may play important roles in modulating parasympathetic responses. It has been reported that both spinal mu and delta opioid receptors are involved in mediating inhibition of gastrointestinal transit induced by opioids (80). Supraspinal pathways have also been implicated in modulating the gastrointestinal transit effects of opioids, but these effects appear to involve primarily mu opioid receptors (80). Other studies demonstrating effects of bilateral microinjections of the opioid antagonist naloxone into the central nucleus of the amygdala to potentiate cold restraint-induced gastric pathological changes significantly in rats (81) provide additional evidence for a role for opioid receptors in modulating stress-induced effects on gastric function. In the opposite fashion, opioid agonists including enkephalin analogs and β-endorphin inhibited stress-induced ulcer formation in a dose-related manner (81).

CRF Receptors

CRF acts within CNS to elicit alterations in autonomic nervous system activity similar to those noted following many forms of stress (82-84). The autonomic effects of CRF are evident in a variety of species including rat, dog, sheep, and monkey and include increases in plasma concentrations of epinephrine, norepinephrine, glucose, glucagon, increases in cardiovascular parameters such as heart rate and mean arterial pressure, and decreases in a variety of gastrointestinal parameters including gastric acid secretion and gastrointestinal motility (for review see 82-84). The distribution of CRF receptors in CNS has been examined in detail using autoradiographic techniques (10). The localization of CRF receptors in brain provides an anatomical basis for some of the observed effects of CRF on autonomic function (see Table 1). CRF may produce some of its effects via receptors in the parabrachial nucleus, medullary reticular formation, nucleus tractus solitarius, and other brainstem areas known to participate in autonomic regulation. CRF binding sites are also present in several forebrain regions reported to affect autonomic outflow. These regions include hypothalamus (especially the paraventricular nucleus), bed nucleus of the stria terminalis, amygdala, septum, hippocampus, and cingulate cortex. Although CRF receptors have been localized in spinal cord, their role in regulating sympathetic outflow is unclear since enrichment of these binding sites in IML is not evident. However, CRF receptors in spinal cord may play important roles in mediating parasympathetic activation, as suggested by effects of intrathecal injections of CRF at the lumbar level to inhibit gastric acid secretion (85).

CRF receptors in locus ceruleus may also play an important role in mediating autonomic responses to stress. Applications of acute and chronic stress produce large increases in the concentration of CRF in locus ceruleus (86) and iontophoretic application of CRF has been demonstrated to increase discharge of locus ceruleus neurons (87). Locus ceruleus efferents project to regions of brainstem involved in control of cardiovascular function, and the locus may represent a relay station projecting to forebrain regions involved in modulating autonomic function.

DISTRIBUTION OF RECEPTORS IN BRAIN AREAS IMPLICATED IN ADAPTIVE RESPONSES TO STRESS: FOCUS ON AMYGDALA AND OLFACTORY SYSTEM

The role of the amygdala in influencing autonomic and endocrine responses to stress has been well characterized. Projections from the amygdala to hypothalamus primarily originate in the central nucleus (88). In addition to modulating endocrine and autonomic function, the central nucleus of the amygdala has been implicated in behavioral responses during arousal, stress, and other emotional behaviors. A surprising finding is that the density of receptors associated with stress responses is less in the central nucleus than in other amygdaloid nuclei. Within the amygdala, there is striking enrichment of CRF, a_2-adrenergic, opioid, and other "stress neurotransmitter" receptors in the basolateral nucleus of the amygdala. The basolateral nucleus may, in turn, influence autonomic, behavioral, and endocrine responses to stress through its connections with the central nucleus of the amygdala. In a similar fashion, other brain regions with high densities of "stress neurotransmitter" receptors such as the cerebral cortex, thalamus, and bed nucleus of the stria terminalis can influence adaptive behaviors through their connections with the amygdala or through direct connections with brainstem and hypothalamic areas involved in autonomic and endocrine regulation, respectively.

The distribution of many "stress neurotransmitters" receptors is striking in the rat olfactory system. For example, CRF binding sites are discretely localized in the glomerular layer, the site of termination of primary olfactory afferent axons, and in the adjacent external plexiform layer where the olfactory output neurons originate (10). Data strongly suggest that sexual, reproductive, social, and feeding behaviors of most mammalian species are affected by olfaction (89). Although the hypothalamus may be the primary anatomical locus for regulating sexual activity and feeding behavior, hypothalamic neuronal activity can be modulated by olfactory impulses relayed through the circuit involving the olfactory bulb, pyriform cortex, amygdala, and subiculum (90). Most "stress transmitters" including catecholamines, CRF, and opioids influence both feeding behavior and sexual activity (91).

BRAIN RECEPTORS INVOLVED IN REGULATING IMMUNE RESPONSES TO STRESS

Increasing evidence suggests a role for the CNS in modulating immune responses to stress (92). In particular, opioids (93) and more recently CRF (94,95) have been demonstrated to modulate immune parameters through actions in CNS. The majority of the evidence suggests that these neurotransmitters influence immune function through their effects on autonomic and/or endocrine systems. The receptors involved in modulating stress-induced alterations in the endocrine axis and autonomic nervous system has been described above.

SUMMARY AND CONCLUSIONS

We have endeavored to describe the distribution of key neurotransmitter receptors in anterior pituitary and CNS that have been implicated in mediating stress responses. These transmitters include CRF, opioid peptides, and catecholamines. The role of other select neurotransmitter receptors involved in endocrine responses to stress has also been addressed. We focused on the distribution of receptors in brain pathways whose role in mediating autonomic, endocrine, and other adaptive responses to stress is well-established. With respect to catecholamines and opioid peptides, we elaborated on the receptor subtype(s) that play primary roles in modulating different aspects of the stress response. However, it should be emphasized that the presence of receptors in a brain area known to mediate stress-induced activity does not necessarily implicate that brain region as playing a seminal role in these responses. Likewise, the failure to detect receptors (due to limitations of technique used) in any given brain region implicated in stress responses does not necessarily preclude its importance in mediating the effects of the neurotransmitter. Future studies utilizing knowledge of the distribution of receptors in combination with well-designated physiological, pharmacological, and neuroanatomical investigations should help to elucidate the role of the various neurotransmitter receptors in modulating stress responses.

ACKNOWLEDGMENTS

We acknowledge Sharon Amos for her help in preparation of the manuscript. We are extremely grateful to Drs. James R. Unnerstall and Michael J. Kuhar for providing figures on the distribution of α_2-adrenergic receptors in CNS.

REFERENCES

1. Selye H. The stress of life. New York: McGraw-Hill, 1956.
2. MacLeod R M. Regulation of prolactin secretion. In Martini L, Ganong WF, eds. Frontiers in neuroendocrinology. New York: Raven Press, 1976; 169–194.
3. Ben-Jonathan N. Catecholamines and pituitary prolactin release. J Reprod Fertil 1980; 58:501–512.
4. Moore K E, Demarest K T, Lookingland K J. Stress, prolactin and hypothalamic dopaminergic neurons. Neuropharmacology 1987; 26:801–808.
5. Creese I, Sibley D R, Hamblin M W, Leff S E. The classification of dopamine receptors: relationship to radioligand binding. Annu Rev Neurosci 1983; 6:43–71.
6. De Souza E B. Serotonin and dopamine receptors in the rat pituitary gland: autoradiographic identification, characterization and localization. Endocrinology 1986; 119: 1534–1542.
7. De Souza E B, Kuhar M J. Dopamine receptors in the anterior lobe of the human pituitary gland: autoradiographic localization. Brain Res 1984; 306: 391–395.
8. De Souza E B, Perrin M H, Rivier J E, Vale W, Kuhar M J. Corticotropin-releasing factor receptors in rat pituitary gland: autoradiographic localization. Brain Res 1984; 296:202–207.
9. De Souza E B, Perrin M H, Whitehouse P J, Rivier J E, Vale W W, Kuhar M J. Corticotropin-releasing factor receptors in human pituitary gland: autoradiographic localization. Neuroendocrinology 1985; 40:419–422.
10. De Souza E B, Insel T R, Perrin M H, Rivier J, Vale W W, Kuhar M J. Corticotropin-releasing factor receptors are widely distributed within the rat central nervous system: an autoradiographic study. J Neurosci 1985; 5:3189–3203.
11. Weiner R I, Ganong W F. Role of brain monoamines and histamine in regulation of anterior pituitary secretion. Physiol Rev 1978; 58:905–976.
12. Müller E E, Nistico G, Scapagnini. Neurotransmitter and anterior pituitary function. New York: Academic Press, 1977.
13. Axelrod J, Reisine T D. Stress hormones: their interaction and regulation. Science 1984; 224:452–459.
14. Vale W, Rivier C. Substances modulating the secretion of ACTH by cultured anterior pituitary cells. Fed Proc 1977; 36:2094–2099.
15. De Souza E B, Kuyatt B L. α_1-Adrenergic receptors in the neural lobe of the rat pituitary: autoradiographic identification and localization. Endocrinology 1987; 120:2227–2233.
16. De Souza E B. β_2-adrenergic receptors in pituitary. Neuroendocrinology 1985; 41:289–296.
17. De Souza E B. Modulation of β-adrenergic receptors in the pituitary gland following adrenelectomy in rats. Neurosci Lett 1987; 73:281–286.
18. Peters J R, Foord S M, Dieguez C, Scanlon M F, Hall R. Alpha$_1$-adrenoreceptors on cultured pituitary cells: correlation with adrenergic stimulation of thyrotropin secretion. Endocrinology 1983; 113:133–140.

19. Chen F M. The adrenergic control of ACTH in the anterior pituitary: possible conversion of β to α-adrenergic responses in culture. Endocrinology 1986; 118 (Annual Meeting Supplement):196.

20. Plotsky P M. Facilitation of immunoreactive corticotropin-releasing factor secretion into the hypophysial–portal circulation after activation of catecholaminergic pathways or central norepinephrine injection. Endocrinology 1987; 121:924–930.

21. Szafarczyk A, Malaval F, Laurent A, Gibaud R, Assenmacher I. Further evidence for a central stimulatory action of catecholamines on adrenocorticotropin release in the rat. Endocrinology 1987; 121:883–892.

22. Rainbow T C, Parsons B, Wolfe B B. Quantitative autoradiography of β_1- and β_2-adrenergic receptors in rat brain. Proc Natl Acad Sci USA 1984; 81:1581–1589.

23. Jones L S, Gauger L L, Davis J N. Anatomy of brain α_1-adrenergic receptors: in vitro autoradiography with [125 I]-HEAT. J Comp Neurol 1985; 231:190–208.

24. Unnerstall J R, Fernandez I, Oresanz J M. The α-adrenergic receptor: radiohistochemical analysis of functional characteristics and biochemical differences. Pharmacol Biochem Behav 1985; 22:859–874.

25. Cummings S, Seybold V. Relationship of alpha-1- and alpha-2-adrenergic-binding sites to regions of the paraventricular nucleus of the hypothalamus containing corticotropin-releasing factor and vasopressin neurons. Neuroendocrinology 1988; 47:523–532.

26. Unnerstall J R, Kopajtic T A, Kuhar M J. Distribution of α_2 agonist binding sites in the rat and human central nervous system: analysis of some functional, anatomic correlates of the pharmacologic effects of clonidine and related adrenergic agents. Brain Res Rev 1984; 7:69–101.

27. Peroutka S J. 5-Hydroxytryptamine receptor subtypes. Annu Rev Neurosci 1988; 11:45–60.

28. Spinedi E, Negro-Vilar A. Serotonin and adrenocorticotropin (ACTH) release: direct effects at the anterior pituitary level and potentiation of arginine vasopressin induced ACTH release. Endocrinology 1983; 112: 1217–1223.

30. Heninger G R, Charney D S, Price L H, Woods S W, Goodman W K. Neuroendocrine and behavioral effects of 5-HT agonists in rhesus monkeys and patients: the effects of lithium. Abstr Am Col Neuropsychopharmacol 1988; 76.

31. Pazos A, Palacios J M. Quantitative autoradiographic mapping of serotonin receptors in the rat brain: I. Serotonin-1 receptors. Brain Res 1985; 346: 205–230.

32. Pazos A, Cortes R, Palacios J M. Quantitative autoradiographic mapping of serotonin receptors in the rat brain: II. Serotonin-2 receptors. Brain Res 1985; 346:231–249.

33. Pfeiffer A, Herz A. Endocrine actions of opioids. Horm Metabol Res 1984; 16:386–397.

34. Akil H, Watson S J, Young E, Lewis M E, Khachaturian H, Walter J M. Endogenous opioids: biology and function. Annu Rev Neurosci 1984; 7: 223–255.
35. Panerai A E, Petraglia F, Sacerdote P, Genazzani A R. Mainly mu-opiate receptors are involved in luteinizing hormone and prolactin secretion. Endocrinology 1985; 117:1095–1099.
36. Pfeiffer A, Herz A, Loriaux D L, Pfeiffer D G. Central kappa- and mu-opiate receptors mediate ACTH release in rats. Endocrinology 1985; 116: 2688–2690.
37. Iyengar S, Kim H S, Wood P L. Kappa opiate agonists modulate the hypothalamic–pituitary–adrenocortical axis in the rat. J Pharmacol Exp Ther 1986; 238:429–436.
38. De Souza E B, Schmidt W K, Kuhar M J. Nalbuphine: an autoradiographic opioid receptor binding profile in the central nervous system of an agonist/antagonist analgesic. J Pharmacol Exp Ther 1988; 244:391–402.
39. Goodman R R, Snyder S H, Kuhar M J, Young W S III. Differentation of delta and mu opiate receptor localization by light microscopic autoradiography. Proc Natl Acad Sci USA 1980; 77:6239–6243.
40. Mansour A, Khachaturian H, Lewis M E, Akil H, Watson S J. Autoradiographic differentiation of mu, delta, and kappa opioid receptors in the rat forebrain and midbrain. J Neurosci 1987; 7:2445–2464.
41. Tempel A, Zukin S. Neuroanatomical patterns of the μ, σ, and κ opioid receptors of rat brain as determined by quantitative in vitro autoradiography. Proc Natl Acad Sci USA 1987; 84:4308–4312.
42. Van Loon G R, De Souza E B, Ho D, Shin S H. β-Endorphin induced prolactin secretion is mediated by suppression of release of newly synthesized hypothalamic dopamine. Can J Physiol Pharmacol 1980; 58: 436–439.
43. De Souza E B. Neuroendocrine effects of benzodiazepines. J Psychiatric Res 1990;
44. Grandison L. Actions of benzodiazepines on the neuroendocrine system. Neuropharmacology 1983; 22:1505–1510.
45. Demeneix B A, Feltz P, Loeffler J P. GABAergic mechanisms and their functional relevance in the pituitary. In: Racagni G, Donoso A O, eds. GABA and endocrine function. New York: Raven Press, 1986; 261–288.
46. Racagni C, Apud J A, Cocchi D, Locatelli V, Muller E E. GABAergic control of anterior pituitary hormone secretion. Life Sci 1982; 31:823–838.
47. Bowery N G, Price G W, Hudson A L, Hill D R, Wilkin G P, Turnbull M J. GABA receptor multiplicity: visualization of different receptor types in the mammalian CNS. Neuropharmacology 1984; 23:219–231.
48. Tallman J F, Paul S M, Skolnick P, Gallager D W. Receptors for the age of anxiety: pharmacology of the benzodiazepines. Science 1980; 207:274–281.

49. Grandison L, Guidotti A. Aminobutyric acid receptor function in rat anterior pituitary: evidence for control of prolactin release. Endocrinology 1979; 105:754–759.

50. Calogero A E, Gallucci W T, Chrousos G P, Gold P W. Interaction between GABAergic neurotransmission and rat hypothalamic corticotropin-releasing hormone secretion in vitro. Brain Res 1988; 463:28–36.

51. D'Eramo J L, Somoza G M, Kertesz E, Libertun C. Baclofen, a GABA derivative, inhibits stress-induced prolactin release in the rat. Eur J Pharmacol 1986; 120:81–85.

52. Bowery N G, Hudson A L, Price G W. GABA$_A$ and GABA$_B$ receptor site distribution in the rat central nervous system. Neuroscience 1987; 20: 365–383.

53. Richards J G, Mohler H. Benzodiazepine receptors. Neuropharmacology 1984; 23:233–242.

54. De Souza E B, Goeders N E, Kuhar M J. Benzodiazepine receptors in rat brain are altered by adrenalectomy. Brain Res 1986; 381:176–181.

55. Sharp B M, Beyer H S, Levine A S, Morley J E, McAllen K M. Attenuation of the plasma prolactin response to restraint stress after acute and chronic administration of nicotine to rats. J Pharmacol Exp Ther 1987; 241:438–442.

56. London E D, Waller S B, Wamsley J K. Autoradiographic localization of [^{3}H]nicotine binding sites in the rat brain. Neurosci Lett. 1985; 53:179–184.

57. Clarke P S, Schwartz R D, Paul S M, Pert C B, Pert A. Nicotinic binding in rat brain: Autoradiographic comparison of [^{3}H]acetylcholine, [^{3}H]nicotine, and [^{125}I]-α-bungarotoxin. J Neurosci 1985; 5:1307–1315.

58. Yamada S, Gehlert D R, Hawkins K N, Nakayama K, Roeske W R, Yamamura H I. Autoradiographic localization of nicotinic receptor binding in rat brain using [^{3}H]methylcarbamylcholine, a novel radioligand. Life Sci 1987; 41:2851–2861.

59. Sharp B M, Nicol S, Cummings S, Seybold V. Distribution of nicotinic binding sites with respect to CRF and neurophysin immunoreactive perikarya within the rat hypothalamus. Brain Res 1987; 422:361–366.

60. Mash D C, Potter L T. Autoradiographic localization of M1 and M2 muscarinic receptors in the rat brain. Neuroscience 1986; 19:551–564.

61. Kaji H, Chihara K, Kita T, Kashio Y, Okimura Y, Fujita T. Administration of antisera to vasoactive intestinal polypeptide and peptide histidine isoleucine attenuates ether-induced prolactin secretion in rats. Neuroenocrinology 1985; 41:529–531.

62. De Souza E B, Seifert H, Kuhar M J. Vasoactive intestinal peptide receptor localization in rat forebrain by autoradiography. Neurosci Lett 1985; 56: 113–120.

63. Besson J, Sarrieau A, Vial M, Marie J C. Rosselin G, Rostene W. Characterization and autoradiographic distribution of vasoactive intestinal peptide binding sites in the rat central nervous system. Brain Res 1986; 398:329–336.

64. Martin J L, Dietl M, Hof P R, Palacios J M, Magistretti P J. Autoradiographic mapping of $[Mono[^{125}I]IODO-Tyr^{10}, MetO^{17}]$ vasoactive intestinal peptide binding sites in the rat brain. Neuroscience 1987; 23: 539-565.

65. Minamitani N, Minamitani T, Lechan R M, Bollinger-Gruber J, Reichlin S. Paraventricular nucleus mediates prolactin secretory responses to restraint stress, ether stress, and 5-hydroxy-L-tryptophan injection in the rat. Endocrinology 1987; 120:860-867.

66. Castagne V, Corder R, Gaillard R, Mormede P. Stress-induced changes of circulating neuropeptide-Y in the rat: comparison with catecholamines. Regul Pept 1987; 19: 55-63.

67. Harstrand A. Brain neuropeptide Y mechanisms. Basic aspects and involvement in cardiovascular and neuroendocrine regulation Acta Physiol Scand Suppl 1987; 565:1-83.

68. Dinarello C A. Biology of interleukin-1. FASEB J. 1988; 2:108-115.

69. Lumpkin M D. The regulation of ACTH secretion by IL-1. Science 1987; 238:452-454.

70. Tracey D E, De Souza E B. Identification of interleukin-1 receptors in mouse pituitary cell membranes and AtT-20 pituitary tumor cells. Soc Neurosci Abstr 1988; 14:1052.

71. Schramm L P. Spinal factors in sympathetic regulation. In: Magro A, Osswald W, Reis P, Vanhoutte P, eds. Central and peripheral mechanism of cardiovascular regulation. New York: Plenum Press, 1986; 303-352.

72. Seybold V S, Elde R P. Receptor autoradiography in thoracic spinal cord: correlation of neurotransmitter binding sites with sympathoadrenal neurons. J Neurosci 1984; 4:2533-2542.

73. Feuerstein G. The opioid system and central cardiovascular control: analysis of controversies. Peptides 1985; 6:51-56.

74. Feuerstein G, Siren A. Cardiovascular effects of enkephalins. ISI atlas of science: Pharmacology 1987; 1:280-283.

75. Pfeiffer A, Feuerstein G, Kopin I J, Faden A I. Cardiovascular and respiratory effect of mu-, delta-, and kappa-opiate agonists microinjected into the anterior hypothalamic brain area of awake rats. J Pharmacol Exp Ther 1983; 225:735-741.

76. Pfeiffer A, Feuerstein G, Zerbe R L, Faden A I, Kopin I J. μ-Receptors mediate opioid cardiovascular effects at anterior hypothalamic sites through sympathoadrenomedullary ad parasympathetic pathways. Endocrinology 1983; 113:929-938.

77. Appel N M, Kiritsy-Roy J A, Van Loon G R. Mu receptors at discrete hypothalamic and brainstem sites mediate opioid peptide-induced increases in central sympathetic outflow. Brain Res 1986; 378:8-10.

78. Kiritsy-Roy J A, Appel N M, Bobbitt F G, Van Loon G R. Effects of mu-opioid receptor stimulation in the hypothalamic paraventricular nucleus on basal and stress-induced catecholamine secretion and cardiovascular responses. J Pharmacol Exp Ther 1986; 239:814-822.

79. Hassen A H, Feuerstein G, Faden A I. Kappa opioid receptors modulate cardiorespiratory function in hindbrain nuclei of rat. J Neurosci 1984; 4: 2213–2221.

80. Porreca F, Mosberg H I, Hurst R, Hruby V J, Burks T F. Roles of mu, delta and kappa opioid receptors in spinal and supraspinal mediation of gastrointestinal transit effects and hot-plate analgesia in the mouse. J Pharmacol Exp Ther 1984; 230:341–348.

81. Ray A, Henke P G, Sullivan R M. Opiate mechanisms in the central amygdala and gastric stress pathology in rats. Brain Res 1988; 442:195–198.

82. Brown M R. Neuropeptide regulation of the autonomic nervous system. In: Tache Y, Morley J E, Brown M R, eds. Neuropeptides and stress. New York: Springer Verlag, 1989; 107–120.

83. Lenz H J, Raedler A, Greten H, Brown M R. CRF initiates biological actions within the brain that are observed in response to stress. Am J Physiol 1987; 252:R34–R39.

84. Tache Y, Ishikawa T. Role of brain peptides in the ulcerogenic response to stress. In: Tache Y, Morley J E, Brown M R, eds. Neuropeptides and stress. New York: Springer Verlag, 1989: 148–157.

85. Hamel D, Tache Y. Intrathecal (I.T.) injections of bombesin and rat CRF inhibits gastric acid secretion in rats. Soc Neurosci Abstr 1984; 10:812.

86. Chappell P B, Smith M A, Kilts C D, et al. Alterations in corticotropin-releasing factor-like immunoreactivity in discrete rat brain regions after acute and chronic stress. J Neurosci 1986; 6:2908–2914.

87. Valentino R J, Foote, S L, Aston-Jones G. Corticotropin-releasing factor activates noradrenergic neurons of the locus coereleus. Brain Res 1983; 270:363–367.

88. Gray T S. Autonomic neuropeptide connections of the amygdala. In: Tache Y, Morley JE, Brown M R, eds. Neuropeptides and stress. New York: Springer Verlag, 1989: 92–106.

89. Whitten W K, Bronson H. The role of pheromones in mammalian reproduction. In: Johnston J W Jr, Moulton D G, Turk A, eds. Communication by chemical signals, vol. 1. New York: Appleton-Century-Crofts, 1970: 309–326.

90. Powell T P S, Cowan W M, Raisman G R. The central olfactory connections. J Anat 1965; 99:791–813.

91. Levine A S, Billington C J. Stress and consummatory behavior. In: Tache Y, Morley JE, Brown M R, eds. Neuropeptides and stress. New York: Springer-Verlag, 1989: 188–198.

92. Dunn A J. Nervous system–immune system interactions: an overview. J Recept Res 1988; 8:589–607.

93. Shavit Y, Depaulls A, Martin F C, et al. Involvement of brain opiate receptors in the immune-suppressive effect of morphine. Proc Natl Acad Sci USA 1986; 83:7114–7117.

94. Irwin M R, Vale W, Britton K T. Central corticotropin-releasing factor suppresses natural killer cytotoxicity. Brain Behav and Immun 1987; 1:81–87.
95. Irwin M, Hauger R L, Brown M, Britton K T. CRF activates autonomic nervous system and reduces natural killer cytotoxicity. Am J Physiol 1988; 255:R744–747.

6

NEUROENDOCRINE MECHANISMS OF ANTERIOR PITUITARY REGULATION IN THE RAT EXPOSED TO STRESS

Catherine Rivier
The Salk Institute, La Jolla, California

Rats exposed to stress show an increase in plasma levels of adrenocorticotropin, β-endorphin, and prolactin, a decrease in luteinizing hormone, thyroid-stimulating hormone, and growth hormone secretion, and usually no measurable changes in follicle-stimulating hormone. We now know that the regulatory system that controls anterior pituitary function is multifactorial, in that stress-induced changes in the secretion of anterior pituitary hormones reflect the interplay of regulatory peptides (corticotropin-releasing factor, vasopressin, oxytocin, atrial natriuretic factor, angiotensin II, and possibly others), neurotransmitters (catecholamines, prostaglandins, acetylcholine, serotonin, gamma-aminobutyric acid [GABA], etc.), as well as opiates and steroids, which act at the level of the brain and the pituitary to modulate anterior pituitary function.

The aim of this chapter is to discuss, with respect to adrenocorticotropic hormone (ACTH), β-endorphin, growth hormone, and gonadotropin, what is presently known of the role of corticotropin-releasing factor (CRF), vasopressin, and catecholamines, in modulating stress-induced changes in pituitary function in the rat. The references quoted are not meant as an exhaustive list of the work discussed, but represent examples of each relevant issue.

ACTH, β-ENDORPHIN: ROLE OF CRF, VASOPRESSIN AND CATECHOLAMINES

The secretion of ACTH and β-endorphin is regulated by several pathways that converge in the basal hypothalamus, where their input is transformed into a multifactorial hypophysiotropic signal composed of CRF, vasopressin, catecholamines, and corticosteroids (for an anatomical description of some of these pathways, see 1, 2). Other secretagogues such as opiates, oxytocin, angiotensin II, and atrial natriuretic factor (ANF) also participate in the regulation of the corticotrophs' activity. The role of corticosteroids is addressed in Chapter 9. For a discussion of the role of opiates, oxytocin, angiotensin II and ANF see (3,4).

The present section will discuss the use of antagonists or antisera to CRF, vasopressin, and catecholamines in investigating the physiological role played by these secretagogues in modulating stress-induced ACTH secretion. Chapter 7 will describe how measurement of secretagogues present in the hypophysial portal system has advanced our knowledge of the effect of stress on the release of CRF, vasopressin, and catecholamines.

Acute Stress

Adult Rats

Under most known circumstances, ACTH and β-endorphin are cosecreted in the rat (5-8). Therefore, what is discussed of ACTH secretion also applies to β-endorphin release. The acute exposure of adult rats to a noxious stimulus causes a rapid increase in plasma ACTH and corticosterone levels (Fig. 1). Following cessation of the stress, the secretion of both hormones returns to baseline values over a period of time that depends primarily on the intensity of the stress.

In the rat, exposure to stress also causes the release of CRF into the portal circulation (9). Consequently, it was anticipated that endogenous CRF played a significant and physiological role in modulating stress-induced ACTH secretion. Indeed, we (10-15) and others (16-18) have observed that the immunoneutralization of endogenous CRF (which follows the injection of anti-CRF serum), the blockade of pituitary CRF receptors by specific CRF antagonists (19) or hypothalamic lesions that markedly reduced CRF-like radioimmunoreactivity in the stalk-median eminence (20), significantly interfered with stress-induced ACTH secretion. These observations supported the hypothesis that endogneous CRF represented a major modulating factor of the effect of stress on ACTH secretion. The removal of the effect of CRF, however, did not always totally abolish the effect of stress (12), which suggested that factors other than CRF also participate in stress-induced ACTH release.

ng ACTH/ml

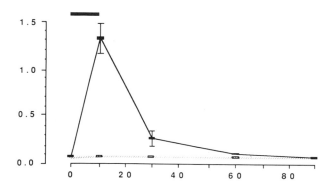

ng corticosterone/ml

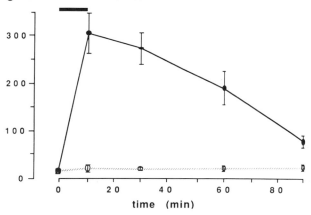

time (min)

FIGURE 1   Effect of a 10 min (bar) mild electroshock on ACTH and corticosterone secretion by intact male rats. Each point represents the mean ± SEM of
6 animals.

Two such factors are vasopressin and catecholamines, secretagogues which represent important modulators of ACTH secretion. Vasopressin (VP) acts on its own or in concert with CRF to stimulate ACTH secretion by the anterior pituitary. Such an interaction is believed to be physiologically relevant in modulating the role of VP during stress. We have shown that the intravenous injection of several doses of vasopressin produced dose-related increases in the plasma levels of intact adult rats (i.e., rats with normal levels of endogenous CRF) (13, 14), but these increases were markedly reduced in the presence of a CRF antiserum or in rats in which the release of CRF had been blocked pharmacologically (21). This suggested the existence of a synergism between VP and CRF. Indeed, this synergism can be demonstrated in the pharmacologically blocked rat. In these animals, VP elicited a significantly lower maximum ACTH response than did CRF, but the concomitant injection of both peptides resulted in a marked potentiation of CRF-induced ACTH secretion (13,14). Is this interaction operative during stress? In rats exposed to stress, it is generally agreed that the role of VP in modulating ACTH secretion is a function of the particular stimulus (22-25). For example, immobilization produces an increase in ACTH secretion that can totally be abolished by removal of endogenous CRF (11). Consequently, ACTH release following this type of stimulus is believed to be exclusively mediated through an increase in endogenous CRF levels. In contrast, exposure of adult rats to the stress of ether vapors or electroshocks causes a marked rise in plasma ACTH levels that is significantly, but not totally, abolished by CRF antisera or antagonists (12). In these models, the administration of vasopressin antagonists or antiserum, which by themselves produce a modest decrease in stress-induced ACTH secretion (12,26), completely abolished the effect of stress when administered concomitantly with a CRF antiserum. It therefore appears that in rats exposed to shocks, VP is a physiological regulator of ACTH secretion. Figure 2 illustrates this discussion by showing the effect of CRF or VP antagonists on ACTH secretion induced by various stresses.

The role of catecholamines in modulating stress-induced ACTH release remains controversial. It is well known that catecholamines are released by stress, and it could therefore be anticipated that these neurotransmitters might modulate ACTH secretion following exposure to a stimulus. Indeed, on the basis of experiments showing that blockage of ganglionic synapses significantly attenuated the stress response, our laboratory proposed an involvement of peripheral catecholamines (which by themselves are powerful stimuli of ACTH secretion [13,27-29]) in the effect of stress (12). A similar role of adrenal catecholamines in the stress response has been proposed by others (30). On the other hand, other investigators have observed that adrenal enucleation (which totally abolished epinephrine, and partially reduced the norepinephrine response to an immobilization stress [31]), did not measurably attenuate the ACTH response (31-34). These authors therefore concluded that catecholamines from the

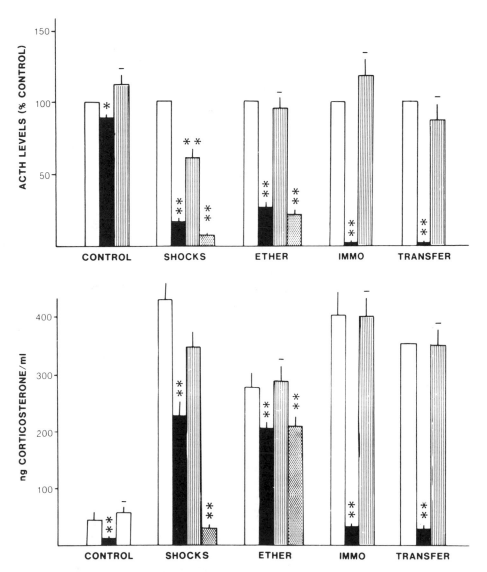

FIGURE 2 Effect of pretreatment of adult male rats with the vehicle ( ), a CRF antiserum (■), a VP antagonist (▥), or both the antiserum and the antagonist (▦) on ACTH and corticosterone secretion following exposure to different stresses. Each bar represents the mean ± SEM of five to six animals. ⁻, p > 0.05 from vehicle; *, p ≤ 0.05; **, p ≤ 0.01 (reprinted by permission from Alan R. Liss, Inc.).

sympathoadrenomedullary systems did not contribute to the acute release of ACTH during this particular stress. At the present time, this controversy is not resolved.

In conclusion therefore, it appears that coding for ACTH release during stress is multifactorial. CRF plays an essential and obligatory role, while vasopressin and catecholamines play roles that may depend upon the type of stimulus.

Infantile Rats

In contrast with adult animals, during the first three weeks of life the neonatal rat exhibits a reduced capacity to secrete ACTH and corticosterone in response to stress (38-41). In theory, the mechanisms responsible for this impaired response could be found at three sites of action: the brain, the pituitary, and the adrenals.

At the brain level, the reduced ability of the pituitary of infantile rats to secrete ACTH might be due to the inability of endogenous CRF to be released and/or to reach the pituitary, or to a defect in the transduction of the stress signal into CRF neurosecretion. We have measured low, but seemingly adequate, amounts of hypothalamic CRF during the first 3 weeks of life. We have similarly observed that the anesthetic urethane, which stimulates ACTH secretion in adult rats, also caused a marked increase in the plasma ACTH levels of rats 3, 5, or 10 days of age (40,41). It therefore appears that the brain possesses an intrinsic ability to secrete CRF at a very early age. Measurements of pituitary CRF receptors, and of pituitary ACTH content, have failed to indicate the possible presence of inadequate function (40). We have also observed that removal of corticosteroid feedback allowed neonatal rats to respond to stress by increased ACTH secretion (41). These results suggested that increased corticosteroid-negative feedback (possibly due to the paucity of transcortin-like receptors, and/or to low concentrations of transcortin, resulting in an increased access of corticosterone to the bioactive receptor [42]) appears to account at least partially for the unresponsiveness of the pituitary of neonatal rats to stress.

Chronic Stress

As discussed above, exposure to an acute stressor produces a rapid increase in plasma ACTH levels. If the stress is prolonged, however, ACTH secretion is often not maintained at this high value (43-45). This is the so-called "adaptation" phenomenon (46), during which plasma ACTH levels return toward baseline levels despite continuous stimulation of the hypothalamic-pituitary axis by the same stimulus.

When we became interested in determining why ACTH secretion was not sustained during some stresses, we realized that an essential requisite for the study of any qualitative aspects of stress was the availability of a stimulus of known and controllable duration and intensity. A large number of stresses have been used over the years, but very few can be adequately quantitated. We there-fore chose mild electroshocks delivered to the paws of the rat as a stress that could be easily manipulated both qualitatively and quantitatively (47-49). We have observed that exposure of adult rats to a 3 h period of electroshocks caused an initial increase in ACTH secretion, followed by a decline (44). Among the mechanisms that might account for this decline, we have considered the role of steroid feedback, desensitization of the pituitary to trophic factors, and the exhaustion of a readily releasable ACTH pool (44). Because adrenalectomized animals, which lack corticosteroids, also showed this decline (albeit to a some-what lesser degree), it does not appear that corticosteroid feedback represents an important mediator of this "adaptation" phenomenon. Measurement of the amount of radioimmunoassayable ACTH present following electroshocks of various intensities and durations indicated both a time- and intensity-dependent decrease in the ACTH pool. The injection of CRF to shocked rats showed no measurable loss of pituitary responsiveness when the pituitary ACTH pool was not significantly depleted, which occurs if the intensity of the shocks remain very low. However, the ability of either CRF or vasopressin to elicit an ACTH response was markedly lost when the ACTH pool of the stressed rats was signifi-cantly decreased. These results indicated that the inability of adult rats to main-tain an increased ACTH release during prolonged exposure to electroshocks appears to be mainly due to a depletion of the readily releasable pool of ACTH.

GROWTH HORMONE

In the rat, the secretion of growth hormone (GH) shows a pulsatile, light-en-trained pattern believed to be controlled by the interplay of two peptides, GH release-stimulating factor (GRF) (50) and GH release-inhibiting factor, or soma-tostatin (SS) (51), as well as opiates, catecholamines, and steroids (52-55). Ex-posure of adult rats to a stressful stimulus results in a marked decrease in GH secretion (56-58). Because passive immunization against SS restored the pulsa-tile pattern of GH release in rats submitted to stress (59-63), it appears that endogenous SS plays a prominent role in mediating stress-induced changes in circulating GH levels. Through what mechanisms is this effect modulated? Two lines of evidence pointed to a possible role of CRF. First, our laboratory had observed that CRF increased the secretion of SS by cultured hypothalamic cells (64). We therefore reasoned that stress-induced CRF release might increase brain SS levels, which in turn would lower plasma GH levels. The second line of evidence was the observation that CRF acts at the level of the brain to inhibit GH release (65). These results led to the hypothesis that endogenous CRF might play a modulating role in the stress-induced inhibition of GH secretion. We tested this hypothesis by injecting a CRF antagonist into the lateral ventricle of the brain of stressed rats, and observed that blockage of CRF receptors counteracted the inhibitory effect of stress (66). This strongly suggested that the increased secretion of endogenous CRF measured during stress modulated the inhibition of GH release by stimulating the release of SS.

LH

The secretion of the gonadotropins (Gn) LH and FSH is regulated by the interplay of factors from brain and peripheral origin. The decapeptide gonadotropin-releasing hormone (GnRH), originally isolated from the hypothalamus of several species (67,68), specifically stimulates the release of LH and FSH from the pituitary. Opiates and catecholamines, as well as ACTH and CRF, exert an inhibitory action on reproductive parameters (69-74). In addition, sex steroids play complex modulating roles at the level of the brain and the pituitary, which result in either a stimulation or an inhibition of GnRH and Gn secretion. In theory, any of these secretagogues could modulate the effect of stress on reproductive parameters.

In most species studied so far, stress exerts a marked deleterious effect on reproductive functions (75-80). However, the mechanisms through which stress interferes with LH and testosterone secretion have long remained elusive. In this chapter, we will discuss a possible role of CRF, ACTH, adrenal steroids (i.e., corticosteroids and progesterone) and opiates.

As in the case of ACTH, it appears that the role of various secretagogues is a function of the type and duration of the stress. We have observed that the subcutaneous administration of CRF to intact male rats for 7 days caused a marked decline in plasma testosterone levels, a result that could be duplicated by the injection of ACTH (81). An interesting finding was that adrenalectomy interfered with the inhibitory effects of both CRF (81) and ACTH (82,83), which suggests that the prolonged exposure to adrenal steroids, rather than ACTH, inhibited androgen production. This hypothesis has been further supported by the observation that glucocorticoids can interfere with GnRH-induced LH secretion (11, 84,85). By contrast, we have shown that removal of the adrenal did not significantly interfere with the effect of *acute* stress on circulating LH values (86). This led to the hypothesis that in contrast with prolonged stress, adrenal steroids did not appear to represent essential mediators of the stress-induced inhibition of LH secretion. What, then, causes the decreases in plasma LH levels observed during acute stress? Because, as mentioned earlier, stress releases CRF (9), we investigated the possibility that this increased CRF might also represent a mechanism through which stress lowered plasma LH levels. We observed that the central (i.e., into the lateral ventricle of the brain), but not the peripheral (i.e., into the jugular vein), injection of CRF markedly inhibited LH (72) and GnRH secretion (87). This observation led to the following question: Is endogenous CRF involved in modulating the inhibitory action of stress on reproductive parameters? To test this hypothesis, we injected a CRF antagonist prior to subjecting the rats to electroshocks. We observed that while the peripheral administration of this antagonist did not alter LH secretion in shocked animals, the central injection of the peptide restored the normal pulsatile pattern of LH release despite the presence of the shocks (86) (see Fig. 3). These results provided evidence that endogenous CRF represents an important mediator of the stress-induced inhibition of LH secretion.

Endogenous opiates are known to alter gonadotropin secretion (88,89). Therefore, their role as modulators of the effect of stress has also to be considered. Opiates exert their effects through at least three classes of receptors, called mu, delta, and kappa (90,91). We had observed that blockade of mu opiate receptors interfered with the ability of CRF to inhibit LH release (92). Consistent with these results, we (92) and others (93) subsequently obtained evidence that a similar blockade totally reversed the effect of stress on LH secretion. These results provided evidence that endogenous opiates also participate in the effect of stress on gonadotropins, a hypothesis supported by functional and anatomical evidence. In particular, there is immunohistochemical evidence that CRF and β-endorphin neurons or nerve terminals are localized in the same areas of the medial basal hypothalamus and in the median eminence (94). Furthermore, β-endorphin is reported to act directly or via noradrenergic pathways (88,95) on GnRH production, while CRF is also known to decrease GnRH levels in the portal vessels (87) and act directly on GnRH production or hypothalamic cells (96). The possibility that CRF exerts an effect on GnRH neurons through the stimulation of catecholamine secretion (97) (hormones known to inhibit the release of this decapeptide [71, 84]), also deserves consideration, but has not been experimentally tested as yet.

Taken together, the results discussed above suggest that in the rat, the inhibition of reproductive functions caused by stress could be modulated by (i) increased levels of circulating corticoids during chronic stress, which may interfere with LH secretion through a pituitary site of action; however, this effect appears to be mainly operative during prolonged stress; or (ii) an increased release of endogenous CRF, which exerts a powerful inhibitory effect on LH secretion. The mechanisms through which CRF is presently believed to exert this effect are illustrated in Figure 4.

CONCLUSION

We have discussed the effects of stress on ACTH, GH, and LH secretion as well as the mechanisms presently believed to mediate these changes. One question that might be asked is: Could there be adaptive advantages to the ability of stress to alter pituitary activity so that the hypothalamic–pituitary–adrenal axis is stimulated, while reproductive functions are inhibited? In a novel approach

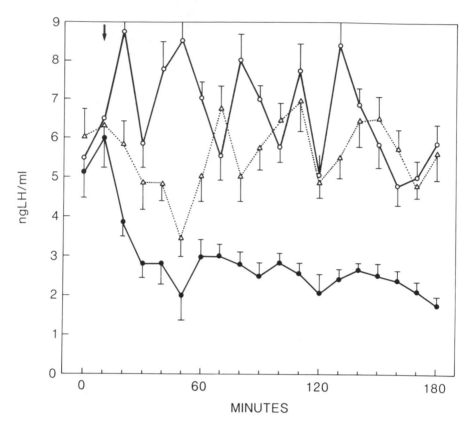

FIGURE 3 Inhibitory effect of mild electroshocks (delivered over the entire course of the experiment on LH secretion by castrated rats, and its reversal by the injection of the CRF antagonist αhel CRF [9-41] into the lateral ventricle of the brain. (o), control; (●) stressed; (Δ) stressed + CRF antagonist. Each point represents the mean ± SEM of six animals (reprinted by permission from Arlene Ennis, American Association for the Advancement of Science)

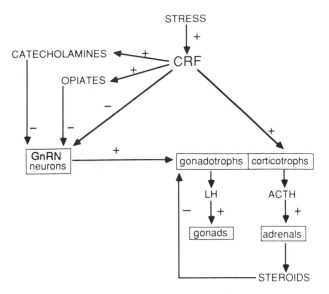

FIGURE 4 Schematic representation of what is presently known of the mechanisms that mediate the inhibitory effect of stress on reproductive functions.

to the study of the effects of glucocorticoids in stress, Munck et al. (99) have proposed that the physiological function of these steroids resided in their ability to "suppress the primary defense reactions." These authors suggest that during stress, elevated levels of glucocorticoids are necessary to influence maximally the cellular processes involved in defense mechanisms (such as immune responses, carbohydrate metabolism, fluid balance, etc.) and required to turn off defense reactions activated by stress, thus preventing them from overshooting. This interesting hypothesis provides a unifying theory for what had until then appeared as a paradox: that glucocorticoids are anti-inflammatory agents and consequently were first thought of as obstacles in the battle of the organism against infection.

Is there an advantage to the inhibition of reproductive functions caused by stress? Studies such as those quoted in (76) suggest that circumstances perceived by the body as stressful (in this case overpopulation possibly resulting in food shortage), result in a decline in fertility that can certainly be regarded as at least temporarily beneficial for the survival of the species. Another adaptive advantage that has been proposed consists of a stress-induced shift from sex steroid to adrenal steroid production, thus allowing the secretion of the glucocorticoids necessary for survival of the organism during stress (98). Consistent with this hypothesis, Bambino and Hsueh (99) have observed that glucocorticoids exerted inhibitory effects on sex steroidogenesis.

ACKNOWLEDGMENTS

This work was supported by NIH grants DK26741 and HD13527. Research was conducted in part by the Clayton Foundation for Research, California Division. C. Rivier is a Clayton Foundation investigator. Dr. Rivier gratefully acknowledges the technical support of David Hutchinson, Rosalia Chavarin, and Leah Gandara and the secretarial assistance of B. Coyne.

REFERENCES

1. Swanson L W. The hypothalamus. In: Bjorklund A, Hokfelt P, Swanson LW, eds. Handbook of chemical Neuroanatomy, vol. 5. Amsterdam: Elsevier, 1987: 1–124.

2. Swanson L W, Sawchenko P E, Rivier J, Vale W W. Organization of ovine corticotropin releasing factor (CRF)-immunoactive cells and fibers in the rat brain: an immunohistochemical study. Neuroendocrinology 1983; 36: 165–186.

3. Antoni F A. Hypothalamic control of adrenocorticotropin secretion: advances since the discovery of 41-residue corticotropin-releasing factor. Endocr Rev 1986; 7:351–378.

4. Rivier C L, Plotsky P M. Mediation by corticotropin-releasing factor (CRF) of adenohypophysial hormone secretion. Ann Rev Physiol 1986; 48:475–494.

5. Berkenbosh F, Vermes I, Tilders F J H. The β-adrenoceptor-blocking drug propranolol prevents secretion of immunoreactive β-endorphin and α-melanocyte-stimulating hormone in response to certain stress stimuli. Endocrinology 1984; 115:1051–1059.

6. Rivier C, Vale W. Interaction between ethanol and stress on ACTH and β-endorphin secretion. Alcoholism Clin Exp Res 1988; 12:206–210.

7. Rivier C, Brownstein M, Spiess J, Rivier J, Vale W. In vivo CRF-induced secretion of ACTH, β-endorphin and corticosterone. Endocrinology 1982; 110:272–278.

8. Rossier J, French E, Guillemin R, Bloom F E. On the mechanisms of the simultaneous release of immunoreactive beta-endorphin, ACTH, and prolactin by stress. Adv Biochem Psychopharmacol 1980; 22:363–375.

9. Plotsky P M, Vale W. Hemorrhage-induced secretion of corticotropin-releasing factor-like immunoreactivity into the rat hypophysial portal circulation and its inhibition by glucocorticoids. Endocrinology 1984; 114: 164–169.

10. Plotsky P M, Bruhn T O, Vale W. Evidence for multifactor regulation of the adrenocorticotropin secretory response to hemodynamic stimuli. Endocrinology 1985; 116:633–639.

11. Rivier C. Involvement of endogenous corticotropin-releasing factor (CRF) in modulating ACTH and LH secretion function during exposure to stress, alcohol or cocaine in the rat. In: Zinder O, Bresnitz S, eds. UCLA symposia

on molecular and cellular biology. New Series, vol. 97. New York: Alan R. Liss, 1989: 31–47.

12. Rivier C, Vale W. Modulation of stress-induced ACTH release by corticotropin-releasing factor, catecholamines and vasopressin. Nature 1983; 305: 325–327.

13. Rivier C, Vale W. Effects of corticotropin-releasing factor, neurohypophyseal peptides, and catecholamines on pituitary function. Fed Proc 1985; 44:189–195.

14. Rivier C, Rivier J, Mormede P, Vale W. Studies of the nature of the interaction between vasopressin and corticotropin-releasing factor on adrenocorticotropin (ACTH) release in the rat. Endocrinology 1984; 115:882–886.

15. Ixart G, Conte-Devolx B, Szafarczyk A, Malaval F, Oliver C, Assenmacher I. L'immunisation passive avec un immunserum anti-oCRF41 inhibe l'augmentation circadienne de l'ACTH plasmatique chez le rat. C R Acad Sci Paris 1985; 301:659–664.

16. Linton E A, Tilders F J H, Hodgkinson S, Berkenbosch F, Vermes I, Lowry P J. Stress-induced secretion of adrenocorticotropin in rats is inhibited by administration of antisera to ovine corticotropin-releasing factor and vasopressin. Endocrinology 1985; 116:966–970.

17. Nakane T, Audhya T, Kanie N, Hollander C S. Evidence for a role of endogenous corticotropin-releasing factor in cold, ether, immobilization and traumatic stress. Proc Natl Acad Sci USA 1985; 82:1247–1251.

18. Ono N, Samson W K, McDonald J K, Lumpkin M D, Bedran DeCastro J C, McCann S M. Effects of intravenous and intraventricular injection of antisera directed against corticotropin-releasing factor on the secretion of anterior pituitary hormones. Proc Natl Acad Sci USA 1985; 82:7787–7790.

19. Rivier J, Rivier C, Vale W. Synthetic competitive antagonists of corticotropin releasing factor: effect on ACTH secretion in the rat. Science 1984; 224:889–891.

20. Bruhn T O, Plotsky P M, Vale W W. Effect of paraventricular lesions on corticotropin-releasing factor (CRF)-like immunoreactivity in the stalk-median eminence: studies on the adrenocorticotropin response to ether stress and exogenous CRF. Endocrinology 1984; 114:57–62.

21. Arimura A, Saito T, Schally A V. Assays for corticotropin-releasing factor (CRF) using rats treated with morphine, chlorpromazine, dexamethasone and nembutal. Endocrinology 1967; 81:235–245.

22. Plotsky P M. Hypophysiotropic regulation of adenohypophyseal adrenocorticotropin secretion. Fed Proc 1985; 44:207–213.

23. Plotsky P M. Central regulation of stimulus-induced ACTH secretion: characterization of hypophysial-portal plasma CRF and AVP concentration profiles. In: Proceedings, Taniguchi foundation's 11th international symposium on brain sciences. Kyoto, Japan: Japan Scientific Societies Press, 1989: 31–48.

24. Plotsky P M. Hypophysiotropic regulation of stress-induced ACTH secretion. In: Chrousos E, Loriaux DL, Gold PW, eds. Advances in experimental biology and medicine, vol. 36. New York: Plenum, 1989: 65–81.

25. Plotsky P M. Regulation of the adrenocortical axis: Hypophysiotropic coding, catecholamines and glucocorticoids. In: Proceedings, Mansell bequest symposium, London, 1989.

26. Ono N, deCastro J B, Khorram O, McCann S M. Role of arginine vasopressin in control of ACTH and LH release during stress. Life Sci 1985; 36: 1779–1786.

27. Dann A J, Kranarch M R. Neurochemical responses in stress: relationships between the hypothalamic–pituitary–adrenal and catecholamine systems. In: Iversen LI, Inversen SD, Snyder SH, eds. Handbook of psychopharmacology, vol. 18. 1984: 455–515.

28. Takao T, Hashimoto K, Ota Z. Central catecholaminergic control of ACTH. Regul Pept 1988; 21:301–308.

29. Tilders F H H, Berkenbosch F, Smelik P G. Adrenergic mechanisms involved in the control of pituitary-adrenal activity in the rat: a β-adrenergic stimulatory mechanism. Endocrinology 1982; 110:114–120.

30. Reisine T, Affolter H-U, Rougon G, Barbet J. New insights into the molecular mechanism of stress. Trends Neurosci 1986; 9:574–579.

31. Tilders F J H, Berkenbosch F. CRF and catecholamines; their place in the central and peripheral regulation of the stress response. Acta Endocrinol 1986; 276:63–75.

32. Culman J, Chiueh C C, Foldes O, Kopin I J. Circulating catecholamines are not involved in immobilization stress-induced plasma ACTH rise in rats with transection of the pituitary stalk. Fourth Symposium on Catecholamines and other Neurotransmitters in Stress, Smolenice Castle, Czechoslovakia, June 22–27, 1987 p. 18 (abstr).

33. Kvetnansky R, Tilders F J H, VanZoest I D, et al. Sympatho-adrenal activity facilitates β-endorphin and a-MSG secretion but not ACTH secretion during immobilization stress. Neuroendocrinology 1987; 45:318–324.

34. Tilders F J H, Berkenbosch F, Vermes I, Linton E A, Smelik P G. Role of epinephrine and vasopressin in the control of the pituitary-adrenal response to stress. Fed Proc 1985; 44:155–160.

35. Bartova A. Functioning of the hypothalamo–pituitary–adrenal system during postnatal development in rats. Endocrinology 1968; 10:235–239.

36. Guillet R, Saffran M, Michaelson S M. Pituitary–adrenal response in neonatal rats. Endocrinology 1980; 106:991–994.

37. Hotta M, Shibasaki T, Masuda A, et al. Ontogeny of pituitary responsiveness to corticotropin-releasing hormone in rat. Regul Pept 1988; 21:245–252.

38. Rivier C. Effect of the age of the rat and the duration of the stimulus on stress-induced ACTH secretion. In: Florin I, Weiner H, Heilhammer D, eds. Neuronal control of bodily function. Toronto/Bern: Hogrefe/Huber, 1989.

39. Schapiro S, Geller E, Eiduson S. Neonatal adrenal cortical response to stress and vasopressin. Proc Soc Exp Biol Med 1962; 109-937–945.

40. Walker C-D, Perrin M, Vale W, Rivier C. Ontogeny of the stress response in the rat: role of the pituitary and the hypothalamus. Endocrinology 1986; 118:1445–1451.

41. Walker C-D, Sapolsky R M, Meaney M J, Vale W W, Rivier C L. Increased pituitary sensitivity to glucocorticoid feedback during the stress nonresponsive period in the neonatal rat. Endocrinology 1986; 119:1816-1821.
42. Sakly M, Koch B. Ontogenesis of glucocorticoid receptors in anterior pituitary gland: transient dissociation among cytoplasmic receptor density, nuclear uptake, and regulation of corticotropic activity in the pituitary gland. Endocrinology 1981; 108:591-596.
43. Cook D M, Kendall J W, Greer M A, Kramer R M. The effect of acute or chronic ether stress on plasma ACTH concentration in the rat. Endocrinology 1973; 93:1019-1024.
44. Rivier C, Vale W. Diminished responsiveness of the hypothalamic–pituitary-adrenal axis of the rat during exposure to prolonged stress: a pituitary-mediated mechanism. Endocrinology 1987; 121:1320-1328.
45. Ruhmann-Wennhold A, Nelson D H. Plasma ACTH levels in stressed and nonstressed adrenalectomized rats. Ann NY Acad Sci 1977; 297:498-508.
46. Armario A, Lopez-Calderon A, Jolin T, Balasch J. Response of anterior pituitary hormones to chronic stress. The specificity of adaptation. Neurosci Biobehav Rev 1986; 10:245-250.
47. Friedman S B, Ader R, Grota L J, Lason T. Plasma corticosterone response to parameters of electric shock stimulation in the rat. Psychosom Med 1967; 29:323-328.
48. Kant G J, Mougey E H, Pennington L L, Meyerhoff J L. Graded footshock stress elevates pituitary cyclic AMP and plasma β-endorphin, β-LPH, corticosterone and prolactin. Life Sci 1983; 33:2657-2663.
49. Rivier C, Smith M, Vale W. Regulation of ACTH secretion by corticotropin-releasing factor (CRF). In: DeSouza EB, Nemeroff CB, eds. Corticotropin-releasing factor: basic and clinical studies of a neuropeptide. Boca Raton, FL: CRC Press, 1989.
50. Rivier J, Spiess J, Thorner M, Vale W. Characterization of a growth hormone-releasing factor from a human pancreatic islet tumour. Nature 1982; 300:276-278.
51. Brazeau P, Vale W, Burgus R, et al. Hypothalamic polypeptide that inhibits the secretion of immunoreactive pituitary growth hormone. Science 1973; 179:77-79.
52. Audet J, Willoughby J O, Brazeau P, Martin J B. Physiologic secretion of growth hormone and prolactin in male and female rats. Clin Endocrinol 1977; 6:19S-28S.
53. Krulich L, Ilner P, Fawcett C P, Guijada M, McCann S M. Control of growth hormone secretion. In: Pecile A, Muller EE, eds. Growth and growth hormones. Amsterdam: Exerpta Medica, 1972: 306.
54. Martin J B, Brazeau P, Tannenbaum G S, et al. Neuroendocrine organization of growth hormone regulation. In: Reichlin S, Baldessarini R J, Martin J B, eds. The hypothalamus New York: Raven Press, 1978: 329.
55. Takahashi K, Daughaday W H, Kipnis D N. Regulation of immunoreactive growth hormone secretion in male rats. Endocrinology 1971; 88:909-917.

56. Dunn J D, Schindler W J, Hutchins M D, Scheving L E, Turpen C. Daily variation in rat growth hormone concentration and the effect of stress on periodicity. Neuroendocrinology 1973; 13:69-78.
57. Krulich L, Hefco E, Illner P, Read C B. The effects of acute stress on the secretion of LH, FSH, prolactin and GH in the normal male rat, with comments on their statistical evaluation. Neuroendocrinology 1974; 16: 293-311.
58. Obonsawin M C, Shin S H, Arrowsmith J. Surgery depresses pulsatile growth hormone release in rats for up to 2 days. Acta Endocrinol 1985; 110:42-45.
59. Arimura A, Smith W D, Schally A V. Blockade of the stress-induced decrease in blood GH by anti-somatostatin serum in rats. Endocrinology 1976; 98:540-543.
60. Chihara K, Arimura A, Chihara M, Schally A V. Studies on the mechanism of growth hormone and thyrotropin responses to somatostatin antiserum in anesthesized rats. Endocrinology 1978; 103:1916-1923.
61. Ferland L, Labrie F, Jobin M, Arimura A, Schally A V. Physiological role of somatostatin in the control of growth hormone and thyrotropin secretion. Biochem Biophys Res Commun 1976; 68:149-156.
62. Tannenbaum G S, Epelbaum J, Colle E, Brazeau P, Martin J B. Antiserum to somatostatin reverses starvation-induced inhibition of growth hormone but not insulin secretion. Endocrinology 1978; 102:1909-1914.
63. Terry L C, Willoughby J O, Brazeau P, Martin J B, Patel Y. Antiserum to somatostatin prevents stress-induced inhibition of growth hormone secretion in the rat. Science 1976; 192:565-567.
64. Peterfreund R A, Vale W W. Ovine corticotropin-releasing factor stimulates somatostatin secretion from cultured brain cells. Endocrinology 1982; 112:1275-1278.
65. Rivier C, Vale W. Corticotropin-releasing factor (CRF) acts centrally to inhibit growth hormone secretion in the rat. Endocrinology 1984; 114: 2409-2411.
66. Rivier C, Vale W. Involvement of corticotropin-releasing factor and somastostatin in stress-induced inhibition of growth hormone secretion in the rat. Endocrinology 1985; 117:2478-2482.
67. Burgus R, Butcher M, Amoss M, et al. Primary structure of the hypothalamic luteinizing hormone-releasing factor (LRF) of ovine origin. Proc Natl Acad Sci USA 1972; 69:278-282.
68. Matsuo H, Baba Y, Nair R, Arimura A, Schally A V. Structure of the porcine LH- and FSH-releasing hormone. I. Proposed animo acid sequence. Biochem Biophys Res Commun 1971; 43:1334-1339.
69. Briski K P, Quigley K, Meites J. Endogenous opiate involvement in acute and chronic stress-induced changes in plasma LH concentrations in the male rat. Life Sci 1984; 34:2485-2493.
70. Kalra S P, Kalra P S. Neural regulation of luteinizing hormone secretion in the rat. Endocr Rev. 1983; 4:311-351.

71. McCann S M. Regulation of secretion of follicle-stimulating hormone and luteinizing hormone. In: Knobil E, Sawyer WH, eds. Handbook of physiology, section 7, vol. 4. Washington, DC: American Physiological Society, 1974: 489-517.

72. Rivier C, Vale W. Influence of corticotropin-releasing factor (CRF) on reproductive functions in the rat. Endocrinology 1984; 114:914-919.

73. Barraclough C A, Wise P M. The role of catecholamines in the regulation of pituitary luteinizing hormone and follicle-stimulating hormone secretion. Endocrine Rev 1982; 3:91-119.

74. Howlett T A, Rees L H. Endogenous opioid peptides and hypothalamo-pituitary function. Annu Rev Physiol 1986; 48:527-536.

75. Blake C A. Effects of "stress" on pulsatile luteinizing hormone release in ovariectomized rats. Proc Soc Exp Biol Med 1975; 148:813-815.

76. Christian J J. Population density and reproductive efficiency. Biol Reprod 1971; 4:248-294.

77. Collu R, Tache Y, Ducharme J R. Hormonal modifications induced by chronic stress in rats. J Steroid Biochem 1979; 11:989-1000.

78. Euker J S, Meites J, Riegle G D. Effects of acute stress on serum LH and prolactin in intact, castrated and dexamethasone-treated male rats. Endocrinology 1973; 96:85-92.

79. Turpen C, Johnson D C, Dunn J D. Stress-induced gonadotropin and prolactin secretory patterns. Neuroendocrinology 1976; 20:339-351.

80. Yonetani S, Jojima M, Suzuki Y. Blockade of ovulation in rats by forced immobilization for surgical treatment. Endocrinol Jpn 1974; 21:68-68.

81. Rivier C, Vale W. Effect of the long-term administration of corticotropin releasing factor on the pituitary-adrenal and pituitary-gonadal axis in the male rat. J Clin Invest 1985; 75:689-694.

82. Mann D R, Evans D, Edoimioya F, Kamel F, Butterstein G M. A detailed examination of the in vivo and in vitro effects of ACTH on gonadotropin secretion in the adult rat. Neuroendocrinology 1985; 40:297-302.

83. Vreeburg J T M, DeGreef W J, Ooms M P, Van Wouw P, Weber R F A. Effects of adrenocorticotropin and corticosterone on the negative feedback action of testosterone in the adult male rat. Endocrinology 1984; 115:977-983.

84. Suter D E, Schwartz N B. Effects of glucocorticoids on responsiveness of luteinizing hormone and follicle-stimulating hormone to gonadotropin-releasing hormone by male rat pituitary cells in vitro. Endocrinology 1985; 117:855-859.

85. Suter D E, Schwartz N B, Ringstrom S J. Dual role of glucocorticoids in regulation of pituitary content and secretion of gonadotropins. Am J Physiol 1988; 254:E595-E600.

86. Rivier C, Rivier J, Vale W. Stress-induced inhibition of reproductive functions: role of endogenous corticotropin-releasing factor. Science 1986; 231: 607-609.

87. Petraglia F, Sutton S, Vale W, Plotsky P. Corticotropin-releasing factor decreases plasma LH levels in female rats by inhibiting gonadotropin-releasing hormone release into hypophysial-portal circulation. Endocrinology 1987; 20:1083–1088.
88. Kalra S P, Simpkins J W. Evidence for noradrenergic mediation of opioid on luteinizing hormone secretion. Endocrinology 1981; 109:776–782.
89. Kalra S P, Kalra P S. Opioid–adrenergic–steroid connection in regulation of luteinizing hormone secretion in the rat. Neuroendocrinology 1984; 38:418–426.
90. Leadem C A, Yagenova S V. Effects of specific activation of mu-, delta- and kappa-opioid receptors on the secretion of luteinizing hormone and prolactin in the ovariectomized rat. Neuroendocrinology 1987; 45:109–117.
91. Paterson S J, Robson L E, Kosterlitz H W. Classification of opioid receptors. Br Med Bull 1983; 39:31–36.
92. Petraglia F, Vale W, Rivier C. Opioids act centrally to modulate stress-induced decrease in luteinizing hormone in the rat. Endocrinology 1986; 119:2445–2450.
93. Hulse G K, Coleman G J. The role of endogenous opioids in the blockade of reproductive function in the rat following exposure to acute stress. Pharmacol Biochem Behav 1983; 19:795–799.
94. Roth K A, Weber E, Barchas J D. Immunoreactive dynorphin-(1-8) and corticotropin-releasing factor in subpopulation of hypothalamic neurons. Science 1983; 219:189–191.
95. Rasmussen D D, Liu J H, Wolf P L, Yen S S C. Endogenous opioid regulation of gonadotropin-releasing hormone from the human fetal hypothalamus in vitro. J Clin Endocrinol Metab 1983; 57:881–884.
96. Gambacciani M, Yen S S C, Rasmussen D D. GnRH release from the mediobasal hypothalamus: in vitro inhibition by corticotropin-releasing factor. Neuroendocrinology 1986; 43:533–536.
97. Brown M R, Fisher L A, Spiess J, Rivier C, Rivier J, Vale W. Corticotropin-releasing factor (CRF): actions on the sympathetic nervous system and metabolism. Endocrinology 1982; 111:928–931.
98. Munck A, Guyre P M, Holbrook N J. Physiological functions of glucocorticoids in stress and their relation to pharmacological actions. Endocr Rev 1984; 5:25–44.
99. Bambino T H, Hsueh A J W. Direct inhibitory effect of glucocorticoids upon testicular luteinizing hormone receptor and steroidogenesis in vivo and in vitro. Endocrinology 1981; 108:2142–2148.

7

NEURAL CODING OF STIMULUS-INDUCED ACTH SECRETION

Paul M. Plotsky

The Salk Institute, La Jolla, California

MEDIAL BASAL HYPOTHALAMUS AND THE FINAL COMMON PATHWAY

It has long been appreciated that secretion of adenohypophysial hormones (adrenocorticotropic hormone [ACTH], follicle-stimulating hormone [FSH], growth hormone [GH], luteinizing hormone [LH], prolactin [PRL], thyroid-stimulating hormone [TSH]) from the pars distalis is dependent upon hypothalamic function (1–3). Removal of the pituitary gland from its normal location in the sella and transplantation to a site distant from the hypothalamus results in hypersecretion of PRL, while secretion of the other hormones is severely attenuated. Because the adenohypophysis is well vascularized but poorly innervated, the nature of hypothalamic regulation presented an enigma for many years.

The hypothalamus, a small heterogeneous structure, plays a critical role in maintaining a constant internal milieu in the face of interoceptive and exteroceptive stimuli. It performs this function by integrating a panoply of afferent inputs to yield coordinated hormonal, autonomic, and behavioral responses necessary for reproduction, growth, feeding, and emotional behavior, and the reponse to stressors. This structure may be divided into multiple regions; however, the periventricular zone is of primary importance for neuroendocrine regulation. It is composed of the median preoptic, anteroventral periventricular preoptic, suprachiasmatic, paraventricular, and arcuate nuclei. Cells within the arcuate nuclei synthesizing dopamine, somatostatin (SRIF), growth-hormone-releasing factor (GRF), and thyrotropin-releasing hormone (TRH) project to the external zone of the median eminence via the tuberoinfundibular tract. The paraventricular nucleus, which lies dorsally along the hypothalamic portion of the third ventricle, contains several anatomically and functionally distinct neuronal groupings (4,5). The magnocellular subdivision is located in the lateral wing of the paraventricular nucleus and contains perikarya that synthesize AVP and oxytocin (OT). These cells send projections to the posterior pituitary via the hypothalamoneurohypophysial tract. The AVP-containing pathways are activated upon body fluid volume loss, whereas OT-containing cells are activated in a phasic manner to complete the efferent limb of the milk ejection reflex. Another group of perikarya give rise to descending projections to other hypothalamic regions as well as to the brainstem and spinal cord. Finally, cells within the dorsal medial portion of the parvocellular subdivision of the paraventricular nucleus synthesize corticotropin-releasing factor (CRF), a 41 amino acid hypophysiotrophic peptide (6,7), as well as other peptide factors (8-10). Projections from this region reach the richly vascularized external zone of the median eminence (11-13) via a retrochiasmatic route, where terminals end in the perivascular space. Because this area contains a fenestrated capillary plexus, it lacks a blood-brain barrier and, thus, is subject to modulatory influences from systemically circulating substances that do not cross the blood-brain barrier. Extending from the median eminence is a bridge of tissue, the infundibular stalk, which carries fibers of the hypothalamoneurohypophysial tract to the posterior lobe and is traversed by 6-10 long portal blood vessels that provide the primary blood supply of the anterior pituitary gland (14-16).

In 1930, Popa and Fielding (17) first described this specialized circulatory system connecting the hypothalamus and adenohypophysis and surmised that the hypophysial-portal circulatory system carried blood from the pituitary gland toward the hypothalamus. This notion was modified by Wislocki and King (16), who observed blood flow in the opposite direction. These observations, coupled with the concept of hypothalamic neurosecretory neurons proposed by Scharrer and Scharrer (18), led to recognition of the unique nature of CNS-adenohypophysial communication by Harris (15), as stated in his portal vessel-chemotransmitter hypothesis. Simply put, this hypothesis suggested that hypophysiotrophic substances are released from nerve terminals within the external zone of the median eminence, diffuse into the blood flowing through the primary capillary plexus, and are carried to receptive cells in the adenohypophysis by the long portal vessels. This neurohemal pathway represents the functional link between the central nervous and endocrine systems and has been referred to as the "final common pathway."

PUTATIVE ACTH SECRETAGOGUES IN THE HYPOPHYSIAL-PORTAL CIRCULATION

The existence of a concentration gradient favoring hypothalamic secretion of putative ACTH secretagogues into the portal vasculature has been demonstrated in a variety of species. An interspecies comparison of hypophysial-portal levels of putative ACTH secretagogues is presented in Table 1. Peripheral plasma levels of these substances are in the range of 2-6 pmol/L. Mimicking the concentration ranges of CRF and AVP found rat hypophysial-portal circulation effectively stimulates secretion of ACTH from in vitro perfused pituitary fragments (19). Indeed, portal plasma CRF concentrations coincide with the steepest portion of the dose-response curve for CRF-stimulated ACTH secretion from in vitro perifused rat anterior pituitary fragments. Finally, with regard to the question of the validity of portal blood collection in anesthesized preparations, it is interesting to note that CRF levels in the portal plasma collected from awake sheep (20) overlap the lower portion of the range reported in the portal plasma of anesthesized rats (21). These observations, together with results of immunohistochemical staining studies (11-13,22) and lesion studies (23-26), support the thesis that CRF, AVP, and OT are specifically secreted from nerve endings in the median eminence into the hypophysial-portal circulatory system.

HYPOPHYSIOTROPIC FACTORS ENCODING ACTH SECRETION

CRF exhibits the highest intrinsic ACTH-releasing activity of the putative ACTH secretagogues (7,27). The other factors are intrinsically weaker secretagogues,

TABLE 1 Neurotransmitter Modulation of CRF Release

Transmitter	CRF	Receptor specificity	References
Acetylcholine	↑	Muscarinic/nicotinic	45–48
Angiotensin II	↑	Saralasin-sensitive	54
Dynorphin 1-13	↓	κ/μ	51
β-Endorphin	↓	μ	51
Epinephrine	↑	$\alpha1$-/β-adrenergic	45,68
GABA	↓	Bicuculline-sensitive	45
Norepinephrine	↑	$\alpha1$-	61,63,65
Norepinephrine	↓	$\alpha2$-/β-adrenergic	63
Serotonin	↑		49,50

although they may elicit additive or nonadditive potentiation of ACTH secretion in the presence of CRF (19,27). Because of these differences in potency, the presence of CRF in the hypophysial–portal circulation is obligatory for the occurrence of stimulus-induced ACTH secretory responses. In addition, CRF appears to be the only factor thus far identified that exerts effects at the genomic level to regulate POMC gene expression.

Basal ACTH secretion at the circadian trough probably represents constitutive secretion from corticotropes (28). The circadian elevation in ACTH secretion may be mediated by several processes including increased CRF tone; increased tone of another ACTH secretagogue such as AVP; enhanced corticotrope sensitivity to a constant secretagogue tone mediated by increased receptor number, affinity, or coupling efficiency; or increased secretagogue presentation rate mediated by a local increase in blood flow. A definitive account of the mechanism(s) contributing to the observed circadian variation in ACTH secretion awaits additional experiments.

Recruitment of these factors occurs in a stimulus-specific and graded manner reflecting stimulus qualities. Major systemic stressors such as rapid hemorrhage evoke activation of all secretagogue systems, resulting in a rapid and high-amplitude ACTH and glucocorticoid secretory response. Experimentally induced arterial hemorrhage, at a rate of 5% of the estimated blood volume/min, elicits a graded increase in ACTH secretion accompanied by graded elevations of CRF, AVP, OT, and epinephrine in anesthetized cats (29) and rats (25,30). The amplitude of this ACTH secretory response is directly and linearly related to hemorrhage magnitude (29,31,32). Pharmacological manipulations confirm the multifactorial regulation of ACTH secretion in response to hemorrhage. Blockade of AVP V1 receptors or reduction of epinephrine release by ganglionic blockade attenuates the ACTH response, while passive immunoneutralization with antiserum to CRF blocks the ACTH secretory response in a dose-related fashion (30). Induction of hypotension by systemic infusion of nitroprusside also evokes an elevation in circulating ACTH levels, which appears to be primarily mediated by increased CRF secretion (21). Reduction of circulating ACTH levels by simulated volume load is associated with a reduction of hypophysial-portal plasma AVP levels without a concomitant reduction in portal CRF (30); indeed systemic clamp of AVP to levels mimicking initial portal levels substantially blunts the reduction in ACTH.

The magnitude of the ACTH response to insulin-induced hypoglycemia is related to the rate of decline in circulating glucose levels. (33). In overnight-fasted rats, the ACTH secretory response to this stimulus is blocked by passive immunoneutralization to CRF and blunted by administration of an AVP antagonist. These observations suggest multifactorial regulation, with a predominant role played by CRF. However, studies of portal plasma ACTH secretagogue concentration profiles reveal that at insulin doses < 0.5 IU/kg body weight (BW) intravenously (iv), which are sufficient to reduce blood glucose levels 50-60% within 20 min, AVP and epinephrine levels increased without a concomitant change in CRF levels (34). At higher insulin doses, the rate of glucose decline increased and changes in portal CRF levels were apparent; however, changes in portal AVP concentrations were far in excess of changes in CRF. These later observations are consistent with other reports demonstrating alterations in CRF release in response to insulin-induced hypoglycemia using insulin doses > 3 IU/ kgBW (20,35). Finally, in awake sheep, the sight and sound of a sheep-dog barking acts as a psychogenic stressor to elicit an ACTH secretory response that appears to be mediated by enhanced CRF and AVP secretion (20).

From these varied observations, the following characteristics of hypophysiotropic coding of stimulus-induced ACTH secretion may be deduced: coding is multifactorial involving at least CRF, AVP, and epinephrine; coding is stimulus-specific, with recruitment of subsets of secretagogues in accordance with the stimulus qualities; the hypophysiotropic signal can be graded to reflect stimulus intensity; and the presence of CRF is obligatory for a stimulus-induced ACTH secretory response, but it may act in the role of a dynamic regulator or as a permissive factor to set corticotrope gain, thereby permitting expression of the weaker ACTH-releasing activity of other factors.

NEURAL MODULATION OF ACTH SECRETAGOGUE RELEASE

Four general classes of pathways provide afferents to the CRF-rich portion of paraventricular nuclei (4,5,32,36–41) and thus may participate in mediation of stimulus-induced ACTH secretion. These inputs include ascending mono- and polysynaptic pathways from brainstem nuclei (nucleus of the solitary tract, locus ceruleus, caudal ventrolateral medulla, etc.); descending pathways from the cortex, hippocampus, and amygdala through the bed nucleus of the stria terminalis; direct and indirect pathways from the subfornical organ; and short intrahypothalamic pathways. Neither the neurotransmitter specificity nor direction of their action on ACTH secretagogue release has been established unambiguously.

Reviews on the effects of putative transmitters on bioactive CRF release may be found in work by Buckingham and Hodges (42) and Jones et al. (43,44), while neurotransmitter effects on CRF release are reviewed by Antoni (55) and in Table 2. With the exception of the actions of the catecholamines, the in vitro and in vivo observations are in substantial agreement. These observations suggest that acetylcholine (45–48) and serotonin (49,50) act as facilitatory agents, while GABA (45) and the opioid peptides (51), β-endorphin and dynorphin, act as inhibitory agents. These latter agents are probably contained in local hypothalamic circuits and maintain a tonic inhibitory tone on function of the hypothalamic–pituitary–adrenal axis.

TABLE 2   Interspecies Comparison of Putative ACTH Secretagogue Levels in
Hypophysial-Portal Circulation (pmol/L)

Species	CRF	AVP	OT	Reference
Cat	113 + 24	1167 + 162	253 + 33	29
Rat	57 + 8	57 + 109	1528 + 275	29,30
Rhesus	29 + 4	610 + 73	2091 + 222	29
Sheep	31 + 7	212 + 29	Not measured	20

Angiotensin II has been implicated in the regulation of ACTH secretion, in
direct modulation of adrenal steroid secretion, and in the regulation of blood
pressure and fluid volume (52). It is present both as a circulating hormone and as
a putative neurotransmitter (52). Although angiotensin II immunopositive terminal fields have been identified in the external zone of the median eminence
(53), there is no direct evidence that it is actually secreted into the hypophysial-
portal circulation (54). An angiotensin II-positive pathway originating in the
subfornical organ projects to the CRF-rich region of the paraventricular nucleus
(38,53), thus providing an anatomical substrate for a neuromodulatory role.
Central administration of exogenous angiotensin II evokes a dose-related and
receptor-specific facilitation of CRF secretion. Furthermore, activation of
endogenous angiotensin II secretion via electrical stimulation of the subfornical
organ also evokes CRF and ACTH secretion, which is blocked by pretreatment
with saralasin, a specific receptor antagonist (54). Therefore, angiotensin II
appears to function at the central rather than adenohypophysial level to modulate ACTH secretion. This system is unique in that systemic levels of angiotensin
II are readily detected by cells within the subfornical organ (52), a circumventricular structure, and then transduced into a neuronal one. This signal is conveyed via an angiotensin-II-positive pathway to the paraventricular nuclei, where
secretion of AVP from both parvocellular and magnocellular regions, and of
CRF from the parvocellular region, is facilitated. Overall, it is likely that this
pathway serves an integrative function in coordinating endocrine, behavioral,
and autonomic responses to situations of hypovolemia or hyperosmolality.

The catecholamines, while exerting facilitatory actions at the adenohypophysial level (27,55), have been generally regarded as inhibitory to ACTH
secretion at the central nervous system level (42,56-59). However, recent studies
have challenged this traditional view. Several groups (60-65) have reported
central stimulatory actions level of both norepinephrine and epinephrine on
hypothalamic-pituitary-adrenal function. The studies by Plotsky (63) that
reported noradrenergic stimulation and inhibition at higher doses via an α1-
adrenergic receptor mechanism and inhibition at higher doses mediated via an

$a2$- and β-adrenergic mechanism bear a striking similarity to noradrenergic actions on supraoptic AVP activity (66). Activation of endogenous amine-containing pathways by electrical stimulation of the ventral noradrenergic ascending bundle also elicit secretion of CRF, which appeared to be at least partially mediated by $a1$-adrenergic mechanisms. Chemical lesions of the catecholaminergic component of this bundle blunt CRF secretion into the portal circulation (65) and attentuate the ACTH response to various stimuli. In humans, the data are consistent with an $a1$-adrenergic-mediated facilitatory effect at the central level (67). Recent in vitro studies also support the concept of catecholaminergic facilitation of CRF secretion (68). The receptor mechanisms by which these stimulatory actions are mediated remain a matter of controversy.

GLUCOCORTICOID FEEDBACK MODULATION OF THE ENCODING PROCESSES

The net secretory response of ACTH can be defined by the modality and qualities of the stimulus and the modulatory effect of glucocorticoid feedback. Feedback activity occurs over multiple time domains at both pituitary and central loci to alter ACTH secretion (69); however, the central loci of this action and identity of hypophysiotropic factors involved in mediating these effects are not yet well defined. The anatomical substrate(s) of central feedback must involve regions containing corticosteroid receptors, which have been mapped by autoradiographic (56,70–74), in situ hybridization (75), and immunocytochemical (76–79) methods. Multiple steroid receptor types appear to be involved in mediating central glucocorticoid feedback actions (69,80). Current understanding of glucocorticoid action dictates that feedback inhibition must be mediated by occupancy of corticosteroid receptors; thus, at the simplest level, one might expect an inverse relationship between corticosteroid receptor occupancy and hypophysial-portal plasma levels of putative ACTH secretagogues. The anatomical distribution of corticosteroid receptors has been mapped; however, the relative importance of various loci to feedback modulation of ACTH secretion and neurotransmitter pathways mediating feedback remains to be evaluated.

In experimental studies, low-dose administration of dexamethasone (25) or corticosterone (21) blocks stimulus-induced but not resting secretion of CRF into the hypophysial-portal circulation. Removal of glucocorticoid feedback via adrenalectomy results in substantial time-dependent alterations in hypothalamic immunostaining (9,12,81,82), CRF messenger RNA levels (83–85), median eminence content (26,82,86,87), and secretion into the hypophysial-portal circulation (62,82,84) of CRF and AVP. The AVP/CRF release ratio shifts dramatically in favor of AVP following adrenalectomy (82,88). Presentation of a variable-amplitude delayed feedback signal to adrenalectomized rats, in the form of a systemic corticosterone infusion, highlights the differential corticosterone threshold for attenuation of stimulus-induced versus initial CRF levels in the portal circulation (21). The threshold dosage for this feedback effect on initial CRF occurred at circulating corticosterone levels of > 25 μg/dl (a level within the physiological range observed during severe stress), while circulating corticosterone levels > 8 μg/dl were sufficient to suppress stimulus-induced CRF secretion. The exquisite sensitivity of this axis to feedback is evident in experiments demonstrating that elevation of systemic glucocorticoid concentrations only slightly above those required for maintenance of body and thymic weight and normal ACTH levels substantially attenuate central secretory drive (69). This sensitivity appears to be encoded at central loci. One may speculate that attenuation of the ACTH secretory response by steroid feedback conserves the response capacity of the hypothalamic–pituitary–adrenal axis to subsequent stressors and acts to limit the duration of total tissue glucocorticoid exposure, thus minimizing catabolic, antireproductive, and immunosuppressive effects (89).

ACKNOWLEDGMENTS

This research was supported by NIH grants DK26741 and DK33093 and conducted in part by the Clayton Foundation for Research, California Division. P. Plotsky is a Clayton Foundation investigator.

REFERENCES

1. Halasz B L, Pupp L, Uhlarik S. Hypophysiotrophic area in the hypothalamus. J Endocrinol 1962; 25:147–154.
2. Harris G W, Jacobson D. Functional grafts of anterior pituitary gland. Proc. R Soc London Ser B 1952; 139:263–276.
3. Nikitovictch-Winer M, Everett J W. Functional restitution of pituitary grafts retransplanted from kidney to median eminence. Endocrinology 1958; 63: 559–566.
4. Swanson L W. Organization of the mammalian neuroendocrine system. In Handbook of Physiology. Washington DC: American Physiological Society 1985: 317–362.
5. Swanson L W, Sawchenko P E. Hypothalamic integration: organization of the paraventricular and supraoptic nuclei. Neuroscience 1983; 36:265–186.
6. Rivier J, Spiess J, Vale W. Characterisation of rat hypothalamic corticotropin-releasing factor. Proc Natl Acad Sci U S A 1983; 80:4851–4855.
7. Vale W Spiess J, Rivier C, Rivier J. Characterization of a 41-residue ovine hypothalamic peptide that stimulates secretion of corticotropin and β-endorphin. Science 1981; 213:1394–1397.
8. Hokfelt T, Fahrenkrug J, Tatemoto K, et al. The PHI (PHI-27)/corticotropin-releasing factor/enkephalin immunoreactive hypothalamic neuron:

possible morphological basis for integrated control of prolactin, cortico-tropin, and growth hormone secretion. Proc Natl Acad Sci USA 1983; 80:895-898.

9. Sawchenko P E, Swanson L W, Vale W W. Coexpression of CRF- and vasopressin-immunoreactivity in paraventricular neurosecretory neurons of the adenalectomized rat. Proc Natl Acad Sci USA 1984; 81:1883-1887.

10. Sawchenko P E, Swanson L W, Vale W W. Corticotropin-releasing factor: co-expression within distinct subsets of oxytocin-, vasopressin-, and neuro-tensin-immunoreactive neurons in the hypothalamus of the male rat. J Neurosci 1984; 4:1118-1129.

11. Kawata M, Hashimoto K, Takahara I, et al. Immunohistochemical demonstration of the localization of corticotropin releasing factor-containing neurons in the hypothalamus of mammals including primates. Anat Embryol 1982; 165:303-313.

12. Merchenthaler I, Vigh S, Petrsz P, Schally A V. The paraventriculo-infundi-bular cortiotropin releasing factor (CRF) pathway as revealed by immuno-cytochemistry in long-term hypophysectomized or adrenalectomized rats. Reg Pep 1983; 5:295-305.

13. Swanson L W, Sawchenko P E, Rivier J, Vale W W. Organization of ovine corticotropin-releasing immunoreactive cells and fibers in the rat brain: an immunohistochemical study. Neuroendocrinology 1983; 36:165-186.

14. Green J D, Harris J W. Observation of the hypophysioportal vessels of the living rat. J Physiol Lond 1949; 108:359-361.

15. Harris G W. Neural control of the pituitary gland. London: Arnold, 1955.

16. Wislocki G B, King L S. The peried observations, the permeability of the hypophysis and the hypothalamus to vital dyes with a study of the hypo-physial vascular system. Am J Anat 1936; 58:421-472.

17. Popa G T, Fielding U. Hypophysial vessels and their colloid accomaniment. J Anat 1933; 67:227-232.

18. Scharrer B. Neurosecretion and its role in neuroendocrine regulation. In: Meites J, Donovan BT, McCann SM, eds. Pioneers in neuroendocrinology. New York: Plenum, 1975: 255-266.

19. Watanabe T, Orth D N. Detailed kinetic analysis of adrenocorticotropin secretion by dispersed rat anterior pituitary cells in a microperfusion system: effects of ovine corticotropin-releasing factor and arginine vaso-pressin. Endocrinology 1987; 121:1133-1145.

20. Engler D, Pham T, Fullerton M J, Ooi G, Funder J W, Clarke, I J. Studies of the secretion of corticotropin-releasing factor and arginine vasopressin into the hypophysial-portal circulation of the conscious sheep. I. Effect of an audiovisual stimulus and insulin-induced hypoglycemia. Neuroendo-crinology 1988; 48:551-560.

21. Plotsky P M, Otto S, Sapolsky R M. Inhibition of immunoreactive cortico-tropin releasing factor secretion into the hypophysial-portal circulation by delayed glucocorticoid feedback. Endocrinology 1986; 119:1126-1130.

22. Whitnall M H. Distributions of pro-vasopressin expressing and pro-vasopressin deficient CRH neurons in the paraventricular hypothalamic nucleus of colchicine-treated normal and adrenalectomized rats. J Comp Neurol 1988; 275:13–28.

23. Bruhn T O, Plotsky P M, Vale W. Effect of paraventricular lesions on corticotropin-releasing factor-like immunoreactivity in the stalk median eminence: stuides on the adrenocorticotropin response to ether stress and exogenous CRF. Endocrinology 1984; 114:57–62.

24. Makara G B, Stark E, Palkovits M. Re-evaluation of the pituitary adrenal response to ether in rats with various cuts around the medial basal hypothalamus. Neuroendorcinology 1980; 30:38–44.

25. Plotsky P M, Vale W. Hemorrhage-induced secretion of corticotropin-releasing factor-like immunoreactivity into the rat hypophysial portal circulation and its inhibition by glucocorticoids. Endocrinology 1984; 114: 164–169.

26. Tilders F J H, Schipper J, Lowry P J, Vermes I. Effect of hypothalamus lesions on the presence of CRF-immunoreactive nerve terminals in the median eminence and on the pituitary–adrenal response to stress. Regul Pept 1982; 5:77–84.

27. Vale W, Vaughan J, Smith M, Yamamoto G, Rivier J, River C. Effects of synthetic ovine corticotropin-releasing factor, glucocorticoids, catecholamines, neurohypophysial peptides, and other substances on cultured corticotropic cells. Endocrinology 1983; 113:1121–1131.

28. Dallman M F, Makara G B, Roberts J L, Levin N, Blum M. Corticotrope response to removal of releasing factors and corticosteroids in vitro. Endocrinology 1985; 117:2190–2197.

29. Plotsky P M. Regulation of hypophysiotropic factors mediating ACTH secretion. N Y Acad Sci 1987; 512:205–217.

30. Plotsky P M, Bruhn T O, Vale W. Evidence for multifactor regulation of the adrenocorticotropin secretory response to hemodynamic stimuli. Endocrinology 1985; 116:633–639.

31. Bereiter D A, Zaid A M, Gann D S. Effect of rate of hemorrhage on release of ACTH in cats. Am J Physiol 1986; 250:E76–E81.

32. Gann D S, Ward D G, Carlson D E. Neural control of ACTH: a homeostatic reflex. Rec Prog Horm Res 1978; 34:357–396.

33. Keller-Wood M E, Shinsako J, Dallman M F. Interaction between stimulus intensity and corticosterone feedback in control of ACTH. Am J Physiol 1984; 247:E489–E494.

34. Plotsky P M, Bruhn T O, Vale W. Hypophysiotropic regulation of adrenocorticotropin secretion in response to insulin-induced hypoglycemia. Endocrinology 1985; 117:323–329.

35. Guillaume V, Grino M, Boudouresque F, Oliver C. Corticotropin-releasing factor secretion increases in rat hypophysial portal blood during insulin-induced hypoglycemia. Neuroendocrinology 1989.

36. Greer M A, Allen C F, Gibbs FP, Gullickson C. Pathways at the hypothalamic level through which traumatic stress activates ACTH secretion. Endocrinology 1970; 86:1404–1409.

37. McKellar S, Loewy A D. Organization of some brainstem afferents to the paraventricular nucleus of the hypothalamus in the rat. Brain Res 1981; 217:351-357.
38. Miselis R R. The efferent projections of the subfornical organ of the rat: a circumventricular organ within a neural network subserving water balance. Brain Res 1981; 230:1-23.
39. Palkovits M. Neural pathways involved in ACTH regulation. Ann N Y Acad Sci (1977; 297:455-476.
40. Sawchenko P E, Swanson L W. Central noradrenergic pathways for the integration of hypothalamic neuroendocrine and autonomic responses. Science 1981; 214:685-687.
41. Sawchenko P E, Swanson L W. The organization of noradrenergic pathways from the brainstem to the paraventricular and supraoptic nuclei in the rat. Brain Res Rev 1982; 4:275-325.
42. Buckingham J C, Hodges J R. Hypothalamic receptors influencing the secretion of corticotropin releasing hormone in the rat. J Physiol 1979; 290:421-431.
43. Jones M T, Gillham B, DiRenzo G, Beckford U, Holmes M C. Neural control of corticotropin secretion. In: Ganong WF, ed. Frontiers in hormone research, vol. 8. Basel: Karger, 1981: 12-43.
44. Jones M T, Hillhouse E W. Neurotransmitter regulation of corticotropin release in vitro. In: Krieger DT, Ganong WF, eds. ACTH and related peptides: structure, regulation, and action. New York: Academic Press, 1977: 536-560.
45. Plotsky P M, Otto S, Sutton S. Neurotransmitter modulation of corticotropin releasing factor secretion into the hypophysial-portal circulation. Life Sci 1987; 41:1311-1317.
46. Suda T, Yajima F, Tomori N, et al. Stimulatory effect of acetylcholine on immunoreactive corticotropin-releasing factor release from the rat hypothalamus in vitro. Life Sci 1987; 40:673-677.
47. Clarke M J O, Gilles G E. Comparison of peptide release from fetal rat hypothalamic neurones cultured in defined media and serum-containing media. J Endocrinol 1988; 116:349-356.
48. Calogero A E, Gallucci W T, Bernardini R, Saoutis C, Gold P W. Chrousos G P. Effect of cholinergic antagonists on rat hypothalamic corticotropin-releasing hormone secretion in vitro. Neuroendocrinology 1988; 47:303-308.
49. Gibbs D M, Vale W. Effect of serotonin uptake inhibitor fluoxetine on corticotropin-releasing factor and vasopressin secretion into hypophysial portal blood. Brain Res 1983; 280:176-179.
50. Nakagami Y, Suda T, Yajima, et al. Effects of serotonin, cyproheptadine and reserpine on corticotropin-releasing factor release from rat hypothalamus in vitro. Brain Res 1986; 386:232-236.
51. Plotsky P M. Opioid inhibition of immunoreactive corticotropin-releasing factor secretion into the hypophysial-portal circulation of rats. Regul Pept 1986; 16:235-242.

52. Reid I A. Actions of angiotensin II on the brain: mechanisms and physiologic role. Am J Physiol 1984; 246:F533–F543.
53. Lind R W, Swanson L W, Bruhn T O, Ganten D. The distribution of angiotensin II-immunoreactive cells and fibers in the paraventriculo-hypophysial system of the rat. Brain Res 1985; 338:81–89.
54. Plotsky P M, Sutton S W, Bruhn T O, Ferguson A V. Analysis of the role of angiotensin II in mediation of adrenocorticotropin secretion. Endocrinology 1988; 122:538–545.
55. Antoni F A. Hypothalamic control of adrenocorticotropin secretion: advances since the discovery of 41-residue corticotropin-releasing factor. Endocr Rev 1986; 7:351–378.
56. Bugnon C, Hadjiyiassemis M, Feldman D, Cardot J. Reserpine-induced depletion of corticoliberin (CRF)-like immunoreactivity in the zona externa of the rat median eminence. Brain Res 1983; 275:198–201.
57. DiRenzo G, Gillham B, Holmes M C, Jones M T. The effect of pretreatment with intraventricular 6-hydroxydopamine on the hypothalamo-pituitary-adrenocortical function of the rat. J Physiol 1975; 293:50–56.
58. Mezey E, Kiss J Z, Skirboll L P, Goldstein M, Axelrod J. Increase of corticotropin-releasing factor staining in rat paraventricular nucleus neurones by depletion of hypothalamic adrenaline. Nature 1984; 310:140–141.
59. Weiner R I, Ganong W F. Role of brain monoamines and histamine in regulation of anterior pituitary secretion. Physiol Rev 1978; 58:904–976.
60. Fehm H L, Voigt K H, Lang R E, Pfeiffer E F. Effects of neurotransmitters on the release of corticotropin releasing hormone (CRH) by rat hypothalamic tissue in vitro. Exp Brain Res 1980; 39:229–234.
61. Guillaume V, Conte-Devolx B, Szafarczyk A, et al. The corticotropin releasing factor release in rat hypophysial portal blood is mediated by brain catecholamines. Neuroendocrinology 1987; 46:143–146.
62. Hary L, Dupouy J P, Chatelain A. Effect of norepinephrine on the pituitary adrenocorticotrophic activation by ether stress and on the in vitro release of ACTH by the adenohypophysis of male and female newborn rats. Neuroendocrinology 1984; 39:105–113.
63. Plotsky P M. Facilitation of immunoreactive corticotropin-releasing factor secretion into the hypophysial–portal circulation after activation of catecholaminergic pathways or central norepinephrine injections. Endocrinology 1987; 121:924–930.
64. Smythe G A, Bradshaw J E, Vining R F. Hypothalamic monoamine control of stress-induced adrenocorticotropin release in the rat. Endocrinology 1983; 113:1062–1071.
65. Szafarczyk A, Malaval F, Laurent A, Gibaud R, Assenmacher I. Further evidence for a central stimulatory action of catecholamines on adrenocorticotropin release in the rat. Endocrinology 1987; 121:883–892.
66. Day T A, Randle J C R, Renaud L P. Opposing α- and β- adrenergic mechanisms mediate dose-dependent actions of noradrenalin on supraoptic vasopressin neurones in vivo. Brain Res 1985; 358:171–179.

67. Al-Damluji S, Perry L, Tomlin S, et al. Alpha-adrenergic stimulation of corticotropin secretion by a specific central mechanism in man. Neuro-endocrinology 1987; 45:68–76.
68. Widmaier E P, Lim A T, Vale W. Secretion of corticotropin-releasing factor from cultured rat hypothalamic cells: effects of catecholamines. Endocrinology 1989; 124:583–590.
69. Keller-Wood M E, Dallman M F. Corticosteroid inhibition of ACTH secretion. Endocrine Rev 1984; 5:1–24.
70. Duncan G E, Stumpf W E. A combined autoradiographic and immunocytochemical study of 3H-corticosterone target neurons and catecholamine neurons in rat and mouse lower brain stem. Neuroendocrinology 1985; 40:262–271.
71. Gerlach J L, McEwen B S. Rat brain binds adrenal steroid hormone: radio-autography of hippocampus with corticosterone. Science 1972; 175:1133–1136.
72. McEwen B S, Weiss J M. The uptake and action of corticosterone: regional and subcellular studies on rat brain. In: deWied D, Weijner JAWN, eds. Progress in brain research, vol. 32. New York: Elsevier, 1970: 200–212.
73. McEwen B S, Weiss S M, Schwartz L S. Uptake of corticosterone by rat brain and its concentration by certain limbic structures. Brain Res 1979; 16:227–241.
74. Stumpf W E, Sar M. Glucocorticosteroid and mineralocorticosteroid hormone target sites in brain: autoradiographic studies with corticosterone, aldosterone, and dexamethasone. In: Jones MT, Dallman MF, Gillman B, Chattapadhyan S, eds. Interactions within the brain–pituitary–adrenocortical system. New York: Academic Press, 1979: 137–147.
75. Arriza J L, Simerly R B, Swanson L W, Evans R M. The neuronal mineralocorticoid receptor as a mediator of glucocorticoid response. Neuron 1988; 1:887–900.
76. Agnati L F, Fuxe K, Yu, Z-Y, et al. Morphometrical analysis of the distribution of corticotropin releasing factor, glucocorticoid receptor and phenylethanolamine-N- methyltransferase immunoreactive structures in the paraventricular hypothalamic nucleus of the rat. Neurosci Letts 1985; 54:147–152.
77. Fuxe K, Harfstrand A, Agnati L F, et al. Immunocytochemical studies on the localization of glucocorticoid receptor immunoreactive nerve cells in the lower brain stem and spinal cord of the male rat using a monoclonal antibody against liver glucocorticoid receptor. Neurosci Letts 1985; 60: 1–6.
78. Fuxe K, Wikstrom A-C, Okret S, et al. Mapping of glucocorticoid receptor immunoreactive neurons in the rat tel- and diencephalon using a monoclonal antibody against rat liver glucocorticoid receptor. Endocrinology 1985; 117:1803–1812.
79. Uht R M, McKelvey J F, Harrison R W, Bohn M C. Demonstration of glucocorticoid receptor-like immunoreactivity in glucocorticoid-sensitive

vasopressin and corticotropin-releasing factor neurons in the hypothalamic paraventricular nucleus. J Neurosci Res 1988; 19:405–411.

80. Reul J M H M, DeKloet E R. Two receptor systems for corticosterone in rat brain: microdistribution and differential occupation. Endocrinology 1985; 117:2505–2511.

81. Kiss J Z, Mezey E, Skirboll L. Corticotropin releasing factor (CRF)-like immunoreactive neurons of the paraventricular nucleus become vasopressin-positive following adrenalectomy. Proc Natl Acad Sci USA 1984; 81: 1854–1858.

82. Plotsky P M, Sawchenko P E. Hypophysial–portal plasma levels, median eminence content, and immunohistochemical staining of corticotropin-releasing factor, arginine vasopressin, and oxytocin after pharmacological adrenalectomy. Endocrinology 1987; 120:1361–1369.

83. Jingami H, Matsukura S, Numa S, Immura H. Effects of adrenalectomy and dexamethasone administration on the level of prepro-corticotropin-releasing factor messenger ribonucleic acid (mRNA) in the hypothalamus and adrenocorticotropin/β-lipotropin precursor mRNA in the pituitary in rats. Endocrinology 1985; 117:1314–1320.

84. Wolfsen B, Manning R W, Davis L G, Arentzen R. Colocalization of corticotropin releasing factor and vasopressin mRNA in neurons after adrenalectomy. Nature 1985; 315:59–61.

85. Young S W III, Mezey E, Siegel R E. Quantitative in situ hybridization histochemistry reveals increased levels of corticotropin-releasing factor: effect on ACTH secretion in the rat. Neurosci Letts 1986; 70:198–203.

86. Suda T, Tomori N, Tozawa F, Mouri T, Demura H, Shizume K. Effects of bilateral adrenalectomy on immunoreactive corticotropin-releasing factor in the rat median eminence and intermediate-posterior pituitary. Endocrinology 1983; 113:1182–1184.

87. Suda T, Tomori N, Tozawa F, Mouri T, Demura H, Shizume K. Effect of dexamethasone on immunoreactive corticotropin-releasing factor in the rat median eminence and intermediate-posterior pituitary. Endocrinology 1984; 114:851–854.

88. Holmes M C, Antoni F A, Catt K J, Aguilera G. Predominant release of vasopressin vs corticotropin-releasing factor from isolated median eminence after adrenalectomy. Neuroendocrinology 1986; 43:245–251.

89. Munck A, Guyre P M, Holbrook N J. Physiological functions of glucocorticoids in stress and their relation to pharmacological actions. Endocr Rev 1984; 5:25–44.

8

REGULATION OF HUMAN PITUITARY RESPONSES TO STRESS

Ashley B. Grossman

St. Bartholomew's Hospital, London, England

In examining the effects of stress on hormone secretion, one immediately comes across an almost insoluble problem. There is no clear consensus as to the meaning of the word *stress* in biological terms, and most authors start by trying to define the word for their own purposes. In reviewing a large body of data, one solution is to include anything that the writers themselves have considered "stressful," accepting that there will be a heterogeneous collection of disparate data that may not easily fall into any clear pattern. As an alternative, clear and distinctive definitions may be used, but these often appear to be so wide-ranging that the intuitive concept of stress (with all its ambiguous connotations of suffering, distress, and biological maladaptation) may be noted for its absence. In this review I will take the latter path to begin with, when it will become apparent that the concept will fragment and the notion of "stress hormones" all but disappear. However, it is then possible to reconstruct the remnants into a more heuristic model that combines general biological concepts of adaptation with more subjective notions of distress.

The starting point for the analysis is the concept of adaptation: an organism will adjust to any change in its environment in such a manner as to maintain its integrity. This applies as much to psychological equilibrium as to glucose homeostasis, but is perhaps most evident in the numerous negative feedback loops that have come to characterize endocrinology. However, the organism is not a passive partner in the world, but acts as an agent in modifying its surroundings and acting upon its relationships. This active modification is also a means of preserving or changing the environment that can maximally ensure the continuation of the organism (or, at a most basic level, its genes). Within this framework, stress can be considered as any alteration in the external situation that impinges on the organism: the latter must then adapt by annulling or coming to terms with the change. For example, a change in environmental temperature may lead to short-term adaptations such as shivering, sweating, vasodilation, or vasoconstriction; medium-term behavioral changes (i.e., moving to a different environment); or more subtle long-term changes (alterations in body fat composition, brown fat, etc.). Crucial to all these changes is that they are adaptive to increase survival. Most biological systems have considerable built-in redundancy, such that a myriad of different mechanisms activate feedback loops to ensure homeostasis. Thus, blood pressure is maintained in the face of considerable insult, such that one is rarely aware of the intrinsically lethal effects of commonplace external stimuli (e.g., standing, walking, running, swimming). Furthermore, different stressors will obviously require differing adjustments in the organism that will be tuned to the specific stimulus. However, the more intuitive interpretation of stress will usually also include subjective (and objective) evidence of severe emotion, usually fear or anger, in response to relatively intense stimuli. Indeed, the objective changes of sympathetic and adrenomedullary activity (tachycardia, perspiration, tremor) are often used as a quantifiable measure of stress activation. Careful analysis of many situations involving such activation, however, suggests that these changes are usually adaptive insofar as they prepare the organism to cope with changing demands. This is most clearly shown in the responses to a stimulus threatening the very existence of the organism. The most appropriate responses in such situations are to flee or destroy the stimulus physically, both of which require considerable physical activity. It is thus not unreasonable to expect metabolic and neuroendocrine adaptations to facilitate these responses. Furthermore, it is now realized that Cannon's concept of generalized sympathetic activation must be replaced by one of sympathetic patterning that is regulated and modulated to be most appropriate to the eliciting situation (1).

Thus, according to either definition discussed, changing environments necessitate responses by the organism, with or without sympathetic activation according to requirements, these responses in turn being patterned and adaptive. According to these interpretations, nonspecific stress becomes biologically meaningless. It is then an interesting task to analyze the pituitary responses to so-called stressors from this vantage point. In this chapter only essential references will be quoted: detailed background literature is available in the reviews quoted in the text.

PROLACTIN

Prolactin is under the dual control of inhibitory (dopamine, and possible GnRH-associated peptide [GAP] and gamma-aminobutyric acid) and excitatory (thyrotropin-releasing hormone [TRH], vasoactive intestinal peptide [VIP]) hypothalamic hormones, although it appears that the predominant control in rat and humans is tonic inhibition by dopamine. While many functions have been suggested for prolactin, in the human female only lactation and the associated amenorrhea are clearly established: in men, prolactin has no established function. It is therefore strange that prolactin is often considered a "stress hormone" par excellence. Serum prolactin levels rise slightly during puberty in the female, probably under the influence of estrogens, and there are also very minor changes during the menstrual cycle. Prolactin levels also rise during severe hypoglycemia induced by exogenous insulin; both these responses may reflect the mild diabetogenic effects of prolactin. During hypoglycemia there is a coordinated rise of all the hypoglycemic hormones, a further example of a redundant (in cybernetic terms) response to a potentially life-threatening event, while the prolactin response is much smaller in intensity and duration. Where stimuli of intense emotional value have been studied, changes in circulating prolactin have been much more variable. First parachute jumps, "swimming" by nonswimmers, and aerial acrobatics apparently cause no change in serum prolactin levels attributable to the mental event, while Brooks et al. (2) could not correlate state or trait anxiety with prolactin levels in a large group of subjects. Acute phobic anxiety elicited by the phobic object does not elevate serum prolactin levels, and neither does gynecological interview or examination in an outpatient setting. Acute surgery will certainly increase circulating prolactin levels, but the responses appear to depend more on the type and site of surgery (general anesthesia is more effective than local anesthesia, thoracotomy more than laparotomy) than the degree of mental upset (3). Furthermore, serum prolactin levels will rise in response to a fall in central venous pressure. Thus, the prolactin response to surgery is more likely to be a response to metabolic, cardiovascular, and local neurogenic cues than a direct reflection of emotional involvement or distress.

Specific emotive situations may induce a rise in prolactin, and it has been suggested that some forms of infertility may result from intermittent hyperprolactinemia induced by sexual problems. However, this too would project the hyperprolactinemia as a specific response (in this context, as an antireproductive hormone) to an environment inimical to reproduction. There is no evidence that prolactin is a nonspecific marker of insult or injury.

GROWTH HORMONE

The data on growth hormone (GH) are in many ways similar to those obtained for prolactin. GH is under the control of two peptides, an excitatory growth-hormone-releasing hormone (GHRH) and an inhibitory somatostatin. GHRH appears to be the predominant peptide: disconnection of the pituitary from the hypothalamus leads to a fall in circulating GH levels. The periodic pulsatile release of GH is dominated by GHRH, although animal studies suggest that GH pulses are also associated with a fall in somatostatin release. Despite the fact that the somatotroph is the most prevalent cell type in the human anterior pituitary, there is little or no evidence that circulating GH plays any major role in the human adult. Like prolactin, GH is diabetogenic, and its levels rise in response to hypoglycemia; it is also more clearly responsive to physical exercise, especially when intense and prolonged. Since GH affects fuel mobilization and utilization, by decreasing tissue glucose uptake but increasing lipolysis, these effects are most likely adaptive changes to long-term energy demands, acting to shift the metabolic balance to reliance on the more calorific fatty acids over carbohydrates. Similar considerations may apply to the transient changes in GH seen during surgery or after severe trauma; there are reports of more prolonged changes in circulating GH levels several months after severe burns, when it may be speculated that GH is required for a long-term anabolic response (4).

However, when one turns to mental stressors there is again little evidence that GH levels change in a predictable determined fashion. We have also recently found that neither prolactin nor GH changes in response to a cold pressor test, involving a harmless but unpleasant and painful immersion of one hand in ice-cold water for 5 min (5). A most interesting finding in one report demonstrated that serum GH levels rose in response to a mental task (mirror drawing) only in subjects with a given (neurotic) personality, thus suggesting a complex interaction between apparent stressor and neuroendocrine response that is dependent on the interpretation of the stimulus (6). This will be returned to later. Nevertheless, there is no substantiation of the concept that circulating GH levels simply reflect the degree of mental stress.

THYROID-STIMULATING HORMONE

The pituitary-thyroid axis is finely tuned to a given set-point, and is highly sensitive to small fluctuations in circulating thyroid hormones in man. Unlike other species, in humans serum thyroid-stimulating hormone (TSH) is relatively resistant to other external influences, and (at least after the neonatal period), varies little with environmental termperature. The conversion of serum thyroxine (T4) to triiodothyronine (T3) falls wth acute surgery, weight loss, or trauma. Since T3 is the principal intracellular regulator of feedback, the failure of TSH levels to rise in this situation suggests that the TRH-TSH axis has also been reset. It would appear that this "sick euthyroid" syndrome is a rather general response to increased metabolic demand ("illness," trauma) or reduced substrate availability (weight loss), which restrains the basal metabolic rate. This may thereby release metabolic substrates for growth and repair that would otherwise be sequestered in less vital tissues. Acute physical exercise or mental stress has little or no effect on circulating TSH levels (3).

GONADOTROPINS

The gonadotropins, luteinizing hormone (LH), and follicle-stimulating hormone (FSH) are under the predominant control of gonadotrophin-releasing hormone (GnRH), which is released in pulsatile bursts by the hypothalamus. It is uncertain whether there is an additional specific FSH-releasing hormone, or whether the variation in LH/FSH ratio in different conditions is merely a consequence of differential feedback sensitivity to gonadal steroids and inhibin. Although acute changes in physical activity, blood glucose levels, or any form of acute stress have little or no effect on the hypothalamopituitary–gonadal axis, it is clear that certain forms of chronic stress may cause profound inhibition of gonadal function, particularly in women. Thus, "hypothalamic amenorrhea" is a well-recognized clinical entity in which absent menstruation is associated with no elevation in FSH (excluding primary gonadal failure) or prolactin levels, in the presence of a normal uterus. Most such cases show abnormalities in the pulsatile release of the gonadotropins, especially LH, and it is assumed that the rhythmic discharge of the GnRH oscillator has been disrupted. Although in some patients this may occur in association with the assumption of an intense exercise training program, or concomitant with a significant weight loss, in others domestic psychological stress is presumed. Cessation of menses during examinations, college entrance, or a move of residence has been clearly recorded. As will be discussed below, these are often the situations that may lead to defects in active coping, in which the pituitary–adrenal axis is also activated, and animal studies have suggested that activation of central corticotropin-releasing factor (CRF) pathways may directly inhibit GnRH release via an opioid mechanism (see below). Some of these patients may respond clinically to naloxone infusion with a resumption of LH pulsatility (7). An open pilot study of these patients has demonstrated the return of ovulatory menses following treatment with oral naltrexone (8). However, the European experience is that many, if not the majority, of patients with such a diagnosis have a low ponderal index and may represent an occult form of anorexia nervosa. These may include patients who have regained lost weight but whose menses have failed to restart: such patients would not be expected to respond to naloxone infusion (9).

Exercise training is an interesting model of reversible hypothalamic amenorrhea, although its relation to chronic stress must remain highly speculative. Prior (10) has argued that mild conditioning exercise produces regular but anovulatory cycles, as a homeostatic adaptation to the high calorie output. The difference in body fat between the average male and female approximately represents the extra energy required to sustain a normal full-term pregnancy and delivery; consequently, any fall in this percentgage due to regular physical exercise would prejudice reproductive fitness, and it is therefore adaptive to inhibit ovulation at this time. The signal that the organism uses to communicate its body mass index to the GnRH pulse generator remains unclear, but we are currently investigating the roles of insulin, insulin-like growth factor-1 (IGF-1), and the newly described IGF small binding protein, BP-28 (11). A similar signal may also be important in mediating the amenorrhea that occurs during weight loss and prepuberty. Excessive exercise training to an elite standard leads to complete amenorrhea, estrogen deficiency, and the risk of long-term osteoporosis. It is interesting that in these usually professional athletes there is evidence of cortisol hypersecretion, indicating increased activity of the CRF–ACTH axis (12). This suggests that exercise-induced amenorrhea may involve components of both loss of body fat (as in pure weight loss) and CRF overactivity (as in "stress-induced amenorrhea"). It would be of considerable interest to dissect out these two components, since our theoretical analysis suggests that the latter, but not the former, may be opiate-mediated. To date, studies of the effects of naloxone infusions in amenorrheic runners have not clearly taken into account changes in body composition as a confounding feature (13). The crucial studies would require the measurement of the gonadotropin responses to opiate antagonists such as naloxone, naltrexone, or nalmefene in amenorrheic runners with preserved body fat composition, ideally in a prospective fashion. Preliminary data suggest that this specific subgroup may indeed demonstrate an increase in opioid tone (14).

In the primate, stress-induced suppression of GnRH may be reversible with naloxone (15), while administration of high doses of CRF-41 intravenously leads to a naloxone-reversible inhibition of gonadotropin pulsatility (16). There is also direct evidence in favour of CRF-induced suppression of GnRH in the rat (17). This suggests that pathways that may activate central CRF-41 may lead to gonadal suppression, and such pathways may be activated during severe stress. In the human, there is only very indirect evidence that this pathway is operative, as, for example, in exercise-induced amenorrhea as cited above. However, in primate colonies in captivity, the social organization into dominant and subordinate animals offers a further model of stress-induced neuroendocrine regulation. Social suppression of female reproduction is found in many species, being most obvious in marmoset and tamarin monkeys. In these species subordinate females exhibit features suggesting hypothalamic inhibition of GnRH release (18). In gonadectomized subordinate females, naloxone induces a more marked rise in serum LH than in dominant females, indicating that at least part of this suppression is due to an increase in opioid tone (19). It is possible that the subordinate female responds to her situation by activation of central CRF-41 and hence inhibition of GnRH. Unfortunately, we were unable to show any effect of intravenous ovine CRF-41 (40 μg/kg) on LH levels in gonadectomized marmosets (D. Abbott, A. Grossman, unpublished observations, 1989), possibly due to poor central penetration of the peptide. Further studies of considerable interest would include investigations of the differential effect of peripheral and central CRF-41 in other species of dominant and subordinate monkeys, and a study of whether the CRF antagonist alpha helical CRF could disinhibit gonadal suppression in subordinate females. Whatever the findings, subordinate inhibition of gonadal function may again be considered as an adaptive response to a complex environment, in this case adaptive on a group, rather than on an individual, basis (20).

The nature of the opiate receptor modulating GnRH release is uncertain in most species, but in the human we have suggested that its high sensitivity to naloxone indicates a μ- or ϵ-receptor (21). We have also been unable to demonstrate any intervening neuramine, such as norepinephrine, dopamine, or acetylcholine, and this together with rat in vitro data suggests a direct interaction between an endogenous opioid and the GnRH neurone, most probably β-endorphin originating from the human homolog of the arcuate nucleus (22; Fig. 1). In

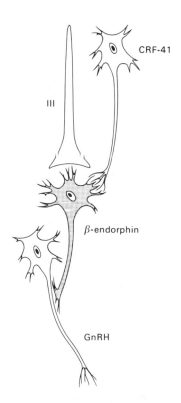

FIGURE 1 Suggested model for the control of GnRH release in the human. GnRH neurons are subject to inhibitory opioid modulation by β-endorphin in the arcuate nucleus, which itself may be stimulated by paraventricular CRF-41.

the rat, there appears to be additional presynaptic modulation of an excitatory noradrenergic input (23).

POSTERIOR PITUITARY

Of the extensive data on the control of vasopressin in humans, there are few suggestions that it may change specifically in response to stress. In the rat, detailed studies by Yagi and his colleagues have demonstrated a differential response of vasopressin to emotional or physical stressors, but this may not necessarily apply to the human situation (24). However, the role of vasopressin in the modulation of adrenocorticotropin release may be more relevant, especially since both peptides are subject to inhibitory opioid regulation (25).

There are even fewer data regarding oxytocin release in the human. Nevertheless, of considerable interest is the finding that birth interval is increased in the parturient rat by "emotional stress," specifically, being placed in a small goldfish bowl: this process is mediated by an opioid-induced suppression of oxytocin release (26). This suggests that certain forms of stress may activate an endogenous opioid system, as for GnRH, although in this instance the endogenous ligand is probably dynorphin rather than β-endorphin (see below).

ADRENOCORTICOTROPIC HORMONE

Cortisol (and corticosterone in the rat) are usually considered the most fundamental stress hormones, and of all the hormones under pituitary control the corticosteroids are the most essential. It is therefore paradoxical that the phsyiological function of the pituitary-adrenal axis is essentially unknown.

Adrenocorticotropic hormone (ACTH) is regulated by a hypothalamic complex of peptides including corticotropin-releasing factor (CRF-41), vasopressin, and at least one other releasing factor, if not more. ACTH-release-inhibiting factors have also been suggested, although not identified. CRF-41 and vasopressin, either coreleased from the same neuron or adjacent terminals, synergize to stimulate the pituitary release of ACTH, which in turn stimulates the adrenal cortex. In the human, there is a free-running circadian rhythm of ACTH of 25 h, which is entrained to the normal 24 h sleep–wake cycle with an acrophase at around 7–8 a.m. Superimposed on this are excursions stimulated by food, exercise, and "stress." Cortisol is one of the counterregulatory responses to hypoglycemia and, like the other endocrine sequelae, it is diabetogenic. However, the defining feature of pituitary-adrenal activity since Selye's time has been its responsiveness to generalized physical and mental stressors.

In an analysis of the effects of mental or psychological stress, many studies have shown that there is a dissociation between corticosteroid and catecholamine release, such that situations eliciting sympathetic activation are not necessarily stressors of the pituitary–adrenal axis. There are also wide interindividual variations, such that responsiveness is as much part of the individual's subjective state as it is a characteristic of the stimulus situation. To rationalize these discordant features, many investigators have embraced the notion of "coping," and have suggested that the defining characteristic of situations associated with corticosteroid release is an actual or projected failure to cope with the apparent threat (27). Thus, while most stressors previously discussed elicit adaptive neuroendocrine and behavioral adaptation, perceived or incipient failure to adapt is associated with a rise in ACTH, and hence cortisol, levels. This concept at once harmonizes otherwise heterogeneous and discrepant data, and emphasizes that it is not the threat per se that is stressful in neuroendocrine terms, but whether the organism considers that it can actively deal with it successfully. It also brings back into play Selye's idea of a general or nonspecific response to stress: most responses to stress are specific and adaptive, but the expectation of a failure to cope may activate a specific neuronal system. Such a system thus reflects the perception of the subjective outcome of a situation rather than the situation itself, that is, it relies upon the interpretation and significance of environmental events. Recent studies in rat and humans suggest that there is a structural and neurochemical substrate for this system.

NEUROTRANSMITTER CONTROL OF ACTH IN HUMANS

There is good evidence for only two classes of neurotransmitters or neuromodulators controlling ACTH in humans: epinephrine and opioid peptides. Early studies in the rat were interpreted as showing an inhibitory adrenergic control of ACTH, but alternative explanations are possible (28). In humans, the specific alpha$_1$-adrenoceptor agonist methoxamine stimulates ACTH and cortisol release, an effect blocked by the alpha$_1$-adrenoceptor antagonist, thymoxamine. Thymoxamine alone slightly but significantly lowers ACTH and cortisol levels during the day and blocks meal-induced rises in ACTH, but has no effect on the circadian rhythm. Since neither epinephrine nor norepinephrine infusions stimulate ACTH, or modify the ACTH response to CRF-41, this adrenoceptor control is apparently regulated at central sites within the blood–brain barrier (28). Under normal circumstances, this control is relatively minor; alpha$_2$-adrenoceptor agonists such as clonidine, which depress adrenergic throughput, cause little or no change in serum cortisol (29). In similar fashion, alpha$_2$-adrenoceptor antagonists such as yohimbine, or the more specific idazoxan, reveal little basal "tone" (30). However, we have suggested that stress-induced activation of the pituitary–adrenal axis is due to an increase in this adrenergic throughput, and indeed the small perturbations in cortisol levels seen in ambulant subjects are lower when they are continuously infused with thymoxamine. There is also evidence in

humans that this adrenergic pathway interacts with an inhibitory opioid regulation. Exogenous opioids and opiates suppress ACTH release at naloxone-insensi-
tive receptors, while high (but not low) doses of naloxone elevate ACTH and
cortisol in normal subjects (21). The naloxone-induced rise in cortisol is blocked
by thymoxamine (31), which suggests that the adrenoceptor control is subject
to opioid inhibition (Fig. 2). If this model is valid, we would predict that naloxone would increase noradrenergic throughput, thereby activating presynaptic
alpha$_2$-adrenoceptors and allowing alpha$_2$-antagonists to elevate cortisol. This
interaction has indeed been proven for both yohimbine (32) and, more recently,
for idazoxan (32a).

A further prediction is that clonidine should attenuate naloxone-induced
cortisol release, but this remains to be validated. Relatively high doses of naloxone are required to demonstrate these changes, 5-20 times greater than are

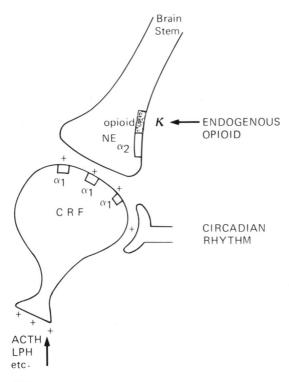

FIGURE 2 Suggested model for the control of ACTH release in humans. An
excitatory noradrenergic input (NE) to corticotropin-releasing factor(s) is
subject to α_2-adrenoceptor presynaptic inhibition, and inhibitory modulation by
an endogenous opioid acting at κ-receptors.

conventionally required to block classic μ-opiate receptors. Since the so-called κ-receptors show a similar order of sensitivity to naloxone, and such receptors are found in high concentrations in human brain, particularly the hypothalamus (33), we would further postulate that endogenous opioids modulate the adrenergic control of ACTH at central κ-receptors.

The precise site(s) of these interactions remains problematic. In the rat, noradrenergic input to CRF neurons in the paraventricular nucleus originates from brain-stem nuclei, principally in the ventral medulla and nucleus tractus solitarius (NTS) in addition to adrenergic inputs. Opiate receptors are present at high concentrations in both the hypothalamus and NTS. Our rat in vitro studies have demonstrated a direct noradrenergic stimulation of CRF-41 release at beta-adrenoceptors (34), although others have apparently shown alpha-adrenoceptor stimulation (35); the reasons for these discrepancies are not obvious. The locus of action of opiates is likewise the subject of discussion. We and others have shown that opioids and opiates block the pituitary ACTH response to exogenous CRF-41 in humans (36), but in the rat no direct effect of opioids on the pituitary release of ACTH has generally been reported; we have also recently found that morphine inhibits stimulated CRF-41 release in vitro (37; Fig. 3). Opioids may act centrally to inhibit the release of both CRF-41 and another part of the CRF complex, such as vasopressin. A crucial experiment, the effect of morphine on ACTH release to CRF-41 and vasopressin in combination, has yet to be carried out, but we are currently investigating the effect of an opioid on the central stimulation of cortisol release with the adrenergic agonist methoxamine.

In summary, in rat and humans there is a potent noradrenergic input to CRF neurons in the hypothalamus, which is apparently stimulatory, although the relative role of alpha- and beta-adrenoceptors remains problematic. Evidence in the human favors an inhibitory opioid modulation of this input, but in the rat current data suggest a direct possibly postsynaptic opioid control of CRF-41 neurons. However, the fact that CRF-41 is only one part of the CRF-complex, and that results dependent on CRF bioassays are often discordant with CRF-41 measurements, must always be born in mind. As discussed above for GnRH, there may be opioid modulation of CRF release at the level of both the presynaptic noradrenergic input and the CRF neuron itself.

No other putative neuroregulators have been as extensively investigated in humans, and those that have been studied have generally given inconsistent results. We have recently reinvestigated the effect of the cholinesterase inhibitor, pyridostigmine, and found that the cholinergic pathway is unlikely to be a major determinant of ACTH release (37a). Modulation of dopamine pathways is also without effect.

Sodium vlaproate, a gamma-aminobutyric acid (GABA)-transaminase inhibitor, does not affect pituitary-adrenal function in normal subjects under basal

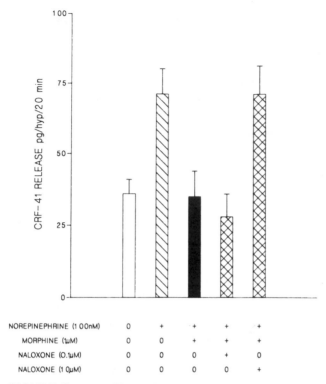

NOREPINEPHRINE (1 OOnM)	0	+	+	+	+
MORPHINE (1μM)	0	0	+	+	+
NALOXONE (O.1μM)	0	0	0	+	0
NALOXONE (1 OμM)	0	0	0	0	+

FIGURE 3 The effect of morphine on the release of CRF-41 from rat hypothalami incubated in vitro. After a period of stabilization, fresh rat hypothalami
were incubated in the presence of various agents for 20 min periods, and the
effects of the agents were compared to parallel control vials. It is apparent that
CRF-41 release is stimulated by norepinephrine, and that this stimulation is
suppressed by morphine. The effect of morphine is itself blocked by a high dose
of naloxone (Ref 37).

conditions (28). Serotoninergic pathways have been implicated in the circadian
rhythmicity of ACTH release in the rat, but the absence until recently of serotonin agonists and antagonists specific for receptor subtypes has hampered
research in humans. Oxytocin and somatostatin have been suggested to inhibit
ACTH release, but we have been unable to demonstrate a direct effect of somatostatin on the corticotroph (39). However, the ACTH response to CRF-41 is
blocked by oxytocin, which suggests that this peptide may act in an opposing
manner to vasopressin in the human (39a).

STRUCTURAL MODEL OF STRESS-INDUCED ACTH
RELEASE

Probably one of the most important recent discoveries in stress research has
been the finding that CRF-41 caused profound behavioral and cardiovascular

changes in the rat when given centrally. These changes were consistent with a response to an acute "stressful" situation. This in turn suggested that there might be a structural system based on CRF-41 as the neuroregulatory peptide that subserved all of the acute changes apparent whenever coping ability was compromised. Various forms of mental illness in the human are also characterized by stress-induced breakdown in adaptation, and it is therefore of considerable interest that many patients with depressive illness have evidence of a hyperactive hypothalamopituitary–adrenal axis, and elevated levels of CRF-41 in their cerebrospinal fluid (CSF) (40). Is it possible to construct a provisional neural model of this process?

Computer-based models of the central nervous system (CNS) are now widespread, although there is no a priori reason for the brain to work in an identical fashion to a digital computer; indeed, the basic unit of the brain is the neuron, which is in no way comparable to a solid-state circuit, and may in some ways be cosidered to be an analog computer itself. However, the conceptual language of computer-derived information processing is clearly applicable to any system in which information is stored and used; an analysis based on concepts of information flow, access, and retrieval may be of great utility in understanding the CNS. These concepts have certainly been fruitfully applied to the brain, in particular, to obviously structured regions such as the cerebellum and hippocampus. The former is essentially a machine for generating smooth physical skills, but the hippocampus has proved more resistant to analysis. There is evidence that it may in some circumstances be considered a mental map of the environment, as first suggested by O'Keefe and Nadel (41). However, our thinking regarding brain structures suffers from rigid compartmentalization into perception, cognition, emotion, and other categories, and it is difficult to ascribe a purely cognitive function to a structure that is clearly part of the emotive–motivational limbic system. Gray and Rawlins (42) have clearly combined these various concepts into their idea that the septohippocampal complex acts as a "comparator" for actual and expected events, activating a behavioral inhibition sequence when there is a "mismatch." This implies that in moving through its environment the organism must compare what it actually experiences with what its previous experience (memories, engrams, neural networks widely disseminated in the neocortex) suggests should come next: it is simplest to consider this in spatial terms, but it can clearly include expectations of social behavior, intended outcome, and so on. The mismatch is then a frustrated expectation that requires the animal to stop and reattend in detail to its immediate surroundings. This checking program proceeds at a rate set by the intrinsic theta rhythm, which is approximately 3–12 times/s. As long as expectation fits with reality, the behavioral program is set by the master plans set down by the frontal cortex (43).

We can combine this model with the CRF concept by postulating that frustrated expectation with no obvious solution, especially when assessed by the organism as being highly significant to its integrity (a function tentatively ascribed to the amygdaloid complex), will activate the CRF complex in the hypothalamic nucleus. This in turn causes sympathoadrenal activation via descending pathways to the locus coeruleus/nucleus tractus solitarius (NTS), increased pituitary–adrenal activity, and behavioral orientation and exploration. As we have discussed, the brainstem noradrenergic nuclei have stimulatory inputs to paraventricular CRF neurons, and may thus "feed forward" to amplify these effects. The ascending diffuse projections from these nuclei to other areas may bias these areas towards attention and behavioral inhibition: in other words, they do not "contain" specific localizing or perceptual information, but sharpen the importance (or increase the signal-to-noise ratio) of the currently attended stimulus. If left to itself, this system will lead to a continuous checking of the environment and a stultification of behavior, similar to patterns seen in patients with free-floating anxiety states and obsessive–compulsive disorders. Gray suggests that the principal therapeutic effect of GABA-enhancing drugs, such as the benzodiazepines, is to block the noradrenergic input to the septohippocampal system, allowing behavior to continue. Unfortunately, this also prevents the individual from learning to cope with the situation such that the development of new coping stratagems deteriorates. I would further suggest that there is a neuronal system that can interpolate into the noradrenergic–CRF–septohippocampal system to damp down or extinguish the feed forward loops and reestablish equilibrium: this is the endogenous opioid network, possibly based on the "reward" areas of the nucleus accumbens. These are either tonically active, as for the pituitary–adrenal axis, or phasically activated during any stressor of the sympathoadrenomedullary system, and counterregulate overactivity in the stress system. Inadequate control leads to excessive frequent excursions in the basic stress axis, while too much control inhibits exploration and the learning of new coping behavior.

Studies of the sympathoadrenomedullary system are fully in agreement with these concepts. Opioids suppress the release of catecholamines basally, and are particularly potent inhibitors of stress-induced catecholamine release, but naloxone has little or no effect on the basal release of epinephrine or norepinephrine (44). However, the stimulated release of epinephrine by hypoglycemia, acute exercise, isometric hand-grip, or the cold pressor test is greatly enhanced by naloxone, with a smaller potentiation of norepinephrine by the more intense stimuli. Only high doses of naloxone are effective (5; Fig. 4), which suggests that the opiate receptors involved are similar to those modulating the pituitary–adrenal axis. Most recently, we have shown that this opioid tone can also be demonstrated in response to a mental stress (44a; Fig. 5). Thus, the endogenous opioids are again involved in attenuating stress hormone responses, but only when the system is activated. The site of this control in humans is presently unknown, but may include both central (NTS) and peripheral (adrenal medulla)

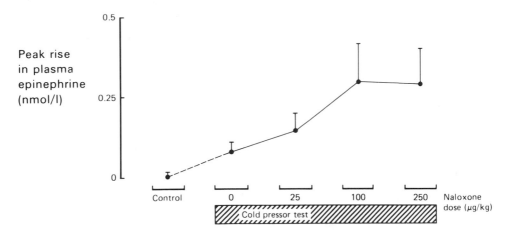

FIGURE 4 The mean peak rise (± SEM) in plasma epinephrine in response to a cold pressor test (5 min immersion of hand in ice-cold water) in eight normal subjects, in the presence of different dosages of naloxone. The rise in epinephrine is potentiated only by the two higher dosages of naloxone: 100 μg/kg and 250 μg/kg (P. Bouloux, A. Grossman, unpublished observations).

loci. It may not be too fanciful to speculate that the induction of opioid counterregulation is reinforcing for too much risk-taking and sympathetic-stimulating behavior. The converse is that an absence of opioid control may predispose to hypertension and ischemic heart disease, since the oscillations in adrenomedullary activity are transmitted in full to the cardiovascular system. In primate models, recurrent emotional stress leads to more labile cardiovascular control, which may in turn increase the rate of formation of atheromatous plaques (15).

If cortisol is ultimately secreted in response to incipient noncoping, what might its function be? High concentrations of corticosteroid receptors are found in the CNS, especially in the hippocampus, and it is the present contention that the principal target for stress-induced cortisol release is the hippocampus. Neuronal networks may produce acute effects of short duration, while a bolus of cortisol may prolong the septohippocampal behavioral inhibition for several hours, acting to keep the organism temporarily more alert to the significance of its environment. Permanently high levels of circulating corticosteroids may generate an exhausting state of continuous alertness and inappropriate ascription of significance, such as may be seen in the paranoia of patients with Cushing's syndrome. Several groups have demonstrated the presence of two types of

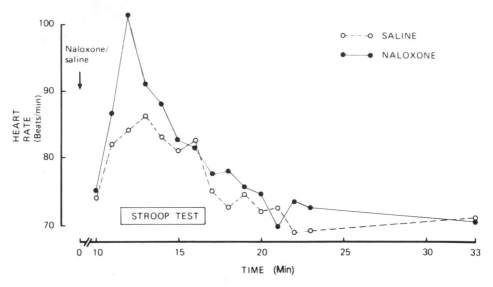

FIGURE 5 Change in mean heart rate in response to a stressful mental task (Stroop test) in eight normal subjects in the presence of saline or 8 mg naloxone. The rise in heart rate was significantly enhanced when naloxone was given (Ref 44a).

corticosteroid receptor in the brain, type 1 or CR, which are particularly prevalent in the septohippocampal complex and are extensively occupied under basal conditions; and a more widespread type 2, or GR, of much lower affinity and occupance (46,47). We would agree that type 2 receptors probably mediate feedback inhibition at high levels of stress-induced arousal, but would argue that the type 1 receptors are not just tonically activated at a plateau level. These receptors are highly sensitive to small fluctuations in corticosteroid levels and are thus ideally situated to amplify hippocampal responses to situational uncertainty. Opioids may antagonize this interaction, while corticoids may block opioid-induced analgesia. These speculations may be tested by assessing the behavioral effects of clamping corticosteroids at different absolute levels, in the face of differing degrees of stress.

In the periphery, corticosteroids have widespread effects, the predominant physiological as well as pharmacological change being a profound suppression of the immune system. It has been suggested that this suppression is to prevent an overexuberant response to exogenous stress stimuli (48), but we would inerpret the data instead as suggesting that in the face of a severe physical stress, vascular volume must be maintained at all costs. The multiple minor and local monocyte-mediated changes in vascular permeability become subsidiary to maintaining vascular integrity, and thus the formation of most immune-derived peptides is inhibited. There must therefore be information flow between the immune and neuroendocrine axes, and recent reports have demonstrated that monocyte-derived interleukin-1 activates the pituitary-adrenal axis: we have shown that this is due to direct activation of CRF-41 release by this peptide (49). Again, an endogenous opioid system is also activated, and this may be the true counterregulatory antistress system postulated by Munck et al. (48).

Thus, it is suggested that a CRF-centered system is activated in the face of stress, particularly when there is the triple burden of unpredictability in a physiologically significant situation where no obvious coping stratagem is apparent (50), that is, in the presence of a threatening challenge. This interacts with brainstem noradrenergic pathways and circulating corticosteroids and eventually self-terminates, possibly with the aid of endogenous opioids. Although adrenocortical activation signals this coping failure, it is also part of the means by which homeostasis is reobtained. Stress-seeking behavior may be a characteristic of individuals who require to be pushed to their limits, being rewarded by their endogenous opioids, but in human terms they may also achieve more. Unfortunately, damage to the cardiovascular and immune systems by such continual adrenocortical and adrenomedullary stimulation may involve a high personal cost.

CONCLUSIONS

Stress is a multifaceted concept that implies harmful interactions with the environment, whereas the majority of responses to situational change are homeostatic and adaptive. However, where coping appears to be compromised, pituitary-adrenal activation occurs simultaneously with the emergence of a finely tuned CRF-dominated system to establish and deal with the situation. Part of this response may include an endorphin-mediated suppression of gonadal function. Chronic hypersecretion of cortisol is clearly pathogenic, but in the short term it may increase attention and aid survival. Feed-forward loops connecting the septohippocampal system with brainstem noradrenergic centers and the pituitary-adrenal axis ultimately require counterregulation, and it is suggested that a network of endogenous opioids supplies this function. These are probably of the dynorphin rather than the endorphin family. Long-term overactivity in these networks, possibly in association with a defect in endogenous opioid control, may be associated with severe psychopathology, as in depressive illness and chronic anxiety states. While this theory is certainly incorrect in many, or even most, details, it is hoped that it can be used to generate experimental predictions which can then be subjected to attempted falsification as we grope towards a more precise understanding of the neuroendocrine mechanisms of stress.

ACKNOWLEDGMENTS

I am most grateful to Miss Alison Platts for secretarial assistance.

REFERENCES

1. Hjemdahl P, Freyschuss U, Juhlin-Dannfelt A, Linde B. Differential sympathetic activation during mental stress evoked by the Stroop test. Acta Physiol Scand (Suppl) 1984; 527: 25–29.
2. Brooks J E, Herbert M, Walder C P, Selby C, Jeffocate W J. Prolactin and stress: some endocrine correlates of pre-operative anxiety. Clin Endocrinol 1986; 24: 653–656.
3. Delitala G, Tomasi P, Virdis R. Prolactin, growth hormone and thyrotrophin-thyroid hormone secretion during stress states in man. In: Grossman A, ed. Baillieres clinical endocrinology and metabolism. vol. 1, no. 2. Neuroendocrinology of stress. London: Bailliere Tindall, 1987: 391–414.
4. Frayn K N. Hormonal control of metabolism in trauma and sepsis. Clin Endocrinol 1986; 24: 577–599.
5. Bouloux P M G, Newbould E, Causon R, et al. The differential effect of high-dose naloxone on the plasma adrenaline response to the cold pressor test. Clin Sci 1989; 76: 625–630.
6. Miyabo S, Asato T, Mizushima N. Prolactin and growth hormone responses to psychological stress. J Clin Endocrinol Metab 1977; 44: 947–951.
7. Khoury S E, Reame N E, Kelch R P, Marshall J C. Diurnal patterns of pulsatile luteinizing hormone secretion in hypothalamic amenorrhoea: reproductivity and responses to opiate blockade and an a_2-adrenergic agonist. J Clin Endocrinol Metab 1987; 64: 755–762.
8. Wildt L, Leyendecker G. Induction of ovulation by the chronic administration of naltrexone in hypothalamic amenorrhoea. J Clin Endocrinol Metab 1987; 64: 1334–1335.
9. Grossman A, Moult P J A, McIntyre H, et al. Opiate mediation of amenorrhoea in hyperprolactinaemia and in weight loss-related amenorrhoea. Clin Endocrinol 1982; 17: 379–388.
10. Prior J C. Physical exercise and the neuroendocrine control of reproduction. In: Grossman A, ed. Baillieres clinical endocrinology and metabolism, vol 1, no 2. Neuroendocrinology of stress. London: Bailliere Tindall, 1987; 299–317.
11. Grossman A. Exercise and the GnRH pulse generator. In Progress in Endocrinology 1988. Amsterdam: Elsevier Science, 1989: 441–448.
12. Ding J-H, Scheckter C B, Drinkwater B L, Soules M R, Bremner W J. High serum cortisol levels in exercise-associated amenorrhea. Ann Int Med 1988; 108: 530–534.

13. Dixon G, Eurman P, Stern B E, Schwartz B, Rebar R W. Hypothalamic function in amenorrheic runners. Fertil Steril 1984; 42: 377–383.
14. Pehrson J. Nalmefene alters LH pulsatility in women runners. Abstract 907, presented at 69th Annual Meeting of the Endocrine Society, Indianopolis, June 10-12, 1987.
15. Sapolsky R M, Krey L C. Stress-induced suppression of luteinizing hormone concentrations in wild baboons: role of opiates. J Clin Endocrinol Metab 1988; 66: 722–726.
16. Gindoff P R, Ferin M. Endogenous opioid peptides modulate the effect of corticotrophin-releasing factor on gonadotrophin release in the primate. Endocrinology 1988; 121: 837–842.
17. Rivier C, Rivier J, Vale W. Stress-induced inhibition of reproductive functions: role of endogenous corticotrophin-releasing factor. Science 1986; 231: 607–610.
18. Abbott D H. Behaviourally mediated suppression of reproduction in female primates. J Zool Lond 1987; 213: 455–470.
19. Abbott D H, Barrett J, Faulkes C G, George L M. Social contraception in naked mole rats and marmoset monkeys. J Zool Lond 1989; 219: 703–710.
20. Herbert J. Neuroendocrine responses to social stress. In: Grossman A, ed. Ballieres clinical endocrinology and metabolism, vol 1, no 2. Neuroendocrinology of stress. London: Balliere Tindall, 1987: 467–490.
21. Grossman A, Moult P J A, Cunnah D, Besser G M. Different opioid mechanisms are involved in the modulation of gonadotrophin and ACTH release in man. Neuroendocrinology 1986; 42: 357–360.
22. Grossman A. Opioid peptides and reproductive function. In: Lobo RA, ed. Seminars in reproductive endocrinology, vol 5, no 2. New York: Thieme Medical Publishers, 1987: 115–124.
23. Karla S P, Simpkins J W. Evidence for noradrenergic mediation of opioid effects on luteinizing hormone secretion. Endocrinology 1981; 109: 776–782.
24. Onaka T, Yagi K, Hamamura M. Vasopressin: physical stress potentiates but emotional stress suppresses its secretion. In: Imura H, ed. Neuroendocrine control of the hypothalamic–pituitary system. Kyoto; Japanese Scientific Societies Press/Karger, 1988: 213–225.
25. Leng G, Mansfield S, Bicknell R J, et al. Stress-induced disruption of parturition in the rat may be mediated by endogenous opioids. J Endocrinol 1987; 114: 247–252.
26. Grossman A, Besser G M, Milles J J, Baylis P H. Inhibition of vasopressin release by an opiate peptide in man. Lancet 1980; 2: 1108–1109.
27. Mason J W. A review of psychoendocrine research on the pituitary-adrenal cortical system. Psychosom Med 1968; 30: 576–607.
28. Al-Damluji S. Adrenergic mechanisms in the control of corticotrophin secretion. J Endocrinol 1988; 119: 5-14.
29. Grossman A, Weerasuriya K, Al-Dmaluji S, Turner P, Besser G M. Alpha$_2$-adrenoceptor agonists stimulate growth hormone secretion, but have no acute effects on plasma cortisol under basal conditions. Horm Res 1987; 25: 65-71.

30. Bouloux P M G, Grossman A, Allolio B, Delitala G, Besser G M. Effects of adrenergic antagonism on the growth hormone, prolactin and cortisol response to a synthetic opioid agonist in man. Horm Res 1986; 23: 83–90.

31. Grossman A, Besser G M. Opiates control ACTH through a noradrenergic mechanism. Clin Endocrinol 1982; 17: 287–290.

32. Charney D S, Henninger G R. α_2-Adrenergic and opiate receptor blockade. Arch Gen Psychiatry 1986; 43: 1037–1041.

32a. Al-Damluji S, Bouloux P, White A, Besser M. The role of alpha-2-adrenoceptors in the control of ACTH secretion; interaction with the opioid system. Neuroendocrinology 1990; 51: 76–81.

33. Pfeiffer A, Pasi A, Mehraien P, Herz A. Opiate receptor binding sites in human brain. Brain Res 1982; 348: 87–96.

34. Tsagarakis S, Holly J M P, Rees L H, Besser G M, Grossman A. Acetylcholine and norepinephrine stimulate CRF-41 release from rat hypothalamus in vitro. Endocrinology 1988; 123: 1962–1969.

35. Calogero A E, Gallucci W T, Chrousos G P, Gold P W. Catecholamine effects upon rat hypothalamic corticotrophin-releasing hormone secretion in vitro. J Clin Invest 1988; 82: 839–846.

36. Grossman A, Delitala G, Coy D H, Manelli M, Al-Damluji S, Besser G M. An analogue of met-enkaphalin attenuates the pituitary-adrenal response to ovine corticotrophin releasing factor. Clin Endocrinol 1986; 25: 421–426.

37. Tsagarakis S, Navara P, Rees L H, Besser G M, Grossman A. Morphine directly modulates the release of corticotrophin releasing factor-41 from rat hypothalamus in vitro. Endocrinology 1989; 124: 2330–2335.

37a. Freeman E, Touzel R, Grossman A, Besser M, Ross R. Pyridostigmine, an acetylcholinesterase inhibitor, stimulates ACTH levels, or on the TSH response to TRH. J Neuroendocrinology 1990 (in press).

38. Abraham R R, Dornhorst A, Wynn V, et al. Corticotrophin, cortisol, prolactin and growth hormone responses to insulin-induced hypoglycaemia in normal subjects given sodium valproate. Clin Endocrinol 1985 22: 639–644.

39. Stafford P, Kopelman P, Davidson K, et al. The pituitary-adrenal response to CRF-41 is unaltered by intravenous somatostatin in normal subjects. Clin Endocrinol 1989; 30: 661–666.

39a. Page SR, Ang VTY, Jackson R, et al. The effect of oxytocin infusion on adenohypophyseal function in man. Clin Endocrinol 1990; 32: 307–313.

40. Nemeroff C B, Widerlov E, Bissette G, et al. Elevated concentrations of CSF corticotrophin-releasing factor-like immunoreactivity in depressed patients. Science 1984; 226: 1342–1344.

41. O'Keefe J, Nadel L. The hippocampus as a cognitive map. London: Oxford University Press, 1978.

42. Gray J A, Rawlins J N P. Comparator and buffer memory: an attempt to integrate two models of hippocampus function. In: Isaacson RL, Pribram KH, eds. The hippocampus, vol 4. New York: Plenum Press, 1986: 159–201.

43. Miller G A, Galanter E, Pribram K H. Plans and the structure of behaviour. New York: Holt Rhinehart and Winston, 1960.

44. Bouloux P M G, Grossman A, Lytras N, Besser G M. Evidence for the participation of endogenous opioids in the sympathoadrenal response to hypoglycaemia in man. Clin Endocrinol 1985; 22: 49–56.

44a. Morris M, Salmon P, Steinberg H, et al. Endogenous opioids modulate the cardiovascular response to mental stress. Psychoneuroendocrinology 1990 (in press).

45. Manuck S B, Kaplan J R, Adams M R, Clarkson T B. Effects of stress and the sympathetic nervous system on coronary artery atherosclerosis in the cynomolgus macaque. Am Heart J 1988; 116:328–333.

46. De Kloet E R, Reul J M H M. Feedback action and tonic influence of corticosteroids on brain function: a concept arising from the heterogeneity of brain receptor systems. Psychoneuroendocrinology 1987; 12: 83–105.

47. Funder J W, Sheppard K. Adrenocortical steroids and the brain. Annu Rev Physiol 1987; 49: 397–411.

48. Munck A, Guyre P M, Holbrook N J. Physiological functions of glucocorticoids in stress and their relation to pharmacological actions. Endocr Rev 1987; 5: 25–44.

49. Tsagarakis S, Gillies G, Rees, L H, Besser G M, Grossman A. Interleukin-1 directly stimulates the release of corticotrophin releasing factor from rat hypothalamus. Neuroendocrinology 1989; 49: 98–101.

50. Rose R M. Endocrine responses to stressful psychological events. Psychiatr Clin North Am 1980; 3(2): 251–276.

9

REGULATION OF ADRENOCORTICAL FUNCTION FOLLOWING STRESS

Mary F. Dallman

University of California School of Medicine, San Francisco, California

Three major factors influence function in the adrenocortical system: stress, the circadian rhythm, and glucocorticoid feedback. Inhibitory feedback clearly interacts with the stimulatory effects of stress and the circadian rhythm, and, possibly through feedback, the two stimulatory effects interact as well; therefore all three factors must be considered when one is attempting to understand the regulation of adrenocortical function following stress.

In this chapter, stress is used in the restricted and dissatisfyingly circular sense as "any stimulus other than the circadian input to basal activity that excites increased activity in the adrenocortical system." It remains difficult to predict which stimuli will activate increased activity in the adrenocortical system, particularly for nonnoxious stimuli.

The chapter is organized into discussions of adrenocortical control after imposition of acute stress and chronic stress. A final section suggests some physiological consequences of glucocorticoid responses to stress.

ACUTE STRESS

What Is It?

State-Dependent Modulation of Stress Responses

Levine and his coworkers have shown elegantly that alterations in the expected schedule of food reinforcement may serve to stress rats (1), and that provision of behavioral outlets to rats that are exposed to stress may reduce the magnitude of, or abolish, adrenocortical responses (2). Thus, whether a given manipulation serves as a stress is determined by the context in which it is presented. In the latter instance, it was shown that rats allowed to fight during a period of foot shock exhibited a marked reduction in the magnitude of the adrenocorticotropic hormone (ACTH) response to the shock paradigm (2). It seems clear in this case that foot-shock constitutes a stress, but that other modulatory neural inputs can damp or extinguish the input to the final common motor output of the adrenocortical system, the corticotropin-releasing factor (CRF) neuron. The neurochemistry and anatomy of such inputs to stress pathways are unknown.

In what may be a similar vein, de Wied et al. (3) and Smelik (4) showed in the 1960s, and we confirmed subsequently (5), that surgical removal of the neurointermediate lobe of the pituitary or provision of 2.5% NaCl as the only source of drinking fluid to rats for at least 5 days produced a novel constellation of effects on adrenocortical system activity and responsiveness to stress. Such rats exhibit a mild increase in basal ACTH and corticosterone concentrations at the trough of the circadian rhythm, responses of normal magnitude to the stimuli of hemorrhage and hypoglycemia, but markedly reduced to no responses to the stimuli of noise, strange environment, or mild heat stress. Treatment of the animals with vasopressin, or with a synthetic vasopressin (V_1) agonist restored the capacity of the neurolobectomized rats to respond to noise stress (Fagin, Verbalis, Dallman, unpublished results 1984). These results suggest strongly that abnormal activity in AVP neurons (induced either by marked salt overloading or by neurointermediate lobectomy) results in inhibition of *specific* stress responses while others are normal in rats. Again, the chemistry and neuroanatomy of such pathways is unknown, although Plotsky has shown that AVP-infused intracerebroventricularly (ICV) inhibits secretion of CRF into the pituitary–portal blood (6).

Noxious Stimuli: Variation From an Internally Defended Set Point?

In contrast to the above examples, acute systemic stresses, such as hemorrhage, hypotension, hypoxemia, or hypoglycemia, or tissue damage by surgery, broken bones, or burns, excite CRFs and ACTH secretion through neural pathways to CRF neurons which are gradually becoming clear. Adrenocortical system responses to burns (7), leg break (8), and surgery (9) are blocked by blocking neural input from the site of damage to the CNS, which shows that the signals are transmitted neurally. In similar fashion, the responses to hemorrhage (10) and hypoxia (11) are blocked by denervation of peripheral baroreceptors and chemoreceptors, which shows that the stimuli are transmitted to CRF neurons through activation of afferents in cranial nerves 9 and 10.

In the case of hemorrhage, Gann and his co-workers have shown that there are electrically responsive, parallel oligosynaptic pathways from the first central synapse in the nucleus of the tractus solitarius to the hypothalamus (10), which includes catecholaminergic cells. Furthermore, with the use of electrochemical detection of catecholamines in situ, norepinephrine secretion in the PVN has been shown to increase during hemorrhage in cats (12). Injection of an alpha-adrenoceptor blocker prior to hypotension blocks the CRF and AVP secretion that normally occurs in rats (13). Therefore, with the stimuli of hemorrhage and hypotension studied under conditions of deep surgical anesthesia, there begins to be considerable information on both the anatomy and the chemistry of the neural pathways that ascend to CRF neurons to mediate the motor response of the adrenocortical system. None of these studies has yet determined the precise neural route(s) taken by stress-induced inputs to CRF secretion, nor has any detemined what structures, in addition to the CRF neurons, might be activated by hemorrhage and act to modulate the response during or after imposition of the stress.

Hypoglycemia is another stress that is used clinically to test neuroendocrine control systems as well as experimentally to decipher neuroendocrine control systems (14). Hypoglycemia alters activity in a multitude of endocrine systems, and appears to act on the hypothalamus to do so. Recently Widmaier et al. (15) have shown that the concentration of glucose in the medium bathing hypothalamic fragments has a marked effect on the secretion rate of CRF. High glucose concentrations inhibited basal CRF secretion, whereas low glucose levels had the converse effect. The effect of glucose was specific to CRF secretion and gonadotropin-releasing hormone (GnRH) and AVP secretion were unchanged. This result shows that hypothalamic glucose sensor activity affects CRF secretion; however, it is not yet clear whether the effect of low glucose is exerted at the CRFs neurons or a more distant site.

Mechanical and Neurotoxin Lesions and Acute Stress

An increasing number of studies has been performed using either mechanical or neurotoxin lesions to study the effect of these on basal and stress-induced adrenocortical activity. Destruction of the ventral noradrenergic bundle using either electrolytic, mechanical, or 6OH-dopamine (6OH-DA) injections results in decreased activity in the adrenocortical system at the circadian peak and after a variety of stresses (16). It seems likely, therefore, that at least some of the noradrenergic input to the system provides an overall tone to, rather than mediating specific, responses of the system. It is probable that the noradrenergic input to the hypothalamus that appears to increase responsiveness in the adrenocortical system is not solely to the CRFs cells in the paraventricular nuclei (PVN), since Assenmacher et al. (17) have shown a greater decrease in ether-induced CRF and ACTH levels after 6OH-DA lesions of the ventral noradrenergic bundle than after injections of 6OH-DA directly into the PVN; although the degree of catecholamine depletion in the PVN was similar after the two lesions.

In a series of studies (18), Feldman and his colleagues have defined lesions that prevent stimulation by a variety of sensory inputs from activating the ACS. The sites of effective lesions are stimulus dependent, suggesting a variety of input pathways to CRF neurons that excite the stress responses.

CRF Neuronal Responses and Secretion

By recording activity of parvocellular cells in PVN, Saphier et al. have shown graded increases in activity from cells coupled to graded increases in stimulation of peripheral nerves or central sites, and has shown that this is inhibited by treatment with corticosterone (19,20). He has not yet identified the cells as CRF-containing, nor is it clear that corticosterone acts directly at the CRF cells in PVN to reduce the responses of these cells to incoming information.

It is clear that a variety of CRFs in different proportions are secreted in response to stress when measured in rats that are anesthetized and acutely prepared for normal responsiveness in the system; the results of immunoneutralization experiments have uniformly revealed that when the action of CRF is damped, the ACS response is also damped. AVP appears to be the other important CRF, and changes in AVP secretion may, in some instances, determine whether a response occurs in this rat preparation. The problem with the preparation is that it is acutely stressed, and thus data are obtained on a background of stimulated activity in the system, a condition that is very different from basal (see below). Tilders and co-workers (22) have devised a system in which small injections of colchicine are made into the 3rd ventricle a few hours prior to stress; they make a reasonable case that the disappearance rates of CRF and AVP from the external layer of the median eminence under these conditions represents the secretion rates of the peptides. Although this approach to the system obviates the acute anesthetic and stress of preparation of the animal for portal blood collection, the preparation has experienced a stress within the preceding 6 h, which has been shown previously to alter the response characteristics of the system (23).

We need to learn a great deal more about the way acute stresses stimulate motor components of the ACS and the way that the state of the animal can modulate the incoming information to the CRF neuron. To date, no single pathway to CRF cells has been implicated as essential for stress-induced activity of the system. Moreover, in attempts to determine what is occurring at the central motor neurons (PVN) of the system, we are confronted with a Heisenberg type of uncertainty problem because it seems clear that preparation of the animal within a few hours of sampling will alter the properties, and perhaps the responses, of the system from normal. It seems likely that we can learn, on a very basic level, the neurochemistry and anatomy of the system by continuing to use the current approaches; however, it is not likely that we will learn how the system really works by continuing to apply these markedly interventional and crude approaches. Another, major problem with the current approaches to measurement of CRFs is the time scale required for the measurement. We are currently limited to collection periods of 15–30 min for measurements of RFs; however, a great deal of important information is lost by these slow collection periods.

What Is Its Effect on Subsequent Control?

What Determines the Magnitude and Duration of ACTH Secretion after Onset of a Stress?

In otherwise normal, conscious animals initial ACTH secretion is proportional to stimulus intensity for the stimuli of hemorrhage, hypotension, hypoxia, electric shock, and hypoglycemia. This may not be so for ACTH secretion induced by hemorrhage in anesthetized rats (24). In general, the duration of ACTH responses appears to be determined by the duration of the stimulus, largely independent of acute corticosteroid responses. The duration of the responses depends on the prior corticosteroid history of the animal. The magnitude of the response appears to be modulated by both acute and chronic corticosteroid secretion.

Rapid Feedback Effects

These are best observed by comparing the effects of bilateral adrenalectomy with those of the sham operation. Within 15–30 min of bilateral adrenalectomy and loss of corticosterone, ACTH secretion is elevated above that in the sham-adrenalectomized group, and is returned to near normal by injection of corticosterone at the time of surgery (25). The sites at which corticosterone acts to inhibit stress-induced ACTH secretion are both brain and pituitary; the magnitude of the inhibition is 50% or less (26).

Intermediate Feedback Effects

These occur within 2–12 h of stress and may be of greater magnitude than the rapid effects. Synthetic or natural corticosteroids, or ACTH infused within 2–8 h prior to stress, have been shown to inhibit responses in proportion to the stimulus intensity and the quantity of steroids administered. In dogs, prior stress has been shown to inhibit the ACTH response to subsequent stress in proportion to the degree of prior stress-induced corticosteroid secretion (27). This effect is not observed in rats unless the stress has been intense and has depleted pituitary stores of ACTH. In rats, prior stress appears to facilitate subsequent stress responses, apparently nullifying the feedback effect of corticosterone secreted in response to the first stress. However, in rats, stress presented 6 h before the circadian rise in adrenocortical activity has been shown to inhibit the magnitude of that rise, as does injection of corticosterone in amounts calculated to match the response to stress (28). A similar phenomenon occurs in humans: adequate-dose

CRF infusions in the evening block the morning rise in ACTH and cortisol in intact, but not in adrenally insufficient humans (29).

Thus, in addition to behavioral inhibition of stress responses, there is clear steroid feedback inhibition of stress responses; however, the degree of stress-induced inhibition of subsequent responses appears to be species dependent. In rats, and possibly in humans, the stress-induced steroid inhibition can be overridden by stress-induced facilitation of some parts of the adrenocortical system. By contrast, in dogs, steroid-induced inhibition of ACTH secretion either by prior stress or by CRF, ACTH, or steroid infusions generally appears to inhibit the responses to subsequent stresses (27). It may be that control in the adrenocortical system of dogs is quite different from that in humans or rat, as a consequence of the fact that dogs appear to have no circadian rhythm in basal ACS function (30,31). Because the phasic daily rhythm in corticosterone appears to be important in rat for control of the magnitude and duration of stress-induced ACTH secretion (see below), it is possible that the organization of the central control of ACS function is different in dogs.

Slow, Long-Term Feedback

To observe the slow feedback effects, animals are manipulated in advance of the experiment and then the effects of these manipulations are compared to the otherwise normal or intact animal. Repeated stress, advanced age, early handling, daily injections of corticosterone, and adrenalectomy with replacement of corticosterone at low, tonic levels all result in rats that exhibit an unusually prolonged ACTH response to stress (32–36). Common to the first four manipulations is a decrease in the numbers of hippocampal neurons and/or corticosteroid receptors. It is probable, but untested, in the case of adrenalectomy with tonic corticosteroid replacement that occupancy of hippocampal corticosteroid receptors is abnormally low. When adrenalectomized rats were treated with a phasic corticosterone signal, allowing a diurnal rhythm in corticosterone of near-normal magnitude, the duration of the ACTH response to stress was normalized, in contrast to the rats treated with the tonic signal (37). Thus, it appears likely that adequate daily occupancy of adequate numbers of brain corticosteroid receptors is a requirement for ACTH responses of normal duration to acute stress. In effect, there is a strong daily interaction between stress and the circadian rhythm, which drives corticosteroids to levels high enough to occupy type II glucocorticoid receptors and thus modulates the duration of stress-induced activation of the adrenocortical system.

Corticosteroid Feedback Receptor Types and Putative Functions

There are two types of corticosteroid receptors: type I, high-affinity receptors ($K_D \sim 0.5$ nM) that in vitro bind aldosterone = corticosterone = cortisol = deoxycorticosterone > dexamethasone; and type II, lower-affinity receptors (K_D 2.5–5 nM) that in vitro bind dexamethasone > cortisol > corticosterone >

deoxycorticosterone > aldosterone. The CNS distribution of the two receptor types is in part overlapping, but generally distinct (38). In situ studies of type I receptor mRNA expression show this to be high in hippocampus, lateral septum, and a variety of other sensory and motor sites outside of the hypothalamus (39). By contrast, type II receptor expression occurs more widely, with high levels of expression in hippocampus, lateral septum, amygdala, cerebral cortex, hypothalamus (including CRF-staining neurons), and monoaminergic cell bodies (40).

Reul and de Kloet have proposed (38), and we have concurred (41-44), that occupancy of type II receptors in brain by corticosterone probably exerts major control of stress-induced ACTH secretion. On the other hand, Reul and de Kloet consider type I receptors to be tonically occupied and irrelevant to the control of ACTH. Our data, from adrenalectomized rats treated with constant low levels of corticosterone, have led us to propose that occupancy of type I corticosteroid receptors probably controls the level of expression of CRF and AVP in neurons in the paraventricular nuclei, thus controlling basal ACTH secretion during the trough of the circadian rhythm (41). More recent pharmacological data suggest that type I receptor occupancy is important in the control of circadian peak ACTH secretion as well (44). Moreover, hypothalamic lesions were shown to elevate ACTH levels in adrenalectomized rats exposed to constant low steroid concentrations that restored ACTH to normal in sham-lesioned adrenalectomized rats (45). We therefore proposed that this feedback control of ACTH, which is probably mediated by association of corticosterone with type I receptors, is mediated transsynaptically from sites outside of the PVN. Since type I receptors are not found, or are found in very low abundance in hypothalamus, it is likely that this type of inhibition is exerted on the CRF neuron through activation or inhibition of extrahypothalamic neural input by increased occupancy of the neuronal receptors by corticosterone.

Two recent publications, considered together, suggest that the proposal of a two-receptor system for the control of ACTH secretion by corticosteroids has merit. Beyer et al. (46) studied CRF mRNA concentrations in adrenalectomized, sham-adrenalectomized, and adrenalectomized B-treated rats 5 days after adrenal surgery. B pellets were provided that elevated plasma B concentrations to 2.5 μg/dl; the rats were killed in the morning by decapitation and the portion of hypothalamus containing CRF cells was taken for measurement of CRF mRNA. This study showed clearly that adrenalectomy resulted in a 2.5-3-fold increase in CRF mRNA and that the low-dose B treatment restored the CRF mRNA concentrations to those seen in sham adrenalectomized controls. In quantitative terms, these results are in good agreement with those showing that bilateral adrenalectomy causes marked increases in CRF mRNA 5-7 days later (47,48), and that low-dose steroid treatment restores basal, nadir activity of the ACS to normal (41).

By contrast, Swanson and Simmons (49) have also examined CRF and mRNA levels after sham or bilateral adrenalectomy in the presence of a variety of concentrations of circulating B, ranging from 0 to 30 μg/dl. The rats were perfused and brains were collected 2–4 hr prior to lights out. There was only a 30% increase in CRF mRNA concentration provoked by adrenalectomy, and the CRF mRNA concentrations were decreased only at B concentrations of 5–10 μg/dl. The quantitative difference in the effects of adrenalectomy and the concentrations of B required to reduce CRF mRNA in the two studies may reside in the fact that the latter studies were performed near the time of the circadian peak in ACS activity; however, it may also be explained by the fact that in the second study the rats were exposed to the intense stress of perfusion prior to brain collection. A marked shift to the right in the sensitivity of ACTH to corticosteroid feedback has been reported in rats (43) between the time of trough and peak basal activity. A similar shift in feedback sensitivity has also been reported to occur in humans (50). Whether the different results are a consequence of the different time of day or of the stress of perfusion imposed on the rats, the data show clearly that there is a shift in feedback efficacy of corticosterone between basal/a.m. conditions and stressed/p.m. conditions. Such a shift is compatible with a shift of predominant corticosteroid control of ACS function from association of steroid with type I, high-affinity receptors to type II, lower-affinity, glucocorticoid receptors.

Can these results and conclusions be reconciled with other studies that show that dexamethasone implants over one PVN reduce CRF immunostaining ipsilaterally in adrenalectomized rats (51,52), and that systemically infused dexamethasone is slightly more effective than corticosterone in inhibiting adrenalectomy-induced increases in CRF and AVP immunostaining in PVN (53)? The results of Swanson and Simmons (49) show that high concentrations of corticosterone for 7 days reduce CRF mRNA to nearly undetectable levels, and that the concentrations of circulating corticosterone required for this effect are compatible with an effect mediated via association with type II receptors. Such receptors are found in high density in CRF neurons (40), and it is logical to suppose that the local implants of dexamethasone provided sufficiently high concentrations of steroid to occupy the type II receptors in CRF cells in PVN. The study showing that dexamethasone was slightly more effective than corticosterone in restoring peptide staining in PVN of adrenalectomized rats (53) used equal quantities of dexamethasone and corticosterone (20 or 50 μg/day) to treat the rats. Because of the markedly different half-lives of the steroids and the fact that dexamethasone is not bound to transcortin, the effective circulating concentration of dexamethasone was probably in the 50 nM range; by contrast, the concentration of corticosterone was probably just measureable, and the free steroid was probably in the subnanomolar range, which suggests that the latter was quantitatively far more effective than the former in inhibiting CRF and AVP.

Much less easy to resolve is the recent report by Kovacs and Makara (54) that bilateral dexamethasone but *not* corticosterone implants over PVN reduced ACTH concentrations in adrenalectomized rats to normal; by contrast, bilateral implants or dexamethasone into dorsal hippocampus were ineffective, but bilateral implants of corticosterone were partially effective in reducing circulating ACTH concentrations in adrenalectomized rats. Because both receptor types bind both steroids, although with differing affinities, these results are difficult to interpret in any context.

Another problem that must be resolved with respect to the steroid-induced inhibition of CRF/AVP-ACTH secretion is the fact that aldosterone and deoxycorticosterone, which bind with high affinity to the type I corticosteroid receptors in vitro (55–57), do not strongly affect adrenalectomy-induced increases in CRF/AVP or ACTH secretion when infused in vivo (53,44). This finding is most at odds with the interpretation that suppression of basal AM ACTH is mediated by association of corticosterone with type I corticosteroid receptors. A mechanism may exist in B-specific type I receptor-containing neurons that serves to metabolize aldosterone and deoxycorticosterone specifically, leaving corticosterone unscathed and free to associate with the receptors. However, this notion is simply raised in analogy to a similar mechanism involving 11B-hydroxysteroid reductase, which preferentially metabolizes cortisol and corticosterone in aldosterone target tissues containing type I receptors (58). There is no evidence for such a mechanism in B-preferring sites.

Acute stress alters the subsequent responsiveness of the adrenocortical system in an unknown fashion. Because chronic stress appears to do the same thing, the detailed description of the alteration is given in the next section. It seems clear that corticosteroids secreted in response to acute stress alter response properties of the adrenocortical system. However, the degree to which this occurs is also unclear because of the apparent concurrent facilitatory effect of the applied stress. Although the localization of corticosteroid receptor types in brain is clear, and although there is evidence favoring feedback effects of corticosteroids mediated by association both with type I and type II receptors, the brain sites at which feedback occurs are unknown. The interaction that may exist between occupancy of type I and type II corticosteroid receptors and the control of CRF secretion also required clarification. In an ideal setting, one would use electrodes that were responsive to specific peptides and others that monitored the degree of occupancy of specific steroid receptor types to begin sorting out the answers to these basic questions. The fact that the preparation of animals for study alters the operating characteristics of the adrenocortical system from basal makes simple questions difficult to answer and a simple description difficult to achieve.

CHRONIC STRESS

Chronic stresses are either those imposed intermittently, but repeatedly over days and weeks, such as electric shock (59), immobilization (60), or a variety of insults repeated multiple times (34), or those that are initiated and maintained such as hypoxia (61), crowding or cold (62,63), chemically induced diabetes (64,65), and, possibly, restricted feeding (66). Overall, the response of the adrenocortical system of rats does not appear to differentiate between chronic intermittent and chronic tonic stresses, and a constellation of responses is observed.

Adrenal weight is increased, as is the rate of the corticosterone response to ACTH (62). There is an increase in the magnitude of the ACTH response to superimposed acute stressors (63), despite the fact that circulating corticosterone concentrations may have been markedly elevated for periods of weeks (62,63). There is decreased sensitivity to the inhibitory effects of prior treatment with glucocorticoids on the magnitude of the ACS response to acute, superimposed stress (64); and stimuli that are subthreshold in control rats are adequate to stimulate ACTH secretion in rats that are chronically stressed (61). Moreover, the number of hippocampal (67), and possibly hypothalamic (65) but not pituitary, corticosteroid receptors is reduced under conditions of chronic stress. Thus, regulation of the adrenocortical system is altered in a major fashion under conditions of chronic stress. The results of these changes yield a system that is highly responsive to new insults under conditions in which there is a high circulating feedback signal.

It has been proposed (67) that the decrease in hippocampal corticosterone receptors observed after weeks of chronic stress or corticosterone treatment is responsible for the changes in adrenocortical activity that occur under these conditions. Although this is a logical hypothesis, it is probably not the entire answer, since all of the changes observed in the responsiveness of elements in the adrenocortical system after chronic stress have also been shown to occur within 2–4 h after imposition of an acute stress (23). It is unlikely that down-regulation of corticosteroid receptors has had time to occur.

The increased capacity and dynamic of the adrenal corticosterone response to ACTH that occur in chronically stressed rats are probably consequences of sustained hypersecretion of ACTH acting to promote adrenal growth and capacity to respond. However, changes in adrenal sensitivity may occur even before the growth- and function-promoting effects of chronically elevated ACTH levels are observed.

How the changes that occur in the central adrenocortical system components are affected after the imposition of acute or chronic stress is unknown. A preliminary study by Rivier et al. (68) showed that chronically shocked rats exhibited a transient increase in CRF, but not AVP mRNA expression that returned to normal with continued days of shock. Little other information is available about the central changes that occur after the institution of chronic stress. With time, decreases in corticosteroid receptor concentration could result in some of the feedback insensitivity that occurs in the chronically stressed system. Bear in mind, however, that there is not yet unequivocal evidence that hippocampal corticosterone receptors play a role in the modulation of CRFs secretion. Also, as pointed out above, the entire system adapts too rapidly to stress for changes in either the level of peptide expression in CRF neurons or the decrease in receptor number to be the only answers.

It seems possible, and even likely, that stress activates other brain systems that interact with the central motor components of the adrenocortical system to cause increased sensitivity of these components to acute stimuli as well as to decrease the influence of inhibitory feedback inputs.

One obvious way in which this could occur is if the ratio of AVP/CRF secreted from CRF neurons increased. Whitnall et al. have provided evidence that ~ 50% of the CRF-containing granules in the axonal endings in the median eminence costain for AVP (69), and that approximately 50% of CRF neurons in the PVN also costain for AVP when studied 2 days after colchicine treatment (70). Initial and chronic stress could activate pathways to CRF neurons that resulted in increased responsiveness of the AVP-containing cells to subsequent stressful inputs. Such a change would act as a switch. Increased secretory ratios of AVP/CRF from the median eminence would not only increase the amount of ACTH secreted from the corticotrope (71) but also confer a degree of steroid resistance at the corticotrope, as shown by Bilizekjian et al. (72). Surgical and chemical adrenalectomy have also been shown to alter the AVP/CRF ratio (73,74) and have been shown to be stresses in addition to acting to remove corticosterone feedback (75).

If, for instance, stress increases the stimulatory input of noradrenergic or adrenergic neurons to the parvocellular CRF- and CRF/AVP-containing neurons, acute stress-induced inputs could reach threshold for action potentials at lower intensity levels, that is, under conditions in which the input normally does not cause neuronal firing. Such a theory could be tested pharmacologically or with selective lesions of the catecholaminergic input system. In addition, the degree of catecholaminergic activity in PVN could be measured in chronically instrumented animals under truly basal conditions and under conditions of chronic stress before and after acute stress is applied.

Although most of the work cited above refers to studies on rats, it is clear that the changes that occur after the chronic stress in rats also occur in humans. Depression (76), particularly in patients with weight loss (77), anorexia nervosa (78), and diabetes mellitus (79) in humans are all accompanied by resistance to the feedback action of dexamethasone. Moreover, the elevated feedback signal conferred by elevated cortisol levels probably is responsible for the diminished ACTH response to acute CRF challange observed in patients with depression and anorexia nervosa (76,78).

After stress, either acute or chronic, all components of the adrenocortical system are more responsive than normal to new stressful inputs, despite elevated circulating glucocorticoids. Although there are hints about how this is achieved, there is little or no information about how any single aspect of this elevated responsiveness operates. This is a major aspect of stress-induced function in the adrenocortical system, and its control is virtually unexplored.

PHYSIOLOGICAL ROLE OF THE STRESS RESPONSE

The fact that even under conditions of chronic stress, when corticosteroid secretion is tonically elevated, mechanisms exist to ensure subsequent acute responsiveness to new stress which suggests that a substantial positive role is played by acute glucocorticoid secretion. The magnitude of the increase in corticosterone after stress (in the range of 10-15 nM available B not bound to CBG) suggests that the stress-induced steroid levels act via association with type II glucocorticoid receptors. Because glucocorticoid receptors grace every cell type in the body, and exert a myriad of tissue-specific effects, it does not seem fruitful to speculate from this basis on the protective action of these steroids. However, when taken from the point of view of physiological systems, some useful and testable generalizations may be put forth.

Early studies on the action of adrenocortical hormones showed that adrenalectomized animals were more fragile than those with adrenal glands, and that in the absence of the adrenals animals were more likely to die after stress (80). Some of the early studies on function in adrenalectomized animals are confounded by the fact that the lack of aldosterone was not compensated for, thus introducing marked volume depletion and electrolyte abnormalities into a preparation that was also debilitated by the lack of glucocorticoids. When adrenalectomized rats were maintained on salt in their drinking water to compensate for the loss of aldosterone, they still were not able to sustain life as well as sham-adrenalectomized or intact controls in the face of a variety of stresses (81,82), and death, or time of death after the onset of an acute stress, was used as an endpoint to determine the efficacy of various adrenal steroid preparations (82).

Acute Role of Glucocorticoids

The systems that appear to exhibit the most profound deficits in adrenalectomized rats maintained on salt, or studied acutely, are the cardiovascular and skeletomuscular systems and systems involved with the maintenance of body heat and glucose. Direct effects of glucocorticoids can be shown on cardiac muscle, vascular smooth muscle, adipose tissue, and skeletal muscle; and it is possible that the life-sustaining property of the glucocorticoids in adrenalectomized rats results from the actions of glucocorticoids on these targets. However, from the results of our recent studies (83–85), we suspect that an acute, primary effect of glucocorticoids, which leads to death after stress in their absence, may be on stress-induced gluconeogenesis and substrate availability.

Darlington and his co-workers have systematically studied the effects of adrenalectomy and replacement of corticosterone on vascular responsiveness and baroreflex sensitivity (83). Minor steroid sensitive-effects were found on mean arterial blood pressure, heart rate, and baroreflex sensitivity in chronically prepared, fed adrenalectomized rats with normal blood volume. Moreover, when adrenalectomized, chronically prepared rats were exposed to 15 ml/kg hemorrhage and hypovolemia for the ensuing 5 h, they were found to restore blood volume as well as, but slightly more slowly than, the sham-adrenalectomized controls. Other neural and hormonal systems that mediate vascular tone hyperresponded to hemorrhage in the adrenalectomized rats and appeared to compensate for the lack of corticosterone (84). However, when we tested the effects of an overnight fast on the cardiovascular response to hemorrhage in adrenalectomized rats, none of the animals was able to sustain adequately its arterial blood pressure or plasma glucose concentrations, and all of the adrenalectomized rats died within 24 h of hemorrhage. By contrast, fasted sham-adrenalectomized rats increased their blood glucose concentrations above initial levels, at the time when blood glucose concentration fell markedly in the adrenalectomized rats. All of these animals restored and maintained arterial pressure after the hemorrhage and lived, as did the fed adrenalectomized rats (85).

The results of these studies suggest that there may be a requirement for elevated blood glucose concentrations after stress in order for animals to survive the insult. The results do not suggest what systems are involved that require glucose, or even that glucose is the essential agent; however, the studies do show that adrenalectomized rats can compensate for a major cardiovascular stress nearly as well as intact rats provided that they are adequately nourished. Stress-induced stimulation of corticosteroid secretion may, in this case, serve to sustain substrate essential for life-maintaining processes to ensue in animals depleted of substrate by fasting, or by prior stress-induced increase in the rate of substrate utilization.

Long-Term Role of Glucocorticoids

Munck and his co-workers (86) have pointed out and provided evidence for the probable physiological utility of the myriad anti-inflammatory actions of glucocorticoids on curtailing action of components of the immune system under conditions of chronic stress. Under more chronic stressful conditions, this effect may also be life-preserving. In this instance, tonically elevated concentrations of glucocorticoids would serve to keep a potentially dangerous endogenous activity in check. Furthermore, examination of the effects of glucocorticoids on other hormonal systems that respond to stress suggests that a persistent elevation in corticosteroids might serve to shape, or tailor, responses in other endocrine systems (87).

In addition, in the absence of concurrent stress, chronically elevated concentrations of corticosterone cause elevated arterial blood pressure in adrenalectomized rats (83). Transcortin concentrations are decreased in such animals (41,43, 45,83), and the increased pressure may be a consequence of increased corticosterone occupancy of renal mineralocorticoid receptors that could occur in the face of decreased buffering of those receptors by transcortin in the renal interstitium (87). The hypersensitive effect that occurs under such conditions in unstressed animals could have definite survival benefits in chronically stressed animals with compromised blood volume.

The behavioral consequences of chronically elevated glucocorticoids are not well described, nor is the site or mechanism by which behavioral changes occur. Nonetheless, there is a clinically well-recognized steroid euphoria (88). In addition, the glucocorticoids have been shown to raise sensory thresholds in glucocorticoid-deficient patients (89). Both of these effects of glucocorticoids could have good survival value in chronically stressed organisms.

Whether these and other potentially beneficial effects of chronic exposure to high steroid concentrations adequately balance the negative effects of glucocorticoids on hippocampal cells (67;Chap. 15)and the other damaging effects of glucocorticoids given chronically in pharmacological quantities (90) probably depends on the type of chronic stress experienced. It seems clear that the response to some stimuli glucocorticoids are life-saving, and their usefulness is unarguable. Under other conditions, possibly those of chronic psychological stress, in which substrate supplies, immune system function, and vascular integrity are not threatened, chronic elevations in glucocorticoids may do more physiological damage than repair.

ACKNOWLEDGMENTS

My gratitude to all who have worked in this laboratory during the last 20 years. Our interactions have shaped to a great extent the way in which my understanding of control in the adrenocortical system has developed. This work was supported by USPHS Grant DK 28172.

REFERENCES

1. Levine S, Goldman L, Coover G D. Expectancy and the pituitary-adrenal system. In Physiology, emotion and psychosomatic illness. Ciba Foundation Symposium 8. Amsterdam: Elsevier-Excerpta Medica North Holland, 1972: 281–296.

2. Levine S, Weinberg J, Brett L P. Inhibition of pituitary-adrenal activity as a consequence of consummatory behavior. Psychoneuroendocrinology 1979; 4:275–286.

3. deWied D. The significance of the antidiuretic hormone in the release mechanism of corticotropin. Endocrinology 1961; 68:956–970.

4. Smelik P G, Gaarenstroom J H, Konijnendijk W, de Wied D. Evaluation of the role of the posterior lobe of the hypophysis in the reflex secretion of corticotropin. Acta Physiol Pharmacol 1962; 11:20–33.

5. Fagin K D, Wiener S G, Dallman M F. ACTH and corticosterone secretion in rats following removal of the neurointermediate lobe of the pituitary gland. Neuroendocrinology 1985; 40:352–362.

6. Plotsky P M, Bruhn T O, Vale W. Central modulation of immunoreactive corticotropin-releasing factor secretion by arginine vasopressin. Endocrinology 1985; 115:1639–1641.

7. Egdahl R H. Pituitary–adrenal response following trauma to the isolated leg. Surgery 1959; 46:9–16.

8. Gibbs F P. Central nervous system lesions that block release of ACTH caused by traumatic stress. Am J Physiol 1969; 217:78–83.

9. Dallman M F, Yates F E. Anatomical and functional mapping of central input and feedback pathways of the adrenocortical system. Mem Soc Endocrinol 1969; 17:39–72.

10. Gann D S, Ward D G, Carlson D E. Neural control of ACTH: a homeostatic reflex. Rec Prog Horm Res 1978; 34:357–400.

11. Raff H, Shinsako J, Keil L C, Dallman M F. Feedback inhibition of adrenocorticotropin and vasopressin responses to hypoxia by physiological increases in endogenous plasma corticosteroids in dogs. Endocrinology 1984; 114:1245–1249.

12. Thrivikraman K V, Bereiter D A, Gann D S. Hemorrhage increases catecholaminergic activity in the caudal paraventricular hypothalamus in cats. Am J Physiol 1989;

13. Plotsky P M. Facilitation of immunoreactive corticotropin-releasing factor secretion into the hypophysial-portal circulation after activation of adrenergic pathways or central norepinephrine injections. Endocrinology 1987; 121:924–930.

14. Keller-Wood M E, Shinsako J, Dallman M F. Interaction between stimulus intensity and corticosteroid feedback in the control of ACTH. Am J Physiol 1983; 245:R53–R59.

15. Widmaier E P, Plotsky P M, Sutton S W, Vale W W. Regulation of corticotropin-releasing factor secretion in vitro by glucose. Am J Physiol 1988; 255:E287–E292.

16. Szafarczyk A, Alonso G, Ixart G, Malaval F, Assenmacher I. Diurnal-stimulated and stress-induced ACTH release in rats is mediated by ventral noradrenergic bundle. Am J Physiol 1985; 249:E219–E226.

17. Szafarczyk A, Guillaume V, Conte-Devolx B, et al. Central catecholaminergic system stimulates secretion of CRH at different sites. Am J Physiol 1988; 255:E463–E468.

18. Feldman S. Neural pathways mediating adrenocortical responses. Fed Proc 1985; 44:169–175.

19. Saphier D, Feldman S. Electrophysiology of limbic forebrain and paraventricular nucleus connections. Brain Res Bull 1986; 17:743–750.

20. Saphier D, Feldman S. Iontophoretic application of glucocorticoids inhibits identified neurones in the rat paraventricular nucleus. Brain Res 1989;

21. Plotsky P M. Hypophyseotrophic regulation of adrenohypophyseal adrenocorticotropin secretion. Fed Proc 1985; 44:207–213.

22. Tilders F J H, Berkenbosch F. CRF and catecholamines; their place in the central and peripheral regulation of the stress response. Acta Endocrinol Supp 1986; 276:63–75.

23. Dallman M F, Yates F E. Anatomical and functional mapping of central neural input and feedback pathways of the adrenocortical system. Mem Soc Endocrinol 1969; 17:39–72.

24. Darlington D N, Shinsako J, Dallman M F. Responses of ACTH, epinephrine, norepinephrine and the cardiovascular system to hemorrhage. Am J Physiol 1986; 251:H612–H618.

25. Dallman M F, Jones M T, Vernikos-Danellis J, Ganong W F. Corticosteroid control of ACTH secretion. Endocrinology 1972; 91:961–968.

26. Keller-Wood M E, Dallman M F. Corticosteroid inhibition of ACTH secretion. Endocr Rev 1984; 5:1–24.

27. Keller-Wood M E, Shinsako J, Dallman M F. Inhibition of the adrenocorticotropin and corticosteroid responses to hypoglycemia after prior stress. Endocrinology 1983; 113:491–496.

28. Zimmerman E, Critchlow V. Suppression of pituitary-adrenal function with physiological levels of corticosterone. Neuroendocrinology 1969; 5:183–192.

29. deBold C R, deCherney G S, Jackson R V, et al. Effect of synthetic ovine corticotropin-releasing factor: prolonged duration of action and biphasic response of adrenocorticotropin and cortisol. J Clin Endocrinol Metab 1983; 57:294–298.

30. Kemppainen R J, Sartin J L. Evidence for episodic but not circadian activity in plasma concentrations of ACTH, cortisol and thyroxine in dogs. J Endocrinol 1984; 103:219–226.

31. Orth D N, Peterson M E, Drucker W D. Plasma immunoreactive proopiomelanocortin peptides and cortisol in normal dogs and dogs with Cushing's syndrome: diurnal rhythm and responsiveness to various stimuli. Endocrinology 1988; 122:1250–1262.

32. Sapolsky R M, McEwen B S. Down-regulation of neural corticosterone receptor by corticosterone and dexamethasone. Brain Res 1985; 339:161–165.

33. Sapolsky R M, Krey L C, McEwen B S. Corticosterone receptors decline in a site-specific manner in the aged brain. Brain Res 1983; 298:235–240.

34. Sapolsky R M, Krey L C, McEwen B S. Stress down-regulates corticosterone receptors in a site-specific manner in the brain. Endocrinology 1984; 114:287–292.

35. Meany M J, Aitken D H, Bodnoff S R, Iny L J, Tatarewicz J E. Early postnatal handling alters glucocorticoid receptor concentrations in selected brain regions. Behav Neurosci 1985; 99:765–770.

36. Akana S F, Jacobson L, Cascio C S, Shinsako J, Dallman M F. Constant corticosterone replacement normalizes basal adrenocorticotropin (ACTH) but permits sustained ACTH hypersecretion after stress in adrenalectomized rats. Endocrinology 1988; 122:1337–1342.

37. Jacobson L, Akana S F, Cascio C S, Shinsako J, Dallman M F. Circadian variations in plasma corticosterone permit normal termination of adrenocorticotropin responses to stress. Endocrinology 1988; 122:1343–1348.

38. Reul J M H M, de Kloet E R. Two receptor systems for corticosterone in rat brain: microdistribution and differential occupation. Endocrinology 1985; 117:2505–2511.

39. Arriza J L, Simerly R B, Swanson L W, Evans R M. The neuronal mineralocorticoid receptor as a mediator of glucocorticoid response. Neuron 1988; 1:887–900.

40. Fuxe K, Wikstrom A-C, Okret S, Agnati L F, Harfstrand A, Yu Z-Y, Granholm L, Zoli M, Vale W, Gustafsson J-A. Mapping of glucocorticoid receptor immunoreactive neurons in the rat tel- and diencephalon using a monoclonal antibody against rat liver glucocorticoid receptor. Endocrinology 1985; 117:1803–1812.

41. Dallman M F, Akana S F, Cascio C S, Darlington D N, Jacobson L, Levin N. Regulation of ACTH secretion: variations on a theme of B. Rec Prog Horm Res 1987; 43:113–173.

42. Levin N, Akana S F, Jacobson L, Kuhn R W, Sliteri P K, Dallman M F. Plasma adrenocorticotropin is more sensitive than transcortin production or thymus weight to inhibition by corticosterone in rats. Endocrinology 1987; 121:1104–1110.

43. Akana S F, Cascio C S, Du J-Z, Levin N, Dallman M F. Reset of feedback in the adrenocortical system: an apparent shift in sensitivity of adrenocorticotropin to inhibition between morning and evening. Endocrinology 1986; 119:2325–2332.

44. Dallman M F, Levin N, Cascio C S, Akana S F, Jacobson L, Kuhn R W. Pharmacological evidence that the inhibition of diurnal adrenocorticotropin secretion by corticosteroids in mediated vita type I, corticosterone-preferring receptors. Endocrinology 1989;

45. Levin N, Shinsako J, Dallman M F. Corticosterone acts on the brain to inhibit adrenalectomy-induced adrenocorticotropin secretion. Endocrinology 1988; 122:694–701.

46. Beyer H S, Matta S G, Sharp B M. Regulation of the messenger ribonucleic acid for corticotropin-releasing factor in the paraventricular nucleus and other brain sites in the rat. Endocrinology 1988; 123:2117–2123.

47. Jingami H, Matsukura S, Numa S, Imura H. Effects of adrenalectomy and dexamethasone administration on the level of preprocorticotropin-releasing factor messenger ribonucleic acid (mRNA) in the hypothalamus and adrenocorticotropin/B-lipotropin precursor mRNA in the pituitary in rats. Endocrinology 1985; 117:1314–1320.

48. Young W S III, Mezey E, Siegel R E. Quantitative in situ hybridization histochemistry reveals increased levels of corticotropin-releasing factor mRNA after adrenalectomy in rats. Neurosci Lett 1986; 70:198–203.

49. Swanson L W, Simmons D M. Differential steroid hormone and neural influences on peptide mRNA levels in CRF cells of the paraventricular nucleus: a hybridization histochemical study in the rat. J Comp Neurol 1989;

50. Angeli A, Fronzo D, Frairia R, Bertello D, Gaidano G, Ceresa F. Proc. Int. Conf. Int. Soc. Chronobiol., 1977: 189–196.

51. Kovacs K, Kiss J Z, Makara G B. Glucocorticoid implants around the hypothalamic paraventricular nucleus prevent the increase of corticotropin-releasing factor and arginine vasopressin immunostaining induced by adrenalectomy. Neuroendocrinology 1986; 44:229–234.

52. Sawchenko P E. Evidence for a local site of action for glucocorticoids in inhibiting CRF- and vasopressin-immunoreactivity parvocellular neurosecretory neurons: anatomic, peptide, and steroid specificity. J Neurosci 1987; 7:1093–1106.

53. Sawchenko P E. Evidence for differential regulation of corticotropin-releasing factor and vasopressin immunoreactivities in parvocellular neurosecretory and autonomic-related projections of the paraventricular nucleus. Brain Res 1987; 437:253–263.

54. Kovacs K, Makara G B. Corticosterone and dexamethasone act at different brain sites to inhibit adrenalectomy-induced adrenocorticotropin hypersecretion. Brain Res 1989;

55. Krowzowsky Z S, Funder J W. Renal mineralocorticoid receptors and hippocampal corticosterone-binding species have identical intrinsic steroid specificity. Proc Natl Acad Sci U S A 1983; 80:6056–6060.

56. Beaumont K, Fanestil D D. Characterization of rat brain aldosterone receptors reveals high affinity for corticosterone. Endocrinology 1984; 113:2043–2051.

57. Veldhuis H D, van Koppen C, van Ittersum M, de Kloet E R. Specificity of the adrenal steroid receptor in rat hippocampus. Endocrinology 1982; 110:2044–2051.

58. Funder J W, Pearce P T, Smith R, Smith I A. Mineralocorticoid action: target tissue specificity is enzyme, not receptor, mediated. Science 1988; 242:583–585.

59. Rivier C, Vale W. Diminished responsiveness of the hypothalamic-pituitary-adrenal axis of the rat during exposure to prolonged stress: a pituitary-mediated mechanism. Endocrinology 1987; 121:1320–1328.

60. Mikulaj L, Kvetnansky R, Murgas K, Parizkova J, Vencel P. Catecholamines and corticosteroids in acute and repeated stress. In: Usdin E, Kvetnansky R, Kopin IJ, eds. Catecholamines and stress. Elmsford, NY: Pergamon Press, 1975; 445–455.

61. Raff H, Sandri R B, Segerson T P. Renin, ACTH, and adrenocortical function during hypoxia and hemorrhage in conscious rats. Am J Physiol 1986; 250:R240–R244.

62. Daniels-Severs A, Goodwin A, Keil L C, Vernikos-Danellis J. Effect of chronic crowding and cold on the pituitary-adrenal system: responsiveness to an acute stimulus during chronic stress. Pharmacology 1973; 9: 348–356.

63. Vernikos-Danellis J, Dallman M F, Bonner C, Katzen A, Shinsako J. Pituitary-adrenal function in rats chronically exposed to cold. Endocrinology 1982; 110:413–420.

64. L'Age M, Langholz J, Fechner W, Salzmann H. Disturbances of the hypothalamo–hypophysial–adrenocortical system in the alloxan-diabetic rat. Endocrinology 1974; 95:760–765.

65. Tornello S, Gridman O, Weisenberg L, Coirini H, De Nicola A F. Differences in corticosterone binding by regions of the central nervous system by normal and diabetic rats. J Steroid Biochem 1981; 14:77–81.

66. Honma K-I, Honma S, Hiroshige T. Critical role of food amount for prefeeding corticosterone peak in rats. Am J Physiol 1983; 245:R339–R344.

67. Sapolsky R M, Krey L C, McEwen B S. Stress down-regulates corticosterone receptors in site-specific manner in the brain. Endocrinology 1984; 114:287–292.

68. Imaki T, Nahon J L, Rivier C, Sawchenko P, Vale W. Effect of chronic stress on the level of corticotropin-releasing factor (CRF) mRNA in rat brain. 18th Ann. Meeting Soc. Neuroscience. Toronto, Canada 1988; abstract 178.17.

69. Whitnall M H, Mezey E, Gainer H. Co-localization of corticotropin-releasing factor and vasopressin in median eminence neurosecretory vesicles. Nature 1985; 317:248–250.

70. Whitnall M II, Gainer H. Major pro-vasopressin-expressing and pro-vasopressin-deficient subpopulation of corticotropin-releasing hormone neurons in normal rats. Neuronedocrinology 1988; 47:176–180.

71. Gillies G E, Linton E A, Lowry P J. Corticotropin releasing activity of the new CRF is potentiated several times by vasopressin. Nature 1982; 299: 355–357.

72. Bilizekjian L M, Blount A L, Vale W W. The cellular actions of vasopressin on corticotrophs of the anterior pituitary: resistance to glucocorticoid action. Mol Endocrinol 1987; 1:451–458.

74. Antoni F A. Hypothalamic control of adrenocorticotropin secretion: advances since the discovery of 41-residue corticotropin-releasing factor. Endocrine Rev 1986; 7:351–378.

74. Plotsky P M, Sawchenko P E. Hypophysial-portal plasma levels, median eminence content, and immunohistochemical staining of corticotropin-releasing factor, arginine vasopressin and oxytocin after pharmacological adrenalectomy. Endocrinology 1987; 120:1361–1369.

75. Jacobson L, Akana S F, Cascio C S, Scribner K, Shinsako J, Dallman M F. The adrenocortical system responds slowly to removal of corticosterone in the absence of concurrent stress. Endocrinology 1989; 124.

76. Gold P W. Loriaux D L, Roy A. Responses to corticotropin releasing hormone in the hypercortisolism of depression and Cushing's disease:

pathophysiologic and diagnostic implications. N Engl J Med 1986; 314: 1329–1355.

77. Pfohl B, Sherman B, Schlecte J, Winokur G. Differences in plasma ACTH and cortisol between depressed patients and normal controls. Biol Psychiatry 1985; 20:1055–1072.

78. Gold P W, Swirtsman H, Avgerinos P, et al. Abnormal hypothalamic–pituitary–adrenal function in anorexia nervosa. Pathophysiologic mechanisms in underweight and weight corrected patients. N Engl J Med 1986; 314:1335–1342.

79. Hudson J I, Hudson M S, Rothschild A J, Bignati L, Schatzberg A F, Melby J C. Abnormal results of dexamethasone suppression tests in nondepressed patients with diabetes mellitus. Arch Gen Psychiatry 1984; 41:1086–1089.

80. Gaunt R. History of the adrenal cortex. In: Blaschko H, Smith AD, eds. Handbook of Physiology: Endocrinology, Vol.VI, Adrenal Gland. Washington, DC: American Physiological Society, 1975: 1–12.

81. Ingle D J. The biologic properties of cortisone:a review. J Clin Endocrinol 1950; 10:1312–1354.

82. Dorfman R I, Shiplley R A, Ross E, Schiller S, Horwitt B N. The relative potencies of adrenal cortical steroids as determined by a cold protection test and by a glycogen deposition test. Endocrinology 1946; 38:189–196.

83. Darlington D N, Kaship K, Keil L C, Dallman M F. Vascular responsiveness in adrenalectomized rats with corticosterone replacement. Am J Physiol 1989; 256:H.

84. Darlington D N, Keil L C, Dallman M F. Potentiation of hormonal responses to hemorrhage and fasting but not hypoglycemia in conscious adrenalectomized rats. Endocrinology 1989;

85. Darlington D N, Keil L C. Fed but not fasted adrenalectomized rats survive hemorrhage. Abstract, Ann. Meetings Endocrine Soc., 1989.

86. Munck A S, Guyre P M, Holbrook N J. Physiologic functions of glucocorticoids in stress and their relations to pharmacological actions. Endocrine Rev 1984; 5:25–44.

87. Dallman M F, Wilkinson C W. Feedback and facilitation in the adrenocortical system and the endocrine responses to repeated stimuli. In Assenmacher I, Farner D S, eds. Environmental endocrinology. New York: Springer Verlag, 1978: 252–259.

88. Baxter J D, Tyrrell L B. The adrenal cortex. In: Felig P, Baxter JD, Broadus AE, Frohman LA, eds. Endocrinology and metabolism, 2nd ed. New York: McGraw-Hill, 1988: 511–650.

89. Henkin R I. Effects of ACTH, adrenocorticosteroids and thyroid hormone on sensory function. In: Stumpf WE, Grant LD, eds. Anatomical neuroendocrinology. Basel: Karger 1975: 298–316.

90. Selye H. A syndrome produced by diverse noxious agents. Nature 1936; 138:32.

10

BRAIN PEPTIDE REGULATION OF AUTONOMIC NERVOUS AND NEUROENDOCRINE FUNCTIONS

Marvin R. Brown
University of California, San Diego, San Diego, California

A stressor is an event, internal or external to an animal, that poses a real or perceived threat to the maintenance of that animal's homeostasis. The interaction between an animal and a stressor results in a constellation of physical and behavioral responses that can be called "stress." Stress responses may play an important role in the optimization of function or may lead to maladaptive changes in biological systems. In animals, chemical messengers, acting as intercellular messengers, involved in the control of homeostasis may participate in these stress responses. Under conditions of excessive perturbation, these regulators of cellular function may exhibit dynamic fluctuations in magnitude or duration in excess of that required to establish homeostasis, resulting in deleterious effects on the animal's physiology.

This chapter discusses the evidence to suggest that peptides present within the central nervous system (CNS) are capable of eliciting complex, integrated neuroendocrine and autonomic nervous system (ANS) responses. The bulk of this evidence is based on pharmacological actions of peptides within the CNS. The possibility that peptides may singularly or collectively mediate changes of neuroendocrine or autonomic function will be discussed.

CNS peptide-mediated regulation of neuroendocrine (i.e., anterior and posterior pituitary and adrenal medullary function) and ANS function can, in a general sense, be viewed to result from two mechanisms: changes of activity that result from peptide involvement in the operation of reflex or feedback systems; and changes of activity that result from peptide actions mediated through command input, in many cases derived from cognitive or sensory systems. For example, the release of pituitary ACTH and vasopressin, and the changes in sympathetic and parasympathetic activity following hemorrhage, may result from a baro- and volume-sensing reflex. Within this sytem there may exist a set-point about which adrenocorticotropic hormone (ACTH) and vasopressin plasma concentrations and sympathetic and parasympathetic activity levels are present for any particular vascular volume or pressure. In contrast, central commands based on input from cognitive or sensory systems may override set points to bring about changes of neuroendocrine or autonomic function. For instance, the visual recognition and rapid interpretation of the significance of viewing a pedestrian walking in front of our automobile while traveling 80 miles/h can result in significant changes in neuroendocrine and autonomic function. Command inputs under basal circumstances do not determine the activity of neuroendocrine or ANS activity.

Is there any reason to believe or doubt that peptides may be candidates for CNS regulators of neuroendocrine and autonomic function? Four major reasons to doubt that peptides may play important roles as CNS regulators of neuroendocrine- and autonomic activities are detailed here.

1. Many different peptides injected into the brain produce changes of autonomic and neuroendocrine function. If the brain works on the basis of unique wiring and synaptic arrangements, it is difficult to imagine how all these peptides might be important.
2. Peptides and their receptors, in many cases, are distributed in different anatomical locations within the brain (1-3). This ligand–receptor mismatch could be interpreted to indicate that peptides are not genuine transmitters within the brain. As an alternative, peptides may act through receptors following their diffusion from sites of release.
3. Changes in neuroendocrine and autonomic function under physiological circumstances are rapidly activated and terminated. Peptide effects are thought to be slow in onset and long in action.
4. Mechanisms for reuptake and inactivation of peptides following their release have, in large part, not been demonstrated.

Reasons to speculate that peptides may play important roles in the regulation of neuroendocrine and autonomic function include the following.

1. Peptides are anatomically distributed in brain areas known to be involved in the regulation of neuroendocrine and ANS function (4).
2. Peptides injected into specific brain regions are capable of eliciting changes in neuroendocrine and ANS function similar to changes observed following exposure of animals to various types of stressors.

3. In several cases, the use of receptor antagonists or passive immunization has demonstrated a role of a peptide in the regulation of either neuroendocrine or ANS function.

A discussion of the peptides that have been evaluated for their CNS action on the regulation of neuroendocrine and ANS activity as may be relevant to stress biology is presented here. This chapter concludes with a brief discussion of the types of methods and experimental approaches necessary to advance an understanding of this area of study.

CORTICOTROPIN-RELEASING FACTOR

Corticotropin-releasing factor (CRF) and its receptors are anatomically distributed in a variety of brain regions suspected of being involved in the control of ANS and neuroendocrine function (5-7). The functional significance of the CNS CRF receptors measured in the brain using autoradiographic and membrane binding studies remains to be determined. Exposure of rats to various stressors or repeated intracerebroventricular (icv) injections of CRF does not significantly change brain CRF receptor binding affinity or number (R. Hauger, unpublished results). Furthermore, it has recently been suggested that some brain CRF receptors may not be functionally linked to postreceptor events (8).

CRF, given icv, acts within the brain to influence pituitary hormone secretion and sympathetic nervous system (SNS) and parasympathetic nervous system (PNS) activity. These changes in neuroendocrine and ANS activity produce alterations in visceral organ function similar to those observed following exposure of animals to some types of stressors. Table 1 lists the changes in neuroendocrine and ANS function observed following icv administration of CRF. It is

TABLE 1 CNS Actions of CRF on Neuroendocrine and ANS Function

System	Effect
Anterior pituitary	Increased ACTH secretion (by increasing release of brain CRF) (9)
	Decreased growth hormone secretion (10)
	Decreased luteinizing hormone secretion (11)
Posterior pituitary	Increased AVP release (in dog, but not rat) (12)
Adrenal medulla	Increase Epi release (13)
Sympathetic nervous	Increase NE and NPY release (13,14)
Parasympathetic nervous	Decrease activity in heart and gut (15,16)

noteworthy that CRF has been suggested to act within the brain to stimulate CRF release, resulting in ACTH secretion (9). This is not to be confused with the action of exogenously administered CRF leaking from the brain to stimulate pituitary ACTH release directly. Table 2 lists the mechanisms by which CRF given icv changes visceral organ function. None of these actions of CRF result from leakage of CRF out of the brain. Table 3 illustrates the results of studies that have used the CRF antagonist, CRF 9-41, to demonstrate physiological participation of CRF in the regulation of stressor-induced changes in visceral organ function. These responses could result in successful adaptation in an animal exposed to a stressor. Initiation of these changes in visceral organ function inappropriately on a day-to-day basis could result in the development of diseases of cardiovascular, metabolic, gastrointestinal, or immune function.

No single CNS site of action of CRF has been identified (33). Introduction of the peptide into several hypothalamic and brainstem areas elicits elevations of

TABLE 2   Mechanism of Effects of CRF on Visceral Organ Function

Observed changes of visceral function	Neuroendocrine or ANS mechanism
Increased plasma concentrations of of glucose and glucagen	Adrenal Epi release
	Possible NE release in the pancreas (13,17)
	Possible decrease of parasympathetic influence on the pancreas
Increased cardiac output	Decreased PNS and increased SNS influence on the heart (15,18–20)
Increased HR	Decreased PNS and increased SNS influence on the heart (15,18–20)
Increased blood pressure	Decreased PNS and increased SNS influence on the heart (15,18-20)
Decreased renal and mesenteric blood flow	Increased SNS outflow (21,22)
Increased interscapular brown fat metabolism	Increased SNS outflow (17)
Decreased gastric acid secretion and motility	Decreased PNS activity (16,23)
	Increased SNS activity
	Pituitary β-endorphin release
Increased duodenal bicarbonate secretion	Increased SNS activity and pituitary β-endorphin release (24)
Decreased natural killer cell function	Increased SNS activity (25)
Inhibition of ovulation	Inhibition of LRF and LH secretion (23,26–28)

TABLE 3 Changes in ANS, Neuroendocrine or Visceral Organ Function
Attenuated by CNS Administration of a CRF Antagonist

Adrenal Epi release induced by ether vapor, insulin-induced hypoglycemia, and
  30% hemorrhage (26,27)
Restraint-induced decrease in gastric acid secretion and gastrointestinal motility
  (23,28–30)
Restraint-induced increase in duodenal bicarbonate secretion (24)
Inhibition of growth hormone and LH secretion (11,31)
Exercise-induced increase in HR, MAP, mesenteric vascular resistance, and iliac
  blood flow (32)

plasma norepinephrine (NE) concentrations. However, multiple brain sites have
been found to be insensitive to CRF.

Detailed descriptions of brain CRF pathways that mediate the changes of
visceral function thus far observed have not been made. We are currently using
electrical and chemical stimulation of CRF-containing brain regions in an
attempt to characterize these pathways.

THYROTROPIN–RELEASING FACTOR

Thyrotropin-releasing factor (TRF) was the first hypophysiotropic factor to be
characterized and was one of the first peptides demonstrated to have CNS
actions (34). Table 4 lists the CNS actions of TRF that affect neuroendocrine
and ANS function. Most of the CNS actions of TRF are qualitatively similar to
those produced by CRF.

Studies have been performed to determine if TRF-induced changes in ACTH
secretion and sympathoadrenal activity are secondary to stimulation of CRF-
containing pathways. In this regard, TRF-induced (given icv) ACTH secretion

TABLE 4 CNS Actions of TRF on Neuroendocrine and ANS Function

System	Effect
Anterior pituitary	Increased ACTH (35)
	Decreased growth hormone (36)
Adrenal medulla	Increased Epi release (37)
Sympathetic nervous	Increased NE release (37)
Parasympathetic nervous	Increased outflow to stomach, pancreas, and thyroid (38–42)

is totally prevented by intravenous (iv) administration of CRF antiserum (43). Icv administration of a CRF receptor antagonist has failed to prevent TRF-induced ACTH secretion, but may not mediate TRF-induced changes of sympathoadrenal activity.

Table 5 shows the mechanism by which icv administration of TRF influences visceral organ function.

A physiological role for TRF within the CNS to regulate the ANS is supported by the observation that icv administration of a TRF antiserum inhibits the spontaneous electrical discharge of the superior laryngeal nerve (119).

SOMATOSTATIN-RELATED PEPTIDES

Somatostatin-related peptides, including the naturally occurring somatostatins (SS), SS-14 and SS-28, and the synthetic octapeptide analog of SS-14, des AA^{1,2,4,5,12,13} D-Trp^8-SS (OD8-SS), have been extensively evaluated for their CNS actions in modifying ANS function (50). SS-28 and ODT8-SS are much more potent that SS-14 in influencing ANS activity.

Table 6 lists the CNS-mediated actions of SS-related peptides on neuroendocrine and ANS function.

Evidence to support a physiological role of SS-28 in the regulation of the ANS has resulted from the demonstration that a putative SS antagonist or depletion of brain SS using cysteamine results in an elevation of plasma epinephrine (Epi) concentrations (58).

Icv administration of SS-28 produces an increase in mean arterial pressure (MAP) and a decrease in heart rate (HR) that are secondary to pituitary vasopressin release (52,53,59). SS-28 given icv also elevates plasma concentrations of

TABLE 5   Mechanisms of the Effects of TRF on Visceral Organ Function

Visceral organ function	Neuroendocrine or ANS Mechanism
Increased plasma glucose concentration	Adrenal Epi release (37)
Increased HR	Decreased PNS and increased SNS outflow to the heart (44,45)
Increased respiratory rate	Mechanism undetermined (46–49)
Increased gastric acid secretion	Increased PNS outflow to stomach (38–42)
Increased duodenal bicarbonate secretion and exocrine pancreatic secretion	Increased PNS outflow (42)

TABLE 6 CNS Actions of Somatostatin-Related Peptides on Neuroendocrine and ANS Function

System	Effect
Anterior pituitary	Inhibits ACTH release (51)
Posterior pituitary	Stimulates oxytocin and AVP secretion (52,53)
Adrenal medulla	Inhibits Epi release (54,55)
Sympathetic nervous	Decreases superior laryngeal nerve activity (56)
Parasympathetic nervous	Increases outflow to the stomach (57)

oxytocin (52). Sawchenko et al. have recently described an SS-containing pathway that projects from the nucleus of the solitary tract (NTS) to vasopressin- and oxytocin-containing cells in the paraventricular and supraoptic nuclei of the hypothalamus (60). Depletion of brain SS using cysteamine attenuates hemorrhage-induced elevation of plasma vasopressin levels (52,53). SS has been demonstrated to inhibit hypothalamic NE release, providing a possible mechanism by which this peptide may stimulate vasopressin release (62). Thus, SS-containing neural pathways may be involved in mediating hemorrhage-induced vasopressin secretion.

Table 7 lists the mechanisms of SS-induced changes of visceral organ function.

BOMBESIN

Several bombesin-like peptides have been isolated and characterized from mammalian gut and brain (63). These peptides all share a common C-terminal

TABLE 7 Mechanisms of the Effects of Somatostatin-Related Peptides on Visceral Organ Function

Visceral organ function	Neuroendocrine or ANS mechanism
Decreased plasma glucose secretion	Inhibition of adrenal Epi concentration (55,61)
Increased blood pressure	Stimulation of AVP secretion (59)
Increased gastric acid secretion	Stimulation of PNS outflow to stomach (57)
Increased duodenal bicarbonate secretion	Stimulation of PNS outflow (41)

decapeptide that imparts biological activity (63,64). The mammalian bombesins exert CNS actions similar to those produced by the frog skin tetradecapeptide, bombesin (63,64). Table 8 lists the CNS actions of bombesin in affecting neuroendocrine and ANS function.

Bombesin influences ANS activity by increasing outflow to the adrenal medulla and parasympathetic innervation to the heart, and decreasing sympathetic outflow to interscapular brown fat. A site of action wherein bombesin increases plasma concentration of Epi has been identified within the brainstem in unanesthetized rats (71). Injection of bombesin (5.7 pM) into the rostral aspect of the NTS produces a dramatic elevation of plasma concentration of Epi; this effect is not observed when bombesin is injected into neighboring or distant brain sites. Injections of bombesin into the fourth ventricle, or 1 mm caudal or rostral to this site, cause much smaller increases in plasma Epi concentration. In the dog, bombesin acts within the dorsal hypothalamic area to elicit adrenal Epi secretion (72). The possibility that bombesin has other additional sites of action to increase plasma Epi concentration in the rat and dog has not been excluded.

The various CNS actions of bombesin to influence ANS activity appear to coordinate metabolic, cardiovascular, and thermoregulatory changes that are observed during nutrient deprivation (73). Whether bombesin is physiologically involved in mediating such adaptive responses to nutrient deprivation remains to be established.

ENKEPHALIN AND β-ENDORPHIN

Current information regarding the CNS actions of opiate peptides and opiate receptor antagonists on the regulation of autonomic function is conflicting and difficult to appraise. Chemical identity of the opiate ligand, dose, site of administration, and presence of anesthesia all modify the response observed. In many instances, the presence of anesthesia drastically alters the cardiovascular response

TABLE 8   CNS Actions of Bombesin in Neuroendocrine and ANS Function

System	Effect
Anterior pituitary	Increased or decreased growth hormone secretion (65)
	Inhibited TSH secretion (66)
Adrenal medulla	Increased Epi release (67)
Sympathetic nervous	Inhibited outflow to interscapular brown fat (68)
Parasympathetic nervous	Increased outflow to heart (69,70)

to opiate peptides administered into the brain (74). This discussion will be limited to studies in unanesthetized animals.

Both the enkephalins and β-endorphin given icv or into discrete brain sites increase plasma concentrations of Epi and NE (75,76). In most cases, leu-enkephalin, acting through a delta opiate receptor in hypothalamic or brainstem sites, increases MAP and HR (74,76). In contrast, β-endorphin administration decreases MAP, HR, and respiratory rate by acting through a mu opiate receptor (77).

β-endorphin, but not leu-enkephalin, decreases gastric acid secretion in both the rat and dog (78,79). This inhibition of gastric acid secretion is mediated by parasympathetic mechanisms (78,79).

Opiate-related peptides have been reported to influence pituitary function, resulting in changes of vasopressin, ACTH, and gonadotropin secretion (80–82).

The most convincing evidence that endogenous brain opiate systems play a physiological role in the regulation of the ANS has been obtained from studies demonstrating that the opiate receptor antagonist, naloxone, increases the MAP of hypotensive animals induced by endotoxin, hemorrhage, spinal cord injury, and anaphylaxis (83,84).

ANGIOTENSIN-II

Angiotensin-II (A-II) has both CNS and extra-CNS actions that subserve an animal's response to volume depletion (85,86). Circulating A-II may act on the brain to modify ANS function by virtue of its effects on the circumventricular organs (85,86). The subject of this discussion, however, is the action of brain A-II within the CNS to modify ANS activity. Icv administration of A-II to rats produces elevations of MAP, ACTH, and vasopressin, and decreases HR (19). Controversy exists over the possible effects of A-II on the CNS to modify sympathoadrenal and parasympathetic activity. The CNS-mediated cardiovascular actions of A-II have been attributed to changes of plasma concentrations of AVP and catecholamines, individually or in combination (86–90). The increase of MAP in awake rats following icv administration of A-II is prevented by systemic treatment with an AVP antagonist, but not with a ganglionic blocker (19). In contrast, when A-II is placed into the NTS of unanesthetized rats, elevations of MAP are not altered by an AVP antagonist (89,90). Based on results in dogs, agreement exists that A-II-induced elevation of MAP is mediated by changes in sympathetic and parasympathetic outflow, as well as changes in AVP secretion (86). However, the role of AVP appears to be more important in the rat than in the dog for A-II-induced changes of MAP (86).

No solid evidence exists in rats to support a physiological role of A-II in the CNS regulation of ANS activity. Evidence does exist to support important roles of peripheral A-II actions on the brain to modify ANS function (85,86).

NEUROPEPTIDE Y

Neuropeptide Y (NPY) has been demonstrated to be codistributed with Epi and NE in neural elements, both inside and outside the brain (91).

Icv administration of NPY has been reported to have no effect (92), to increase (93,94), or to decrease MAP and HR in rats (95). The explanation for the lack of agreement among different investigators is not apparent at this time. In our own studies, NPY produced a significant reduction of HR when injected icv or into the NTS (96). This change in HR resulted from decreased sympathetic outflow to the heart. In these studies, NPY did not alter plasma concentrations of Epi or NE. In the context of stress-related physiology, NPY release from peripheral sympathetic nerves may be of great importance. NPY released from sympathetic nerves may act to increase MAP and possibly decrease cardiac output (97,98).

SUBSTANCE P

Icv administration of substance P (SP) increases splanchnic, renal, and adrenal nerve activity (99,100), plasma concentrations of Epi, NE, and glucagon (99, 101), and MAP, HR, and respiratory rate (99,100,102). No specific CNS sites of action of SP have been identified, with the exception of the NTS, where SP may mediate afferent baroreceptor and/or chemoreceptor information (76). SP-induced increases of HR have been suggested to be mediated by modulation of parasympathetic outflow to the heart (76).

Evidence for a physiological role of SP in the regulation of ANS activity is supported by several observations. The sympathetically mediated elevations of MAP and HR produced by bicuculline or kainic acid injection into the ventral medulla are reversed by intrathecal injection of SP antagonists (102,103). Consistent with these observations is the finding that SP release from perfused spinal cord in vivo increases during kainic-acid-induced sympathetic excitation (104).

VASOPRESSIN

Vasopressin (AVP) given icv to rats has been reported to increase plasma concentrations of Epi and NE, and MAP and HR (105–108). The mechanisms involved in mediating the changes of MAP and HR are not known. Intrathecal administration of AVP has also been reported to produce antidiuresis by a neural mechanism (106,108). In these studies, peripheral administration of an AVP antagonist did not prevent the antidiuresis produced following intrathecal administration of AVP (109). Gruber et al. and Pittman et al. have suggested that brain AVP-containing pathways may mediate changes of sympathoadrenal function during stress (105,110).

CALCITONIN GENE-RELATED PEPTIDE

Calcitonin gene-related peptide (CGRP) given icv to rats increases plasma concentrations of NE but not Epi, and increases MAP and HR (111). CGRP is the only peptide demonstrated to increase plasma concentrations of NE selectively without also increasing plasma Epi levels. CGRP given icv to rats and dogs decreases gastric acid secretion and duodenal bicarbonate secretion (112–115). CGRP-induced decrease from changes of sympathetic nervous activity and increases of plasma concentrations of AVP. To date, a CNS site of action of CGRP has not been identified. No data exist to support a physiological role of CGRP in the regulation of the ANS.

INTERLEUKIN-1

Interleukin-1 (Il-1) acts within the CNS and at the pituitary level to stimulate ACTH secretion (116–118). The CNS actions of Il-1 to stimulate ACTH secretion results from CRF release. Recent studies have demonstrated that Il-1 given icv or iv increases plasma levels of NE (M. Brown and C. Rivier, unpublished results). These results are most consistent with two actions of Il-1 on sympathetic activity: one mediated by central CRF release and a second by an action of Il-1 peripherally.

ATRIAL NATRIURETIC PEPTIDE

Atrial natriuretic peptide (ANP) is released from cardiac myocytes (119,120). It is not suprising that this peptide and its receptors have been identified in the CNS. ANP outside the CNS inhibits most all of the known effects of angiotensin. ANP administered into the cerebroventricles of rats inhibits A–II-induced vasopressin release and elevation of arterial pressure (121–125). In contrast to these studies, ANP injected into the anteroventral third ventricle region of the rat brain elevates arterial pressure (126). Like many peptides, ANP is capable of exerting effects both within and outside the brain that result in a collectively coordinate series of actions.

SUMMARY OF PEPTIDE ACTIONS

Each peptide discussed above has a pharmacologically unique pattern of responses that it is capable of stimulating. Whether these responses result from single or multiple sites of action, and/or modification of afferent information to produce diverse efferent neuroendocrine and ANS responses, is unclear at this time. It is clear, in general, that the patterns of response produce coordinated signals to visceral organs that mimic those responses observed in normal animal physiology. Several peptides, CRF, TRF, SP, enkephalin, and AVP, produce generally qualitatively similar ANS responses. Such redundancy exists in other regulatory systems and may be important under circumstances of brain development or impaired brain function. An alternative explanation is that each of these peptides may subserve the regulation of ANS function by different brain areas. For example, the ANS response to certain types of emotional stress and exposure to cold may have similar gross ANS responses regulated by different brain systems utilizing different neuropeptides, but using the same efferent hard-wired neurocircuitry.

No unequivocal evidence exists to implicate any neuropeptide, by acting within the brain, in the physiological regulation of neuroendocrine or ANS activities. At least five peptides have been demonstrated to exert potentially physiologically relevant actions on ANS functions: CRF, SP, β-endorphin, SS, and TRF (Table 9). Once researchers are equipped with the appropriate pharmacological tools, animal models, and neurobiological techniques, the biological role of these and other neuropeptides to regulate ANS function will no doubt be identified.

FUTURE DEVELOPMENTS NECESSARY TO UNDERSTAND THE BIOLOGICAL ROLES OF PEPTIDES WITHIN THE CNS

The rich peptide pharmacology that has unfolded over the past 20 years is ripe to be tested for its relevance to physiology. This task is unfortunately limited

TABLE 9   Evidence to Support Physiological Actions of Peptides on the CNS Regulation of the Autonomic Nervous System

Peptide	Action	Evidence
CRF	Increased adrenal Epi secretion	CRF antagonist blocks stress-induced increase of plasma Epi levels and changes of gastrointestinal function (23,24,26–30)
SP	Increased sympathetic outflow	SP antagonist blocks sympathetic outflow (102, 103)
β-endor	Decreased MAP	Naloxone increases MAP in hypotensive animals (83,84)
SS	Decreased adrenal Epi secretion	SS antagonist, or depletion of brain SS with cysteamine, increases adrenal Epi secretion (58)
TRF	Increased sympathetic outflow	TRF antiserum inhibits electrical discharge of the superior laryngeal nerve (119) and gastric acid secretion (127)

by the complexity of the organism and questions to be answered, as well as by limitations of methodology. Following the simplistic concept of Koch's postulates leads one to recognize immediately at least some of the obvious developmental requirements that will be needed to assess adequately the physiological role of peptides in biological systems.

Regulation of Peptide Synthesis and Release

In the next few years, it is hoped that molecular biotechnology will be developed to allow biologists to manipulate selectively the transcriptional, translational, and posttranslational events that lead to the generation of a particular peptide in a specific anatomical cellular site. For instance, the ability to shut off CRF expression within a particular brain nucleus would be an unprecedented and powerful tool for studying the role of CRF within that brain area. As an alternative, and perhaps more powerful and important, will be the development of methods to modify selectively the secretion of a peptide. Such methods should ideally be rapid in onset, reversible, and devoid of nonspecific effects. To date, this goal has never been achieved. The closest approximation has been the use of capsaicin and cysteamine to study the physiology of SP and SS, respectively. Capsaicin depletes cellular stores of SP in primary sensory neurons (120). This methodology has been used to demonstrate a physiological role of SP in this system (120). Cysteamine depletes cellular stores and inhibits the synthesis of SS (121). Through the use of cysteamine, brain SS has been demonstrated to be involved in the regulation of adrenal Epi and pituitary AVP secretion (53,58). Despite the successful use of capsaicin and cysteamine as tools to study SP and SS, these substances are not without problems and controversy concerning their use.

Measurement of Peptide Release In Vivo

Measurement of peptides in discrete brain areas using radioimmunoassay or immunocytochemistry is useful; however, these methods are severely limited by sensitivity, specificity, and ability to test dynamic changes. In situ collection methods, especially the use of in vivo microdialysis, may prove useful, although these methods are extremely laborious (122). In vivo electrochemistry for peptides has been of little value. Future development of probes capable of dynamic sensing of the release of peptides within a discrete region may solve many of our problems. Coupling antibodies or peptide receptors to transducing membranes encasing microchips may provide this methodology.

Receptor Characterization

Two areas in receptor characterization would provide methods that would extend our current investigational ability. First would be the isolation and biochemical characterization of individual peptide receptors. This would aid a variety of investigators including, but not limited to, the study of the interactions between ligands and receptors to aid in analog design, evaluation of receptor interaction with postreceptor proteins, and development of antibodies against receptors to facilitate receptor localization and their use to inhibit ligand binding to receptors as a tool to study physiology.

The second area of receptor characterization will be to develop methods that can identify and segregate the functionally significant peptide receptors in the brain from those that may be artifact, receptors not coupled to postreceptor events, or receptors in transit. The apparent difficulties in showing functional changes of brain peptide receptors under different physiological conditions or following the sustained administration of their respective ligand may result from the inability to measure truly relevant receptors.

Peptide Analog and Antagonist Development

Receptor antagonists have provided powerful tools in the study of the history of numerous biologically important ligands such as catecholamines, histamine, acetylcholine, and others. The potency and specificity of these peptide antagonists vary; however, these analogs have been important in the development of an understanding of the biology of their respective peptide agonists. Development of peptide antagonists has largely been an empirical effort directed at optimizing regions of peptide binding while eliminating those residues involved in the generation of intrinsic activity. Several investigators have devoted efforts to analysis of peptide confirmation with the goal of predicting changes in structure that might result in higher receptor affinity and/or intrinsic activity (123).

An ultimate goal in peptide analog design is to characterize predictable ways to synthesize nonpeptide ligands that act as agonists or antagonists by binding to peptide receptors. The future of pharmacotherapeutics based on actions through peptide receptors will depend on the success of this venture. Such an achievement will provide ligands capable of binding to specific peptide receptors in or outside the brain, based on their controlled entrance into the brain resulting from differences in analog size, charge, or other physiochemical characteristics.

An extension of analog development is the coupling of peptides to cytotoxic agents. Conjugate of peptides to toxins such as ricin or gelonin may result in products capable of binding to and destroying cells possessing a particular receptor type (124,125). These compounds can be used as functional antagonists to prevent the action of a peptide, and also as tools to identify brain cellular elements that contain these receptors and to determine the neuroanatomic relationship of these sites to other cell structures.

CONCLUSION

In addition to the development of new methods, future efforts in the study of brain peptide regulation of neuroendocrine and ANS functions should include development of a conceptual framework in which peptides are thought to operate. It may be that these new pictures of peptide biology will be necessary before current and future facts can be seen in a different perspective (128-135).

Peptide biology has reached a point in its developmental history to allow the formulation of general concepts regarding their chemistry, cellular mechanisms of action, and general roles as transmitters of intercellular information. It will, as in all areas of science, be important to use information derived from reductionist analysis to form a method of predictable constructionalism that leads to an understanding of the role of peptides in biology.

REFERENCES

1. Shults C W, Quirion R, Chronwall B, Chase T N, O'Donohue T L. A comparison of the anatomical distribution of substance P and substance P receptors in the rat central nervous system. Peptides 1984; 3:1097–1128.
2. Herkenham M, McLean S. Mismatches between receptor and transmitter localizations in the brain. In: Boast CA, Snowhill EW, Alter CA, eds. Quantitative receptor autoradiography. New York: Alan R. Liss, 1986; 137–171.
3. Kruger L, Mantyh P W, Sternini C, Brecha N C, Manthy C. Calcitonin generelated peptide (CGRP) in the rat central nervous system: patterns of immunoreactivity and receptor binding sites. Brain Res 1985; 463:223–244.
4. Palkovits M. Distribution of neuropeptides in the brain: a review of biochemical and immunohistochemical studies. In: Negro-Villar A, Conn PM, eds. Peptide hormones: effects and mechanism of action, vol. 1. Boca Raton, FL: CRC Press, 1988; 3–67.
5. Bloom F F, Battenberg E L, Rivier J, Vale W. Corticotropin releasing factor (CRF): immunoreactive neurons and fibers in rat hypothalamus. Regul Peptides 1982; 4:43–48.
6. Swanson L W, Sawchenko P E, Rivier J, Vale W. Organization of ovine corticotropin-releasing factor immunoreactive cells and fibers in the rat brain: an immunohistochemical study. Neuroendocrinology 1983; 36:165–186.
7. DeSousa E B. Corticotropin-releasing factor receptors in the rat central nervous system: characterization and regional distribution. J Neurosci 1987; 7:88–100.
8. Insel T, Battaglia G, Fairbanks D W, DeSousa E B. Ontogeny of brain receptors for corticotropin releasing factor and development of a functional association with adenylate cyclase. J Neurosci 1988; 4151–4158.

9. Cunningham J J, Meara P A, Lee R Y, Bocle H H. Chronic intracerebroventricular CRF infusion attenuates ACTH-corticosterone release. Am J Physiol 1988; 255: E213–E217.

10. Ono N, Lumpkin M D, Samson W K, McDonald J I, McCann S M. Intrahypothalamic action of corticotropin-releasing factor (CRF) to inhibit growth hormone and LH release in the rat. Life Sci 1984; 35:1117–1123.

11. Rivier C, Rivier J, Vale W. Stress-induced inhibition of reproductive functions: role of endogenous corticotropin-releasing factor. Science, 1986; 231:607–609.

12. Brown M R, Fisher L A. Central nervous system effects of corticotropin releasing factor in the dog. Brain Res 1983; 280:75–79.

13. Brown M R, Fisher L A, Spiess J, Rivier C, Rivier J, Vale W. Corticotropin-releasing factor: actions on the sympathetic nervous system and metabolism. Endocrinology 1982; 111:928–931.

14. Hauger R L, Irwin M, Britton K T, Lorang M, Brown M R. Autonomic nervous system (ANS) modulation of immune responses to corticotropin releasing factor (CRF). The Endocrine Society, in press, 1989

15. Fisher L A, Jessen G, Brown, M R. Corticotropin-releasing factor (CRF): mechanism to elevate mean arterial pressure and heart rate. Regul Peptides 5:153–161.

16. Tache Y, Goto Y, Gunion M W, Vale W, Rivier J, Brown M. Inhibition of gastric acid secretion in rats by intracerebral injections of corticotropin-releasing factor. Science 1983; 222: 935–937.

17. Brown M R, Fisher L A. Corticotropin-releasing factor: effects on the autonomic nervous system and visceral systems. Fed. Proc. 1985; 44:243–248.

18. Fisher L A, Brown M R. Corticotropin-releasing factor: central nervous system effects on the sympathetic nervous system and cardiovascular regulation. In: Ganten D, Pfaff D, eds. Current topics in neuroendocrinology, vol. 3. Heidelberg: Springer Verlag, 1983; 87–101.

19. Fisher L A, Brown M R. Corticotropin-releasing factor and angiotensin II: comparison of CNS actions to influence neuroendocrine and cardiovascular function. Brain Res 1984; 296:41–47.

20. Fisher L A. Corticotropin-releasing factor: central nervous system effects on baroreflex control of heart rate. Life Sci 1988; 42: 2645–2649.

21. Overton J M, Fisher L A. Differentiated regional hemodynamic responses to peripheral and central administration of corticotropin-releasing factor. FASEB J 1989; 3:A1015, no 4583.

22. Grosskreutz C L, Brody M J. Regional hemodynamic responses to central administration of corticotropin-releasing factor (CRF). Brain Res 1988; 442:363–367.

23. Durge G, Raedler A, Greten H, Lenz H J. Pathways mediating CRF-induced inhibition of gastric acid secretion in rats. Am J Physiol 1989; 256:G214–G219.

24. Lenz H J. Regulation of duodenal bicarbonate secretion during stress by corticotropin-releasing factor and β-endorphin. Proc Natl Acad Sci USA 1989; 86:1417–1420.

25. Irwin M, Hauger R L, Brown M, Britton K T. CRF activates autonomic nervous system and reduces natural killer cytotoxicity. Am J Physiol 1988; 255:R744-R747.

26. Brown M R, Fisher L A, Webb V, Vale W W, Rivier J E. Corticotropin-releasing factor: a physiologic regulator of adrenal epinephrine secretion. Brain Res 1985; 328:355-357.

27. Brown M R, Gray T S, Fisher L A. Corticotropin-releasing factor receptor antagonist: effects on the autonomic nervous system and cardiovascular function. Regul Peptides 1986; 16:321-329.

28. Williams C L, Peterson J M, Villar R G, Burks T F. Corticotropin releasing factor directly mediates colonic responses to stress. Am J Physiol 1987; 253: G582-G586.

29. Lenz H J, Raedler A, Greten H, Vale W W, Rivier J E. Stress-induced gastro-intestinal secretory and motor responses in rats are mediated by endogenous corticotropin-releasing factor. Gastroenterology 1988; 95:1510-1517.

30. Stephen R L, Yang H, Rivier J, Tache Y. Intracisternal injections of CRF antagonist blocks surgical stress-induced inhibition of gastric secretion in the rat. Peptides 1988; 9:1067-1070.

31. Rivier C, Vale W. Involvement of corticotropin-releasing factor and somato-statin in stress-induced inhibition of growth hormone secretion in the rat. Endocrinology 1985; 117:2478-2482.

32. Kregel K C, Overton J M, Fisher L A, Taylor J A, Tipton C M, Seals D L. Influence of central CRF 9-41 injection on the cardiovascular responses to exercise in the rat. FASEB J 1988; 2:A1318, no 5944.

33. Brown M. Corticotropin releasing factor: central nervous system sites of action. Brain Res 1986; 399:10-14.

34. Segal D S, Mandell A J. Differential behavioral effects of hypothalamic polypeptides. In: Prange AJ, Jr, ed. The thyroid axis, drugs, and behavior. New York: Raven Press, 1974; 29-133.

35. Brown M R, Rivier C, Gray T S. Thyrotropin-releasing factor (TRF) effects on pituitary ACTH release and autonomic function. Soc Neurosci Abstr 1988; 14:1287, no 515.7.

36. Brown M, Vale W. Growth hormone release in the rat: effects of somato-statin and thyrotropin releasing factor. Endocrinology 1975; 97:1151-1156.

37. Brown M R. Thyrotropin releasing factor: a putative CNS regulator of the autonomic nervous system. Life Sci 1981; 28:1789-1795.

38. Tache Y, Vale W, Brown M. Thyrotropin-releasing hormone—CNS action to stimulate gastric acid secretion. Nature 1980; 287:149-151.

39. Kato Y, Kanno T. Thyrotropin-releasing hormone injected intracerebro-ventricularly in the rat stimulates exocrine pancreatic secretion via the vagus nerve. Regul Peptides 1983; 7:347-356.

40. Tonoue T. Stimulation by thyrotropin-releasing hormone of vagal outflow to the thyroid gland. Regul Peptides 1982; 3:29-39.

41. Lenz H J, Forquignon I, Druge G, Greten H. Effects of neuropeptides on gastric acid and duodenal bicarbonate secretion in freely moving rats. Regul Peptides, 1989, 24:293-300.

42. Lenz H J, Vale W W, Rivier J E. TRH-induced vagal stimulation of duodenal HCO₃ mediated by VIP and muscarine pathways. Am J Physiol, 1989; 257:G677–682.

43. Brown MR, Carver-Moore K, Gray TS, Rivier C. Thyrotropin-releasing factor-induced adrenocorticotropin secretion is mediated by corticotropin-releasing factor. Endocrinology 1989; 125:2558–2562.

44. Koivusalo F, Paakkari I, Leppauluoto J, Karppanen H. The effect of centrally administered TRH on blood pressure, heart rate and ventilation in the rat. Acta Physiol Scand 1979; 106:83–86.

45. Diz D I, Jacobowitz D M. Cardiovascular effects produced by injections of thyrotropin-releasing hormone in specific preoptic and hypothalamic nuclei in the rat. Peptides 1984; 5:801–808.

46. Myers R D, Metcalf G, Rice J C. Identification by microinjection of TRH-sensitive sites in the cat's brain stem that mediate respiratory, temperature and other autonomic changes. Brain Res 1977; 126:105–115.

47. Feuerstein G, Hassen A H, Faden A I. TRH: cardiovascular and sympathetic modulation in brain nuclei of the rat. Peptides 1983; 4:617–620.

48. Hedner J, Hedner T, Wessberg P, Lundberg D, Jonason J. Effects of TRH and TRH analogues on the central regulation of breathing in the rat. Acta Physiol. Scand 1983; 117:427–437.

49. Niewoehner D E, Levine A S, Morley J E. Central effects of neuropeptides on ventilation in the rat. Peptides 1983; 4:277–281.

50. Brown M R, Fisher L A. Brain peptide regulation of adrenal epinephrine secretion. Am J Physiol 1984; 247:E41–E46.

51. Brown M R, Rivier C, Vale W. Central nervous system regulation of adrenocorticotropin secretion: role of somatostatins. Endocrinology 1984; 114: 1546–1549.

52. Brown M R, Crum R, Sawchenko P. Somatostatin-28 (SS-28) stimulation of vasopressin (AVP) and oxytocin (OT). Endocrinology (Suppl) 1988; 122:660.

53. Brown M R, Mortrud M, Crum R, Sawchenko P. Role of somatostatin in the regulation of vasopressin secretion. Brain Res 1988; 452:212–218.

54. Brown M, Rivier J, Vale W. Somatostatin-28: selective action on the pancreatic β-cell and brain. Endocrinology 1981; 108:2391–2393.

55. Fisher D A, Brown M R. Somatostatin analog: plasma catecholamine suppression mediated by the central nervous system. Endocrinology 1980; 107:714–718.

56. Somiya H, Tonoue T. Neuropeptides as central integrators of autonomic nerve activity: effects of TRH, SRIF, VIP and bombesin on gastric and adrenal nerves. Regul Peptides 1984; 9:47–52.

57. Tache Y, Rivier J, Vale W, Brown M. Is somatostatin or a somatostatin-like peptide involved in central nervous system control of gastric secretion? Regul Peptides 1981; 1:307–315.

58. Brown M, Fisher L, Mason R T, Rivier J, Vale W. Neurobiological actions of cysteamine. Fed Proc 1985; 44:2556–2560.

59. Brown M R. Somatostatin-28 effects on central nervous system regulation of vasopressin secretion and blood pressure. Neuroendocrinology 1988; 47: 556–562.

60. Sawchenko P E, Benoit R, Brown M R. Somatostatin 28-immunoreactive inputs to the paraventricular and supraoptic nuclei: principal origin from non-aminergic neurons in the nucleus of the solitary tract. J Chem Neuroanat 1988; 1:81–94.

61. Gothert M. Somatostatin selectively inhibits noradrenaline release from hypothalamic neurones. Nature 1980; 288:86–88.

62. Brown M, Rivier J, Vale W. Somatostatin: central nervous system actions on glucoregulation. Endocrinology 1979; 104:1709–1715.

63. Walsh J H. Bombesin-like peptides. In: Krieger D T, Brownstein M J, Martin J B, eds. New York: Wiley, 1983: 941–960.

64. Brown M, Marki W, Rivier J. Is gastrin releasing peptide mammalian bombesin? Life Sci 1980; 27:125–128.

65. Tache Y, Brown M, Collu R. Central nervous system actions of bombesin-like peptides. In: Collu R, Ducharme J R, Barbeau A, Tollis G., eds. Brain peptides and hormones. New York: Raven Press, 1982; 183–196.

66. Brown M, Vale W. Peptides and thermoregulation. In Cox B, Lomax P, Milton A S, Schonbaum E, eds. Thermoregulatory mechanisms and their therapeutic implications. Basel: S. Karger, 1980: 186–194.

67. Brown M, Tache Y, Fisher D. Central nervous system action of bombesin: mechanism to induce hyperglycemia. Endocrinology 1979; 105:660–665.

68. Brown M R, Allen R, Fisher L. Bombesin alters the sympathetic nervous system response to cold exposure. Brain Res 1987; 400:35–39.

69. Fisher L A, Brown M R. Bombesin-induced stimulation of cardiac parasympathetic innervation. Regul Peptides 1984; 8:335–343.

70. Fisher L A, Cave C R, Brown M R. Central nervous system cardiovascular effects of bombesin in conscious rats. Am J Physiol 1985; 248:H425–H431.

71. Carver K, Brown M R. Bombesin central nervous system site of action to increase plasma concentrations of epinephrine. Soc Neurosci Abstr 1987; 204.8.

72. Brown M R. Central nervous system sites of action of bombesin and somatostatin to influence plasma epinephrine levels. Brain Res 1983; 276:253–257.

73. Brown M R, Carver K, Fisher L A. Bombesin: central nervous system actions to affect the autonomic nervous system. Ann NY Acad Sci 1989; 547:174–182.

74. Pfeiffer A, Feuerstein G, Kopin I J, Faden A I. Cardiovascular and respiratory effects of mu-, delta- and kappa-opiate agonists microinjected into the anterior hypothalamic brain area of awake rats. J Pharmacol Exp Ther 1983; 225:735–741.

75. VanLoon G R, Appel N M, Ho D. Beta-endorphin-induced stimulation of central sympathetic outflow: beta-endorphin increases plasma concentrations of epinephrine, norepinephrine and dopamine in rats. Endocrinology 1981; 109:46–53.

76. Lang R E, Gaida W, Ganten D, Hermann K, Kraft K, Unger T. Neuropeptides and central blood pressure regulation. In: Ganten D, Pfaff D, eds. Central cardiovascular control. Basic and clinical aspects. New York: Springer Verlag, 1983: 103–123.

77. Sitsen J M, Van Fee J M, DeJong W. Cardiovascular and respiratory effects of beta-endorphin in anesthetized and conscious rats. J Cardiovasc Pharmacol 1982; 4:883–888.

78. Morley J E, Levine A S, Silvis S E. Endogenous opiates inhibit gastric acid secretion induced by central administration of thyrotropin-releasing hormone (TRH). Life Sci 1981; 29:293–297.

79. Lenz J H, Brown M R. Central nervous system actions of β-endorphin on gastric acid secretion. Brain Res 1987; 413:1–9.

80. Plotsky P M. Opioid inhibition of immunoreactive CRF secretion into the hypophysial-portal circulation of rats. Regul Peptides 1986; 16:235–242.

81. Grossman A, Moult P J A, Cunnah D, Besser G M. Different opioid mechanisms are involved in the modulation of gonadotropin and ACTH release in man. Neuroendocrinology 1986; 42:357–360.

82. Forsling M L. Opioid peptides and vasopressin release. In: Schrier RW, ed. Vasopressin. New York: Raven Press, 1985: 425–434.

83. Holaday J W, Faden A I. Naloxone reversal of endotoxin hypotension suggests a role of endorphins in shock. Nature 1978; 275:450–451.

84. Faden A I, Holaday J W. Opiate antagonists: a role in the treatment of hypovolemic shock. Science 1979; 205:317–318.

85. Gannong W. The brain renin angiotensin system. In: Krieger D T, Brownstein M J, Martin J B, eds. Brain Peptides. New York: Wiley 1983: 806–826.

86. Reid I A. Actions of angiotensin II on the brain: mechanisms and physiologic role. Am J Physiol 1984; 246:F533–F543.

87. Bickerton R K, Buckley J P. Evidence for a central mechanism in angiotensin induced hypertension. Proc Soc Exp Biol Med 1961; 106:834–836.

88. Ferrario C M, Gildenberg P L, McCubbin J W. Cardiovascular effects of angiotensin mediated by the central nervous system. Circ Res 1972; 30: 257–262.

89. Casto R, Phillips M I. Mechanism of pressor effects by angiotensin in the nucleus tractus solitarius of rats. Am J Physiol 1984; 247:R575–R581.

90. Rettig R, Healy D P, Printz M P. Cardiovascular effects of microinjections of angiotensin II into the nucleus tractus solitarii. Brain Res 1986; 364: 233–240.

91. O'Donohue T L, Chronwall B M, Pruss R M, et al. Neuropeptide Y and peptide YY neuronal and endocrine systems. Peptides 1985; 6:755–768.

92. Petty M A, Dietrick R, Lang R E. The cardiovascular effects of neuropeptide Y (NPY). Clin Exp Hypertens 1984; [A] 6:1889–1892.

93. Fuxe K, Agnati L F, Harfstrand A, et al. Central administration of neuropeptide Y induces hypotension, bradypnea and EEG synchronization in the rat. Acta Physiol Scand 1983; 118:189–192.

94. Carter D A, Vallejo M, Lightman S L. Cardiovascular effects of neuropeptide Y in the nucleus tractus solitarius of rats: relationship with noradrenaline and vasopressin. Peptides 1985; 6:421–425.

95. Vallejo M, Lightman S L. Pressor effect of centrally administered neuropeptide Y in rats: role of sympathetic nervous system and vasopressin. Life Sci 1986; 38:1859–1866.

96. Scott N A, Webb V, Boublik J H, Rivier J, Brown M R. The cardiovascular actions of centrally administered neuropeptide Y. Regul. Peptides, in press, 1989.

97. Maisel A S, Scott N A, Motulsky H J, et al. Elevation of plasma neuropeptide Y levels in congestive heart failure. Am J Med 1989; 86:43–48.

98. Brown M R, Scott N A, Boublik J, et al. Neuropeptide Y: biological and clinical studies. In: Mutt V, Fuxe K, Hokfelt T, eds. Nobel conference on NPY. New York, Raven Press, 2989.

99. Unger T, Becker H, Petty M, et al. Differential effects of central angiotensin II and substance P on sympathetic nerve activity in conscious rats. Circ Res 1985; 56:563–575.

100. Unger T, Rascher W, Schuster C, et al. Central blood pressure effects of substance P and angiotensin II: role of the sympathetic nervous system and vasopressin. Eur J Pharmacol 1981; 70:33–42.

101. Iguchi A, Matsunaga H, Nomura T, Gotch M, Sakamoto N. Glucoregulatory effects of intrahypothalamic injections of bombesin and other peptides. Endocrinology 1984; 114:2242–2246.

102. Keeler J R, Charton C G, Helke C J. Cardiovascular effects of spinal cord substance P: studies with a stable receptor agonist. J Pharmacol Exp Ther 1985; 233:755–760.

103. Loewy A D, Sawyer W B. Substance P antagonist inhibits vasomotor responses elicted from ventral medulla in rat. Brain Res 1982; 245:379–383.

104. Takano Y, Martin J E, Leeman S E, Loewy A D. Substance P immunoreactivity released from rat spinal cord after kainic acid excitation of the ventral medulla oblongata: a correlation with increases in blood pressure. Brain Res 1984; 291:168–172.

105. Pittman Q J, Lawrence D, McLean L. Central effects of arginine vasopressin on blood pressure in rats. Endocrinology 110: 1982; 1058–1060.

106. Riphagen C L, Bauce L, Veale W L, Pittman Q J. The effects of intrathecal administration of arginine–vasopressin and substance P on blood pressure and adrenal secretion of epinephrine in rats. J Autono Nerv Syst 1986; 16:91–99.

107. Zerbe R L, Kirtland S, Faden A I, Feuerstein G. Central cardiovascular effects of mammalian neurohypophyseal peptides in conscious rats. Peptides 1983; 4:627–630.

108. Zerbe R L, Feverstein G. Cardiovascular effects of centrally administered vasopressin in conscious and anesthetized rats. Neuropeptides 1985; 6: 471–484.

109. Riphagen C L, Pittman Q J. Vasopressin influences renal function via a spinal action. Brain Res 1985; 336:346–349.

110. Gruber K A, Eskridge S L, Callahan M F. Activation of the central vasopressin system: a potential factor in the etiology of hypertension. Klin Wochenschr (Suppl. VIII) 1987; 65:82–86.

111. Fisher L A, Kikkawa D O, Rivier J E, et al. Stimulation of noradrenergic sympathetic outflow by calcitonin gene-related peptide. Nature 1983; 305:534–536.

112. Lenz H J, Mortrud M T, Vale W W, Rivier J E, Brown M R. Calcitonin gene-related peptide acts within the central nervous system to inhibit gastric acid secretion. Regul Peptides 1984; 9:271–277.

113. Tache Y, Gunion M, Lauffenberger M, Goto Y. Inhibition of gastric acid secretion by intracerebral injection of calcitonin gene related peptide in rats. Life Sci 1984; 35:871–878.

114. Hughes J J, Levine A S, Morley J E, Gosnell B A, Silvis S E. Intraventricular calcitonin in gene-related peptide inhibits gastric acid secretion. Peptides 1984; 5:665–667.

115. Lenz H J. Calcitonin and CGRP inhibit gastrointestinal transit via distinct neuronal pathways. Am J Physiol 1989; 254:

116. Bernton E W, Beach J E, Holaday J W, Smallridge R C, Fern H G. Release of multiple hormones by a direct action of interleukin-1 on pituitary cells. Science 1988; 238:519–520.

117. Katsuura G, Gottschall P E, Dahl R R, Arimura A. Adrenocorticotropin release induced by intracerebroventricular injection of recombinant human interleukin-1 in rats: possible involvement of prostaglandin. Endocrinology 1988; 122:1773–1779.

118. Berkenbosch F, Van Oers J, del Rey A, Tilders F, Besedovsky H. Corticotropin-releasing factor-producing neurons in the rat activated by interleukin-1. Science 1987; 238:524–526.

119. Zamir N, Skofitsch G, Eskay R L, Jacobowitz D M. Distribution of immunoreactive atrial natriuretic peptides in the central nervous system of the rat. Brain Res 1986; 363:105–111.

120. Quirion R, Dalpe M, DeLean A, Gutkowska J, Cantin M, Genest J. Atrial natriuretic factor (ANF) binding sites in brain and related structures. Peptides 1984; 5:1167–1172.

121. Itake K, Share L, Crofton J T, Brooks D P, Ouchi Y, Baline E H. Central atrial natriuretic factor reduces vasopressin secretion in the rat. Endocrinology 1986; 119:438–440.

122. Yamada T, Nakao K, Morii N, et al. Central effect of atrial natriuretic polypeptide on angiotensin II-stimulated vasopressin secretion in conscious rats. Eur J Pharmacol 1986; 125:453–456.

123. Samson W K, Aguila M C, Martinovic J, Antunes-Rodrigues J, Norris M. Hypothalamic action of atrial natriuretic factor to inhibit vasopressin secretion. Peptides 1987; 8:449–454.

124. Shimzu T, Katsuura G, Nakamura M, Nakao K, Morii N, Itoh Y, Shiono S, Imura H. Effect of intracerebroventricular atrial natriuretic polypeptide on blood pressure and urine production in rats. Life Sci 1986; 39: 1263-1270.

125. Casto R, Hilbig J, Schroeder G, Stock G. Atrial natriuretic factor inhibits central angiotensin II pressor response. Hypertension 1987; 9:473-477.

126. Sills M A, Nguyen K Q, Jacobowitz D M. Increases in heart rate and blood pressure produced by microinjections of atrial natriuretic factor into the AV3V region of rat brain. Peptides 1985; 6:1037-1042.

127. Tonoue T, Somiya H, Matsumoto H, Ogawa N, Leppaluoto J. Evidence that endogenous thyrotropin-releasing hormone (TRH) may control vagal efferents to thyroid gland: neural inhibition by central administration of TRH antiserum. Regul Peptides 1982; 4:293-298.

128. Burks T F, Buck S H, Miller M S. Mechanisms of depletion of substance P by capsaicin. Fed Proc 1985; 44:2531-2534.

129. Arimura A, Szabo S. Selective depletion of somatostatin in rat brain by cysteamine. Brain Res 1982; 240:178-180.

130. Westerink B H C, Damsma G, Rollema H, DeVries J B, Horn A S. Scope and limitations of *in vivo* dialysis: a comparison of its application to various neurotransmitter systems. Life Sci 1987; 41:1763-1776.

131. Hagler A, Osguthorpe D, Dauber-Osguthorpe P, Hempel J. Dynamics and conformational energetics of a peptide hormone: vasopressin. Science 1985; 227:1309-1315.

132. Oeltmann T N, Heath E C. A hybrid protein containing the toxic subunit of ricin and the cell-specific subunit of human chorionic gonadotropin. J Biol Chem 1979; 254:1022-1028.

133. Stirpe F, Olsnes S, Phil A. Gelonin, a new inhibitor of protein synthesis, nontoxic to intact cells. J Biol Chem 1980; 255:6947-6952.

134. Eldredge N, Gould S J. Punctuated equilibrium: an alternative to phyletic gradualism. In: Schopt TJM, ed., Models in paleobiology. San Francisco: Freeman, Cooper and Co, 1972: 82-115.

135. Hernandez D E, Jennes L, Emerick S G. Inhibition of gastric acid secretion by immunoneutralization of endogenous brain thyrotropin-releasing hormone. Brain Res 1987; 401:381-384.

11

SYMPATHOADRENAL CATECHOLAMINE STORAGE AND RELEASE IN HUMANS
Insights from the Study of Chromogranin A

Daniel T. O'Connor, M. A. Takiyyuddin, R. J. Parmer,
J. H. Cervenka, J. A. Barbosa, R. J. Hsiao, and Y. M. Chang
*University of California and Veterans Administration Medical Center,
San Diego, California*

Catecholamines in adrenal medullary chomaffin cells are sequestered from the cytosol in membrane-limited organelles known as chromaffin granules (chromaffin vesicles, catecholamine storage vesicles) (1-4). The soluble core of such vesicles contains numerous components in addition to catecholamines (1-4): ATP, ascorbic acid, calcium, dopamine beta-hydroxylase, and the chromogranins/secretogranins, a family of acidic, soluble proteins (5) whose functions are not clearly established. The best-studied chromogranin, known as chromogranin A, is a 48 kilodalton protein whose primary structure has recently been elucidated (6-13). Chromogranin A occurs not only in sympathoadrenal vesicles (14-17) but also in a widespread distribution in secretory vesicles throughout the neuroendocrine system (17-22) and in brain (17,22).

ROLE OF THE CHROMOGRANINS

The functional role (if any) of the chromogranins has been debated without clear consensus to date. Some frequently discussed putative activities or functions are listed in Table 1.

Evidence has been presented for actions of chromogranin A within secretory vesicles, including calcium binding (23-25), catecholamine binding (15,26-29), an ion exchanger (28-29), an inhibitor of prohormone/propeptide processing enzymes (30), complexing of ATP (31-33), and an osmotic pressure stabilizer (34).

TABLE 1   Putative Actions or Functions of Chromogranin

Within the cell of origin
  Binding (perhaps electrostatic) or osmotic inactivation of hormone storage
    vesicle soluble core constitutents
    H^+ buffering (1)
    Ca^{2+} (23–25)
    Catecholamines (15,26–29)
    Adenosine triphosphate (31–33)
    Osmotic pressure stabilizer (34)
  Modulator or inhibitor of prohormone processing enzymes (30)
  "Helper" protein in targeting peptides to secretory vesicles (8)
After release from the cell of origin
  Precursor of biologically active neuropeptides (8–10 paired basic sites)
    Pancreastatin, diminishing insulin secretion (13,35,36)
    Fragments, diminishing chromaffin cell secretion (37)

Putative actions of chromogranin A after its release from chromaffin cells include the generation of biologically active peptides such as pancreastatin (13, 35,36), or chromogranin A fragments that may suppress nicotinic-agonist-mediated catecholamine release from chromaffin cells (37).

Chromogranin A itself has no direct effects upon blood pressure when administered peripherally into the bloodstream or centrally into the subarachnoid space (38).

STRUCTURE

The primary structures of bovine (7,8), human (9,10), porcine (13), and rat (11, 12) chromogranin As have been deduced from the sequences of their cDNAs. Figure 1 shows a domain map based on the primary structure of bovine chromogranin A (7,8). Chromogranin A's putative structural/functional domains include a hydrophobic N-terminal signal peptide, which is cleaved from the mature protein; two cysteine residues toward the N-terminus, which may form an intramolecular disulfide loop (39); several sites of paired basic residues (8–10, depending upon the species), which may represent cleavage sites for prohormone processing enzymes; short oligoglutamic acid residue clusters; and areas with homology to known calcium-binding proteins.

Chromogranin A is apparently processed to a variety of fragments within the chromaffin granule (40), and one processing site is at the most N-terminal-paired basic site (41).

CHROMOGRANIN A RELEASE IN VITRO

Chromogranin A is coreleased along with catecholamines and dopamine beta-hydroxylase from chromaffin cells in the isolated perfused adrenal gland (42, 43) and chromaffin cells in primary monolayer culture (44) as well as PC-12 pheochromocytoma cells in culture (45). Chromogranin A and dopamine beta-hydroxylase are also coreleased with catecholamines from noradrenergic neurons in the isolated perfused spleen (46). The corelease of chromogranin A and dopamine beta-hydroxylase with catecholamines was and is the biochemical evidence underlying the hypothesis that exocytosis (all-or-none release of soluble constituents from the storage vesicle core) is the mode of catecholamine release from the sympathoadrenal system (42,43).

CHROMOGRANIN A RELEASE DURING ALTERATIONS OF SYMPATHOADRENAL ACTIVITY IN HUMANS

Figure 2 illustrates the stability of plasma chromogranin A and catecholamines in grouped data over time, and the lack of perturbation of either by an intravenous placebo.

Within the human sympathoadrenal system, selective provocation of catecholamine secretion both from the adrenal medulla (47,48) and from sympathetic neurons (49) results in corelease of chromogranin A with increases in plasma CgA.

Chromogranin A

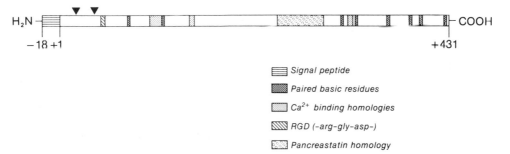

FIGURE 1 Putative structural/functional domains in the primary structure of chromogranin A, as deduced from the bovine adrenal cDNA sequence (7,8). The triangles mark cysteine residues that may form an intramolecular disulfide loop (39).

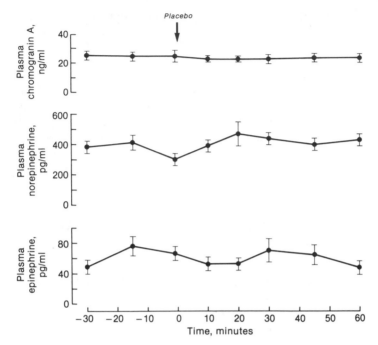

FIGURE 2 Stability of plasma chromogranin A and plasma catecholamines before and after the intravenous injection of placebo (normal saline) into 11 normal human subjects. The results are grouped data, shown as the mean value ± 1 SEM.

Figure 3 illustrates the response of plasma epinephrine and chromogranin A to selective stimulation of adrenal medullary secretion by insulin (0.15 U regular insulin/kg body weight, as an intravenous bolus) (47,48). Plasma epinephrine rose ~ 20-fold, by 30 min after the stimulus. Plasma chromogranin A rose ~ twofold, but the rise was not maximal until 90–120 min. Although the relative rise in chromogranin A was far less than that of epinephrine (~ twofold versus ~ 20-fold), its absolute rise was far greater (~ 20 ng/ml versus ~ 1 ng/ml).

The lag in appearance of chromogranin A suggests that chromogranin A takes an indirect route from the chromaffin granule to the bloodstream. Other evidence supporting this hypothesis includes the lack of a "step-up" in plasma chromogranin A in the adrenal vein compared with the inferior vena cava in humans, and the observation that chromogranin A is transported from the adrenal medulla at least in part by the lymphatics (thoracic duct) after hypoglycemia in the cat (50).

Selective, intense stimulation of sympathetic postganglionic axons by vigorous dynamic bicycle exercise (12 min, up to 200 W) increased plasma norepinephrine

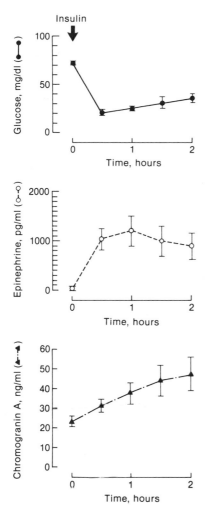

FIGURE 3 Time course of the response of plasma epinephrine and plasma chromogranin A to insulin-induced hypoglycemia in five normal human adults. The stimulus (secretagogue) was 0.15 units of regular insulin/kg body weight, given as an intravenous bolus at time zero. The results are shown as the mean value ± 1 SEM.

by $\sim$ 300%, but chromogranin A by only $\sim$ 20% (49). A lesser change in plasma chromogranin A after sympathetic neuronal than adrenal medullary stimulation is consistent with the relative tissue abundances of chromogranin A. Sympathetic axons contain $\sim$ 97-fold (in humans) to $\sim$ 5000-fold (in the cow) less immunoreactive chromogranin A than does the adrenal medulla (17,51). Thus, the mechanism of physiological sympathoadrenal catecholamine release in humans would appear to be exocytosis.

Only very intense stimulation of the adrenal medulla (hypoglycemia) or sympathetic axons (high-intensity dynamic exercise) measurably perturbs plasma chromogranin A (47–49,51). Less intense stimuli to the adrenal medulla (caffeine) or sympathetic axons (standing, smoking, low-intensity exercise) elevate the appropriate plasma catecholamine level without change in levels of plasma chromogranin A (47–49,51). The lack of change in chromogranin A levels does not preclude exocytosis during modest sympathoadrenal stimulation, but is consistent with the small expected changes in chromogranin A levels (based upon the measured catecholamine changes and the known catecholamine/chromogranin A ratio in storage vesicles) on top of its rather high basal value (normal plasma chromogranin A level, $\sim$ 20–50 ng/ml, versus $\sim$ 200–500 pg/ml for total plasma catecholamines).

The specificity of chromogranin A release for exocytosis is indicated in Figure 4. Tyramine, a weak base that may release catecholamines by diffusion as a consequence of alkalinization of the chromaffin granule interior (3), raises systolic blood pressure and plasma norepinephrine levels when infused into humans, but leaves chromogranin A levels unaltered. Thus, chromogranin A release is specific for exocytosis, and its measurement therefore yields information about the *mechanism* as well as the extent of sympathoadrenal catecholamine release.

Although both chromogranin A and dopamine beta-hydroxylase are core-leased along with catecholamines from storage vesicles (42,43,46), their basal plasma concentrations do not correlate in humans (Fig. 5). Thus, different factors (possibly differences in rates of removal) govern the relative concentrations of chromogranin A and dopamine beta-hydroxylase after their arrival in the circulation.

We have also been able to dissociate responses of plasma catecholamines, plasma chromogranin A, blood pressure, and heart rate pharmacologically in humans with agents such as reserpine (impairs vesicular storage of catecholamines), desipramine (blocks high-affinity neuronal reuptake of catecholamines), pargyline (inhibits monoamine oxidase), and amantadine (impairs protein endocytosis); thus, measurement of plasma chromogranin A yields a very different kind of information about the sympathoadrenal system than does measurement of catecholamines.

A modest increase in plasma chromogranin A levels in untreated essential hypertension suggests an excess of exocytotic sympathoadrenal activity in this

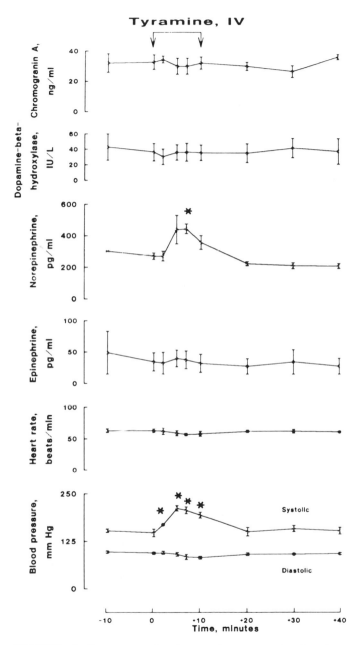

FIGURE 4 Response of plasma chromogranin A, plasma catecholamines, blood pressure, and heart rate to the intravenous infusion of tyramine hydrochloride into three human subjects for 10 min. The tyramine infusion rate was adjusted to raise systolic blood pressure by at least 20 mmHg. The results are shown as the mean value ± 1 SEM.

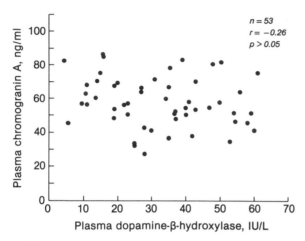

FIGURE 5   Basal (resting) plasma chromogranin A and dopamine beta-hydroxy-lase concentrations in 53 healthy adults (26 men, 27 women), aged 19–75 years. Dopamine beta hydroxylase was assayed spectrophotometrically (61).

disorder (52). Plasma chromogranin A levels are elevated in most subjects with pheochromocytoma, which suggests that exocytosis is one mode of catechol-amine secretion by the tumor, and yields a new diagnostic tool for this disease (52,53).

CHROMOGRANIN A RELEASE FROM OTHER ENDOCRINE SITES

Chromogranin A has a widespread if not universal occurrence in secretory ves-icles throughout the neuroendocrine system (1,17-22).

Chromogranin A is coreleased along with the usual resident peptide hormone by a variety of endocrine neoplasia with electron-dense core secretory vesicles, including pancreatic islet cell tumor, parathyroid adenoma and hyperplasia, oat cell lung carcinoma, medullary thyroid carcinoma, and C-cell hyperplasia (54-56). Dense core-granule-bearing endocrine tumors such as pheochromocytoma, carcinoid tumor, and neuroblastoma also secrete chromogranin A, even though no other peptide hormone is classically used as a daignostic test for the presence of these neoplasia (54,55,57-59). Measurement of plasma chromogranin A may be a valuable diagnostic tool for such tumors.

Other neoplasia, such as nonendocrine tumors or endocrine tumors not associated with peptides or dense core secretory vesicles, do not produce chromogranin A (54-57). Thus, secretion of chromogranin A by a neoplasm suggests that the tumor has neuroendocrine character. By contrast, several neoplasia with disputed neuroendocrine character or lineage, such as malignant melanoma, thymoma, choriocarcinoma, or renal cell carcinoma, did not secrete chromogranin A (59).

Normal neuroendocrine sites other than the adrenal medulla and sympathetic neurons (i.e., anterior pituicytes, pancreatic islet cells, gut enteroendocrine cells, parathyroid chief cells, thyroid parafollicular C-cells) when individually stimulated by appropriately selective secretagogues (e.g., hypothalamic-releasing hormones) measurably release the usual resident hormone(s) but do not perturb plasma chromogranin A (47).

Thus, under physiological or pharmacological perturbation, plasma chromogranin A responds primarily to alterations in sympathoadrenal activity, rather than other potential neuroendocrine sites. This finding is consistent with radioimmunoassay data documenting that among the endocrine tissues, the adrenal medulla is by far the major source of chromogranin A (17,18,60).

CONCLUSION

Measurements of chromogranin A have yielded insight into the exocytotic component of sympathoadrenal catecholamine release in humans.

ACKNOWLEDGMENTS

We appreciate the technical assitance of Ms. Annie Chen and the secretarial support of Ms. Ann Chavez.

This work was supported by the Veterans Administration, The National Institutes of Health, the American Heart Association, and the National Kidney Foundation.

REFERENCES

1. Winkler H, Apps D K, Fischer-Colbrie R. The function of adrenal chromaffin granules: established facts and unresolved topics. Neuroscience 1986; 18: 261-290.
2. Winkler H, Carmichael S W. The chromaffin granule. In: Poisner AM, Trifaro JM, eds. The secretory granule. Amsterdam: Elsevier Biomedical Press, 1982: 3-79.
3. Phillips J H. Dynamic aspects of chromaffin granule structure. Neuroscience 1982; 7:1595-1609.
4. Carmichael S W, Winkler H. The adrenal chromaffin cell. Sci Am 1985; 253 (2):40-49.
5. Eiden L, Huttner W, Mallet J, O'Connor D T, Winkler H, Zanini A. A nomenclature proposal for the chromogranin/secretogranin proteins. Neuroscience 1987; 21:1019-1021.

6. Kruggel W, O'Connor D T, Lewis R V. The amino terminal sequences of bovine and human chromogranin A and secretory protein I are identical. Biochem Biophys Res Commun 1985; 127:380–383.

7. Iacangelo A, Affolter H U, Eiden L E, Herbert E, Grimes M. Bovine chromogranin A sequence and distribution of its messenger RNA in endocrine tissues. Nature 1986; 323:82–86.

8. Benedum U M, Baeuerle P A, Konecki D S, et al. The primary structure of bovine chromogranin A, a representative of a class of acidic secretory proteins common to a variety of peptidergic cells, EMBO J 1986; 5:1495–1502.

9. Konecki D S, Benedum U M, Gerdes H H, Huttner W B. The primary structure of human chromogranin A and pancreastatin. J Biol Chem 1987; 262: 17026–30.

10. Helman L J, Ahn T G, Levine M A, et al. Molecular cloning and primary structure of human chromogranin A (secretory protein I) cDNA. J Biol Chem 1988; 263:11559–11563.

11. Iacangelo A, Okayama H, Eiden L E. Primary structure of rat chromogranin A and distribution of its mRNA. FEBS Lett 1988; 227:115–121.

12. Parmer R J. Koop A H, Handa M T, O'Connor D T. Molecular cloning of chromogranin A from a rat pheochromocytes cDNA library provides insight into functional domains. Am J Hypertens 1988; 1:65A (abstr).

13. Iacangelo A, Fischer-Colbrie R, Koller K J, Brownstein M J, Eiden L E. The sequence of porcine chromogranin A messenger RNA demonstrates chromogranin A can serve as the precursor for the biologically active hormone, pnacreastatin. Endocrinology 1988; 122:2339–2341.

14. Smith A D, Winkler H. Purification and properties of an acidic protein from chromaffin granules of the adrenal medulla. Biochem J 1967; 103:483–492.

15. Smith W J, Kirshner N. A specific soluble protein from catecholamine storage vesicles of bovine adrenal medulla. Purification and chemical characterization. Mol Pharmacol 1967; 3:52–62.

16. De Potter W P, Smith A D, DeSchaepdryver A F. Subcellular fractionation of splenic nerve: ATP, chromogranin A, and dopamine-beta-hydroxylase in noradrenergic vescles. Tissue Cell 1970; 2:529–546.

17. O'Connor D T, Frigon R P. Chromogranin A, the major catecholamine storage vesicle soluble protein. J Biol Chem 1984; 259:3237–3247.

18. O'Connor D T. Chromogranin: widespread immunoreactivity in polypeptide hormone producing tissues and in serum. Regul Peptides 1983; 6:263–280.

19. O'Connor D T, Burton D W, Deftos L J. Chromogranin A: immunohistology reveals its universal occurrence in normal polypeptide hormone producing endocrine glands. Life Sci 1983; 33:1657–1653.

20. Lloyd R V, Wilson B S. Specific endocrine tissue marker defined by a monoclonal antibody. Science 1983; 222:628–630.

21. Cohn D V, Elting J J, Frick M, Elde R. Selective localization of the parathyroid secretory protein I/adrenal medulla chromogranin A protein family in a wide variety of endocrine cells of the rat. Endocrinology 1984; 114: 1963.

22. Somogyi P, Hodgson A J, De Potter R W, et al. Chromogranin immunoreactivity in the central nervous system: immunochemical characterization, distribution and relationship to catecholamine and enkephalin pathways. Brain Res Rev 1984; 8:193-230.

23. Reiffen F U, Gratzl M. Chromogranins, widespread in endocrine and nervous tissue, bind calcium. FEBS Lett 1986; 195:327-330.

24. Reiffen F U, Gratzl M. Calcium binding to chromaffin vesicle matrix proteins: effect of pH, magnesium, and ionic strength. Biochemistry 1986; 25:4402-4406.

25. Mezger M S, O'Connor D T. Electrostatic interaction between calcium and adrenal catecholamine storage vesicle soluble proteins (chromogranins). Clin Res 1985; 33:365A (abstr).

26. Slotkin T A, Ferris R M, Kirshner N. Compartmental analysis of amine storage in bovine adrenal medullary granules. Mol Pharmacol 1971; 7:308-316.

27. O'Connor D T, Mezger M S, Chang Y M. Catecholamines interact with chromogranins, the major catecholamine storage vesicle soluble core proteins. Kidney Int 1987; 30:305 (abstr).

28. Uvnas B, Aborg C-H. The ability of ATP-free granule material from bovine adrenal medulla to bind inorganic cations and biogenic amines. Acta Physiol Scand 1977; 99:476-483.

29. Uvnas B, Aborg C-H. In vitro studies on a two-pool storage of adrenaline and noradrenaline in granule material from bovine adrenal medulla. Acta Physiol Scand 1980; 109:345-354.

30. Seideh N G, Hendy G N, Hamelin J, et al. Chromogranin A can act as a reversible processing enzyme inhibitor. Evidence from inhibition of the IRCM-serine protease 1 cleavage of proenkephalin and ACTH at pairs of basic amino acids. FEBS Lett 1987; 211:144-150.

31. Helle K B. Some chemical and physical properties of the soluble protein fraction of bovine adrenal chromaffin granules. Mol Pharmacol 1966; 2: 298:310.

32. Daniels A J, Williams R J P, Wright P E. The character of the stored molecules in chromaffin granules of the adrenal medulla: a nuclear magnetic resonance study. Neuroscience 1978; 3:573-585.

33. Sharp R R, Richards E P. Molecular mobilities of soluble components in the aqueous phase of chromaffin granules. Biochim Biophys Acta 1977; 497:260-271.

34. Helle K B, Reed R K, Pihl K E, Serck-Hansson G. Osmotic properties of the chromogranins and relation to osmotic pressure in catecholamine storage granules. Acta Physhiol Scand 1985; 123:21-33.

35. Eiden L E. Is chromogranin a prohormone? Nature 1987; 325:301.
36. Huttner W B, Benedum U M. Chromogranin A and pancreastatin (letter). Nature 1987; 325:305.
37. Simon J P, Bader M F, Aunis D. Secretion from chromaffin cells is controlled by chromogranin A derived peptides. Proc Natl Acad Sci 1988; 85: 1712–1716.
38. O'Connor D T. Chromogranin A: implications for hypertension. J Hypertension 1984; 2(Suppl):145–150.
39. Benedum U M, Lamouroux A, Konecki D S, et al. The primary structure of human secretogranin I (chromogranin B): comparison with chromogranin A reveals homologous terminal domains and an intervening variable region. EMBO J 1987; 6:1203–1211.
40. Wohlfarter T, Fischer-Colbrie R, Hogue-Angeletti R, Eiden L E, Winkler H. Processing of chromogranin A within chromaffin granules starts at C- and N-terminal cleavage sites. FEBS Lett 1988; 231:67–70.
41. Peirce J, Gill B, DeGuire M, Dinh T, Garrod S, O'Connor D T. Secretory vesicle processing of chromogranin A. Presented, Federation of American Societies for Experimental Biology (FASEB) (abstract), 1989.
42. Schneider F H, Smith A D, Winkler H. Secretion from the adrenal medulla: evidence for exocytosis. Br J Pharmacol Chemother 1967; 31:94–104.
43. Sage J K, Smith W J, Kirshner N. Mechanism of secretion from adrenal medulla. I. A microquantitative immunologic assay for bovine adrenal catecholamine storage vesicle protein and its application to studies of the secretory process. Mol Pharmacol 1967; 3:81–98.
44. Eiden L E, Iacangelo A, Hsu C M, Hotchkiss A J, Bader M F, Aunis D. Chromogranin A synthesis and secretion in chromaffin cells. J Neurochem 1987; 49:65–74.
45. Schubert D, Klier F G. Storage and release of acteylcholine by a clonal cell line. Proc Nat Acad Sci USA 1977; 74:5184–5188.
46. Smith A D, De Potter W P, Moerman E H, de Schaepdryver A F. Release of dopamine-beta-hydroxylase and chromogranin A upon stimulation of the splenic nerve. Tissue Cell 1970; 2:547–568.
47. O'Connor D T, Pandian M R, Cervenka J, Mezger M, Parmer R J. What is the source and disposition of chromogranin A in normal human plasma? Clin Res 1987; 35:605A (abstr).
48. Takiyyuddin M A, Cervenka J, Pandian M R, O'Connor D T. Selective adrenal medullary stimulation releases chromogranin A in man. Am J Hypertension 1988; 1:52A (abstr).
49. Takiyyuddin M A, Sullivan P, Cervenka J, O'Connor D T. Exocytotic catecholamine and chromogranin A corelease during selective stimulation of the sympathetic nervous system in man. Kidney Int 1989; 35:335 (abstr).
50. Stoddard S, O'Connor D T, Tyce G M, Yaksh T L, Carmichael S. The secretion of catecholamines, chromogranin A, and neuropeptide Y from the feline adrenal medulla in situ. Presented, Am Soc Anatomists (abstract), 1988.

51. Takiyyuddin M A, Cervenka J H, Sullivan P A. Pandian M R, O'Connor D T. Is physiologic catecholamine release exocytotic in man? Circulation 1990; 81:185–195.

52. O'Connor D T. Plasma chromogranin A: initial studies in human hypertension. Hypertension 1985; 7:176–179.

53. O'Connor D T, Bernstein K N. Radioimmunoassay of chromogranin A in plasma as a measure of exocytotic sympathoadrenal activity in normal subjects and patients with pheochromocytoma. N Engl J Med 1984; 311: 764–770.

54. O'Connor D T, Deftos L J. Secretion of chromogranin A by peptide producing endocrine neoplasms. N Engl J Med 1986; 314:1145–1151.

55. O'Connor D T, Deftos L J. How sensitive and specific is measurement of plasma chromogranin A for the diagnosis of neuroendocrine neoplasia? Ann NY Acad Sci 1987; 493:379–386.

56. Sobol R E, O'Connor D T, Addison J, Suchocki K, Royston I, Deftos L J. Elevated serum chromogranin A concentrations in small cell lung carcinoma. Ann Intern Med 1986; 105:698–700.

57. Cooper M J, Helman L, Evans A, Swamy S, O'Connor D T, Israel M. Chromogranin A expression in childhood peripheral neuroectodermal tumors. Adv Neuroblast. Res 1988; 2:175–184.

58. Hsiao R J, Seeger R C, Yu A L, O'Connor D T. Chromogranin A in children with neuroblastoma: plasma concentration parallels disease stage and predicts survival. J Clin Invest 1999; (in press).

59. O'Connor D T, Pandian M R, Carlton E, Cervenka J, Hsiao R J. Rapid measurement of circulating human chromogranin A: in vitro stability, exploration of the neuroendocrine character of neoplasia, and assessment of the effects of organ failure. Clin Chem 1989; 35:1631–1637.

60. O'Connor D T, Burton D W, Parmer R J, Deftos L J. Human chromogranin A: detection by immunohistochemistry in C-cells and diverse polypeptide hormone producing tumors. In: Cohn DV, Fujita T, Potts JT, Talmadge RV, eds. Endocrine control of bone and calcium metabolism. Amsterdam: Elsevier, 1984: 187–190.

61. Nagatsu T, Udenfriend S. Photometric assay of dopamine-beta-hydroxylase in human blood. Clin Chem 1972; 18:980–983.

12

HYPOTHALAMIC CONTROL AND PERIPHERAL CONCOMITANTS OF THE AUTONOMIC DEFENSE RESPONSE

Susan L. Stoddard

Indiana University School of Medicine, Fort Wayne, Indiana

DEFENSE RESPONSE IN THE CAT

In 1943 Hess and Brügger described the "Abwehrreaktion," or defense response in the cat (1). This purposeful, organized behavioral pattern consists of alerting, turning of the head, pupillary dilatation, flattening of the ears, piloerection, growling, hissing, and baring the claws; these actions frequently culminate in a sudden, directed attack. This response is familiar not only to psychologists and physiologists but also to any observer of cat behavior. This "Halloween cat" display is classically linked to confrontation with a dog, but it is seen in numerous other social situations: between unacquainted cats and in protection of food or young. Because this behavior appears to indicate some degree of fear on the part of the cat, we have anthropomorphically characterized the defense response as an example of "emotional" behavior in animals, and have conducted countless experiments based on the truth of this wholly unprovable assumption. As one of many such investigators, this author accepts the premise that the feline defense response is an emotional response, and can thus be used to examine aspects of emotional stress. Although there are extensive reports concerning defensive behavior in other animals, especially rodents, the following discussion will focus primarily on this behavior in the cat. This animal has been most frequently used both in identification of the neural control of defense and in characterization of the physiological concomitants of the behavior.

Hypothalamic Stimulation and the Central Nervous System: Anatomy of the Defense Response

The defense response occurs frequently in a cat's real world. However, dependable evocation of a consistent response in the laboratory is elusive. Therefore, hypothalamically elicited affective aggressive behavior has been used as a model for the naturally occurring defense response. Wasman and Flynn (2) first reported that electrical stimulation of hypothalamic regions could evoke aggressive behavior with affective (emotional) qualities indicative of autonomic arousal. These observations were extended to include the model of hypothalamically elicited affective defense, that is, defensive behavior directed at another cat (3,4). In this paradigm, electrical stimulation of, particularly, the ventromedial nucleus and the perifornical region (3,5) elicits a highly organized and directed behavioral pattern. Such a hypothalamically stimulated experimental cat, tested in an observation box in the presence of a second "target" cat, will alert at the onset of stimulation; the pupils dilate and the ears retract as the cat fixes its gaze on the target cat. Piloerection and growling or hissing are followed by the launching of a well-directed attack in which the experimental cat strikes with unsheathed claws at the target cat (3). Other hypothalamic electrodes may elicit a similar behavior in which the cat, rather than attacking, cowers in the corner of the observation box (4,5). (The active and passive aspects of these two hypothalamically stimulated behaviors led Adams [4] to suggest that these behaviors would be more accurately defined as defense and submission, and were associated with different patterns of neuronal firing in the ventromedial hypothalamic nucleus. This is an important distinction in the ethological and phylogenetic development of behavior, but will not be explored further in the present context.) At the termination of stimulation in both instances the attention of the experimental cat wanders from the target cat and the autonomic symptoms subside. There is little disagreement that centrally evoked affective defensive behaviors are empirically similar to those that occur naturally. Such resemblance between evoked and natural behavior prompted Leyhausen to state that "This procedure [electrostimulation of the brain] is without any doubt more valuable to ethologists at present than any other neurophysiological method" (6, p. 199).

In anatomical terms, the hypothalamus is critical to the organization of all the behavioral elements of affective defense into a coordinated, well-organized pattern. Portions of this behavior, such as hissing or paw striking, can be obtained by electrical stimulation more caudally along the neuraxis, as in the mesencephalic periaqueductal gray. However, the hypothalamus is the only region from which electrical stimulation will elicit an integrated, directed, purposeful behavior (Malcolm MacDonnell, personal communication). Thus, studies that have sought to understand affective defensive behavior, or the defense response, have focused on the hypothalamus.

In the approximately 25 years that have followed Wasman and Flynn's initial report, the neuroanatomy of affective defense has been intensely studied. A comprehensive review of these investigations, many of which were undertaken by colleagues of Flynn, is presented by Siegel and Edinger (7). These investigations have not only thoroughly mapped the hypothalamus to identify sites from which affective defensive behavior may be elicited but extensive studies have also identified modulatory sites, both facilitatory and inhibitory to this behavior, throughout the limbic system, cortex, and brainstem. Although the initial tools for these anatomical studies were electrical stimulation and lesions, more recently microinjection of glutamic acid (8) and neurotransmitter agonist and antagonists (9,10), in addition to [^{14}C] 2-deoxyglucose and tritiated amino acid autoradiography (11), have been used. Thus, an excellent understanding of the central neural control and modulation of affective defensive behavior is developing.

Physiological Concomitants of the Defense Response

In contrast to the extensive literature on the neuroanatomical bases of the feline defense response, with a few notable exceptions there has been a paucity of information obtained on the concomitant peripheral physiological correlates of affective defensive behavior. Cannon proposed a linkage between the defense response and the sympathetic nervous system in his description of the "fight or flight" response (12). Investigation into the cardiovascular concomitants of defense followed logically from Cannon's proposal since cardiovascular function is indeed modulated by sympathetic activation. The seminal study of Adams et al. in 1969 (13) reported the cardiovascular changes that accompanied naturally elicited fighting in cats. Their work led to a broader investigation of the cardiovascular concomitants of feline emotional behavior by Zanchetti and his colleagues (cf. 1 for review). Since cholinergic vasodilatation in the hind limb muscles was shown to result from stimulation of the same hypothalamic areas that, in the awake animal, elicit the defense response (14), this parameter was also investigated in the behaving animal (15). Along a somewhat different line, but related to the descriptive physiology of the defense response, Smith and co-workers (16), in an elegant series of experiments, identified a specific region in the anterior hypothalamus that controls the pattern of cardiovascular responses to a conditioned emotional response in chair-restrained baboons.

SYMPATHETIC ACTIVATION AND THE CENTRAL NERVOUS SYSTEM

It may be of use at this point to clarify the term *sympathetic activation*. For the purposes of the following discussion, the sympathetic nervous system will be arbitrarily classified into two components: the peripheral sympathetic nerves and the adrenal medulla. Thus, measurement of sympathetic activation becomes measurement of the "sympathoadrenal" response. All of the studies discussed in the previous section focused on cardiovascular function, which is the result of complex interactions between both the sympathetic and parasympathetic nervous systems. Because of the intricate interactions between these two systems, evaluations of cardiovascular changes during behavior become particularly complex; considerable evidence both from our lab and those of others (cf. below) has indicated that cardiovascular parameters may not be the best measure of the activity of the sympathetic nervous system.

Thus, in deciding to determine some of the physiological parameters of defensive behavior, we chose what we thought would be a more direct measurement of sympathetic activation: measurement of the plasma catecholamines norepinephrine (NE) and epinephrine (EPI). In fact, in 1914, Cannon reported that ". . . when a cat is frightened by a barking dog the blood in the cat's vena cava close in front of the opening of the adrenal veins gave definite evidence of the presence of adrenalin (relaxation of the rhythmically contracting intestinal strip), whereas blood from the same region previous to the excitement was ineffective" (17, p. 357). This observation encouraged us to focus particularly on adrenal medullary function in relation to defensive behavior.

Central Nervous System Control of the Adrenal Medulla

The literature on the central nervous system (CNS) control of the adrenal medulla, although not particularly extensive, is both complex and bewildering. The complexity of this literature is due to the use of different animals, anesthetic agents, measurement techniques and experimental paradigms. Table 1 presents a selective summary of research in this field over the past 35 years, including variations in procedures and results. Further aspects of the CNS control of autonomic function are discussed in other chapters in this voume (cf. particularly the contributions by Sawchenko, Gray, and Loewy).

The studies that preceded our own investigations could not, for several reasons, be directly translated to our problem: description of the sympathoadrenal response associated with defensive behavior. First, and perhaps foremost, previous studies had not specifically linked stimulation sites in the CNS with behavior. Second, various anesthetic agents were employed across studies. Various types of anesthesia are known to affect adrenal medullary output differentially (34), and it seems reasonable that any anesthesia, by affecting the CNS, would produce physiological responses not identical to those elicited in the awake animal. Last, variation in the patterns of adrenal medullary secretion in response to the same physiological stimulus exist between species. Critchley and colleagues (35) demonstrated that in the pentobarbital anesthetized cat, chemoreceptor or baroreceptor tests changed the resting ratio of 1:1 for NE/EPI to, respectively, 1:6 and 3:1. In contrast, the resting ratio of 1:4 (NE/EPI) in the cloralose–urethane- or pentobarbital-anesthetized dog was not altered by these stimuli.

Measurement of Plasma Catecholamines in the Hypothalamically Stimulated, Awake Cat

Since we were unable to find any previous studies that had measured plasma catecholamine levels in relation to CNS stimulation in the awake animal, this was our first step in investigating sympathoadrenal activation during the defense response. Electrodes were lowered into the hypothalamus in 19 stereotaxically prepared, head-holder-restrained, unanesthetized cats, permitting the stimulation of 131 hypothalamic sites for 5 s at standard stimulus parameters (biphasic, square-wave pulses; 1 ms half-cycle duration; 0.4 mA peak-to-peak; 60 Hz) (28). Peripheral plasma was collected from the femoral vein and levels of free NE and EPI were measured by radioenzymatic assay (36). In this experimental paradigm the greatest increases in peripheral NE and EPI occurred following stimulation of sites in the ventromedial nucleus, perifornical area, and medial forebrain bundle. It is of note that the ventromedial nucleus and perifornical areas are also the hypothalamic regions from which affective defensive behavior is most reliably evoked (3,5). Our data also indicated, in agreement with other reports (Table 1), that preferential increases in plasma NE or EPI could be elicited by hypothalamic stimulation.

Whereas this study provided much-needed information about sympathoadrenal activity in the awake cat, certain weaknesses were apparent. We observed considerable variability in the responses of the individual animals; this variability in the feline adrenal medullary response has been extensively confirmed (37,38). We also could not be certain of the source of NE in the peripheral plasma. EPI is derived primarily or wholly from the adrenal medulla; there is no evidence of catecholamine secretion from extraadrenal chromaffin tissue (39). Peripheral NE, however, may be secreted from the adrenal medulla, or may be the overflow of neurotransmitter from noradrenergic sympathetic nerves that has not been reclaimed by the presynaptic terminal, and has diffused into the circulation. Kvetnansky et al. (40) convincingly demonstrated that in the rat approximately 70% of the peripheral NE is derived from sympathetic nerves, thus permitting the level of peripheral NE to serve as an index of sympathetic neural function. However, if one considers both the variation noted among individual cats and the established species differences in the ratio of NE to EPI secreted from the adrenal medulla, there is no a priori reason to expect the results of Kvetnansky et al. in the rat to be applicable to the cat.

TABLE 1   Selective Summary of Studies Investigating the CNS Control of
Adrenal Medullary Secretion

Year	Authors	Animal	Anesthesia	Blood collection site
1953	Redgate and Gellhorn (18)	Cat	Chloralose	None
1954	Folkow and von Euler (19)	Cat	Chloralose and urethane	L adrenal vein
1958	von Euler and Folkow (20)	Cat	Chloralose and urethane	Adrenal vein
1958	Grant et al. (21)	Cat	Dial or chloralose and urethane	L adrenal vein
1962	Goldfien and Ganong (22)	Dog	Pentobarbital	Adrenal vein
1965	Matsui (23)	Cat	Pentobarbital	L adrenal vein
1979	Matsui (24)	Rat	Pentobarbital	L adrenal vein
1981	Matsui (25)	Rat	Pentobarbital	L adrenal vein
1982	Francke et al. (26)	Cat	Dial-urethane	Bilateral adrenal vein
1983	Robinson et al. (27)	Cat	Dial-urethane	L adrenal vein
1983	Stoddard-Apter et al. (28)	Cat	Awake	Femoral vein

CA measurement	Active areas and number of sites investigated	Results and comments[a]
Autologous bioassay	Anterior hypothalamus, posterior hypothalamus	↑ NE in anterior hypothalamus ↑ EPI in posterior hypothalamus
Bioassay	Preoptic area, posterior hypothalamus, thalamus, dorsal pons, midbrain (32 sites)	↑ in both NE and EPI most common; evidence for selective secretion of both NE and EPI
Bioassay	Orbital cortex	Selective change in EPI secretion; ↓ EPI from ventral cortex, little effect on NE
Bioassay	Dorsomedial nucleus and paraventricular n. in anterior hypothalamus (14 sites)	Sites selected to elicit cholinergic vasodilation in hind limb caused ↑ % EPI > ↑ % NE
Ethylenediamine	Dorsomedial and posterior nuclei and in caudally-laterally extending band (66 sites)	↑ EPI alone most common; ↑ NE always accompanied by ≥ ↑ EPI; adrenal medullary pathways bilateral
Fluorometric	Dorsal medulla via floor IV ventricle (23 sites)	↑ NE and EPI both alone and together; ↓ NE
Fluorometric	Dorsal medulla via floor IV ventricle (25 sites)	↑ EPI; ↓ NE with and without ↓ EPI; no ↑ NE
Fluorometric	Dorsolateral pons and midbrain near nucleus of V (29 sites)	↑ EPI with and without ↑ NE
Fluorometric	Anterior and posterior hypothalamus, rostral mesencephalic tegmentum (27 sites)	Bilateral ↑ NE and EPI most common with ipsilateral predominance; evidence of selective secretion of both NE and EPI
Fluorometric	Throughout hypothalamus (355 sites)	Differential facilitation and inhibition of both NE and EPI; no consistent relation between MAP and catecholamine changes
Radioenzymatic	Throughout hypothalamus (131 sites)	Greatest ↑ NE and EPI from vm, MFB and perifornical area; differential activation of both NE and EPI; HR and MAP changes inconsistent with ↑ CAs

TABLE 1   (Continued)

Year	Authors	Animal	Anesthesia	Blood collection site
1986	Katafuchi et al. (29)	Rat	Ketamine	L adrenal vein
1986	Stoddard et al. (5,30)	Cat	Pentobarbital	Bilateral adrenal vein and atrial appendage
1987	Matsui (31)	Rat	Pentobarbital	L adrenal vein
1987	Bereiter et al. (32)	Cat	Chloralose and urethane	L adrenal vein
1988	Bereiter and Gann (33)	Cat	Ketamine and chloralose	L adrenal vein

[a]All studies employed electrical stimulation, except Bereiter and Gann (33) who stimulated via microinjections of glutamic acid.

CA, catecholamines; EC, electrochemical detection; HPLC, high performance liquid chromatography; HR, heart rate; L, left; MAP, mean arterial blood pressure; MFB, medial forebrain bundle; n., nucleus; vm, ventromedial nucleus of the hypothalamus.

Adrenal Medullary Secretion Related to Stimulation of Hypothalamic Defense Sites

Having confirmed that peripheral NE could be preferentially increased by stimulation at certain hypothalamic sites, we chose to measure directly the outflow from the adrenal gland itself; comparison of levels of catecholamines in adrenal venous plasma with levels in the peripheral venous plasma would, we believed, clarify the source of peripheral NE related to hypothalamic stimulation. Numerous other investigators had measured catecholamine levels in adrenal venous blood; however, we were not aware at that time of any studies that had compared adrenal and peripheral venous catecholamines, or that had used behaviorally identified hypothalamic sites. The major drawback of our experimental design was that collection of blood from bilateral adrenal veins required the use of an acute, anesthetized preparation.

Hypothalamic sites were identified in the freely moving cat (n = 20), that elicited affective defensive behavior (5). The following day, the cat was

CA measurement	Active areas and number of sites investigated	Results and comments[a]
HPLC	Lateral hypothalamic area (10 sites)	Selective ↑ EPI or ↓ NE or combined ↓ EPI and NE
Radioenzymatic	Medial hypothalamus (60 behaviorally identified sites)	Bilateral ↑ NE and EPI most common with ipsilateral predominance; preferential ↑ of both NE and EPI
Fluorometric	Zona incerta (10 sites)	↑ EPI and ↓ NE and EPI
HPLC + EC	Pars caudalis of spinal nucleus of V and ventrolateral medulla (36 sites)	↑ EPI with burst pattern of stimulation of nucleus V; ↑ NE with burst or continuous stimulation of nucleus V or ventrolateral brainstem
HPLC + EC	Marginal layers, pars caudalis of spinal nucleus V (22 sites)	↑ EPI > ↑ NE; mainly ipsilateral effect; no correlation with MAP or HR

anesthetized with sodium pentobarbital and cannulae placed to collect blood samples simultaneously from both adrenal veins and the right atrial appendage. Cardiovascular parameters were continuously monitored through another cannula in the femoral artery. Three consecutive 1 min blood samples were collected concurrently from the three sources, two prior to stimulation and the third commencing with the onset of stimulation. Hypothalamic sites that had evoked affective defensive behavior in the awake animal were stimulated for a period of 30 s at the same intensity (0.2-0.8 mA) that had elicted the behavior. A total of 31 behaviorally identified hypothalamic sites were investigated, 24 with bilateral adrenal venous samples and 7 with unilateral adrenal venous samples, ipsilateral to the side of hypothalamic stimulation. The most common adrenal medullary response, following 58% of the stimulations, was a bilateral increase in the secretion of both NE and EPI $\geq$ 10 ng/min (Fig. 1). Furthermore, the increases in EPI from the adrenal gland ipsilateral to the hypothalamic stimulation site were significantly greater than the increases from the contralateral gland. In similar fashion, NE increases were greater from the ipsilateral gland, but the differences from the contralateral gland were not significant. Other specific responses included both preferential increases and decreases in either NE or EPI. Hypothalamic stimulation at the behaviorally identified sites also significantly altered the ratio of catecholamines secreted by the adrenal medulla.

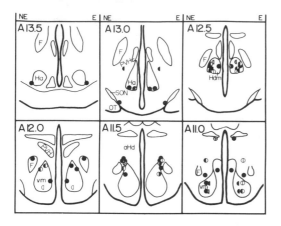

FIGURE 1 Composite map of the stimulation sites that elicited defensive behavior when the freely moving experimental cat was presented with a second cat as a target. Sites are plotted on drawings of coronal sections from the atlas of Jasper and Ajmone-Marsan (41). Symbols indicate the type of adrenal medullary response elicited by stimulation of each site in the anesthetized cat at the intensity that elicited behavior in the freely moving animal. Changes in NE secretion are on the left of each drawing; changes in epinephrine (E) secretion are on the right. Shaded circle: increase in catecholamine (CA) output $\geqslant$ 10 ng/min; clear circle: increase in CA secretion $\geqslant$ 0 but $<$ 10 ng/min; circle with dots: decrease in CA secretion. Each circle is divided into halves: the left shows the response from the adrenal medulla ipsilateral to the side of hypothalamic stimulation; the right half shows the response from the contralateral adrenal medulla. Half circles show the adrenal medullary responses in cats in which blood samples were collected from only the ipsilateral adrenal vein. F, fornix; Ha, anterior hypothalamic area; PVH, paraventricular nucleus; SON, supraoptic nucleus; OT, optic tract; Hdm, dorsomedial nucleus; vm; ventromedial nucleus; aHd, dorsal hypothalamic area. (from ref. 5).

The baseline ratio of 2.6:1 for NE/EPI decreased to 1.4:1 following stimulation of hypothalamic defense sites.

Activation of the peripheral noradrenergic sympathetic nerves was estimated by comparing levels of catecholamines in the bilateral adrenal venous samples to levels in blood samples collected simultaneously from the atrial appendage. These comparisons permitted us to estimate that under baseline conditions (and anesthesia), approximately 67% of the NE in the peripheral plasma was contributed by the sympathetic nerves. It is of considerable interest that this proportion is in close agreement with that measured in the rat by Kvetnansky et al. (40). The proportion of NE derived from the sympathetic nerves increased to 75% following stimulation of hypothalamic defense sites. Although stimulation of hypothalamic defense sites increased peripheral NE, suggesting activation of the sympathetic nervous component of the sympathoadrenal system, the concomitant increases in heart rate and blood pressure were small and did not reliably reflect the increased activity of the sympathetic nerves.

At about the same time, Bereiter and colleagues (42) demonstrated that peripheral catecholamine responses best reflected large increases in adrenal medullary secretion. Furthermore, they showed that the correlation between adrenal secretion and peripheral levels was related to the time after CNS stimulation when concurrent samples were drawn. In light of these observations it is possible that our concurrent adrenal and peripheral venous samples (5,30) were collected too early to allow us to evaluate fully the effect of adrenal NE secretion on peripheral NE levels.

We concluded that hypothalamically elicited defensive behavior in the cat is accompanied most often by activation of both the adrenal medullary and sympathetic nervous components of the sympathoadrenal system. The hypothalamic sites that elicit defensive behavior are distributed throughout the medial hypothalamus; although there was a predominant sympathoadrenal response, the responses did indeed vary among stimulation sites. Thus, these results led us to question seriously the efficacy of using hypothalamically stimulated defensive behavior as a true "model" for the defense response. Although the evoked and natural behaviors are empirically very similar, as discussed above, our findings on the variability of one physiological concomitant—the sympathoadrenal response—questions the reliability of using the brain-stimulated behavior as a means for investigating the physiology of defensive behavior.

Sympathoadrenal Activation in the Behaving Cat

Having established the paradigm of hypothalamically stimulated behavior as a means to investigate the physiological concomitants of defense, and then reporting data that we believed substantively weakened our original premise, we were left with only one avenue: to undertake the description of the sympathoadrenal response in the naturally behaving animal. The primary weakness of this approach (cf. above) was that only peripheral catecholamines could be measured. Plasma NE and EPI were measured in blood collected from the atrial appendage in 12 cats in which natural defensive behavior was elicited (43). Cardiovascular parameters were concurrently monitored through a second cannula placed in the aortic arch. Our experimental paradigm was very similar to that used by Adams et al. (13). The experimental cat was placed in the larger portion of a divided observation box (Fig. 2); defensive behavior was evoked in this animal by both intraspecies and interspecies stimuli. The intraspecies stimulus was another cat with a hypothalamic electrode placed to elicit affective defensive behavior. For testing, the partition between the two sides of the box was opened, and the

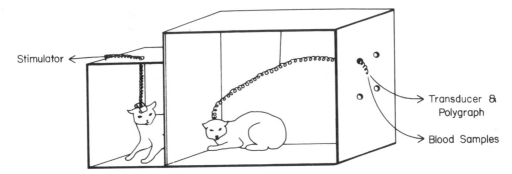

FIGURE 2   Schematic representation of the experimental paradigm used to test naturally elicited defensive behavior. The experimental cat was placed in the larger portion of the observation box. The hypothalamically stimulated cat was placed in the smaller side, or a large, barking dog was brought to the front of the larger side. Cannulae for the collection of blood samples and the monitoring of cardiovascular parameters from the experimental cat were enclosed in a spring and led out of the observation box.

hypothalamically stimulated cat pulled on a leash toward the experimental cat to elicit an exhibition of defensive behavior. The interspecies stimulus was a large dog that was trained to jump up in front of the observation box and bark. Each stimulus was presented for 15 s; three trials were run on one day with at least 30 min elapsing between trials. Two baseline blood samples were taken prior to the presentation of the stimulus, at 15 s intervals during the first minute following the presentation of the stimulus, and at 2 and 3 min after stimulus onset. Since the half-lives of EPI and NE in the plasma are comparatively short (1-4 min) (44,45), we wished to maximize our opportunity to observe changing levels of plasma catecholamines related to defensive behavior.

Several unexpected observations resulted from this study. The increases in both plasma NE and EPI, as well as in heart rate and blood pressure, were significantly greater in the first trial with the dog than in the first trial with another cat. A chi-square analyses was used to compare that trial (of three) in which the greatest increase in NE or EPI occurred (Table 2). In general, the largest increases in NE and EPI were coincident when the behavioral stimulus was a dog. However, when the behavioral stimulus was another cat, the patterns of occurrence of the greatest increases in NE and EPI were significantly different, with the greatest increase in NE generally occurring later in the series of three trials. We concluded that defensive behavior evoked by a dog (Fig. 3A) was accompanied by primarily adrenal medullary activation; the peak levels of NE and EPI were generally coincident. Defensive behavior evoked by a cat was accompanied by a different pattern of sympathoadrenal activity, as suggested by levels of plasma catecholamines. Intraspecies defensive behavior appeared to be associated initially with EPI release from the adrenal medulla. However, in later trials (Fig. 3B) increased NE responses and a lack of coincidence between the peaks of NE and EPI suggested increased involvement of the sympathetic nerves as the source for plasma NE.

We believe the most notable result of this study is the observation that defensive behaviors, which appear similar if not identical in many instances, are different physiological events in terms of sympathoadrenal responsiveness. In support of our observations are the studies of Zanchetti and colleagues (46,47), who found that changes in iliac blood flow are, at least in part, dependent on the emotional stimulus. Thus, while exhibiting similar somatic and autonomic reactions, some cats showed muscle vasoconstriction, while others exhibited cholinergic vasodilatation when presented with various "emotional" stimuli, including a barking dog and fire. Williams et al. (48) likewise reported that in the rat the sympathetic response to stress is not an all-or-none response, but is a patterned activation that depends upon the behaviors available to the animal.

Our investigations of the characteristics of the sympathoadrenal response that accompanies not only defense but also other forms of aggressive behavior, such as flight (escape) and offense, have only begun to define the extent of the

TABLE 2 Natural Defensive Behavior Elicited by a Barking Dog or a Hypothalamically Stimulated Cat

Cat no.	Dog NE (trial no.)			Dog EPI (trial no.)			Stimulus cat NE (trial no.)			Stimulus cat EPI (trial no.)		
	1	2	3	1	2	3	1	2	3	1	2	3
1137	X			X					X	X		
1133	X			X				X			X	
1154	X			X					X	X		
1135	X			X					X	X		
1131	X			X				X		X		
1132	X			X			X				X	
1130			X		X		X			X		
1153	X			X				X		X		
1150	X			X			X				X	
1148			X		X				X	X		
1149	X			X					X		X	
1156								X			X	

The trial in which the maximal change from baseline of norepinephrine (NE) or epinephrine (EPI) occurred with each behavioral stimulus is indicated by an "X."
Source: Ref. 43.

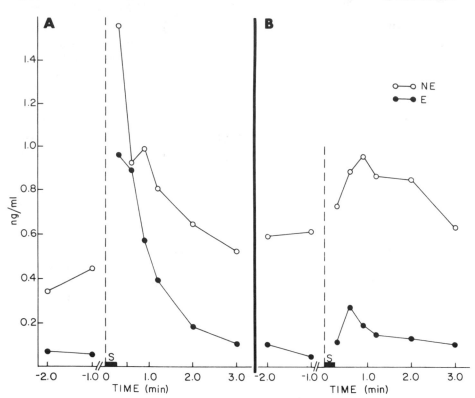

FIGURE 3 Absolute levels of plasma NE (open circles) and epinephrine (E; solid circles) in ng/ml during representative defensive behavior trials for a single cat (#1149). A. First trial with a dog. B. Third trial with a cat. Bar with "S" indicates the duration of the behavioral stimulus. Baseline values for NE and E are shown to the left of time = 0, in relation to negative time values (from ref. 43).

problem rather than provide definitive answers. Certain conclusions can be drawn from our studies, but perhaps more importantly, our work raises numerous questions and suggests diverse lines of further investigation. Using the author's prerogative of speculation, several of these options will be discussed below.

HYPOTHESES AND SUGGESTED LINES OF FUTURE INVESTIGATION

Centrally Elicited Behavior and the Sympathoadrenal System

The studies discussed above and the results from numerous other laboratories (cf. Table 1) convincingly demonstrate that the CNS can selectively evoke the secretion of both NE and EPI from the adrenal medulla. There also appear to be discrete, but at least partially overlapping, regions in the CNS for the control of the adrenal medulla, the peripheral noradrenergic sympathetic nerves, and the cardiovascular system. We have shown that while discrete hypothalamic sites may elicit similar patterns of defensive behavior, the patterns of sympatho-adrenal activation may vary. This observation suggests that a single sympatho-adrenal response is not a prerequisite for the expression of defensive behavior. Evidence suggests that the defense response is a CNS-initiated event, in part because of this lack of a standard sympathoadrenal response associated with the behavior. Additional support for this point of view comes from the observation that intravenous injections of NE into human subjects do not elicit the subjective symptom of anger, although NE has been linked to naturally occurring aggressive feelings in humans (49). However, we realize intuitively that knowledge gained through evaluation of hypothalamically stimulated behavior can be used only as a guide to the responses that occur naturally. Our expectation that hypothalamically elicited defensive behavior, which consists of certain stereotyped actions, would be accompanied by a similar stereotyped sympathoadrenal response was incorrect. Electrical stimulation of the brain, by exciting both cell bodies and fibers of passage, and by the unavoidable spread of current, must necessarily activate portions of the neuraxis that are not essential for the elicitation of a behavior. In similar fashion, physiological events may be triggered by the stimulus that are not concomitants of the natural behavior. One line of investigation that might clarify the role of the CNS in defining the integral physiological concomitants of a behavior is the use of glutamic acid and neurotransmitter agonists and antagonists. The actions of these neurochemicals is limited to cell bodies (glutamic acid) or to specific populations of neurons with certain classes of receptors. Thus elicitation of defensive behavior by chemical means accompanied by measurement of the sympathoadrenal response would help to identify neuronal populations that mediate the autonomic components of the defense response.

Defense and Related Behaviors are Associated with a Range of Sympathoadrenal Responses

We suggest that different forms of aggressive behavior, to use the term somewhat loosely, are associated with qualitatively different sympathoadrenal responses, although the boundaries among the response characteristics are not clear. We have described some of the characteristics of both hypothalamically and naturally elicited defensive behavior in the cat, and have noted that in naturally occurring behavior, two stimuli that evoke empirically similar patterns of defensive behavior are accompanied by different patterns of sympathoadrenal activation. Flight, or escape, behavior may also be elicited by stimulation of discrete hypothalamic sites. There are both similarities and differences between the sympathoadrenal responses that accompany stimulation of hypothalamic sites that elicit either defensive or escape behavior in the awake animal (30). Hypothalamic escape sites, similarly to defense sites, most often elicited bilateral increases in the secretion of NE and EPI from the adrenal medulla and significantly altered the ratio of NE/EPI. However, escape sites showed more selectivity for the control of adrenal NE, did not activate the peripheral sympathetic nerves to as great a degree as defense sites, and elicited increases in cardiovascular parameters that were significantly correlated with increases in adrenal catecholamines, which suggested concomitant activation of the adrenal medullary and cardiovascular subsystems of the sympathoadrenal system. Pure attack behavior, or offense, is a unique form of aggression found, in cats, only between males (6). Both our experience and that of others (Robert Adamec, personal communication) has shown that this behavior is particularly difficult to elicit in the laboratory. Preliminary data from our laboratory, however, suggests that offense in the cat is accompanied by a decrease in EPI secretion from the adrenal medulla (50); this is yet another separate, distinctive pattern of sympathoadrenal activation. It is of interest in this regard that the author knows of no report in which the unique pattern of feline offense has been elicited by hypothalamic stimulation, an observation also made by Bandler (8).

Significance of Adrenal Blood Flow in Describing the Sympathoadrenal Response

While investigating the sympathoadrenal responses related to hypothalamically elicited defensive and escape behaviors, we identified 13 hypothalamic sites (9 defense and 4 escape) that increased the rate of adrenal venous blood flow 20% or more from the baseline rate of 0.83 ± 0.02 ml/min (51). These sites were located primarily in the ventromedial nucleus and the anterior hypothalamic area (Fig. 4). The lack of correlation between changes in mean arterial pressure and adrenal venous flow rate elicited by stimulation at those sites suggested that the increased adrenal venous flow was not merely a reflection of a generalized increase in blood pressure. However, the mean increase in the adrenal secretion of EPI at these sites was significantly greater than the mean increase at all other behaviorally identified hypothalamic sites. These data suggest an overlap between CNS sites that stimulate the selective secretion of EPI from the adrenal and those that increase adrenal venous blood flow. More important is that this study emphasizes the importance of considering the variable of adrenal blood flow rate in any evaluation of evoked adrenal secretion. Unrecognized changes in blood flow can artificially produce alterations in the plasma concentration of catecholamines, which thus suggests modified adrenal medullary secretion that may be inaccurate.

Role of CNS Areas that Modulate Defensive Behavior

It is well established that the limbic system can modulate hypothalamically elicited defensive behavior. Separate, discrete sites in the septal area and amygdala,

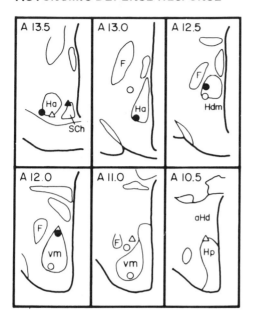

FIGURE 4 Composite map of behaviorally identified hypothalamic sites that elicited an increase ≥ 20% the baseline mean in adrenal venous flow rate. Sites are plotted on coronal sections from the atlas of Jasper and Ajmone-Marsan (41). Circles indicate sites that elicited affective defensive behavior in the freely moving cat; triangles indicate sites that elicited escape behavior. Open symbols indicate sites where hypothalamic stimulation evoked an increase in blood flow from the adrenal vein ipsilateral to the side of stimulation; filled symbols indicate sites that evoked increases in blood flow both adrenal veins. (from ref. 51).

for example, have been shown both to facilitate and inhibit hypothalamically elicited defense (52). However, the effects of combined stimulation of behaviorally identified hypothalamic sites and limbic modulatory sites on the accompanying sympathoadrenal response, or specifically on adrenal medullary secretion, have not been investigated in detail. Dual stimulation of behaviorally active sites together with modulatory sites is an obvious line of investigation to explore how CNS structures interact in adrenal medullary or sympathoadrenal control.

Differentiation of the Adrenal Medullary and Sympathetic Neural Responses

Another apparent line of inquiry in defining the sympathoadrenal response that accompanies natural defensive behavior is to use separately adrenalectomized and sympathectomized animals. Each procedure, in theory, would remove one of the two components of the sympathoadrenal system. Thus the activity of the remaining component could be evaluated. We have done preliminary experiments with both these techniques (Stoddard and Bergdall, unpublished observations). Acute guanethidine administration in cats did not, in our hands, reliably result in convincing sympathectomy. Adrenalectomized cats, in our experience, evidenced increased levels of peripheral NE, which suggested compensatory hyperactivity of the peripheral sympathetic nerves. The defensive behaviors evoked in these animals by a barking dog or a hypothalamically stimulated cat appeared similar. However, stress-induced death, resulting from a steady decline in heart rate and mean arterial blood pressure, was observed in several adrenalectomized cats; death was associated only with defensive behavior directed at another cat. These observations support our observations in the intact animal that the physiological mechanisms underlying interspecies and intraspecies behaviors are different. However, the use of surgically altered animals may only serve to provide additional perturbances to the system and further obscure whatever common characteristics may exist among sympathoadrenal responses and defensive behavior.

The Ideal Experimental Paradigm

The best model for defensive behavior is unequivocally the naturally behaving cat in which behavior is elicited by a standard, constant stimulus. The potential for such a model exists through the use of a stimulus cat with the perfectly placed (of ever so many) hypothalamic electrodes; the pattern of hypothalamically elicited affective defensive behavior with a stable hiss latency has been reported (3). The perfect experimental cat would then be an awake, behaving animal with unilaterally (or bilaterally) placed adrenal venous cannulae, in addition to peripheral venous and arterial cannulae. Our experience with the placement of adrenal venous lines that continue to function in the awake, behaving animal has been less than remarkably successful. However, the use of Teflon intravenous placement units connected to Silastic tubing, which are placed in the adrenolumbar vein from a lateral approach, may facilitate this procedure (37). Other possible techniques might involve concentric cannulae placed through the superior into the inferior vena cava such that the smaller, interior line is positioned below the input from the adrenal veins, while the larger, exterior portion is positioned above the level of the diaphragm. Although the bilateral adrenal vein cannulation would provide more direct information, the use of concentric cannulae has been shown to be effective in exercising dogs (53) and, to a degree, in the behaving cat (54). To complete the ideal experiment, it would also be necessary to measure the blood flow through the adrenal medulla. Thus, it would be possible to determine whether changes in catecholamine concentration were due to an actual increase in secretion from the adrenal medulla or were merely a byproduct of changes in the rate of blood flow through the adrenal gland.

SUMMARY

This discussion has considered many aspects of the defense response in the cat. Hypothalamically elicited defensive (and perhaps the subset of submissive) behavior is directed at another cat, that is an animal of the same species. In contrast, naturally occurring defensive behavior may be directed either at same-species animals under a variety of conditions (*intra*species behavior), or may be focused on a member of another species (*inter*species behavior). These various forms of defensive behavior, together with escape behavior and pure intermale offense, may each be looked upon as a subset of aggression. We compare this group of behaviors in the cat subjectively to our own experiences, and thus assign them the designation of "emotional" or "stressful" behavior. Whether the animal can or is indeed experiencing emotion we shall probably never discern. However, calling these behaviors a form of stress is less controversial, since continued aggressive behavior can provoke the greatest stress: death of the animal.

Work in our laboratory has described the sympathoadrenal response, as determined by the measurement of plasma catecholamines, primarily in relation to the defense response, while a number of other laboratories have explored the cardiovascular concomitants of this behavior. This author believes that the observations resulting from these studies have only identified the "tip of the iceberg" of physiological concomitants of the defense response. We conclude that there is a range of both sympathoadrenal and cardiovascular responses that accompany various expressions of the defense response, and suggest that this behavior is not "hard-wired" to an inherent physiological pattern. Behaviors related to defense, such as escape and offense, at least in the cat, appear to have related but unique patterns of sympathetic activation. Although these conclusions are indeed gross generalizations, they are more than we had before Adams (4) and Zanchetti and colleagues (1) began their studies. Perhaps the development of more precise experimental paradigms and more sophisticated instrumentation will permit us to describe the sympathoadrenal activation related to expression of the defense response more precisely. It is an area of investigation that would indeed benefit from the contributions of more investigators.

REFERENCES

1. Zanchetti A, Baccelli G, Mancia G, Ellison G D. Emotion and the cardiovascular system in the cat. In Physiology, emotion and psychosomatic illness. Ciba Found Symp, vol. 8. Amsterdam: Elsevier, 1972: 201–223.

2. Wasman M, Flynn J P. Directed attack elicited from hypothalamus. Arch Neurol 1962; 6:220–227.
3. MacDonnell M F, Fessock L, Brown S H. Ethanol and the neural substrate for affective defense in the cat. Q J Stud Alcohol 1971; 32:406–419.
4. Adams D B. Brain mechanisms for offense, defense, and submission. Behav Brain Sci 1979; 2:201–241.
5. Stoddard S L, Bergdall V K, Townsend D W, Levin B E. Plasma catecholamines associated with hypothalamically-elicited defense behavior. Physiol Behav 1986; 36:867–873.
6. Leyhausen P. Cat behavior. New York: Garland STPM Press, 1979.
7. Siegel A, Edinger H. Neural control of aggression and rage behavior. In: Morgan PJ, Panksepp J, eds. Handbook of the hypothalamus, vol. 3, Part B. Behavioral studies of the hypothalamus. New York: Marcel Dekker, 1981: 203–240.
8. Bandler R. Neural control of aggressive behaviour. Trends Neurosci 1982; 5:390–394.
9. Barrett J A, Shaikh M B, Edinger H, Siegel A. The effects of intrahypothalamic injections of norepinephrine upon affective defense behavior in the cat. Brain Res 1987; 426:381–384.
10. Shaikh M B, Siegel A. GABA-ergic modulation of feline aggression elicited from the midbrain periaqueductal gray. Soc Neurosci Abstr 1988; 14:1261.
11. Fuchs S A G, Edinger H M, Siegel A. The organization of the hypothalamic pathways mediating affective defense behavior in the cat. Brain Res 1985; 330:77–92.
12. Cannon W B. Bodily changes in pain, hunger, fear and rage. New York: Appleton, 1915.
13. Adams D B, Baccelli G, Mancia G, Zanchetti A. Cardiovascular changes during naturally elicited fighting behavior in the cat. Am J Physiol 1969; 216:1226–1235.
14. Abrahams V C, Hilton S M, Zbrozyna A. Active muscle vasodilatation produced by stimulation of the brain stem: its significance in the defence reaction. J Physiol (London) 1960; 154:491–513.
15. Ellison G D, Zanchetti A. Diffuse and specific activation of sympathetic cholinergic fibers of the cat. Am J Physiol 1973; 225:142–149.
16. Smith O A, DeVito J L, Astley C A. The hypothalamus in emotional behavior and associated cardiovascular correlates. In: Morrison AR, Strick PL, eds. Changing concepts of the nervous system. New York: Academic Press, 1982: 569–584.
17. Cannon W B. The emergency function of the adrenal medulla in pain and the major emotions. Am J Physiol 1914; 23:356–372.
18. Redgate E S, Gellhorn E. Nature of sympathetico-adrenal discharge under conditions of excitation of central autonomic structures. Am J Physiol 1953; 174:475–480.
19. Folkow B, von Euler U S. Selective activation of noradrenaline and adrenaline producing cells in the cat's adrenal gland by hypothalamic stimulation. Circ Res 1954; 2:191–195.

20. von Euler U S, Folkow B. The effect of stimulation of autonomic areas in the cerebral cortex upon the adrenaline and noradrenaline secretion from the adrenal gland in the cat. Acta Physiol Scand 1958; 42:313-320.

21. Grant R, Lindgren P, Rosen A, Uvnäs B. The release of catechols from the adrenal medulla on activation of the sympathetic vasodilator nerves to the skeletal muscles in the cat by hypothalamic stimulation. Acta Physiol Scand 1958; 43:135-154.

22. Goldfien A, Ganong W F. Adrenal medullary and adrenal cortical response to stimulation of diencephalon. Am J Physiol 1962; 202:205-211.

23. Matsui H. Effect of myelencephalic stimulation on the secretion of noradrenaline and adrenaline of the adrenal gland of the cat. Tohoku J Exp Med 1965; 87:332-337.

24. Matsui H. Adrenal medullary secretory response to stimulation of the medulla oblongata in the rat. Neuroendocrinology 1979; 29:385-390.

25. Matsui H. Adrenal medullary secretory response to pontine and mesencephalic stimulation in the rat. Neuroendocrinology 1981; 33:84-87.

26. Francke P F, Culberson J L, Carmichael S W, Robinson R L. Bilateral secretory responses of the adrenal medulla during stimulation of hypothalamic or mesencephalic sites. J Neurosci Res 1982; 8:1-6.

27. Robinson R L, Culberson J L, Carmichael S W. Influence of hypothalamic stimulation on the secretion of adrenal medullary catecholamines. J Auton Nerv Syst 1983; 8:89-96.

28. Stoddard-Apter S L, Siegel A, Levin B E. Plasma catecholamine and cardiovascular responses following hypothalamic stimulation in the awake cat. J Auton Nerv Syst 1983; 8:343-360.

29. Katafuchi T, Yoshimatsu H, Oomura Y, Sato A. Responses of adrenal catecholamine secretion to lateral hypothalamic stimulation and lesion in rats. Brain Res 1986; 363:141-144.

30. Stoddard S L, Bergdall V K, Townsend D W, Levin B E. Plasma catecholamines associated with hypothalamically-elicited flight behavior. Physiol Behav 1986; 37:709-715.

31. Matsui H. Effect of subthalamic stimulation on adrenal epinephrine and norepinephrine secretion in the rat. Brain Res 1987; 417:158-160.

32. Bereiter D A, Engeland W C, Gann D S. Adrenal secretion of epinephrine after stimulation of trigeminal nucleus caudalis depends on stimulus pattern. Neuroendocrinology 1987; 45:54-61.

33. Bereiter D A, Gann D S. Adrenal secretion of catecholamines evoked by chemical stimulation of trigeminal nucleus caudalis in the cat. Neuroscience 1988; 25:697-704.

34. Roizen M F, Moss J, Henry D P, Weise V, Kopin I J. Effect of general anesthetics on handling- and decapitation-induced increases in sympathoadrenal discharge. J Pharmacol Exp Ther 1978; 204:11-18.

35. Critchley J A J H, Ellis P, Ungar A. The reflex release of adrenaline and noradrenaline from the adrenal glands of cats and dogs. J Physiol (London) 1980; 298:71-78.

36. Levin B E, Triscari J, Sullivan A C. Abnormal sympatho-adrenal function and plasma catecholamines in obese Zucker rats. Pharmacol Biochem Behav 1980; 13:107–113.

37. Gaumann D M, Yaksh T L, Tyce G M, Lucas D L. Opioids preserve the adrenal medullary response evoked by severe hemorrhage: studies on adrenal catecholamine and met-enkephalin secretion in halothane anesthetized cats. Anesthesiology 1988; 68:743–753.

38. Hubbard J W, Buchholz R A, Keeton T K, Nathan M A. Plasma norepinephrine concentration reflects pharmacological alteration of sympathetic activity in the conscious cat. J Auton Nerv Syst 1986; 15:93–100.

39. Mascorro J A. The extraadrenal chromaffin "paraneuron." Anat Rec 1987; 218:88A.

40. Kvetnansky R, Weise V K, Thoa N B, Kopin I J. Effects of chronic guanethidine treatment and adrenal medullectomy on plasma levels of catecholamines and corticosterone in forcibly immobilized rats. J Pharmacol Exp Ther 1979; 209:287–291.

41. Jasper H H, Ajmone-Marsan C A. Sterotaxic atlas of the diencephalon of the cat. Ottawa: National Research Council of Canada, 1954.

42. Bereiter D A, Engeland W C, Gann D S. Peripheral venous catecholamines versus adrenal secretory rates after brain stem stimulation in cats. Am J Physiol 1986; 251:E14–E20.

43. Stoddard S L, Bergdall V K, Conn P S, Levin B E. Increases in plasma catecholamines during naturally elicited defensive behavior in the cat. J Auton Nerv Syst 1987; 19:189–197.

44. Whitby L G, Axelrod J, Weil-Malherbe H. The fate of H^3-norepinephrine in animals. J Pharmacol Exp Ther 1961; 132:193–201.

45. Axelrod J, Weil-Malherbe H, Tomchick R. The physiological disposition of H^3-epinephrine and its metabolite metanephrine. J Pharmacol Exp Ther 1959; 127:251–256.

46. Baccelli G, Ellison G D, Mancia G, Zanchetti A. Opposite responses of muscle circulation to different emotional stimuli. Experientia 1971; 27:1183–1184.

47. Mancia G, Baccelli G, Zanchetti A. Hemodynamic responses to different emotional stimuli in the cat: patterns and mechanisms. Am J Physiol 1972; 223:925–933.

48. Williams R B Jr, Eichelman B S, Ng L K Y. The effects of peripheral chemosympathectomy and adrenalectomy upon blood pressure responses of the rat to footshock under varying conditions: evidence for behavioral effects on patterning of sympathetic nervous system responses. Psychophysiology 1979; 16:89–93.

49. Frankenhaeuser M, Järpe G, Matell G. Effects of intravenous infusions of adrenaline and noradrenaline on certain psychological and physiological functions. Acta Physiol Scand 1961; 51:175–186.

50. Stoddard S L, Wilson P E, Bergdall V K. Sympathoadrenal activation related to aggressive behavior. Aggress Behav 1987; 13:296.

51. Bergdall V K, Levin B E, Townsend D W, Stoddard S L. Increases in blood flow from the adrenal gland following medial hypothalamic stimulation in the cat. J Auton Nerv Syst 1986; 15:263–268.

52. Stoddard-Apter S L, MacDonnell M F. Septal and amygdalar efferents to the hypothalamus which facilitate intraspecific aggression and associated hissing in the cat. An autoradiographic study. Brain Res 1980; 193:19–32.

53. Peronnet F, Nadeau R A, de Champlain J, Magrassi P, Chatrand C. Exercise plasma catecholamines in dogs: role of adrenals and cardiac nerve endings. Am J Physiol 1981; 241:H243–247.

54. Stoddard-Apter S L, Bergdall V, Levin B E. Adrenal catecholamine secretion associated with natural aggressive behavior in the cat. Soc Neurosci Abstr 1985; 11:1267.

13

BEHAVIORAL RESPONSES TO STRESS
Focus on Corticotropin-Releasing Factor

George F. Koob

*Research Institute of the Scripps Clinic, La Jolla and
University of California, San Diego, San Diego, California*

Stress is a hypothetical construct that pervades physiology, psychology, and medicine and often eludes precise definition. Selye conceptualized stress as a nonspecific response to any demand (usually noxious) upon the body, or anything that causes an alteration in homeostatic processes. Exposure of rats to acute nonspecific noxious agents resulted in a typical "general adaptation syndrome," the symptoms of which were hypothesized to be independent of the nature of the damaging agent (1). This syndrome consisted of three stages; the first stage occurred during the first 48 h and consisted of a rapid decrease in the size of endocrine organs, formation of gastrointestinal erosions, loss of adrenal cortical lipids and chromaffin substance from the adrenal glands, and other behavioral signs such as exophthalmos, lacrimation, and salivation. The second stage is reflected in enlarged adrenals, atrophy of the gonads, and a decrease in body growth. With continued treatment, eventual exhaustion represents the third stage. One of the most fundamental parts of the general adaptation syndrome was that the functional changes elicited by various systems stressor agents were the same regardless of the specific nature of the elicitor's stimulus. Thus, stress was defined as a nonspecific response and the wide number of stimuli capable of producing nonspecific responses were defined as stressors.

In a reevaluation of Selye's concept of the nonspecificity of stress theory, Mason (2) has elaborated a crucial role for what he called "the psychological approaches involved in emotional or arousal reactions to threatening or unpleasant factors in the life situation as a whole." Mason points out that psychological stimuli are among the most potent stimuli affecting a response to the pituitary adrenal system, and indeed in many cases without a concomitant psychological reaction or arousal, subjects show little pituitary adrenal response to a stressor (2). Mason further argues that adrenal cortical responses occur ubiquitously to a wide variety of stimuli because emotional reactions occur ubiquitously in a wide variety of situations in which subjects are exposed to physical stress. Thus the "nonspecific" response of Selye is primarily behavioral or psychological in nature and "the interpretive processes underlying the 'non-specific' bodily responses to stressors probably involve a *higher level* of central nervous function than was previously realized" (2). This revisionist conceptualization of the non-specificity of the stress response fits well with more modern definitions of stress. Stress here is defined as "anything which causes an alteration of psychological homeostatic processes" (3).

When such a definition is used, one of the most reliable and sensitive measures of a state of stress is an increase in the production of corticotropin-releasing factor (CRF). Internal or external demands are conveyed in the form of stimuli to the anterior pituitary via neurohumoral means (presumably CRF), and the pituitary responds with a secretion of adrenocorticotropic hormone ACTH. ACTH, in turn, stimulates the adrenal cortex to secrete glucocorticoids, which have widespread effects on metabolism such as gluconeogenesis, hyperinsulinemia, lysis of lymphoid tissue, increased gastric secretion, and reduced inflammatory and antibody responses. These widespread physiological responses can then feed back to modulate central nervous function and ultimately perhaps the psychological variables originally eliciting the stress response.

The importance of psychological variables in the stress response requires a neurological substrate to process the interaction of sensory stimuli with this ultimate neuroendocrine response. The presumed substrate for the afferent limb of the stress response is the brain system classically involved in the processing and expression of emotion: the limbic system. Under this conceptualization, activation of the pituitary–adrenal axis (ACTH and corticosteroids) should reflect activation or the expression of limbic system activity.

However, recent evidence showing a central nervous system neurotropic role for corticotropin-releasing factor (CRF) has led to the hypothesis of an alternative means for contributing to the behavioral state of stress. Thus, just as psychological stimuli elicit emotional responses via the limbic system that activate the CRF–pituitary–adrenal axis, this afferent limb may also activate a central nervous system (CNS) CRF system and this CNS CRF action may contribute significantly both to behavioral responses to stress and emotional behavior itself.

NEUROTROPIC ACTION FOR CNS CRF

Corticotropin-releasing factor has been localized to the CNS both in the hypothalamus and in extrahypothalamic structures. Immunoreactive fibers staining for CRF were found in rat, sheep, dog, and monkey hypothalamus using anti-bodies to ovine CRF (4–7). Cell bodies located in the paraventricular nucleus project a dense fiber plexus to the median eminence and other hypothalamic and mesencephalic loci. Subsequent work using an ovine antibody on untreated sheep brain (8) and on colchicine-treated rat brain (9) revealed this same hypo-thalamic–median eminence projection and a more extensive extrahypothalamic distribution. CRF-stained cells were also found in the central nucleus of the amygdala, bed nucleus of the stria terminalis, parabrachial nucleus, laterodorsal tegmental nucleus, substantia inominata, and some neocortical areas, and a few cells were observed in the hippocampus. The most densely stained number of CRF fibers were seen in the median eminence and neurohypophysis. High-density staining was also seen in the medial preoptic area, central and dorsal medial nuclei of the amygdala, the substantia inominata, and the parabrachial nuclei. Thus, the majority of CRF-stained cell groups and pathways are associa-ted predominantly with the hypothalamus and brainstem and with limbic parts of the telencephalon. A system of CRF-stained pathways appears to interrelate several systems in the basal forebrain, pons, and medulla that are involved in the integration of autonomic and neuroendocrine responses (9,10).

When directly administered intracerebroventricularly (ICV) or intracerebrally CRF appears to activate CNS function. CRF ICV produces a profound dose-dependent activation of the electroencephalogram (EEG) (11). Doses of 0.015–0.15 nmol produce a long-lasting activation of EEG. At the cellular level, CRF produces increases in the firing rate of cells within the locus ceruleus (12), a system thought to be of importance in the mechanisms by which the brain is able to attend selectively to changes in internal and external events. CRF also has been shown to produce a significant depolarization and excitation of hippo-campal pyramidal cells. (13). With the use of an in vitro hippocampal slice preparation, CRF applied by superfusion depolarized by 3–12 mV all CA1 and CA3 cells tested. This depolarization was accompanied by significant increases in action potential discharge, but no apparent decrease in input resistance. Intracel-lular recordings showed that the excitation arose from reduction of the after-hyperpolarizations that followed bursts of spikes (14). It was hypothesized that CRF may alter potassium conductance either directly or by a change in calcium conductances. These changes may provide a cellular basis for the EEG changes observed following ICV injection.

BEHAVIORAL EFFECTS OF CRF ACTIVATION

The electrophysiological activation produced by central administration of CRF is paralleled by a dose-dependent activation of behavior. Both ovine and rat CRF were equally active in stimulating locomotor activity of rats in a familiar environment (Fig. 1) (15-17). These effects appear to be independent of direct mediation by the pituitary–adrenal system, since they were observed in

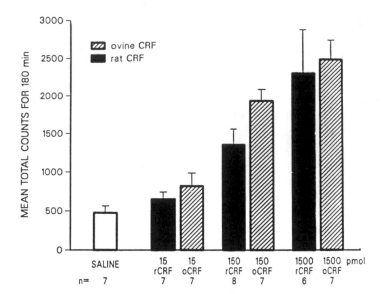

FIGURE 1 Effects of ovine and rat CRF on locomotor activity in the rat. Results represent the total activity counts over 3 h (mean ± SEM) N = 7 in each group except for the 10 μg of rat CRF for which was N = 6. A two-factor analysis of variance (ANOVA) revealed no overall significant difference between rat or ovine CRF (p > 0.05) and no dose X peptide interaction (p > 0.05).

hypophysectomized and dexamethasone-treated rats (see Fig. 2) (18–20). Given that this activation is not seen with systemic administration, these observations suggested that CRF exerted its effects within the CNS on CRF receptors independent of the pituitary–adrenal axis.

The locomotor activation caused by CRF was not antagonized by the opiate antagonist, naloxone, or by low doses of a dopamine receptor antagonist (15). Nor was this activation reversed by 6-hydroxydopamine lesions of the region of the nucleus accumbens, which reverse the locomotor-stimulated effects of indirect sympathomimetics such as amphetamine and cocaine (21).

To examine further the site of action for this activating effect, experiments were conducted examining lateral ventricular and cisterna magna injections of CRF combined with obstruction of the cerebral aqueduct. Rats injected ICV with CRF in the lateral ventricle or cisterna magna showed a dose-dependent increase in locomotor activity. The increase in locomotor activity resulting from injections of CRF into the cisterna magna was blocked by a cold cream plug in the cerebral aqueduct (22). A similar plug failed to block the increase in locomotor activity produced by CRF injected into the lateral ventricle. These results suggest that the activating effects of CRF are more dependent on forebrain CRF receptors than on hindbrain CRF receptors.

In a subsequent study, rats were surgically implanted with cannulae aimed at the lateral ventricle, frontal cortex (FC), nucleus accumbens (NAC), amygdala centralis (AC), substantia innominate/lateral preoptic area (SI/LPS), or pedunculopontine nucleus (PPN). Injection of 0.5 µg rat CRF into discrete brain regions produced increases in locomotor activity that were higher the closer the injection site to the SI/LPO. Activation was least intense when produced by CRF injection into the FC and PPN, and most intense when produced by CRF injection into the SI/LPO and lateral ventricle (22). These results together suggest some localization for the neural substrates of CRF-induced behavioral activation to a region near the SI/LPO or lateral ventricle.

Low doses of CRF (0.003 and 0.015 nmoles) administered ICV also potentiated amphetamine-induced stereotyped behavior as measured by a rating scale and behavioral observations (44). CRF enhanced the tendency for the rats to sniff with their heads down 20 min after injection and induced licking behavior later during testing. These results suggest that low doses of CRF can potentiate behavioral responses associated with arousal and that CNS CRF may form an arousal system parallel to but independent of the brain dopamine system that innervates the extrapyramidal motor system.

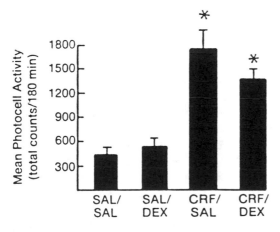

FIGURE 2 The interaction of CRF (1.0 µg, ICV) and dexamethasone (100 µg/ kg, intraperitoneally) on locomotor activity in photocell cages. Results represent total activity counts over 3 h (mean ± SEM). N = 12 saline and n = 15 for other groups. *Significantly different from saline-treated group, p < .05 (from ref. 19, with permission).

BEHAVIORAL RESPONSES TO STRESS
Unconditioned

While exogenous administration of CRF produced behavioral activation in animals in a familiar, presumably non- or less stressful environment, administration of CRF in behavioral tests designed to reflect changes in stress or designed to reflect increased behavioral responsiveness to stress showed that CRF had the opposite behavioral effect. This is reflected in behavioral inhibition and a suppression or decrease in activity. For example, when mildly food-deprived rats are exposed to an open field situation where food is available, they will eventually approach the food and eat. Increases in stress level are usually reflected in increased latency to eat and decreases in eating. Decreases in stress level are reflected in decreased latency to eat and increased eating (24). Rats previously injected ICV with CRF showed a significant decrease in exploratory and ingestive behavior and stayed close to the corners of the open field (25). In contrast, untreated animals made increasingly frequent forays into the center of the field to consume food. CRF also decreased food intake in the home cage and muscimol-, norepinephrine-, dynorphin-, and insulin-induced feeding, effects attributed to a stress-related suppression of food intake (26,27). Similar effects were observed after sauvagine and urotensin I treatment (28).

Similar stresslike results were observed with nondeprived animals tested in a novel open field without food (17). Rats tested in the open field following ICV injection of CRF (0.0015–0.15 nmoles) showed decreases in locomotion and rearing (17), which are consistent with increased emotionality. In this test, a typical saline-injected rat rapidly circled the outer squares of the open field during the first 3–4 min of the 5 min test. During the last few minutes of the test these saline-injected animals then made some forays into the center of the open field, usually accompanied by rearing on their hind legs. Typically a rat injected with 0.15 nmole of CRF and placed 60 min later in the open field moved slowly to the outer squares and then either circled the open field, remaining close to the floor and to the edge, or remained in one of the corners, grooming or hesitantly moving forwards and backwards (17). These behavioral changes are consistent with increased sensitivity to the presumably stressful aspects of the test, or with the induction of a stresslike state.

Similar effects have been observed in other tests of unconditioned exploratory behavior. CRF administered ICV to mice exposed to a novel multicompartment chamber significantly reduced the time mice spent in contact with novel stimuli, an effect similar to that observed with restraint stress (30,31). In rats tested in an environment consisting of a large open field that contained a small chamber, CRF administered ICV also inhibited open field exploration and facilitated a pattern of defensive withdrawal into the chamber (32). CRF also enhanced shock-elicited "freezing" behavior, an adaptive response often produced by fear-elicited stimuli (33); this enhanced freezing was not accompanied by increased sensitivity to pain.

Stressors can also have response-enhancing properties as well as response-suppressing properties and in these situations CRF ICV also appeared to enhance behavioral responsiveness to stress. The acoustic startle reflex is an easily quantified muscular contraction in response to an intense acoustic stimulus. CRF (0.15 nmoles ICV) significantly increased the acoustic startle amplitude (23,34). Pretreatment with the benzodiazepine chlordiazepoxide in doses that did not by themselves lower startle baseline reversed this effect.

Mild uncontrollable foot shock to rats exposed together as pairs produces characteristic behavioral responses such as boxing (upright postures) or fighting (upright postures followed by physical contact) within a few sessions. The frequency of fighting responses increases gradually with shock intensity, presumably as a consequence of the gradual physiological changes accompanying the increased stress. CRF ICV at low doses (0.0015 and 0.015 nmole) facilitated stress-induced fighting (35).

At higher doses, CRF can clearly disrupt organized behavior. Rhesus monkeys injected ICV with 180 μg of CRF showed behavioral changes associated with arousal when restrained but in their home cages they withdrew into a combination of huddling and lying down (36). Other disruptive effects of CRF administered at higher doses include a suppressive effect on female sexual behavior (37).

Conditioned

A variety of operant procedures have been developed to determine the effects of antianxiety drugs or as measures of conditioned fear (psychological stress, no direct physical stressor). In an operant conflict test, CRF produced a significant decrease in punished and unpunished responding, an effect opposite to that observed with benzodiazepines (38). However, this increased sensitivity to aversive events was not accompanied by an obvious increased sensitivity to pain as measured by tail flick or hot plate analgesia tests. These effects also appear to be independent of the pituitary-adrenal axis: dexamethasone treatment failed to alter the suppression in operant behavior produced by CRF (19).

CRF injected ICV in rats also produced further suppression during the conditioned stimulus (CS) presentation part of a conditioned suppression task (Fig. 4). There was a significant decrease in the suppression rate measure which emphasizes that the decrease in performance was more pronounced during the CS period that signalled impending shock. These results using a psychological stressor suggest that the enhanced sensitivity to stress associated with excess CRF does not depend on the presence of an actual physical stressor and support the hypothesis that CRF might act to potentiate behavioral responses normally expressed during states of enhanced fear or anxiety (see Table 1).

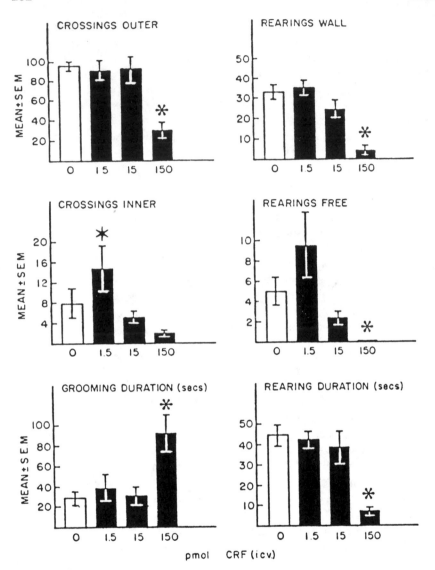

FIGURE 3 Effects of CRF injected ICV on behavior of rats in an open field.
Values represent mean ± SEM of the total number of observations during the 5
min test. 1.5, 15, and 150 pmoles of CRF correspond to 0.01, 0.1, and 1.0 μg/
rat. *Significantly different from saline-injected rats, Newman-Keuls test (p <
0.05 following ANOVA) (adapted from ref. 17).

TABLE 1 Summary of Behavioral Effects of CRF

Injected ICV in doses of 0.1–10μg (15–1500 pmoles) increases locomotor activity in a familiar photocell cage environment (17)
Facilitates the acoustic startle response (34)
Facilitates acquisition of a visual discrimination task (39)
Produces increased responsiveness to "stress" in an open field test (17)
Enhances behavioral effects of novelty (25)
Suppresses exploration similar to restraint stress (30)
Has an "anxiogenic-like" effect in an operant conflict test (38)
Enhances stress-induced freezing behavior (33)
Enhances conditioned fear in a conditioned suppression test (41)
Facilitates stress-induced fighting (35)
Suppresses food intake (27)
Disrupts sexual behavior in female rats (37)

A possible site of action for the effect of CRF to enhance sensitivity to stress was elaborated in a recent experiment in which propranolol was found to reverse the effects of CRF on CS responding in a conditioned suppression test (41). Similar effects were found with central (ICV) administration of a nonlipophilic alpha-2-agonist, suggesting an effect on central noradrenergic systems. Other recent work suggests that the locus ceruleus (site of origin of forebrain norepinephrine) may be particularly sensitive to the suppression of exploratory behavior observed with central administration of CRF (42). The reversal of response inhibition by blockade of nonadrenergic receptors may have some behavioral specificity in that propranolol does not reverse but actually potentiates CRF-induced locomotion (41).

BEHAVIORAL EFFECTS OF CRF ANTAGONIST

Until recently, work with CRF has succeeded only in characterizing a behavioral action of the peptide administered exogenously in amounts of possible dubious physiological relevance (it is estimated that the total hypothalamic content of CRF is 600-700 pg or 0.1 pmol) (43). Nevertheless, given that CRF is a large molecule (41 amino acids) and that the specific site of action for these effects remains largely unexplained, it is still possible that at some distant point from the ventricular injection, particularly when it is administered at the lower dose, the effects of exogenously administered CRF do represent the hypothesized exaggeration of normal function.

More important for the hypothesis that endogenous CNS CRF has a role in behavioral responses to stress, recent work has demonstrated behavioral actions of an intraventricularly administered CRF antagonist, alpha helical CRF 9-41. This CRF antagonist injected ICV at a dose of 50 μg partially reversed the attenuation of feeding induced by stress (29). Alpha helical CRF injected ICV also attenuated stress-induced fighting (35). A slightly higher shock level (0.6 mA) produced a higher fighting frequency in control animals (not pretreated with CRF) and this fighting was reversed by administration of 5 and 25 μg/rat of αHEL CRF (9-41) (see Fig. 5).

Alpha-helical CRF in mice in doses of 10 μg ICV reversed the suppression in exploratory behavior produced by restraint stress (31). In rats subjected to an environment consisting of a large open field that contained a small chamber it produced a more rapid emergence from the chamber into the open field and more exploration of the unfamiliar open field (32). This CRF antagonist also inhibits stress-induced freezing behavior in rats (40).

In operant studies alpha-helical CRF has not produced a significant release of punished responding in a Geller-Seiffer conflict test nor has it reversed the suppression responding produced by the CS in a conditioned suppression task (Koob, Britton, and Cole, unpublished results). However, alpha-helical CRF does appear to attenuate the acquisition of conditioned suppression task Cole, Britton Rivier et al., unpublished observation. Food-deprived rats were trained to respond on a random interval 60 s (RI-60) schedule for food reinforcement. The

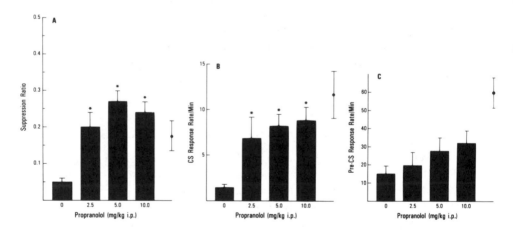

FIGURE 4 Effects of systemic dl-propranolol on the response to 0.5 μg of CRF (ICV) in the conditioned emotional response paradigm. (A) mean ± SEM suppression ratios; (B) mean ± cs response rate/min; (C mean ± SEM pre-CS response rate/minute. The data point on the right of each panel shows base-line performance from the session preceding the onset of the drug studies. Note the suppression in responding produced of CRF alone. *Significantly different from ICV CRF and IP saline (P < .01) (from ref. 41 with permission).

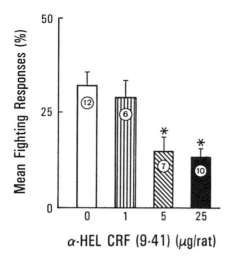

α-HEL CRF (9-41) (μg/rat)

FIGURE 5   Acoustic startle amplitude in rats. Animals received ICV infusion of alpha helical CRF (0,1,5 or 25 μg) and were exposed to a startle stimulus alone, or in the presence of a cue (CS) previously associated with shock. An asterisk indicates $p < 0.05$, within-subject comparison of startle amplitude following tone alone versus amplitude following tone + CS, by Newman-Keuls following significant ANOVA (from ref. 23, with permission).

effects of alpha-helical CRF on the acquisition of a conditioned emotional response were examined by infusing the antagonist (0, 1, 5, 25 μg/5 μl) into the lateral ventricle 30 min before each test session. During these test sessions, four pairings of a conditioned stimulus (CS) (light) and a 0.5 s, 2.1 mA (biphasic, direct, constant current) footshock were presented while the animals were responding for food reinforcement. The control animals showed a significant decrease in response rate during the presence of the CS in the nine test sessions, demonstrating acquisition of a conditioned emotional response. However, this response suppression was significantly attenuated by alpha-helical CRF, at all of the doses studied. Alpha-helical CRF also facilitates acquisition of tail-pinch-induced feeding (Cole and Koob, unpublished observations) whereas alpha-helical CRF at high doses suppresses tail-pinch-induced feeding. Finally, alpha-helical CRF has been shown to reverse CRF and fear potentiated startle (23) (Fig. 6).

Although most of the behavioral effects of alpha-helical CRF are clearly opposite to those produced by CRF itself (see Table 2), there is always the possibility that alpha-helical CRF has a pharmacological effect independent of any action on endogenous CRF systems. However, the CRF antagonist has been

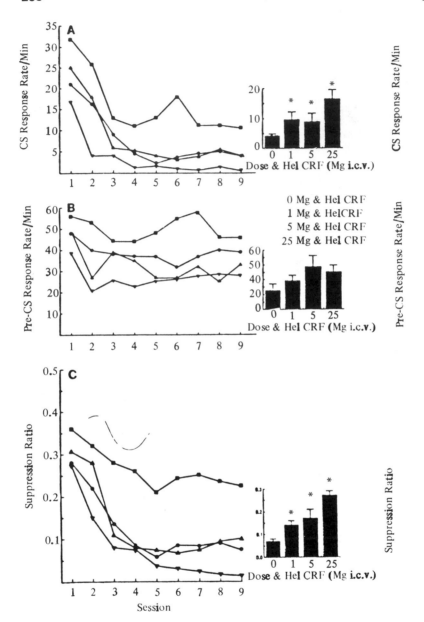

FIGURE 6 Effects of ICV alpha-helical CRF on the acquisition of a conditioned emotional response. A. Mean ± SEM suppression ratios. B. Mean ± SEM pre-CS response rate/min. C. Mean ± SEM suppression ratios. On the right of each panel, the mean effects of alpha-helical CRF on the different measures, collapsed across sessions, are shown. *Significantly different from ICV vehicle alone (from ref. 23 with permission).

TABLE 2 Summary of Behavioral Effects of the CRF Antagonist, Alpha Helical CRF

Reverses CRF- and stress-induced suppression of feeding (29)
Blocks development of stress-induced fighting in rats (35)
Reverses stress-induced changes in exploratory behavior in mice (31)
Attenuates stress-elicited freezing in the rat (40)
Blocks the acquisition of a conditioned emotional response (Cole, Britton, Rivier, Rivier, and Koob, unpublished)
At low doses facilitates acquisition of tail-pinch-induced feeding at high doses suppresses tail-pinched-induced feeding (Cole, Rivier, and Koob, unpublished)
Blocks fear potentiated startle (23)

---

shown to decrease baseline release of ACTH both in vitro and in vivo, as well as ether-induced ACTH secretion (45). At the behavioral level, alpha-HEL CRF (9-41) has been shown to block the activating and "anxiogenic" actions of CRF in the rat (46). These observations, while pointing to the involvement of CRF-receptors in such effects, did not specify a behavioral role for endogenous CRF released during stress. The present results, however, suggest that under certain conditions of high arousal and stress endogenous CRF systems may play a role in mediating behavioral responses to stress.

CONCLUSIONS

These results describing neuronal activation, general behavioral activation, and stress-enhancing actions of exogenous CRF all suggest a possible role for CRF as a fundamental activating system (see Table 1). However, the results with the CRF antagonist suggest that endogenous CNS CRF systems may become active in situations involving response inhibition, particularly when the situation is novel or where the contingencies are novel and, most importantly for the hypothesis under test, where some degree of stress in involved (see Table 2). The possibility that endogenous CRF systems are involved in the activating properties of stress needs further exploration.

Preliminary results also indicate that the sites of action for CRF in the response-activating compared with the response-inhibiting effects of stress may be different. The response-activating effects may involve an action in the forebrain (cold cream plug experiment) whereas the response-inhibiting properties of CRF may involve an action in the pons, possibly associated with activation of central noradrenergic systems (propranolol and locus ceruleus experiments).

Thus, the functional significance of an endogenous CNS CRF neuronal network may have developed as a means for an organism to mobilize not only the pituitary adrenal system but also the CNS in response to environmental challenge. Some hypothetical CNS activation system definitively linked to the pituitary adrenal system, which can activate behavioral responses at low levels of output but inhibit behavioral responses at high levels of output, would certainly be of survival value. It is not difficult either to imagine a possible role for over-activation of such a system in clinical disorders such as anxiety, affective disorders, and other psychopathology.

ACKNOWLEDGMENTS

This work was supported by NIH grant AM26741. This is publication 5847BCR from the Research Institute of Scripps Clinic, La Jolla, California.

REFERENCES

1. Selye H. A syndrome produced by diverse noxious agents. Nature 1936; 32:138.
2. Mason J W. A re-evaluation of the concept of "non-specificity" in stress specificity in stress theory. J Psychiatr Res 1971; 8:323–333.
3. Burchfield S. The stress responses: a new perspective. Psychosom Med 1979; 41:661–671.
4. Bloom F E, Battenberg E L F, Rivier J, Vale W. Corticotropin-releasing factor (CRF): immunoreactive neurons and fibers in rat hypothalamus. Regul Pept 1982; 4:43–48.
5. Bugnon C, Fellman D, Gouget A, Cardot J. Corticoliberin in rat brain: immunocytochemical identification and localization of a novel neuro-glandular system. Neurosci Lett 1982; 30:25–30.
6. Olschowka J A, O'Donohue T L, Mueller G P, Jacobowitz D M. Hypo-thalamic and extrahypothalamic distribution of CRF-like immunoreactive neurons in the rat brain. Neuroendocrinology 1982; 35:305–308.
7. Paull W K, Scholer J, Arimura A, et al. Immunocytochemical localization of CRF in the ovine hypothalamus. Peptides 1982; 3:183–191.
8. Battenberg E L F, Bloom F E, Rivier J, Vale W. Corticotropin releasing factor (CRF): immunoreactive neurons and fibers in rat and primate hypo-thalamus. Neurosci Abstr 1982; 8:110.
9. Swanson L W, Sawchenko P E, Rivier J, Vale W W. Organization of ovine corticotropin-releasing factor immunoreactive cells and fibers in the rat brain: an immunohistochemical study. Neuroendocrinology 1983; 36: 165–186.
10. Sawchenko P E, Swanson L W. Localization, co-localization and plasticity of corticotropin-releasing factor immunoreactivity in rat brain. Fed Proc 1985; 44:221–227.
11. Ehlers C L, Henriksen S J, Wang M, Rivier J, Vale W, Bloom F E. Cortico-tropin releasing factor produces increases in brain excitability and convul-sive seizures in the rat. Brain Res 1983; 278:332–336.

12. Valentino R J, Foote S L, Aston-Jones G. Corticotropin-releasing factor activates noradrenergic neurons of the locus coeruleus. Brain Res 1983; 270:363–367.

13. Aldenhoff J B, Gruol D L, Siggins G R. Corticotropin releasing factor decreases postburst hyperpolarizations and excites hippocampal neurons. Science 1983; 221:875–877.

14. Siggins G R, Gruol D, Aldenhoff J, Pittman Q. Electrophysiological actions of corticotropin-releasing factor in the central nervous system. Fed Proc 1985; 44:237–242.

15. Koob G F, Swerdlow N, Seeligson M, et al. CRF-induced locomotor activation is antagonized by alpha flupenthixol but not naloxone. Neuroendocrinology 1984; 39:459–464.

16. Sherman J E, Kalin N H. The effects of ICV–CRH on novelty-induced behavior. Biochem Biophys 1987; 26:699–703.

17. Sutton R E, Koob G F, Le Moal M, Rivier J, Vale W. Corticotropin releasing factor (CRF) produces behavioral activation in rats. Nature 1982; 297: 331–333.

18. Britton D R, Varela M, Garcia A, Rivier J. Dexamethasone suppresses pituitary-adrenal but not behavioral effects of centrally administered CRF. Life Sci 1986; 38:211–216.

19. Britton K T, Lee G, Dana R, Risch S C, Koob G F. Activating and "anxiogenic" effects of CRF are not inhibited by blockade of the pituitary-adrenal system with dexamethasone. Life Sci 1986; 39:1281–1286.

20. Eaves M, Britton K T, Rivier J, Vale W, Koob G F. Effects of corticotropin releasing factor in locomotor activation in hypophysectomized rats. Peptides 1985; 6:923–926.

21. Swerdlow N R, Koob G F. Separate neural substrates of the locomotor-activating properties of amphetamine, caffeine and corticotropin releasing factor (CRF) in the rat. Pharmacol Biochem Behav 1985; 23:303–307.

22. Tazi A, Swerdlow N R, Le Moal M, Rivier J, Vale W, Koob G F. Behavioral activation of CRF: evidence for the involvement of the ventral forebrain. Life Sci 1987; 41:41–50.

23. Swerdlow, N R, Britton K T, and Koob G F. Potentiation of acoustic startle by corticotropin-releasing factor (CRF) and by fear are both reversed by a-helical CRF (9-41) Neuropsychopharmacology 1989; 2:285–292.

24. Britton D R, Britton K T. A sensitive open field measure of anxiolytic drug activity. Pharmacol Biochem Behav 1981; 15:577–582.

25. Britton D R, Koob G F, Rivier J, Vale W. Intraventricular corticotropin-releasing factor enhances behavioral effects of novelty. Life Sci 1982; 31: 363–367.

26. Levine A S, Rogers B, Kneip J, Grace M, Morley J E. Effect of centrally administered corticotropin releasing factor (CRF) on multiple feeding paradigms. Neuropharmacology 1983; 22:337–339.

27. Morley J E, Levine A S. Corticotropin-releasing factor, grooming and ingestive behavior. Life Sci 1983; 81:1459–1464.

28. Britton D R, Hoffman D K, Lederis K, Rivier J. A comparison of the behavioral effects of CRF, sauvagine, and urotensin I. Brain Res 1984; 304: 201–205.

29. Krahn D D, Gosnell B A, Grace M, Levine A S. CRF antagonist partially reverses CRF- and stress-induced effects on feeding. Brain Res Bull 1986; 17:285–289.

30. Berridge C W, Dunn A J. Corticotropin-releasing factor elicits naloxone sensitive stress-like alterations in exploratory behavior in mice. Regul Pept 1986; 16:83–93.

31. Berridge C W, Dunn A J. A corticotropin-releasing factor antagonist reverses the stress-induced changes of exploratory behavior in mice. Horm Behav 1987; 21:393–401.

32. Takahashi L K, Kalin N H, Vandenburgt J A, Sherman J E. Corticotropin-releasing factor modulates defensive withdrawal and exploratory behavior in rats. Behav Neurosci 1989; 103:648–654.

33. Sherman J E, Kalin N E. ICV–CRH alters stress-induced freezing behavior without affecting pain sensitivity. Pharmacol Biochem Behav 1988; 30: 801–807.

34. Swerdlow N R, Geyer M A, Vale W W, Koob G F. Corticotropin releasing factor potentiates acoustic startle in rats: blockade by chlordiazepoxide. Psychopharmacology 1986; 88:142–152.

35. Tazi A, Dantzer R, Le Moal M, Rivier J, Vale W, Koob G F. Corticotropin-releasing factor antagonist blocks stress-induced fighting in rats. Regul Pept 1987; 18:37–42.

36. Kalin N H, Shelton S E, Kraemer G W, McKinney W T. Corticotropin-releasing factor administered intraventricularly to rhesus monkeys. Peptides 1983; 4:217–220.

37. Sirinathsinghji D J S, Rees L H, Rivier J, Vale W. Corticotropin-releasing factor is a potent inhibitor of sexual receptivity in the female rat. Nature (London) 1983; 305:230–235.

38. Britton K T, Morgan J, Rivier J, Vale W, Koob G F. Chlordiazepoxide attenuates CRF-induced responses suppression in the conflict test. Psychopharmacology 1985; 86:170–174.

39. Koob et al. In Tache Y, Morley JE, Brown MR, eds. Neuropeptides and stress. New York: Springer, 1989: 49–60.

40. Kalin N H, Sherman J E, Takahashi L K. Antagonism of endogenous CRH systems attenuates stress-induced freezing behavior in rats. Brain Res 1988; 457:130–135.

41. Cole B J, Koob G F. Propranolol antagonizes the enhanced conditioned fear produced by corticotropin releasing factor. J Pharmacol Exp Ther 1988; 247:902–910.

42. Butler P D, Weiss J M, Stout J C, Kilts C D, Cook L L, Nemeroff C B. Corticotropin-releasing factor produces anxiogentic and behavioral activating effects following microinfusion into the locus coeruleus. J. Neurosci. 1990; 10:176–183.

43. Fischman A J, Moldow R L. Extrahypothalamic distribution of CRF-like immunoreactivity in the rat brain. Peptides 1982; 1:149–153.
44. Cole B J, Koob G F. Low doses of corticotropin releasing factor potentiate amphetamine-induced stereotyped behavior. Psychopharmacology 1989; 99:27–33.
45. Rivier J, Rivier C, Vale W. Synthetic competitive antagonists of corticotropin-releasing factor: effect on ACTH secretion in the rat. Science 1984; 224:889–891.
46. Britton K T, Lee G, Vale W, Rivier J, Koob G F. Corticotropin releasing factor antagonists block activating and "anxiogenic" actions of CRF in the rat. Brain Res 1986; 369–303.

Role of Homeostatic Processes in the Development of Pathophysiology Following Stress

14

CHARACTERIZATION OF BRAIN ADRENAL STEROID RECEPTORS AND THEIR INVOLVEMENT IN THE STRESS RESPONSE

Bruce S. McEwen, Helen M. Chao, Maureen N. Gannon, and Robert L. Spencer
Rockefeller University, New York, New York

The adrenal cortex is essential for the long-term survival of a mammal and particularly for challenges to homeostasis including those described as "stress." This is true of both the mineralocorticoids, which regulate salt balance, and the glucocorticoids, which have diverse effects related to the diurnal rhythm and the response to stress. Thus, in spite of the negative effects that can be attributed to glucocorticoids, such as immunosuppression and neuronal death, these hormones and their mineralocorticoid counterparts are essential for the survival of the organism.

The brain is an important target organ for adrenal steroids and contains receptors for glucocorticoids and mineralocorticoids. Examination of the conditions under which glucocorticoids and mineralocorticoids are secreted and of the binding characteristics of receptors for these hormones is important for understanding the diverse response of the brain to adrenal steroids. This chapter summarizes the current status of work on the adrenal steroid receptors in the brain and the effects they mediate that are related to adaptive processes. The chapter by Sapolsky deals with the pathological aspects of glucocorticoid action with regard to cell death.

ADRENAL STEROID RECEPTORS IN THE BRAIN

Uptake of Corticosterone by Hippocampus

In 1968, we reported that tracer doses of [³H] corticosterone in adrenalectomized rats accumulated in the hippocampus (1). Subsequent studies revealed uptake sites in septum, amygdala, and scattered regions throughout the brain (2,3). Other work revealed that soluble cytosol receptors for adrenal steroids occur throughout the brain, with the hippocampus not having higher levels than other brain areas (4), suggesting that receptors in hippocampus were only part of the story. Radioimmunoassay of corticosterone (CORT) in cell nuclei isolated from different brain regions under different hormone conditions showed that at low CORT levels the hippocampus had the predominant concentration of hormone, whereas under stress conditions all brain regions contained cell nuclear CORT, with the hippocampus having only slightly higher levels than other brain areas (4).

Type I and Type II Receptors

The discrepancy between the distribution of CORT uptake during different physiological conditions began to be resolved when DeKloet and co-workers in The Netherlands showed that there are two types of adrenal steroid receptors in hippocampus (5). Their work followed the original demonstration of two receptor types in kidney by Funder et al. (6). These receptors, which will be referred to as type I ("mineralocorticoid") and type II ("glucocorticoid"), differ in affinity for CORT as well as other steroids. Type I receptors show a higher affinity for CORT than type II and possess equally high affinity for aldosterone (ALDO). Type II receptors have a lower affinity for ALDO than type I and a higher affinity for the synthetic glucocorticoid, dexamethasone (DEX) (Table 1).

Corticosterone and Aldosterone

In keeping with differences in affinity for CORT, type I receptors are more extensively occupied by CORT than type II receptors as hormone levels increase (7; 7a). Since the blood levels of CORT are 100–1000-fold higher than ALDO (8), the type I receptors normally bind CORT unless other factors intervene. In other words, the type I receptors are normally receptors for CORT and not for ALDO. However, type I receptors appear to function as mineralocorticoid receptors in the kidney, where it is now believed that the enzyme 11 beta steroid dehydrogenase may act to metabolize CORT and allow ALDO access to the type I receptors (9). We are currently investigating whether a similar mechanism may operate in the brain (10), since we know that [^{3}H] ALDO does gain access to type I receptors in some brain areas even in the presence of CORT (11). Moreover, radioimmunoassay (RIA) for ALDO in cell nuclei reveals concentrations of this steroid in the hypothalamus–preoptic area even in the presence of CORT (12). Finally, ALDO's effects on salt appetite are not mimicked by CORT, nor are they blocked, thus indicating that in vivo recognition systems for CORT and ALDO are separate (11).

TABLE 1   Binding Affinities (K_I) of Some Glucocorticoids and Mineralocorticoids for Type I and Type II Receptors in Rat Brain

Competitor	K_I (nM)	
	Type I	Type II
Aldosterone	0.18 (0.09)	2.50
Corticosterone	0.17 (0)	0.59
Dexamethasone	1.29 (0.09)	0.42
RU26988	–	0.39
RU26752	<0.10	5.94

Studies of competition of cytosolic receptor binding were performed on 3 day ADX rats. Type I binding of hippocampal cytosol was measured with [^{3}H]aldosterone (3 nM) in the presence of 0.5 μM RU26988, a selective type II agonist. Type II binding of frontal cortex cytosol was measured with [^{3}H]dexamethasone (3.5 nM). Less than 10% of the glucocorticoid receptor-binding sites in the frontal cortex are of the type I variety. Competition curves were based on eight concentrations of each competitor ranging from $10^{-10.5}$ M to 10^{-6} M. K_I values reported for type I binding are the mean (SEM) of two to three separate experiments. Due to a Hill coefficient much less than 1, the type I K_I for RU26752 (a selective type I ligand) could only be estimated. K_I values for type II binding are the result of one experiment.

Receptor Occupancy in Stress and During the Diurnal Rhythm

As implied by the lower affinity of the type II receptor for CORT, this receptor is not extensively occupied by CORT except at very high hormone concentrations (5). In contrast, type I receptors are extensively occupied by the range of CORT levels occurring during the diurnal cycle (5). In fact, it is not always possible to find a time in the cycle when more than a small percentage of type I receptors are available and unoccupied by endogenous CORT (7), although we have recently had some success in demonstrating unoccupied type I receptors at the low point of serum CORT levels (7a, 13).

REGULATION OF ADRENAL STEROID RECEPTORS

The regulation of adrenal steroid receptors in brain tissue has become an important topic of investigation since it was shown that the hippocampal receptors are more sensitive to regulation than those in other brain areas and pituitary gland (11). Adrenalectomy-induced increases in total cytosol glucocorticoid receptor levels are greater in hippocampus both in absolute and percentage terms than those in other brain areas (14), and elevated CORT levels produce decreases in receptor levels that are larger in hippocampus than in other brain areas (4,15). The significance of such receptor regulation is open to speculation. It may be regarded as a means of reducing target cell sensitivity to circulating hormones, which may have deleterious effects if present in high concentrations for too long (16). This may be important for the hippocampus, which is particularly vulnerable to damage evoked by hypoxia, excitatory amino acids, and age that can be exacerbated by circulating glucocorticoids (17-19).

The original observations regarding adrenal steroid receptor regulation did not differentiate between effects on type I and type II receptor populations. Subsequent studies have indicated that the two receptor subtypes are regulated in different ways. Type II receptors, which are in the majority, even in the hippocampus, show a sustained upregulation after adrenalectomy and a sustained downregulation after CORT replacement (7,20,21). These changes in cytosol receptor number are not accompanied by significant changes in receptor mRNA levels in whole hippocampus (13). Type I receptors show a more rapid increase after adrenalectomy (ADX), which may reflect either a rapid regulation of receptor number or the level of steroid occupancy of a fixed population of receptors (20,21). There are no significant changes in hippocampal type I receptor mRNA levels accompanying ADX or CORT replacement, nor are there differences in hippocampal type I mRNA levels during the diurnal variations in serum CORT, despite measurable changes in type I receptor-binding activity (13).

Beyond the fact that type I and type II receptor mRNA levels do not change in parallel with changes in binding activity, it is important to reemphasize that binding assays only measure the number of receptors able to bind labeled steroid, including those that can exchange labeled for unlabeled steroid. However, unlike estrogen, progestin, and androgen receptors, type I and type II adrenal steroid receptors lack the ability to exchange labeled for unlabeled steroid after they have been activated to the DNA-binding form (22,23). Therefore, binding data obtained on tissue containing unlabeled steroid indicate nothing about the number of activated receptors that may be present in the cytosol or the number of nuclear receptors bound to DNA. As a result, additional tools are needed, such as quantitative immunoassays with antireceptor antibodies, to estimate the true number of receptors under various conditions.

The differential regulation of type I and type II receptors by glucocorticoids may explain some peculiar observations. For example, dexamethasone (DEX) treatment failed to reduce hippocampal cytosol receptor levels, whereas it did produce a reduction in the hypothalamus (24). When type I and type II receptors are measured separately, it turns out that type II receptor levels decrease in both hippocampus and hypothalamus after DEX treatment, but type I receptor levels, which are richer in hippocampus, actually increase or do not change (5), thus accounting for no overall change in the total (type I plus type II) hippocampal receptor population.

Brain, especially hippocampal, glucocorticoid receptors are subject to other types of regulation than those produced directly by glucocorticoids. These include the decline in hippocampal receptors due to the congenital absence of vasopressin in the Brattleboro rat (25,26) and the decline in hippocampal receptors with aging in the rat (26-29). The former deficit is reversed by vasopressin therapy (26), whereas the age-related deficit in type I receptors is reversed by therapy with an adrenocorticotropic hormone (ACTH) analog (30). Age-related deficit in type II receptors is unaffected by this analog (30) and may reflect the loss in neurons that accompanies aging in hippocampus (see above).

Finally, regulation of type I and/or type II receptors by neural inputs to hippocampus and other brain regions is a very real possibility that should be examined in view of evidence that neurotransmitter drugs can alter receptor levels for other steroid-receptor systems (31,32). In a later section we will return to the question of receptor regulation in relation to some of the feedback effects that glucocorticoids have on the brain.

ROLE OF GLUCOCORTICOIDS IN BRAIN FUNCTION

Modes of Operation of HPA Axis and the Puzzle of How the Brain Differentiates Between Them

The hypothalamopituitary–adrenal (HPA) axis has two modes of operation: diurnal and stress. The diurnal mode is driven by an endogenous clock located somewhere in the vicinity of the suprachiasmatic nucleus, and the glucocorticoid secretion acts as a chemical signal to coordinate activities of various tissues, organs, and brain regions according to the time of day (Fig. 1). Glucocorticoid feedback on the brain in relation to diurnal secretion patterns is responsible for facilitating the waking state, increasing hunger and food-seeking, increasing cognitive function, and delaying sleep (33). The stress mode of glucocorticoid secretion is driven by experiences and traumatic events that threaten or challenge homeostasis. Glucocorticoid secretion in relation to stress plays a role in the adaptation of the organism to the stressful event or situation. Some of the actions of glucocorticoids may be regarded as promoting adaptation, whereas others are contrary to successful adaptation (15,33).

Since the hormonal output of the HPA axis appears to be qualitatively similar in both stress and diurnal modes of secretion, there must be some means by which the target tissues respond to these signals and "recognize" them. There are at least three possible means by which the stress and diurnal signals may be

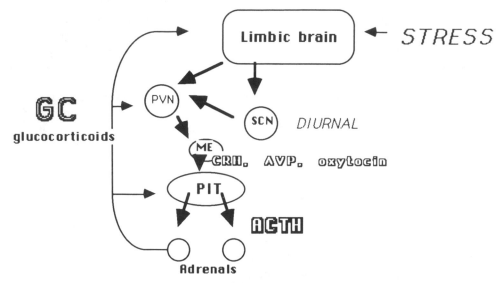

FIGURE 1 Schematic diagram of relationships between brain structures and inputs of stress and the diurnal clock in controlling hypothalamic–pituitary–adrenal function.

discriminated. First, the levels of glucocorticoid and peptide hormones are generally higher in stress than in the diurnal mode, and therefore the occupation of the type I and type II receptor systems differs between the two modes. Second, the frequency and duration of glucocorticoid secretion during the two modes differ in various ways, as discussed below. Finally, there may be quantitative or even qualitative differences in the secretion of hormones other than glucocorticoids between the stress and diurnal modes, which can be discriminated by the organism. We discuss below the evidence relating to the first two possibilities.

Glucocorticoid Feedback on HPA Function

Glucocorticoid feedback affecting the HPA axis has been classified into fast, intermediate, and delayed feedback (34), and this feedback maintains glucocorticoid levels within a narrow range of concentrations compatible with normal levels of body and thymus weight and ACTH levels (35). The diurnal rhythm involves a quiescent phase (in the rat, the a.m.) in which the pituitary corticotroph is not being driven by corticotropin-releasing factor (CRF) from the hypothalamus and an active phase (in the rat, the p.m.) in which the hypothalamus is secreting CRF in response to signals from the circadian pacemaker (36).

During the quiescent phase, the low levels of glucocorticoid hold in check ACTH release from the pituitary, and type I receptors are implicated in this action because of the low level of CORT involved (36).

Contrary to what has been thought about the termination of the response of the HPA axis to stress, the elevation of glucocorticoid levels in the stress response is not a requirement. Instead, diurnally varying levels of CORT in the low to moderate range set the HPA axis to shut off ACTH secretion after restraint stress in rats (37). This same series of experiments showed that normal shut-off persisted when stress-induced levels of glucocorticoids were attenuated by cyanoketone treatment, which does not eliminate diurnal variations of corticosterone and basal CORT secretion (37). On the other hand, treatment of ADX rats with low, constant levels of glucocorticoid in subcutaneous pellets led to prolonged ACTH secretion after a variety of stressors (38).

Thus low and diurnally varying levels of corticosterone determine the normal shut-off of the HPA axis's stress response (Fig. 2). Shut-off of ACTH secretion after stress can occur in a normal fashion even in the absence of a surge of glucocorticoid induced by stress. This important finding implies that a priming by glucocorticoids activates a neurochemical mechanism that operates neurally to terminate ACTH secretion, and it raises several questions. First, what kind of mechanism can be activated by discontinuous hormone and not by continuous hormone treatment in the same dose range, or vice versa? Second, which receptors, type I or type II, are likely to be involved? Third, in which brain regions is the hormone priming taking place? These are all questions for further research.

BASIC FACTS ABOUT GLUCOCORTICOID NEGATIVE FEEDBACK

1. System normally operates within narrow range of hormone concentrations
2. In AM, pituitary corticotroph is on its own – CRH signal is held in check by AM CORT via Type I receptors
3. In PM, brain drives corticotroph via CRH, AVP, etc
4. Shut-off of ACTH after stress can occur independently of CORT and requires prior discontinuous exposure to circulating CORT
5. Continuous CORT or deficiency of receptors may result in deficient shut-off

FIGURE 2 Summary of operating characteristics of HPA axis, based on discussion in text.

Involvement of Brain Regions in Glucocorticoid Negative Feedback

Suppression of ACTH secretion with glucocorticoid treatment after adrenalectomy involves a brain site and not the pituitary. The pituitary is only sensitive to very high levels of corticosterone (36). Local implants of glucocorticoids in the vicinity of the paraventricular nuclei (PVN), where CRF and vasopressin-containing cell bodies are located, suppress ACTH levels but these effects are not likely to be involved in the dynamics of a stress response, which are more rapid and do not necessarily involve measurable changes in levels of CRF and vasopressin in PVN.

However, brain structures that feed neural input into the PVN also play a role in ACTH secretion and glucocorticoid negative feedback. We know this because glucocorticoid implants into extrahypothalamic structures affect glucocorticoid secretion and lesions of these brain regions also modify adrenocortical activity (see 39 for review). The hippocampus has been of interest in this connection for several reasons. First, it contains high levels of type I adrenal steroid receptors, as noted. Second, lesions of hippocampus have been found to produce basal as well as stress-related hypersecretion of corticosterone (for review, see 16). Recent work indicates that dorsal or total hippocampal ablation increased levels of CRF mRNA in PVN (40) and that corticosterone implants in dorsal hippocampus suppress a.m. levels of ACTH in ADX rats (41). Furthermore, lesions of the lateral septum, which is a way-station from the hippocampus to the hypothalamus, potentiate the ADX-induced elevation in expression of vasopressin mRNA in the PVN (42). Taken together, these results implicate the hippocampus as an important site of modulation of the CRF and AVP control of ACTH secretion.

What is the role of glucocorticoid receptors in the hippocampus in this modulation? Suspicion that the hippocampus is involved in shut-off of the stress response was raised by the finding that aging rats are deficient in hippocampal neurons, glucocorticoid receptors, and the ability to shut off rapidly the glucocorticoid response to restraint stress (16). A similar defect was caused by glucocorticoid-induced downregulation of hippocampal glucocorticoid receptors (43–45). At the time those studies were done, the type I/type II receptor distinction was not clear, and only now do we know that aged rats are deficient in type I as well as type II receptors (30). In light of the new information reviewed above, how are we to view an attenuation of shut-off of the stress response such as occurs in aging rats? Rather than this being the consequence of failed negative glucocorticoid feedback at the time of stress, the work of the Dallman group (37) strongly suggests that this defect is the result either of fewer type I (and possibly type II) receptors or receptor-containing neurons in the aging hippo-campus or the consequence of the more constant secretion of corticosterone during the diurnal cycle, or both. As to the receptors involved, only further studies can determine the extent to which type I and type II receptors and the hippocampus itself may be involved in the priming effect of diurnally varying glucocorticoids that apparently sets the shut-off mechanism.

Glucocorticoid Actions on Food Intake

Glucocorticoids enhance food intake and food-seeking behavior, which can be seen during the diurnal rhythm (46,47), after exogenous glucocorticoid treat-ment (48,49), and in ventromedial hypothalamus-damaged animals (50) (see Fig. 3). During the diurnal cycle, presentation of food for restricted times during the day leads to an anticipatory surge of glucocorticoids prior to food presentation that can be shifted away from the normal diurnal rise (51,52).

In other words, glucocorticoids are a powerful stimulus to feeding, and more than one mechanism may be involved. This is indicated by the fact that moderate to high levels of glucocorticoids are associated with the diurnal elevation of feeding and with the potentiation of norepinephrine-induced feeding (47,49), whereas very low levels of glucocorticoids are sufficient to maintain hyperphagia and obesity in VMN-damaged rats (50). The low levels of corticosterone involved in the latter situation is suggestive of the involvement of type I receptors (50).

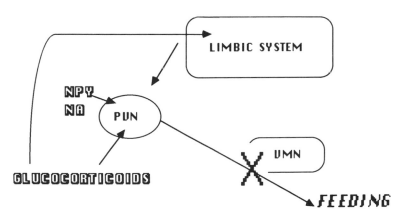

FIGURE 3 Schematic diagram of hypothesized role of limbic glucocorticoid targets in mediating adrenal steroid effects of feeding and body weight in rats with VMH lesions, based on discussion in text.

Study of glucocorticoid effects as permissive agents for norepinephrine (NE)-induced feeding have focused on the PVN, where glucocorticoids induce a rapid increase in alpha-2 adrenergic receptors that are implicated in NE action (46). The PVN sends descending projections that pass near the VMN and which are believed to be disrupted by VMN lesions that cause hyperphagia and obesity (53). Therefore glucocorticoids act in PVN to potentiate NE's effects, thus suppressing an inhibitory system that normally inhibits feeding.

However, the dependency of VMN lesioned rats' hyperphagia and obesity on low levels of glucocorticoids implicates another pathway in the control of feeding, since the VMN lesions have effectively removed the PVN influence (53). The low levels of corticosterone that maintain the hyperphagia of the VMN-lesions rats implicate the type I receptors, whereas a rapid and possibly direct membrane action of glucocorticoids is a distinct possibility in the case of the glucocorticoid effect on NE-induced feeding. It remains to be determined to what degree both receptor types are involved and whether the hippocampus plays an important role.

RESPONSE OF THE BRAIN TO STRESS AND THE ROLE OF GLUCOCORTICOIDS IN ADAPTATION

Stress induces adaptive responses that help the organism to adjust to a changed environment. What used to be called "homeostasis" may also be called "allostasis," referring to the concept that the new state into which the adaptation takes the organism is not the same as the initial state (54). In particular, changes in the brain take place as a result of stress. The initial alterations in neurotransmitter (e.g., NE) turnover that accompany stress are transient and dependent on whether the animals are able to cope (55). However, if stress is repeated or prolonged, there are changes in the noradrenergic and other systems that are long-lasting. These include increased tyrosine hydroxylase (TOH) activity (56,57) and TOH messenger RNA (58), and decreased NE-stimulated cAMP formation in cerebral cortical and hippocampal slices (59–61). One way of looking at these changes is as checks and balance on NE activity, with the decreased responsiveness to NE counteracting the increased capacity for making NE. Other systems change as well. Serotonin responsiveness increases as a result of repeated stress (62), and tryptophan hydroxylase activity is increased by stress (63,64).

What is the role of glucocorticoids in these changes? For tyrosine hydroxylase, there is no evidence that glucocorticoids play an important role in its induction by stress, although they may have some influence during development (65) and in the autonomic nervous system of the adult (66). As for NE-stimulated cAMP accumulation, glucocorticoids appear to mediate the decline produced by stress (67–69) in both cerebral cortex and hippocampus (61). In cortex, this appears to be due to a suppression by glucocorticoids of the alpha-adrenergic facilitation of the beta-adrenergic receptor-mediated response (68). Paradoxically, however, the adrenal glands may also facilitate the NA cAMP response, at least in hippocampus, during the diurnal rhythm, possibly through glucocorticoids (69).

Manipulations of the HPA axis also influence calcium-dependent adenylate cyclase (AC) catalytic activity (61). Long-term, repeated daily stress for 21 days decreased calmodulin-stimulated AC activity by approximately 45% in cerebral cortex, but not in hippocampal, membrane preparations. This decrease appeared selective for the calcium-calmodulin form of adenylate cyclase, since basal and forskolin stimulated activities were not changed. Daily corticosterone injection (50 mg/kg intraperitoneally) mirrored the effects of stress, while carrier injection had no significant effect. A smaller decline was achieved by adding CORT to the drinking water (400 μg/ml). Since both routes of CORT administration caused a similar decrease in body weight, the larger decrease observed with injection of this steroid may reflect glucocorticoid potentiation of a stress (injection) response. In contrast to these long-term effects, adrenalectomy (6 days) selectively decreased calmodulin-stimulated adenylate cyclase activity in hippocampal, but not cortical, membranes. In general, these changes mirror the attenuation of NE-responsive cAMP accumulation in brain slices. These observations suggest that glucocorticoids may modulate a common, postreceptor, calcium-dependent component of cAMP-generating systems in brain. However, the stress- and/or corticosterone-induced decrease in the hippocampal NE cAMP response is not paralleled by a change in calmodulin-stimulated adenylate cyclase activity, which suggests a regionally specific dissociation of these two responses.

As for serotonin, glucocorticoid treatment decreases serotonin receptor density in some regions of hippocampus (70,71), and it also reduces central responsiveness to serotonergic drugs (72). These effects appear to counteract the effects of stress per se to increase serotonergic activity. Thus, glucocorticoids may have a similar role in reducing responsiveness to both NE and serotonin (73). At the same time, glucocorticoids appear to have a permissive role in facilitating the stress-induced increase in tryptophan hydroxylase activity (64).

Are these changes in NE and serotonin responsiveness adaptive or maladaptive, and is the role of glucocorticoids to improve or inhibit the process of adaptation? With regard to NE, it can be argued that glucocorticoid effects are "antidepressant" in that they reduce the NE–cAMP response just like tricyclic antidepressant drugs do (68). However, for serotonin, the suppression of the serotonin responsiveness by glucocorticoids appears to be counterproductive for behavioral adaptation to repeated restraint stress in the rat (60,74). Thus the role of glucocorticoids in adaptation to stress may not be uniformly beneficial, and what may be more important are the time courses of the responses of individual neurochemical systems in relation to the severity and duration of the stressor, as well as the ratio of noradrenergic to serotonergic activity in a particular individual. We are describing only several neurotransmitters in the brain; changes in the other systems, including the many neuropeptide systems, deserve more extensive study before we can begin to understand the nature of the brain's adaptation to stress, as well as its meaning for maladaptation, as in depressive illness.

The overall significance of glucocorticoids for the process of allostasis may be as follows. The body has a set of initial responses to stress and trauma that can cause harm if allowed to go unchecked (75). Glucocorticoids tend to counteract many of these initial reactions, which is why they are useful in suppressing inflammatory and immune responses and counteracting edema (75). The same general phenomenon may underlie the postulated role of glucocorticoids in NE and 5HT responses to stress, even though it is not yet clear how glucocorticoid suppression of their activity may ultimately be beneficial.

CONCLUSIONS

The brain contains receptors for adrenal steroids, which represent the products of two different genes and respond to two different hormone classes: glucocorticoids and mineralocorticoids. Yet behind this deceptively simple statement, we have seen that there is considerable complexity: one receptor, known as "type I" or "mineralocorticoid" functions as a receptor for both hormone classes depending on the presence of extrinsic factors such as enzymes that metabolize the glucocorticoid. In other words, type I receptors in the hippocampus see CORT rather than ALDO because CORT levels are much higher and the metabolizing enzymes are absent; type I receptors in the kidney see ALDO rather than CORT because 11 beta steroid dehydrogenase activity eliminates CORT and allows ALDO access to the receptors (8).

With regard to glucocorticoids such as CORT, type I and type II receptors function as a two-level recognition system in hippocampus, with type I receptors being occupied at lower levels of CORT than type II receptors. This recognition system provides the beginnings of the ability of the brain to recognize and perhaps discriminate between the two different modes of glucocorticoid secretion, namely, the diurnal mode and stress. It is important to acknowledge the importance of the feedback by diurnally varying glucocorticoids on the brain as a signal that coordinates behavior and neuroendocrine function with the time of day. Included in this may also be the efficiency with which the glucocorticoid stress response is terminated, since we have seen that constant glucocorticoid levels contribute to inefficient shut-off.

As to the receptor mechanisms that respond to stress-induced glucocorticoid secretion, we presume that type II receptors are principally involved. These receptors are found throughout the brain, both in neurons and in glial cells, and they are likely to be involved in many of the long-term changes that glucocorticoids produce, including the suppression of myelin formation and glial cell proliferation (76,77) and the long-term effect described above on sensitivity of the CNS serotonergic and noradrenergic systems. Future research will help to determine the exact mechanisms involved, including the genes that are modulated up or down by glucocorticoid–receptor complexes.

ACKNOWLEDGMENTS

Research in the authors' laboratory described in this chapter is supported by NIMH Grant MH41256 and NIMH Grant NS07080. Mr. Philip Choo, Ms. Melissa Adaniel, and Ms. Maryse Aubourg provided important technical assistance.

REFERENCES

1. McEwen B S, Weiss J, Schwartz L. Selective retention of corticosterone by limbic structures in rat brain. Nature 1968; 220:911–912.
2. Warembourgh M. Radioautographic study of the rat brain after injection of $1,2^3$H corticosterone. Brain Res 1975; 89:61–70.
3. Stumpf W, Sar M. Glucocorticosteroid and mineralocorticosteroid hormone target sites in the brain: autoradiographic studies with corticosterone, aldosterone and dexamethasone. In: Jones M, Gillham B, Dallman M, Chattopaohyay S, eds. Interactions within the brain–pituitary–adrenocortical system. London: Academic Press, 1979: 137–147.
4. McEwen B S, DeKloet E R, Rostene W. Adrenal steroid receptors and actions in the nervous system. Physiol Rev 1986; 66:1121–1188.
5. Reul J M, DeKloet E R. Two receptor systems for corticosterone in rat brain: microdistribution and differential occupation. Endocrinology 1985; 117:2505–2511.
6. Funder J, Feldman D, Edelman I. The roles of plasma binding and receptor specificity in the mineralocorticoid action of aldosterone. Endocrinology 1973; 92:994–1004.
7. Reul J M, VanDenBosch F R, DeKloet E R. Relative occupation of type I and type II corticosteroid receptors in rat brain following stress and dexamethasone treatment: functional implications. J Endocr 1987; 115:459–467.
7a. Spencer, R., Young, E., Choo, P and McEwen, B.S. Glucocorticoid type I and type II receptor binding: estimates of in vivo receptor number occupancy and activation with varying levels of steroid. Brain Res 1990 in press.
8. Eilers E, Peterson R. Aldosterone secretion in the rat. In: Baulieu EE, Robel P, eds. Aldosterone. Oxford: Blackwell, 1964; 251–264.
9. Funder J, Pearce P, Smith R, Smith A. Mineralocorticoid action: target tissue specificity is enzyme, not receptor, mediated. Science 1988; 242: 583–585.

10. Coirini H, Schulkin J, McEwen B S. Behavioral and neuroendocrine regulation of mineralocorticoid and glucocorticoid action. Abstr Soc Neurosci 1988; 14:528.15, p 1322.

11. McEwen B S, Lambdin L, Rainbow T, DeNicola A. Aldosterone effects on salt appetite in adrenalectomized rats. Neuroendocrinology 1986; 43:38–43.

12. Yongue B, Roy E. Endogenous aldosterone and corticosterone in brain cell nuclei of adrenal-intact rats: regional distribution and effects of physiological variations in serum steroids. Brain Res 1987; 436:49–61.

13. Chao H M, Choo P H, McEwen B S. Glucocorticoid and mineralocorticoid receptor mRNA expression in rat brain. Neuroendocrinology, 1989: 50: 365–371.

14. Olpe H-R, McEwen B S. Glucocorticoid binding to receptor-like proteins in rat brain and pituitary: ontogenetic and experimentally-induced changes. Brain Res 1976; 121–128.

15. Tornello S, Fridman O, Weisenberg L, Coirini H, DeNicola A. Differences in corticosterone binding by regions of the central nervous system in normal and diabetic rats. J Steroid Biochem 1981; 14:77–81.

16. Sapolsky R, Krey L, McEwen B S. The neuroendocrinology of stress and aging: the glucocorticoid cascade hypothesis. Endocr Rev 1986; 7:284–301.

17. Sapolsky R, Pulsinelli W. Glucocorticoids potentiate ischemic injury to neurons: therapeutic implications. Science 1985; 229:1397–1399.

18. Sapolsky R. A mechanism for glucocorticoid toxicity in the hippocampus: increased neuronal vulnerability to metabolic insults. J Neurosci 1985; 5: 1228–1232.

19. Sapolsky R. Glucocorticoid toxicity in the hippocampus: temporal aspects of synergy with kainic acid. Neuroendocrinology 1986; 43:440–444.

20. Reul J M, VanDenBosck F, DeKloet E R. Differential response of type I and type II corticosteroid receptors to changes in plasma steroid level and circadian rhythmicity. Neuroendocrinology 1987; 45:407–412.

21. Stephenson G, Funder J. Hippocampal and renal type I receptors are differentially regulated. Am J Physiol 1987; 252:E525–E529.

22. Chou Y-C, Luttge W G. Activated type II receptors in brain cannot rebind glucocorticoids: relationship to progesterone's antiglucocorticoid actions. Brain Res 1988; 440:67–78.

23. Mendel D, Bodwell J, Munck A. Glucocorticoid receptors lacking hormone-binding activity are bound in nuclei of ATP-depleted cells. Nature 1986; 324:478–480.

24. Sapolsky R, McEwen B S. Down-regulation of neural corticosterone receptors by corticosterone and dexamethasone. Brain Res 1985; 339: 161–165.

25. Veldhuis H, DeKloet E R. Vasopressin related peptides increase the hippocampal corticosterone receptor capacity of diabetes insipidus (Brattleboro rat). Endocrinology 1982; 110:153–157.

26. Sapolsky R, Krey L, McEwen B S, Rainbow T. Do vasopressin-related peptides induce hippocampal corticosterone receptors? Implications for aging. J Neurosci 1984; 4:1479–1485.

27. Angelucci L, Valeri F, Grossie E, Veldhuis H, Bohus B, DeKloet E R. Involvement of hippocampal corticosterone receptors in behavioral phenomena. In: Brambilla F, Racagni G, DeWied D, eds. Progress in psychoneuroendocrinology. Amsterdam: Elsevier, 1980; 177–185.

28. Rigter H, Veldhuis H, DeKloet E R. Spatial learning and the hippocampal corticosterone receptor system of old rats: effect of the ACTH 4-9 analogue ORG 2766. Brain Res 1984; 309:393–398.

29. Sapolsky R, Krey L, McEwen B S. Corticosterone receptors decline in a site-specific manner in the aged rat brain. Brain Res 1983; 289:235–240.

30. Reul J, Tonnaer J, DeKloet E R. Neurotropic ACTH analogue promotes plasticity of type I corticosteroid receptor in brain of senescent male rats. Neurobiol Aging 1988; 9:253–260.

31. Nock B, Feder H. a1-Noradrenergic regulation of hypothalamic progestin receptors and guinea pig lordosis behavior. Brain Res 1984; 310:77–85.

32. Kitayama I, Janson A, Cintra A, et al. Effects of chronic imipramine treatment on glucocorticoid receptor immunoreactivity in various regions of rat brain. J Neurol Transm 1988; 73:191–203.

33. McEwen B S, Brinton R. Neuroendocrine aspects of adaptation. In: DeKloet E R, Wiegant V, DeWied D, eds. Progress in brain research. Amsterdam: Elsevier, 1987: 11–26.

34. Keller-Wood N M, Dallman M. Corticosteroid inhibition of ACTH secretion. Endocr Rev 1984; 5:1–24.

35. Akana S, Cascio C, Shinsako J, Dallman M. Corticosterone: narrow range required for normal body and thymus weight and ACTH. Am J Physiol 1985; 249:R527–R532.

36. Dallman M, Akana S, Cascio C, Darlington D, Jacobson L, Levin N. Regulation of ACTH secretion: variations on a theme of B. Rec Prog Horm Res 1987; 43:113–172.

37. Jacobson L, Akana S, Cascio C, Shinsako J, Dallman M. Circadian variations in plasma corticosterone permit normal termination of adrenocorticotropin responses to stress. Endocrinology 1988; 122:1343–1348.

38. Akana S, Jacobson L, Cascio C, Shinsako J, Dallman M. Constant corticosterone replacement normalizes basal adrenocorticotropin (ACTH) but permits sustained ACTH hypersecretion after stress in adrenalectomized rats. Endocrinology 1988; 122:1337–1342.

39. McEwen B S. Adrenal steroid feedback on neuroendocrine tissues. Ann NY Acad Sci 1977; 297:568–579.

40. Herman J, Schafer M, Young E, et al. Evidence for hippocampal regulation of neuroendocrine neurons of the hypothalamus-pituitary adrenocortical axis. J Neurosci 1988; 9:3072–3082.

41. Kovacs K, Makara G. Corticosterone and dexamethasone act at different brain sites to inhibit adrenalectomy-induced adrenocorticotropin hypersecretion. Brain Res 1988; 474:205–210.

42. Baldino F, Kane T, Fitzpatrick-McElligott S, Wolfson B. Coordinate hormonal and synaptic regulation of vasopressin messenger RNA. Science 1988; 241:978–981.

43. Meaney M, Sapolsky R, McEwen B S. The development of the glucocorticoid receptor system in the rat limbic brain. I. Ontogeny and autoradiographic study. Brain Res 1985; 18:159–164.

44. Meaney M, Sapolsky R, McEwen B S. The development of glucocorticoid receptor system in the rat limbic brain. II. An autoradiographic study. Dev Brain Res 1985; 18:165–168.

45. Sapolsky R, Meaney M, McEwen B S. The development of the glucocorticoid receptor system in the rat limbic brain. III. Negative feedback regulation. Dev Brain Res 1985; 18:169–174.

46. Jhanwar-Uniyal M, Leibowitz S. Impact of circulating corticosterone on α2- and α2-noradrenergic receptors in discrete brain areas. Brain Res 1986; 368: 404–408.

47. Jhanwar-Uniyal M, Leibowitz S. Diurnal rhythm of $alpha_2$-noradrenergic receptors in the paraventricular nucleus and other brain areas: relation to circulating corticosterone and feeding behavior. Life Sci 1985; 38:473–482.

48. Von Zerssen D. Mood and behavioral changes under corticosteroid therapy. In: Util T, Landahn G, Herrman W. eds. Psychotropic action of hormones. New York: Spectrum, 1976: 195–222.

49. Roland C, Chakthavatsalam P, Leibowitz S. Interaction between corticosterone and $alpha_2$-noradrenergic system of the paraventricular nucleus in relation to feeding behavior. Neuroendocrinology 1986; 42:296–305.

50. King B. Glucocorticoids and hypothalamic obesity. Neurosci Biobehav Rev 1988; 12:29–37.

51. Krieger D. Food and water restriction shifts corticosterone, temperature, activity and brain amine periodicity. Endocrinology 1974; 95:1195–1201.

52. Honma K-I, Honma S, Hiroshige T. Feeding-associated corticosterone peak in rats under various feeding cycles. J Physiol 1984; 246:R72–R726.

53. Kirchgessner A, Sclafani A. PVN-hindbrain pathway involved in the hypothalamic hyperphagia-obesity syndrome. Physiol Behav 1988; 42:517–528.

54. Sterling P, Eyer J. ALlostasis: a new paradigm to explain arousal pathology. In: Fisher S, Reason J, eds. Handbook of life stress, cognition and health. John Wiley and Sons, London 1988; 631–651.

55. Tsuda A, Tanaka M. Differential changes in noradrenaline turnover in specific regions of rat brain produced by controllable and uncontrollable shocks. Behav Neurosci 1985; 99:802–817.

56. Musacchio J, Julou L, Kety S, Glowinski J. Increase in rat brain tyrosine activity produced by electroconvulsive shock. Proc Natl Acad Sci USA 1969; 63:1117–1119.

57. Thoenen H. Induction of TH in peripheral and central adrenergic neurons by cold exposure of rats. Nature 1970; 228:861–862.

58. Richard F, Faucon-Biguet N, Labatut R, Rollet D, Mallet J, Buda M. Modulation by tyrosine hydroxylase gene expression in rat brain and adrenals by exposure to cold. J Neurosci Res 1988; 20:32–37.

59. Stone E, Slucky A, Platt J, Trullas R. Reduction of the cyclic adenosine 3'5'-monophosphate response to catecholamine in rat brain slices after repeated restraint stress. J Pharmacol Exp Ther 1985; 233:382–388.

60. Stone E, Platt J, Herrera A, Kirk K. Effect of repeated restraint stress, desmethylimipramine or adrenocorticotropin on the alpha and beta adrenergic components of the cyclic AMP response to norepinephrine in rat brain slices. J Pharmacol Exp Ther 1986; 237:702–707.

61. Gannon M, and McEwen B S. Calmodulin involvement in stress- and corticosterone- induced down-regulation of cyclic AMP generating systems in brain J Neurochem 1990 in press.

62. Kennett G, Dickinson S, Curzon G. Central serotonergic responses and behavioral adaptation to repeated immobilization: the effect of the corticosterone synthesis inhibitor metyrapone. Eur J Pharmacol 1985; 119:143–152.

63. Azmitia E, McEwen B S. Corticosterone regulation of tryptophan hydroxylase in rat midbrain. Science 1969; 166:1274–1276.

64. Azmitia E, McEwen B S. Adrenocortical influence on rat brain tryptophan hydroxylase activity. Brain Res 1974; 78:291–302.

65. Markey K, Towle A, Sze P. Glucocorticoid influence on tyrosine hydroxylase activity in mouse locus coeruleus during postnatal development. Endocrinology 1982; 111:1519–1523.

66. Stachowiak M, Rigual R, Lee P, Viveros O, Hong J. Regulation of tyrosine hydroxylase and phenylethanolamine N-methyltransferase mRNA levels in the sympathoadrenal system by the pituitary-adrenocortical axis. Mol Brain Res 1988; 3:2675–286.

67. Mobley P, Manier D, Sulser F. Norepinephrine-sensitive adenylate cyclasc system in rat brain: role of adrenal corticosteroids. J Pharmacol Exp Ther 1983; 226:71–77.

68. Stone E, McEwen B S, Herrera A, Carr K. Regulation of alpha and β components of noradrenergic cyclic AMP response in cortical slices. Eur J Pharmacol 1987; 141:347–356.

69. Duman R, Strada S, Enna S. Effect of imipramine and adrenocorticotropin administration on the rat brain norepinephrine-coupled cyclic nucleotide generating system:alterations in alpha and beta adrenergic components. J Pharmacol Exp Ther 1985; 234:409–414.

70. Biegon A, Rainbow T, McEwen B S. Corticosterone modulation of neurotransmitter receptors in rat hippocampus: a quantitative autoradiographic study. Brain Res 1985; 332:309–314.

71. DeKloet E R, Sybersma H, Reul H. Selective control by corticosterone of serotonin receptor capacity in raphe-hippocampal system. Neuroendocrinology 1986; 42:513–521.

72. Dickinson S, Kennett G, Curzon G. Reduced 5a-hydroxytryptamine-dependent behavior in rats following chronic corticosterone treatment. Brain Res 1985; 345:10–18.

73. McEwen B S. Glucocorticoid-biogenic amine interactions in relation to mood and behavior. Biochem Pharmacol 1987; 36:1755–1763.

74. Kennett G, Dickinson S, Curzon G. Corticosteroid inhibition of ACTH secretion. Endocr Rev 1985; 5:1–24.
75. Munck A, Guyre P, Holbrook N. Physiological functions of glucocorticoids in stress and their relation to pharmacological actions. Endocr Rev 1984; 5:25–44.
76. Meyer J. Biochemical effects of corticosteroids on neural tissues. Physiol Rev 1985; 65:946–1020.
77. Yehuda R, Fairman K, Meyer J. Early adrenalectomy promote brain cell proliferation in rats. Soc Neurosci Abstr 1985; 11:262.6.

15

EFFECTS OF STRESS AND GLUCOCORTICOIDS ON HIPPOCAMPAL NEURONAL SURVIVAL

Robert M. Sapolsky

Stanford University School of Medicine, Stanford, California

For the neurologist, the hippocampus provokes exasperation and despair. It is a pleasing structure: no one could fail to be charmed by its cytoarchitecture. It is an important structure: it appears to be critical to various aspects of cognition. But for those concerned with neurological disorders and neuron death, the overriding fact of the hippocampus is its profound vulnerability to neurological insult. It is either the primary or among the primary brain regions damaged by global ischemia (following cardiac arrest), various forms of sustained epileptic seizures, Alzheimer's dementia, hypoglycemia, organometal toxicity, and alcoholic dementia (1). The vulnerability of the hippocampus, especially to anoxic or hypoxic injury, was originally thought to be a vascular problem. This view, which held sway earlier this century, was based on the vascularization in the region; the hippocampus is at a "watershed" between a number of sparse vascular beds. In most regards, this vascular emphasis has not held up, and a more cellular emphasis has predominated since then; the hippocampus is viewed as being particularly vulnerable because its cells are intrinsically vulnerable (2). As will be discussed below at length, the current and credible version of this view concentrates on the excitatory neurotransmitters that predominate in the hippocampus.

Why should the hippocampus and its neurotoxic vulnerability have a place in a volume on stress? This chapter will review a frightening literature that has emerged in recent years suggesting that stress, via excessive secretion of glucocorticoids (GCs), can also damage the hippocampus. I will first consider the evidence that GCs damage hippocampal neurons as a normal part of aging, and can exacerbate the hippocampal damage induced by some of the neurological insults mentioned above. I will then consider, at length, the cell biology of how GCs might be endangering hippocampal neurons, because considerable information is beginning to emerge on that question. Then I will consider whether this information allows us to design rational therapies that might protect the hippocampus. Finally, I will discuss whether any of this information might apply to the primate or human.

GLUCOCORTICOIDS AS PACEMAKERS OF HIPPOCAMPAL AGING

A theme that emerges from this volume is that GCs are hormones that should not be taken lightly. They are obviously critical in order for organisms to survive major, acute physical stressors, and the fragility of the addisonian patient in the face of physical demands underlines the importance of these steroids. All of this makes sense in the context of the physiological effects of GCs throughout the body: the mobilization of energy at the cost of energy storage, the potentiation of cardiovascular tone, and the inhibition of long-term, anabolic processes for more auspicious times. Just as clear, however, is that an overabundance of the highly catabolic GCs is damaging, and many of the stress-related pathological conditions discussed in this volume (steroid diabetes, myopathy, hypertension, ulceration, reproductive and immunosuppression) can be thought of as arising, at least in part, from overexposure to GCs. These hormones are essential for life, but are, in excess, highly pathogenic.

In this context GC neurotoxicity in the hippocampus must be considered. First, why should the hippocampus be sensitive to any GC actions, whether deleterious or not? As will be discussed in this volume and in previous reviews by McEwen and his colleagues (3), the hippocampus is a primary target site in the brain for GCs. The clearest support for this view is the sheer number of corticosteroid receptors in the structure. It has by far the highest concentration of type I receptors of any brain region; and at least as plentiful concentrations of type II receptors as any region. From an electrophysiological and neurochemical standpoint, the hippocampus is extremely responsive to GCs. A number of hippocampal-dependent behaviors are also sensitive to GCs. Thus in viewing the relationship between GCs and hippocampal aging, it was no surprise that GCs should have an impact on the hippocampus, but it was surprising that it should be so deleterious.

The first evidence that GCs could damage the aging hippocampus was essentially correlative. With age, basal GC concentrations rise in the male rat (4-12). This effect is not as strong in the aging female rat, but is still apparent (11,13, 14). In parallel with this, the aging hippocampus loses neurons (cf. 15). This is most pronounced among the pyramidal neurons of Ammon's horn, and is accompanied by the glial hyperplasia and infiltration that typically accompany neurological damage. Landfield and colleagues (8) demonstrated that the higher an aged rat's basal GC concentrations, the more reactive gliosis is found in their hippocampus postmortem.

A few years after that, Landfield et al. (16) showed that this correlation between GC hypersecretion and hippocampal degeneration is more than correlative. By adrenalectomizing rats at midage (12 months) and maintaining them GC-free until senescence (approximately 2 years), they showed that the "normal" degenerative aging of the hippocampus can be prevented. They also showed that some of the cognitive deficits that normally emerge during aging in the rat are prevented when the hippocampal neurodegeneration is prevented. Thus, some humoral factor from the adrenals appears to play a role in bringing about the degeneration typical of hippocampal aging. At that point, we examined whether the factor is, indeed, GCs. In somewhat of an inverse from the Landfield experiment, we determined whether prolonged exposure to *elevated* GC concentrations would cause hippocampal degeneration and thus accelerate the aging of the structure. More than a decade before, it had been demonstrated that extremely high, pharmacological concentrations of GCs damage the hippocampus in the guinea pig (17). We were interested in seeing whether high GC concentrations that were still in the physiological range (i.e., equivalent to the circulating concentrations typical of major stressors) could also be damaging. We found that after 3 months of near-constant exposure to GCs in the upper physiological range, hippocampi showed many indices of accelerated aging (18). Total cell number was decreased, and the size class of cells lost corresponded to pyramidal neurons. This was accompanied by glial infiltration, was most pronounced in the Ammon's horn region, and autoradiographic analysis revealed that surviving neurons were those with few corticosteroid receptors. All of these features matched those seen in the aging hippocampus (18,19). Moreover, such rats had impaired spatial memory (19a). Following that, it was demonstrated that chronic stress, itself, will accelerate some of these aspects of hippocampal aging (20).

Thus, GCs appear capable of damaging hippocampal neurons, and this seems to play a role in hippocampal aging. These studies, however, left some uncertainty as to the sensitivity of the phenomenon. The demonstration that complete removal of GCs (by adrenalectomy) prevented senescent degeneration suggests that even basal, nonstressed concentrations of GCs can eventually damage the hippocampus. However, it was not clear whether relatively subtle fluctuations in GC concentrations over the lifespan alter the rate of hippocampal neurodegeneration, or if protection is only afforded by the dramatic decrease seen after adrenalectomy.

A recent study of ours suggests that subtle alterations in GC concentrations will also influence the aging of the system. We took advantage of a phenomenon long-recognized in the developmental psychobiology literature. If rats are handled daily for brief periods during their immediate neonatal period (the first few weeks of life) a variety of behavioral and endocrine changes are induced that are extremely persistent throughout the lifetime. Among these is a long-lasting reduction in basal GC concentrations. Thus, we studied a population of male rats that had been handled neonatally. First, we found that the effects on GC secretion are indeed life-long, and that handled animals do not have the progressive rise in basal GC concentrations that normally occurs during aging. Instead, levels remain fairly unchanged throughout the lifespan. If the hippocampus is sensitive to relatively small changes in cumulative life-long GC exposure, instead of only to the large differences due to adrenalectomy or (possibly unphysiological) GC administration, handled rats should have less degenerated hippocampi in old age than normal aged controls. This is precisely what we observed (21). Handled animals show less of the progressive neuron loss and of the deficits in hippocampal-dependent spatial learning typical of normal old rats. We have recently replicated this finding with female rats (Meaney et al., in press). Thus, the rate of GC exposure over the lifespan can act as an important determinant of the rate of hippocampal neuron death, and the structure appears to be sensitive to relatively small changes in the amount of GC exposure. How, then, do GCs damage hippocampal neurons?

GLUCOCORTICOIDS IMPAIR THE ABILITY OF NEURONS TO SURVIVE METABOLIC INSULTS

In considering how GCs might damage hippocampal neurons during aging, it seemed possible that the hormones might not really be directly toxic themselves; to use a very concrete metaphor, what if they did not actually push neurons off a cliff? Instead, they might merely be catabolic (as they certainly are in peripheral tissue), and endanger neurons, leaving them on the edge of a cliff. Under such conditions, were heavy GC exposure to occur by itself, the neurons would be pushed to the edge of that cliff but, with the abatement of the steroid effect, would recover from the threat. However, if the period of exposure coincided with some other challenge, the two might combine to push neurons over the edge. This idea suggested that GCs, over the lifespan, impair the capacity of neurons to withstand the intermittent metabolic challenges to which they are no doubt exposed; the odds of a neuron surviving any given crisis thus declines.

This notion of GC endangerment of neurons generated an easily testable hypothesis. Were this the case, concentrations of GCs that were, themselves, not damaging to hippocampal neurons, should make other hippocampal insults more toxic. Considerable data now show that the more GCs hippocampal neurons are exposed to, the more damaging are the effects of a variety of neurotoxins, including kainic acid, 3-acetylpyridine, hypoxia–ischemia, and paraquat (22–29a). This was first shown for the glutamatergic excitotoxin kainic acid, which induces status epilepticus seizures and preferentially damages the CA3 hippocampal region (22). In this instance, elevated GC concentrations in the upper physiological range for a week before and after kainic acid microinfusion into the hippocampus causes a significant increase in the amount of damage induced by the toxin. Two weeks of such GC administration alone do not damage the structure. Conversely, adrenalectomizing a rat and keeping it GC-free for a week before and after kainic acid infusion decreases the amount of hippocampal damage typically produced by the excitotoxin. A similar synergy between GCs and kainic acid is not observed in the cerebellum (a region with ample kainic acid receptors and a vulnerability to the toxicity of kainic acid, but few corticosteroid receptors), or the hypothalamus (an area with ample corticosteroid receptors but few kainic acid receptors).

A similar GC/toxin synergy occurs with the antimetabolite 3-acetylpyridine, which uncouples electron transport and, much like hypoglycemia, preferentially damages the dentate gyrus region of the hippocampus (22). Elevated GC concentrations increase while adrenalectomy decreases the damaging effects of hypoxia–ischemia, which preferentially damages the CA1 region of the hippocampus.

Do GCs induce a vulnerability in the neurons, or do they make the toxins intrinsically more toxic? To return to the earlier metaphor, are GCs impairing the ability of neurons to withstand being pushed when they are at the edge of the cliff, or are the GCs helping the toxins push harder? For example, might GCs make kainic acid "push harder" by inducing more kainic acid receptors in hippocampal neurons, or increasing the efficacy with which kainic acid diffuses through the hippocampus? That is not the case (22). Similar examination of the other toxins suggests that a broad and general vulnerability is being induced in the neurons themselves, rather than the GCs somewhat enhancing the intrinsic toxicity of the toxins; this makes sense, given the broad range of mechanisms of actions by which these toxins work. It is difficult to imagine specific mechanisms by which the GCs could interact with all these different insults.

Are GCs themselves the agents that act upon the neurons to induce this vulnerability? The hormones obviously have an enormous number of physiological effects, and the hippocampal endangerment could be secondary to GC-induced changes in rates of cerebral bloodflow, in concentrations of any of an array of hormones, of energy substrates, so on. By all logic, it seems reasonable that the GCs should be the agents that directly endanger the hippocampal neurons: why else should the hippocampus, with its high concentrations of corticosterone receptors, be so vulnerable to GCs' actions? More direct evidence also supports this view. Recent work has shown that the GC/toxin synergy also occurs in vitro, with primary cultures of fetal rat hippocampal neurons. In these studies, cultures are exposed to the various toxins, with or without prior exposure to GCs and the efflux of lactate dehydrogenase into the media from lysed cells is used to measure the extent of damage. With these conditions, a synergy has now been shown between GC concentrations in the nanomolar to micromolar range and kainic acid, 3-acetylpyridine, and the oxygen radical generator paraquat (27). The GC/toxin synergy is not seen with cerebellar or hypothalamic cultures, and non-GC steroids do not have the same effects on hippocampal cultures. Finally, use of specific receptor antagonists suggests that the endangerment is mediated through both the type I and II corticosteroid receptors (30).

Thus, the GCs appear to act directly on hippocampal neurons to induce a broad metabolic vulnerability. Subsequent study has shown that whatever the mechanism is, it is a relatively rapid one: the GC/insult synergy can occur both in vivo and in vitro with as little as 48 hr of steroid exposure bracketing the application of the insult. Moreover, the GC effect is persistent: exposure only during the period prior to the insult still compromises neuronal viability (25). Also, it appears as if sheer numbers of corticosteroid receptors are not the sole determinant of which neurons will be vulnerable to the synergy. Certainly, a neuron must be sensitive to GC actions, and thus presumably have a reasonable complement of receptors; however, it must also be vulnerable to the insult with which the GCs are synergizing. Thus, the GC synergy with kainic acid is most pronounced in the CA3 cell field, the area most sensitive to the kainic acid toxicity itself. In similar fashion, the CA1 neurons are most vulnerable to hypoxia–ischemia, as well as to the synergy between hypoxia–ischemia and GCs, while the dentate gyrus is most sensitive to either 3-acetylpyridine or the antimetabolite/GC/synergy. All of those cell regions have plentiful concentrations of corticosteroid receptors.

These observations have some striking clinical implications for the possible role of GCs in exacerbating various neurological insults; these will be considered at the end of this chapter. When it comes to understanding how GCs are endangering hippocampal neurons, the most salient point in these observations is just how broadly endangered the neurons are by the hormones. Insults as different as hyperexcitation, oxygen radical generation, oxygen deprivation, and disruption of energy production all are made worse by GCs. What exactly are GCs doing to these neurons? In the following section, I will review the growing evidence that these various insults all damage hippocampal neurons through a single, convergent cascade. I will then present evidence for how GCs worsen this cascade both through disruption of neuronal energy stores and by nonenergetic means.

POSSIBLE MECHANISMS OF GLUCOCORTICOID ENDANGERMENT

A Common Pathway Underlying Hippocampal Damage?

A tremendous amount of excitement has run through the neurological literature in recent years concerning the roles of excitatory amino acid (EAA) neurotransmitters, and/or calcium in mediating neuron death. Each has gained considerable credibility as a mediator of neuronal damage, and the two together form an interactive cascade that is quite convincing.

The EAAs appear to be used as excitatory signalers in a substantial percentage of CNS synapses; this is particularly so in the hippocampus (31). While the precise endogenous transmitter is somewhat of a matter of controversy, glutamate, aspartate, or the dipeptide N-acetyl-L-aspartyl-1-glutamate appear as the best candidates for endogenous neurotransmitters. The EAAs interact with a class of receptors that include the N-methyl-D-aspartate (NMDA) receptor, and non-NMDA receptors (the kainate and quisqualate receptors). All three are found in high concentrations, although with differing anatomical distributions, within the hippocampus (31).

The NMDA receptor is of particular interest. Normally, it appears to play an important role in phenomena of electrophysiological plasticity, such as long-term potentiation. As evidence, this model of learning can be prevented by administration of NMDA-receptor antagonists (31). In addition to this physiological role, NMDA-receptor activation is now being seen as mediating numerous forms of damage to hippocampal neurons. The EAAs, such as glutamate, NMDA, and kainic acid, have long been recognized as neurotoxic at high concentrations, and their toxicities can all be reversed with NMDA-receptor antagonists (the most convincing mechanism for how this occurs with kainic acid, which bind to the kainate, rather than NMDA receptor, is that the kainate receptors are presynaptic and, when binding kainic acid, release glutamate, which then binds to post-synaptic NMDA receptors (32) (33,34). A broader range of neurological insults is now being shown to involve NMDA receptor activation. As correlative evidence, insults such as hypoxia–ischemia, hypoglycemia, and epileptic seizures all lead to EAA release from neurons. This can be shown with tissue slices of dispersed cultured cells, in which EAA concentrations rise in the media, or in vivo, as measured by dialysis perfusion of the extracellular space (35–41). Moreover, all of these insults lead to a period of neuronal excitation, presumably due to the release of these excitatory neurotransmitters (42–45). As more direct evidence that the EAAs mediate the neurotoxicity of these insults, damage induced by hypoxia–ischemia, incomplete ischemia, anoxia (in cultured neurons), excitotoxic seizures, hypoglycemia, and electron transport uncouplers can all be prevented with NMDA receptor antagonists or by destruction of glutamatergic projections to the hippocampus (46–54). Thus, the view has emerged that a number of different hippocampal insults all lead to exposure of neurons to damaging levels of the powerfully excitatory EAAs, whose proximal effects are mediated by their interaction with the NMDA receptor.

NMDA receptor activation, in turn, is viewed as provoking an excessive and damaging increase in levels of free cytosolic calcium in the postsynaptic neuron. The receptor is coupled to a calcium channel; under physiological resting conditions, the channel is typically blocked with magnesium; with prolonged or strong depolarization, the voltage-dependent magnesium block is released and receptor occupancy leads to calcium influx (55,56). The elevated cytosolic levels of calcium are also viewed as arising from release from intracellular stores. Receptor activation also leads to sodium influx, which releases calcium from sequestering sites such as the endoplasmic reticulum or mitochondria (57). A considerable amount of evidence supports this next step in the cascade. First, EAAs lead to an increase in calcium conductance (58) and a decrease in extracellular calcium concentrations (59–61), with the calcium presumed to move into the intracellular compartment. This is shown more directly with the evidence that EAAs cause intracellular calcium accumulation (61–63), which can be blocked with NMDA receptor antagonists. These studies have typically used either histological techniques for visualizing intracellular calcium or have examined movement of calcium (46). A causative role for calcium in EAA-induced neurotoxicity is supported by the finding that the toxicity of various EAAs is decreased or prevented under culture conditions in which there is no calcium available (64–67). If numerous neurological insults are damaging via NMDA-receptor activation, and such activation produces calcium overload in the postsynaptic neuron, these various insults should produce predictable fluxes in calcium, and their toxicity should be calcium-dependent. This has been observed. For example, ischemia leads to reduction of extracellular calcium concentrations and accompanying inflow and accumulation of calcium into neurons; furthermore, some of the disruptive effects of ischemia on ATP levels can be prevented with calcium channel blockers (60,38–72). Thus, considerable evidence supports the cascade of various insults producing EAA overflow and, subsequently, calcium overload.

Calcium, in turn, has long been among everyone's leading suspects for damaging cells. Numerous proteases, lipases, and endonucleases are dependent on calcium, and most researchers view extremely high cytosolic concentrations of calcium as a guarantee of cellular dysfunction and damage (cf. 73). To give one of many possible examples of theoretical routes by which calcium can damage neurons: the enzyme xanthine dehydrogenase is irreversibly converted to xanthine oxidase in the presence of high calcium concentrations; the latter enzyme is a potent generator of damaging oxygen radicals (74). Most of the adherents to the idea of a cascade involving EAAs, the NMDA receptor, and subsequent calcium overload do not, as yet, speculate much on the precise events subsequent to excessive calcium levels. Nevertheless, the feeling in the field is that there are ample ways in which ionic perturbation can push a neuron over the edge.

NMDA/Calcium Cascade of Damage is Sensitive to Energy Availability

A critical point in understanding where GCs might fit into this cascade of damage is that numerous steps in this cascade are likely to be worsened in neurons that are depleted of energy. The most direct evidence in support of this arises from pathological conditions of energy failure. As noted, both hypoglycemic damage (induced by insulin administration) and damage induced by uncoupling of electron transport (with 3AP) can be prevented with NMDA receptor antagonists. (see above). This implies that the energy failure induces either more EAAs to reach the postsynaptic NMDA receptors and/or an impaired ability to withstand the EAAs. The enhanced EAA signal has been shown in a number of cases. For example, hypoglycemia leads to enhanced EAA outflow in vivo and in vitro, as well as failure of high-affinity EAA reuptake (37, 75). Evidence also suggests that neurons are less capable of withstanding the EAAs when they are deprived of energy. For example, in cerebellar cultures, glutamate, acting via the NMDA receptor, becomes more toxic when glucose concentrations are decreased, or when sublethal concentrations of cyanide are applied to the culture (76).

How might the various steps in the cascade be sensitive to energy failure? A variety of the components of EAA movement are extremely sensitive to energy state. The initial release of glutamate or aspartate in the axon terminal is, of course, contingent upon an action potential allowing an influx of calcium, which triggers the vesicles to release the EAA (77–79). After interaction with the postsynaptic receptor, the EAA is disposed of, in general, through one of two routes. Reuptake can occur directly into the presynaptic terminal. This is accomplished with a bidirectional transporter that cotransports EAAs along with sodium. Conditions normally favor the transporter working in the direction of reuptake: as long as the Na^+-K^+-ATPase is working optimally, intracellular sodium concentrations will be low, and the concentration gradient will favor the inflow of EAAs along with the sodium (77). A second route of removing of the EAAs out of the synapse is via uptake into glia. A potent uptake system exists there (75), and EAAs taken up via that route (specifically glutamate) are then eventually recycled from the glia back to the presynaptic neuron for repackaging in vesicles and ultimate reuse. The relative contributions of direct neuronal reuptake and the loop via the glia are uncertain, but a large percentage of glutamate being used in synapses travels via the glial route (80) (this entire glial component of EAA communication will be considered below in far more detail).

A paucity of energy will disrupt all of the steps outlined.

1. Enhanced release of vesicular EAAs. With energy failure, efficacy of the Na^+-K^+-ATPase will decline and the membrane will depolarize. This should lead to enhanced voltage-gated calcium influx at the presynaptic terminals and increased calcium-dependent release of EAAs. In addition, the increased intracellular concentrations are likely to release calcium from intracellular sites, and thus trigger calcium-dependent EAA release.

2. Failure of neuronal reuptake. This step is also likely to be highly vulnerable to energy depletion, since the reuptake is dependent upon maintaining a very steep extracellular/intracellular sodium gradient. As the gradient is lost with prolonged depolarization and sodium entering in through voltage-gated sodium channels, the drive for pulling EAAs back into the neuron is lost. The consequences of loss of this neuronal reuptake compartment are considerable: the toxicity of EAAs is greatly enhanced when reuptake is blocked (either by poisoning the pump, or destruction of presynaptic neurons) (81–83). Moreover, this seems to be a fairly vulnerable component of the system. For example, in the case of the ischemia-induced accumulation of synpatic EAAs, failure of reuptake appears to be what initially brings about this state (39). With the failure of reuptake comes an additional source of elevated EAAs. As noted, the reuptake pump is bidirectional. Thus, as intracellular sodium concentrations rise with depolarization, the cotransport of sodium and EAAs should be favored to flow outward. Thus, there should be an increase in the calcium-independent release of nonvesicular EAAs from the terminal: this has been found to occur at a precise point of ATP depletion (79,84).

3. Failure of glial uptake of EAAs. The glial component of this system is also sensitive to energy depletion, and uptake appears to fail at that point (75, 85). The glial uptake component is particularly vulnerable to failure for a number of reasons. First, disruption of either glycolysis alone or electron transport alone is sufficient to disrupt glutamate uptake. (85). Second, the uptake of glutamate into glia is dependent not only upon cotransport of sodium with the EAA but also with antiport movement of potassium from out of the glia; in fact, a rise in extracellular potassium concentrations very effectively halts uptake (86). Thus, high levels of excitation or energy failure in neurons (producing increased extracellular potassium concentrations) will impair neighboring glia. The glial route of glutamate uptake is not only vulnerable but is also likely to be quantitatively important (since its Vmax for uptake is even higher than in neurons [87]). Therefore, removal of the glial component of uptake (via energy failure) should have a large and deleterious impact on the system. In support of this view, the toxicity of anoxia upon cultured neurons is decreased when they are cocultured with astrocytes. The speculated mechanisms include the idea that the glial reuptake mechanism serves as a protective sponge for the EAAs (88).

Once the EAAs interact with the postsynaptic NMDA receptor, the calcium component of the story is also likely to have many points of metabolic vulnerablity. As noted, the initial elevation of free cytosolic calcium levels can come from two sources: from extracellular pools (once the voltage-dependent magnesium block of the NMDA-gated calcium channel is removed), and from intracellular sequestering sites such as the ER or mitochondria (with an influx of sodium triggering the calcium release). Once free cytosolic calcium concentrations rise and exert their biological signal, neurons must rapidly remove the calcium from the cytosol, and a variety of mechanisms are available for this. The first is extrusion of the ion out of the cell, and this can be accomplished with a sodium–calcium exchanger, or with a calcium–ATPase pump. The second option is to sequester the calcium into intracellular sites such as the endoplasmic reticuluum or mitochondria; a calcium-ATPase pump can accomplish this in both cases. Third, the cytosolic calcium can be bound by various calcium-binding proteins, such as calmodulin, calcineurin, or calbindin. In this case, it is a matter of some interest whether these proteins exist to transduce a biological signal (as is clearly the case with, e.g., calmodulin), or to act as a calcium "sponge," merely containing the ion. Which particular mechanism predominates in any given neuron is likely to vary, but the routes of containment, collectively, are highly efficient: in the giant squid, it has been estimated that perhaps only 0.1–1% of the cytosolic calcium escapes these various mechanisms and exerts a biological effect (56).

An efficient, yet energetically costly system of control such as this is going to be vulnerable to energy depletion at a number of points:

1. The initial influx of calcium should be enhanced in neurons starved of energy. Because the Na^+-K^+-ATPase pump will be failing, cells will be tending towards depolarization. This will release the calcium channel from its magnesium blockade to a certain extent, allowing a greater influx of the former ion with each activation by NMDA. As evidence, glutamate toxicity in cerebellar cultures increases when Mg^+ is omitted from the medium, even in the presence of large amounts of glucose (76); conversely, NMDA toxicity is inhibited by magnesium (89). In addition, the energy failure and prolonged depolarization will lead to elevated intracellular sodium concentrations, and this will lead to the release of greater amounts of calcium from intracellular sequestering sites. In agreement with this prediction, glutamate becomes more toxic in cultures when ouabain is used to poison the sodium-potassium-ATPase pump, even in the presence of large amounts of glucose and magnesium (76).

2. Once free cytosolic calcium levels have risen, it will be more difficult to contain them. Most obviously, the efficacy of any pumps that are directly dependent upon ATP will decline and that route of removal or sequestering will be limited. In addition, extrusion via the sodium–calcium exchanger should be impaired as the sodium–ATPase fails and intracellular sodium concentrations

rise. In fact, much as with the problem of glutamate reuptake with energy failure, the exchanger should even begin to run backwards, importing even more calcium into the neuron. Furthermore, the sodium should trigger the release of even more calcium from sequestering sites. With prolonged energy deprivation, protein synthesis declines and the levels of the various calcium-binding proteins in the cytosol should gradually decline, leading to even more free cytosolic calcium. This, however, seems a rather minor and indirect route of serious damage to the cell, compared to these other potential routes.

Glucocorticoids Disrupt Glucose Utilization in Hippocampal Neurons

Thus, to the extent that EAA excess, NMDA receptor activation, and elevated intracellular calcium concentrations form a final common cascade of neurological damage to the hippocampus, numerous steps in this pathological chain are going to be worsened by energy depletion. It appears possible that GCs induced just such a state.

Indirect support for this view emerges in a pair of studies from this laboratory. In considering the synergy between GCs and excitotoxins, antimetabolites, and hypoxia–ischemia, it seemed that the theme common to all the latter neurological insults was the induction of an energy crisis. In the case of hypoxia-ischemia and exposure to antimetabolites, the primary insult involves disruption of energy *production*. In the case of excitotoxic seizures with prolonged depolarization, the primary insult involves a pathologically elevated *demand* for energy: with sustained seizures, the glucose utilization soars, substrate delivery falls below the metabolic demand, and tissue stores of glucose and high-energy phosphates decline, and lactate accumulates (90–92). Moreover, increased glucose availability at the time of certain types of seizures decreases the hippocampal damage (93). This seemed a strong theme among the insults, and if GCs induce a broad and general vulnerability in neurons facing these insults, it might involve a depletion of energy. The precedent that motivated this idea was a standard feature of GC action in peripheral tissue: the inhibition of glucose uptake. This is one of the most rapid of GC actions and involves a decrease in the numbers of glucose transport molecules in cell membranes. The precise mechanism is interesting: it involves GC-induced synthesis of a protein that promotes the translocation of the glucose transporter from functional sites on the membrane to inactive intracellular storage sites. The scale of the GC inhibition of glucose utilization in the periphery can be high, in the 40–60% range (94).

Thus, precedent existed for GCs to disrupt energy availability in peripheral tissue, and this was certainly consonant with the general catabolic nature of the hormone. Could GCs also be disrupting energy availability in the hippocampus? In the first study, the in vivo synergy between GCs and the various neurotoxins was studied. I found that when rats are supplemented heavily with additional energy sources, the synergy can be decreased. Extra quantitites of glucose are somewhat protective, while mannose, a saccharide that can be used by the brain and whose transport appears to be mediated by a different system than for glucose, is highly protective. The ketone, beta-hydroxybutyrate, which neurons can utilize, is also protective. In contrast, fructose, which does not penetrate the blood–brain barrier, does not protect the hippocampal neurons. The pattern of protection suggested that supplementation with the extra energy substrates decreases the GC component of the synergy, rather than the neurotoxin component (24). In a subsequent study, we have shown that a similar protection by additional energy substrates can occur with the GC/toxin synergy in vitro (26).

Thus, the endangering of hippocampal neurons by GC seems to involve an energy problem. Considerable clarification of this picture has emerged in the last year. A trio of studies have demonstrated that, essentially, GCs appear to disrupt glucose transport in the hippocampus, much as in peripheral tissue. First, it was shown with 2-deoxyglucose autoradiography of the whole brain that adrenalectomy causes a significant increase in glucose utilization and that this is reversible with dexamethasone. This was observed in a number of brain regions, with one of the strongest effects occurring in the hippocampus (95). This suggestion of GC inhibition of CNS glucose utilization is in agreement with an earlier, somewhat methodologically eccentric report (96). A more recent study replicated this effect and showed that GCs could prevent catecholamine-induced increases in glucose utilization in the brain (97). These studies did not clarify some of the mechanisms of the effect, however. Working with hippocampal cultures in vitro, we have observed a similar GC inhibition of ^{14}C2-deoxyglucose transport. The inhibitory effects of corticosterone are half maximal at 10^{-8} M; dexamethasome also works, at a concentration an order of magnitude lower. Other steroids do not inhibit glucose transport, and the effect appears to be mediated by the type II GC receptor. The effect does not occur in cultures from other brain regions. Finally, the effect is protein synthesis dependent, and appears to occur in both the neuronal and glial compartments (98).

Thus, both in vivo and in vitro, GCs appear to inhibit glucose utilization in the hippocampus. In both systems, the scale of effect is somewhere between 15 and 30% of the glucose transport being inhibited. What does this magnitude of effect mean? It is not yet clear; there are many cell types in which a 30% reduction in glucose availability is not likely to have a major effect. My view is that few cells in the body are more vulnerable to this sort of disruption than a neuron: neurons have enormously high rates of energy demands. In addition, they have very few substrates other than glucose to subsist on. Finally, their capacity to store energy (as glycogen) is limited (1). It will be critical to now determine how much a 30% inhibition of glucose utilization disrupts the energy charge of a hippocampal neuron, but I suspect it will be shown to have a significant impact on these cells.

If GCs are leading to a substantial impairment of energy sources in these hippocampal neurons, a number of predictions should immediately be generated concerning routes of toxicity. First, the strength of an excitatory glutamate signal in hippocampal synapses should be enhanced. This could be due, as outlined above, to increased release of glutamate and/or persistence of the glutamate in the synapse. At present, there are only limited data on this prediction. Some studies have examined the effect of GCs on total tissue glutamate levels (with some showing a decrease in glutamate levels after stress [99,100] and others showing the opposite, namely a decrease in glutamate levels after adrenalectomy [101]). However, it is difficult to evaluate what total tissue levels of glutamate mean when the component that has neurotransmitter function is extremely small. One recent study reported that GCs inhibit a component of [^{3}H] glutamate binding that is thought to represent the presynaptic reuptake sites (102); if this tentative interpretation holds, it suggests that GCs should cause EAAs to persist in the synapse longer. As a second prediction, if GCs exacerbate the whole neurodegenerative cascade outlined above, GC exposure should be associated with enhanced calcium levels in the cytoplasm of hippocampal neurons. As outlined, this could be due to enhanced influx, enhanced release from intracellular stores, and/or impaired capacity to extrude and sequester the ion. We are currently testing all of these predictions. Some data already support them. We observe that glucocorticoids enhance the magnitude and the duration of the moiblization of free cytosolic calcium induced in hippocampal neurons by kainic acid. We have observed this in cultured neurons using calcium-sensitive dyes (102a). This is in agreement with a prior report that glucocorticoids enhance the influx of calcium[45] into hippocampal neurons (103). Furthermore, GC concentrations rise with age in the rat, and aged rats have prolonged calcium-dependent afterhyperpolarizations in hippocampal neurons (104) and prolonged retention of calcium in cortical synaptosomes (105); of critical importance is that this afterhyperpolarization is dependent on GC. Aged rats, when adrenalectomized, lost this calcium-dependent trait while GC administration to young rats prolonged the afterhyperpolarizations (106). Although preliminary, these data support the idea that GCs can influence the cellular pathway that seems the best candidate for mediating hippocampal neurotoxicity. As discussed below, there is an additional, nonenergetic way in which GCs can influence this pathway very powerfully.

Glucocorticoids and the Glutamate/Glutamine Cycle

As discussed above, an important route for removal of glutamate from the synapse (after interacting with the postsynaptic receptor) is via the glia, after which the glutamate is eventually recycled back to the presynaptic neuron. As one would predict, the actual process is more complicated, since the glutamate undergoes a transformation in the glia to glutamine. In the form of glutamine the transfer occurs back to the presynaptic neuron, at which point the glutamine is converted back to glutamate. The critical step in this shuttle is the conversion of glutamate to glutamine in the glia. This is accomplished by the enzyme glutamine synthetase, and return of the glutamine to the presynaptic neuron is contingent upon the generation of the glutamine for export (80). The glutamate/glutamine cycle seems to be a means to get the glutamate out of the synapse the instant it has done its job, to get it to somewhere far away to deactivate it (i.e., in the glia), and to then return it to the presynaptic neuron in a safe, deactivated form. "Rearming" it as glutamate occurs only at the last instant, at the presynaptic terminal. The glutamate/glutamine shuttle can probably best be thought of as a complicated system for dealing with a frightening but necessary biohazard.

Thus, the shuttling of glutamine to glutamatergic neurons should potentially be able to exacerbate EAA-induced damage. This was shown in a recent study in which glutamine augmented anoxic damage to cortical cultures, and this exacerbation was NMDA-receptor-dependent, implying a potentiation of the glutamate signal (107). The shuttle also appears to be of considerable importance: some have estimated that as much as 80% of glutamate used as neurotransmitter cycles through this shuttle (80). The importance of this route is shown in excellent recent studies. In one, the release of glutamate and aspartate from striatal slices was monitored. When glucose concentrations in the media were dropped from 5 mM to 0.2 mM, the efflux of the EAAs increased dramatically. This observation certainly fits with the discussion above, showing the ways in which energy deprivation should lead to EAA release. An important factor was that the neurons were limited in just how long they could maintain this dramatic release of the EAAs, probably because they were becoming depleted of the neurotransmitter. In support of this, when glutamine was supplied to the media, as a precursor for the glutamate regeneration, the low-glucose state led to far more release of EAAs. (75). In a similar vein, when the glutamine synthetase is poisoned (with the compound methionine sulfoximine), neurons are quickly unable to release adequate glutamate; supplementation with glutamine reverses the glutamate failure (108). Thus, to the extent that a state of energy depletion will lead to augmented release of EAAs, the cascade will be fueled even more when the neurons have a steady supply of glutamine as a precursor. Given that glutamine synthetase is the rate-limiting step in the glutamate/glutamine shuttle, the level and activity of the enzyme can be critical determinants in any neurodegenerative cascades built around glutamate neurotoxicity.

With this background one can appreciate the observation that GCs stimulate the synthesis of glutamine synthetase. This is among the most powerful of genomic effects observed to be triggered in the brain by GCs (109–114). Synthesis of the enzyme is induced rapidly in astrocytes and this induction is reflected in increased enzymatic activity. The bulk of these studies have concentrated on the effects of GCs on glutamine synthetase in the developing brain; in vitro studies have typically utilized neonatal or perinatal tissue, while in vivo studies have usually manipulated GC concentrations in neonates. However, we have examined this issue in the adult hippocampus, and we observe that glucorticoids do not induce hippocampal glutamine sythetase activity under physiological circumstances (114a).

The sequence outlined here is, when viewed together, somewhat plausible. It suggests that GCs may exacerbate the glutamate/NMDA/Ca^{2+} cascade of damage. By disrupting energy availability, the GCs can potentially enhance the release of EAAs and cause them to persist in the synapse, via inhibition of presynaptic or glial uptake. Next, they may enhance the influx of calcium into the postsynaptic neuron and impair the ability of the neuron to dispose and sequester the ion. None of these steps need be inevitably damaging, and glutamate release and interaction with the NMDA receptor appear to have important and advantageous consequences for the nervous system (i.e., long-term potentiation). However, these GC effects can bias the system towards more excitation, more calcium influx, and thus increase the probability that the line will be crossed into the area in which this system becomes damaging.

What should be apparent is the extremely speculative nature of this synthesis. The roles of glutamate, the NDMA receptor, and calcium in this cascade are fairly credible. The impact of GCs upon this cascade is tentative, at best. The data are very few, although supportive; however, the magnitude of the effects they reveal is not yet clear. For example, it is not yet known whether the GC inhibition of glucose uptake into hippocampal neurons has a considerable impact on the energy profiles of these neurons under either resting or challenged conditions. Considerable research must be done to examine the plausibility of the model proposed here.

WAYS IN WHICH GLUCOCORTICOIDS DO NOT ENDANGER NEURONS

Before discussing the possible clinical relevance and implications of the ideas outlined above, it is important to mention at least one way in which the steroid is not likely to endanger hippocampal neurons. An attractive and clear mechanism by which GCs damage another class of cells has been uncovered in recent years, and it is important to show that this mechanism does not seem to apply to neurons.

As emphasized in this volume, one of the hallmarks of GC action is their suppressive effects upon the immune system. These include such global effects as thymic involution and narrow actions as inhibition of production and/or cellular responsiveness to various lymphokines. Among the most interesting immunosuppressive actions of GCs are actual killing of lymphocytes in some species (115). Such lymphocytolysis has attracted attention in recent years, no doubt in part for the sheer drama of actual destruction of cells but also because knowledge is emerging concerning the precise mechanisms underlying this case of programmed cell death. Glucocorticoids appear to interact with the receptor and induce synthesis of a protein(s) that leads to enhanced endonuclease activity in the lymphocyte. The precise mechanism of that enhancement is not understood now. Some view the protein induced as being itself an endonuclease, while others hypothesize that the induced protein somehow promotes a calcium influx into the nucleus that activates preexisting calcium-dependent endonucleases. In either scenario, the result is inappropriate endonuclease activity, leading to DNA cleavage and, inevitably, cell death. A few different types of evidence support this dramatic cascade. The cleavage of the DNA appears to occur at internucleosomal sites, leading to regularly spaced cleavage products. Thus, DNA on GC-treated lymphocytes, when run on an agarose gel, shows a characteristic "ladder" pattern of bands that are multiples of 180 base pairs, in contrast to the single band from DNA-intact, control cells. In support of the view of the DNA degradation as a cause rather than consequence of the cell lysis, the ladder pattern is noted prior to cell death (as determined by exclusion of viability stains). As a second piece of evidence, it appears as if a lymphocyte attempts to repair its DNA as it is being fatally cleaved by activating poly(ADP-ribosyl)ation. Thus, poisoning of this repair process (with the poly(ADP-ribose)synthetase inhibitor benzamide) should exacerbate GC-induced lymphocytolysis, which has been observed (116,117).

This represents an exciting, well-understood mechanism of "apoptosis": programmed and stereotypical cell death. This immediately suggested that a similar GC-induced attack on DNA integrity might be occurring on hippocampal neurons. This would certainly consitute a broad and general form of insult, which should compromise neuronal viability in the face of a very wide range of challenges. We have recently tested this idea, however, and found no evidence for it. The DNA from cultured hippocampal neurons does not form the ladder pattern when exposed to either damaging concentrations of GCs alone or concentrations of GCs that would synergize with kainic acid. Furthermore, we do not observe that benzamide augments the toxicity of GC in these hippocampal cultures (117a).

Thus, the first approach to this question suggests that GCs endanger hippocampal neurons with a mechanism that differs from the apoptosis of lymphocytes. In hindsight this seems reasonable, since the whole neuronal phenomenon seems less stereotyped and all-or-none than the immunosuppressive phenomenon.

IMPLICATIONS AND INTERVENTIONS

The body of data outlined above strikes me as more than slightly terrifying. It suggests that the endangerment of neurons and perhaps even the destruction of neurons, may come to be viewed as stress-related pathological conditions. For the gerontologist, these data indicate that the extent of cumulative exposure to GCs over the lifespan can act as a major determinant of the rate of hippocampal neuronal degeneration. Landfield and colleagues (16) showed that even basal concentrations of GCs can damage the system; all that stress can do is exacerbate the situation. For the neurologist, these data have two important implications. First, in the aftermath of a neurological crisis such as hypoxia–ischemia or epileptic seizure, exogenous GCs will worsen the extent of hippocampal damage. Second, following such insults, if you *decrease* GC concentrations (e.g., by adrenalecomy), you decrease hippocampal damage. Following neurological crises such as these, very substantial GC stress responses are triggered and the endogenous hypersecretion is apparently enough to add to the neuronal endangerment. Thus, what is viewed as the "normal" amount of hippocampal damage following cardiac arrest or seizure may, in fact, be the normal damage being made worse by the concurrent GC stress-response.

Can anything be done about this? For the neurologist, the potential interventions are easier than those for the gerontologist. The most obvious advice possible for the neurologist is that in the aftermath of insults such as global ischemia or seizure, exogenous GCs be administered only with the greatest of caution. While this seems logical and simple from the perspective of GCs and their putative effects upon hippocampal neuronal metabolism, it runs counter to much of neurological wisdom. GCs are, in fact, frequently given in the aftermath of these insults to control cerebral edema. The steroids appear to be effective at controlling the edema that frequently accompanies brain tumor. However, the data regarding the efficacy in controlling postischemic edema is conflicting and, if anything, balances on the side of no salutary effect (cf. 26). In addition, alternative, non-GC agents are available to control edema, such as mannitol. Thus, we have urged strongly that the use of GCs in such circumstances be eliminated (26).

Can anything be done to minimize the endangering effects of the endogenous GCs secreted in the stressful aftermath of cardiac arrest or seizure? The intervention already discussed is obviously not applicable in a clinical setting: patients cannot be adrenalectomized. A number of options are available, however.

1. Block the secretion of the endogenous GCs. While it is not possible to adrenalectomize individuals after, for example, a seizure, reversible chemical adrenalectomies can be accomplished pharmacologically, with inhibitors of steroidogenesis. Metyrapone is such a compound and has been in long clinical use for treatment of adrenocortical abnormalities. The drug will, for example, completely block a major adrenocortical stress response in rats. We have recently observed that if metyrapone is administered to rats who have had intrahippocampal microinfusion of kainic acid, there are substantial reductions in the volume of hippocampal damage. In these studies, we gave ourselves the clinical

constraint of not knowing in advance that the seizure was going to occur: metyrapone was administered only at the onset of electroencephalographic indices of seizure (118). We are currently examining whether metyrapone can protect the hippocampus from some of the other clinically relevant insults discussed.

2. If it is too late to block GC secretion, block GC access to its hippocampal corticosteroid receptors. Highly specific antagonists for both the type I and II corticosteroid receptor have been developed, and have been administered to humans for research purposes (119). Although these have not yet been tested in the context of reducing hippocampal damage in the aftermath of various neurological insults, it seems logical, a priori, that they should be helpful. In fact, they should be somewhat more helpful than trying to inhibit adrenal steroidogenesis, since the strategy gives more time for intervention. While it may be too late for metyrapone to block synthesis and release of GCs, there still may be the opportunity to block the receptors with the antagonists before the GCs reach there.

3. If it is too late to block GC access to hippocampal receptors, counteract the metabolic disruption of GCs. This has already been shown in the experiments discussed, in which the endangering effects of GCs (in synergizing with kainic acid or 3-acetylpyridine) were decreased by administering large quantities of glucose, mannose, or ketones to rats (25). This is akin to the numerous studies in which various insults that activate the glutamatergic cascade are made less toxic when there is plentiful energy available for the neuron. Thus, supplementary energy substrates might protect neurons from some of the disruptive effects of GCs (although probably not all, given the nonenergetic nature of the GC effect upon glutamine synthetase). A complication in this idea arises with trying to use glucose (or other substrates) to decrease the GC synergy with hypoxia-ischemia. This insult has the paradoxical trait of being made worse by glucose pretreatment. For example, hippocampal damage tends to be worse in ischemic crises following meals, or when there is still a trickle of bloodflow sufficient to deliver glucose to neurons. This is thought to be due to the anaerobic metabolism that occurs during the hypoxia-ischemia. With substantial glucose preloading, large amounts of the substrate are available to neurons at the onset of the ischemic anaerobic metabolism (stored as glycogen). This allows for increased lactic acid production, with the resulting acidosis being damaging (thus, in this instance, the neuron would fare better being a bit more deprived of ATP, than obtaining ATP at the cost of acidosis) (120,121). However, manipulating glucose concentrations after hypoxia-ischemia, during reperfusion, does not worsen the damage. Therefore, during the time-span being discussed here (interventions in the aftermath of these insults), using glucose to attenuate the GC component of damage will not be at the cost of exacerbating the acidotic component.

4.   If it is too late to prevent the energetic disruption of GCs, counteract the consequences of energetic disruption. This is, at present, the most speculative of these suggestions. The preceding pages have outlined ample ways in which things can go wrong in a neuron is being challenged while it is short of energy. The question becomes, of course, which dysfunctions are the most damaging ones? What goes most wrong most quickly? This is not yet clear, nor what can be done with the knowledge that, say, the excessive free cytosolic levels of Ca^{2+} induced by GCs are mostly due to failure of the mitochondrial sequestering component. Considerably more research is needed before this option produces any perscriptions for realistic interventions.

It is even more difficult to design interventions for the gerontologist. In the model that I find most plausible for understanding how GCs might cumulatively damage the aging hippocampus, the steroids are not directly toxic. Instead, they sensitize the neurons to various challenges that might be quite subtle: transient periods of hypoglycemia, hyperexcitation, and so on. None has a high likelihood of being damaging, but collectively, with the neurons closer to the edge, more damage gradually occurs: the system is chipped away at. If it is not feasible to adrenalectomize a patient following an overt single seizure, it is even less feasible to do so with these more subtle insults. Moreover, with this scenario, it does not seem feasible to attempt to administer metyrapone, receptor antagonists, and so on, to counteract GC secretion coinciding with subtle microinsults that may not even be readily apparent.

A more plausible route of intervention, for the gerontologist, is to find ways to damp the overall activity of the adrenocortical axis throughout the lifespan. As discussed (21), we have shown one way in which to accomplish that: by taking advantage of neonatal handling of rats and its decrease in basal GC concentrations for the rest of the lifespan. By this manipulation, the hippocampus is exposed to less cumulative GCs over the lifespan and the neurodegenerative impact of aging of this system is lessened. I suspect that other environmental or psychological manipulations are available to alter the intensity of stressors, the perception of them, so on. As a physiologist, it seems most striking that these are interventions in the realm of the psychologist. When it comes to the gradual impact of GCs upon age-related neurodegeneration, I suspect that acute and dramatic interventions in the aftermath of insults will not be as helpful as interventions of a more preventive nature.

CAN GLUCOCORTICOIDS DAMAGE THE PRIMATE HIPPOCAMPUS?

Does any of this story apply to the primate hippocampus? Many of the experiments carried out on rodents are not ethically acceptable in primates or humans. Studies involving assessing whether certain environmental or experiential manipulations have an impact upon aging could take years to carry out. It is often difficult to obtain postmortem tissue, and analysis of the tissue is often confounded by variation in time after death or coincident diseases. Nevertheless, bits of information available on this question tend to support an endangering action of GCs in the primate.

First, the catabolic array of GC actions through the body is fairly similar among all mammals. Moreover, the primate hippocampus appears to be a principal neural target site for GCs, at least as evidenced by its being as relatively rich in corticosteroid receptors as the rat hippocampus (cf. 3). But can stress and/or GCs damage the primate hippocampus?

A number of studies of humans suggest that stress can be neurodegenerative, although the evidence is indirect. In a study of a human population that has gone through, arguably, the most severe of stressors conceivable—concentration camp survivors—rates of dementia are elevated (122). Moreover, political prisoners who had undergone torture were found to have cerebral atrophy, and ventricular enlargement, although these conditions do not appear to be permanent (123). Long-term psychotic depressives, who are among the most likely of affective disorder patients to hypersecrete GCs, show cerebral atrophy at postmortem (124). These data, however, are very circumstantial in suggesting that stress might damage the hippocampus or impair hippocampal-dependent aspects of cognition. We have recently found more direct evidence for this link in the primate.

We examined a population of vervet monkeys who, after becoming agricultural pests in the wild in Kenya, had been caught and housed in a primate center in Nairobi. Vervets develop dominance hierarchies when in social groups. When this occurs in the confines of a cage, socially subordinate animals have the disadvantages of being limited in how far they can move away from dominant individuals. Thus, under captive conditions, various forms of social aggression and harassment appear to be more severe than in the wild. In accordance with this, a subpopulation of vervets at the primate center developed fatal gastric ulcers. They appeared to be socially subordinate (with atypically high incidences of canine-tooth punctures and bite wounds) and under sustained stress (with hyperplastic adrenal cortices). When examined neuropathologically, we found that these ulcerated animals had hippocampal damage. This was apparent both on a qualitative level (with dispersed Nissel bodies, atrophic dendritic branches, shrunken perikarya, decreased vesicle number, depletion of mossy fiber terminals, and glial infiltration) and on a quantitative level, with neuron loss most pronounced in the CA3 region. The damage in ulcerated animals could not have been due to different postmortem times from the healthy control animals (who had been euthanized for other research purposes), nor was there any damage in nonhippocampal regions (125). This observation suggests that the stress of sustained social subordinance in this captive setting could have been neurodegenerative. My opinion is that such stress must be very extreme to produce this sort of damage. We have recently examined the brains of dominant and subordinate monkeys from stable captive social groups housed in large outdoor corrals, in which there was no evidence of sustained harassment of social subordinates, nor of peptic ulceration. Among these animals, we found no indications of neurological damage (Uno, Kaplan, and Sapolsky, unpublished findings).

Could GCs be the damaging agents in these cases? The simplest way of determining this might be to examine whether there is neurodegeneration and/or dementia among cushingoid individuals, with their pathological hypersecretion of GCs. However, it has been a long time since cushingoid patients were not treated in some manner to attenuate their GC secretion. If one goes back to 40-year-old literature, however, there are small, tantalizing hints of "limbic atrophy" of such brains at postmortem (126). We are currently examining whether there is neurodegeneration in the brains of individuals exposed long-term to exogenous GCs to treat autoimmune disorders, asthma, brain tumors, and so on. Somewhat more direct evidence has arisen from a recent study of fetal rhesus monkeys. These animals were exposed to high concentrations of dexamethasone during fetal days 132-135. When examined as late as 3 months after birth, there was substantial depletion of neurons in the hippocampus, but not in other brain regions. The age at which the animals were exposed to the steroids was past the point of most hippocampal neurogenesis, suggesting that the depletion of neurons is due to destruction of preexisting cells rather than prevention of the formation of new ones (126). We have tested this idea more directly. We recently implanted either cortisol- or cholesterol-secreting pellets into the hippocampi of vervet monkeys and allowed them to remain for a year. This is a relatively short time for a primate; the equivalent for a rat would be roughly 4–6 weeks, a time in which GC overexposure has not yet been shown to cause hippocampal damage. Under these conditions, cortisol-treated hippocampi sustain preferential damage (128).

In conclusion, many decades after the work of Cannon and Selye, we have come to view a variety of pathological conditions as being exacerbated by stress and sensitive to the perturbations of our environment and how we view them. This chapter gives us reason to think that neurological damage might also be among the pathological conditions sensitive to stress. The importance of the hippocampus for various aspects of cognition, and the emerging evidence that GCs might be neurodegenerative to the primate hippocampus, lend urgency to our acquiring an understanding of the cellular mechanisms by which GCs endanger these neurons.

REFERENCES

1. Siesjo B. Cell damage in the brain: a speculative synthesis. J Cereb Blood Flow Metab 1981; 1: 155.

2. Pulsinelli W. Selective neuronal vulnerability: morphological and molecular characteristics. Prog Brain Res 1985; 63:29.
3. McEwen B, de Kloet E, Rostene W. Adrenal steroid receptors and actions in the nervous system. Physiol Rev 1986; 66:1121.
4. Angelucci L, Valeri P, Grossi E. Involvement of hippocampal corticosterone receptors in behavioral phenomena. In Brambilla G, Racagni G, de Wied D, eds. Progress in psychoneuroendocrinology. Amsterdam:Elsevier, 1980: 186.
5. Britton G, Rotenberg S, Freeman C. Regulation of corticosterone levels and liver enzyme activity in aging rats. Adv Exp Med Biol 1975; 61:209.
6. deKosky S, Scheff S, Cotman C. Elevated corticosterone levels: a mechanism for impaired sprouting in the aged hippocampus. Neuroendocrinology 1984; 38:33.
7. Hess G, Riegle G. Adrenocortical responsiveness to stress and ACTH in aging rats. J Gerontol 1970; 25:354.
8. Landfield P, Waymire J, Lynch G. Hippocampal aging and adrenocorticoids: a quantitative correlation. Science 1978; 202:1098.
9. Rapaport P, Allaire Y, Bourliere F. Reactivite au "stress" et capacité d'adpatation a une situation inhabituelle chez le rat jeune, adulte et agé. 1964; Gerontology 10:20.
10. Sapolsky R, Krey L, McEwen B. The adrenocortical stress-response in the aged male rat: impairment of recovery from stress. Exp Gerontol 1983; 18:55.
11. Sencar-Cupovic I, Milkovic S. The development of sex differences in adrenal morphology and responsiveness in stress of rats from birth to end of life. Mech Ageing Dev 1976; 5:1.
12. Tang G, Phillips R. Some age-related changes in pituitary-adrenal function in the male laboratory rat. J Gerontol 1978; 33:377.
13. Hess G, Riegle G. Effects of chronic ACTh stimulation on adrenocortical function in young and aged rats. Am J Physiol 1972; 222:1458.
14. Riegle G. Chronic stress effects on adrenocortical responsiveness in young and aged rats. Neuroendocrinology 1973; 11:1.
15. Coleman P, Flood D. Neuron numbers and dendritic extent in normal aging and Alzheimer's disease. Neurobiol Aging 1987; 8:521.
16. Landfield P, Baskin R, Pitler T. Brain–aging correlates: retardation by hormonal–pharmacological treatments. Science 1981; 214:581.
17. Aus der Muhlen K, Ockenfels H. Morphologische Verander ungen in Diencaphlon und Telencephalon nach Storngen des regelkreises Adenohhypophyse-Nebennierenrinde: III. ERgebnisee beim Meerschweinchen nach Verabrerichung von Cortison und Hydrocortison. Z Zellforsch 1979; 93: 126.
18. Sapolsky R, Krey L, McEwen B. Prolonged glucocorticoid exposure reduces hippocampal neuron number: Implications for aging. J Neurosci 1985; 5: 1221.
19. Sapolsky R, Krey L, McEwen T. Do vasopressin-related peptides induce

hippocampal corticosterone receptors? Implications for aging. J Neurosci 1984; 4:1479.

19a. Meaney M, Aitken D, Sapolsky, R. Postnatal handling attenuates neuro-endocrine, anatomical and cognitive dysfunctions associated with aging in female rats. Neurobiol Aging in press.

20. Kerr D, Applegate M, Campbell L, Goliszek A, Brodish A, Landfield P. Chronic stress-induced accelerationg of age-related hippocampal neuro-physiological changes. Soc Neurosci Abstr 1986; 12:274.

21. Meaney M, Aitken D, Bhatnager S, van Berkel C, Sapolsky R. Effect of neonatal handling on age-related impairments associated with the hippo-campus. Sciences 1988; 239:766.

22. Sapolsky R. A mechanism for glucocorticoid toxicity in the hippocampus: increased neuronal vulnerability to metabolic insults. J Neurosci 1985; 5: 1227.

23. Sapolsky R. Glucocorticoid toxicity in the hippocampus: temporal aspects of neuronal vulnerability. Brain Res 1985; 359:300.

24. Sapolsky R. Glucocorticoid toxicity in the hippocampus: synergy with kainic acid. Neuroendocrinology 1986; 43:386.

25. Sapolsky R. Glucocorticoid toxicity in the hippocampus: reversal by sup-plementation with brain fuels. J Neurosci 1986; 6:2240.

26. Sapolsky R, Pulsinelli W. Glucocorticoids potentiate ischemic injury to neurons: therapeutic implications. Science 1985; 229:1397.

27. Sapolsky R, Packan D, Vale W. Glucocorticoid toxicity in the hippocam-pus: in vitro demonstration. Brain Res 1988; 453:367.

28. Koide T, Wieloch T, Siesjo B. Chronic dexamethasone pretreatment aggra-vates ischemic neuronal necrosis. J Cereb Blood Flow Metab 1986; 6:395.

29. Theoret Y, Caldewell-Kenkel J, Krigman M. The role of neuronal metabolic insult in organometal neurotoxicity (abstr). Toxicologist 1985; 6:491.

29a. Morse J, Davis J. Chemical adrenalectomy protects hippocampal cells following ischemia. Soc Neurosci (Abstr) 1989; 15:149.4.

30. Packan D, Sapolsky R. Glucocorticoid endangerment in the hippocampus: tissue, sterod and receptor specificity. Neuroendocrinology 1990: in press.

31. Cotman C, Monaghan D, Otterson O, Storm-Mathisen J. Anatomical organi-zation of excitatory amino acid receptors and their pathways. Trends Neurosci 1987; 10(7):273.

32. Collingridge G, Bliss T. NMDA receptors—their role in long-term potentia-tion. Trends Neurosci 1987; 10:288.

33. Kohler C, Schwarcz R, Fuxe K. Perforant path transections protect hippo-campal granule cells from kainate lesion. Neurosci Lett 1978; 10:241.

34. Rothman S, Olney J. Excitotoxicity and the NMDA receptor. Trends Neurosci 1987; 10:299.

35. Benveniste H, Drejer J, Schousboe A, Diemer N. Elevation of extracellular concentrations of glutamate and aspartate in the rat hippocampus during transient cerebral ischemia monitored by intracerebral microdialysis. J Neurochem 1984; 43:1369.

36. Dodd P, Bradford H. Release of amino acids from the maturing cobalt-induced epileptic focus. Brain Res 1976; 111:377.
37. Dodd P, Bradford H, Abdul-Ghani A, Cox D, Continho-Netto J. Release of amino acids from chronic epileptic and subepileptic foci in vivo. Brain Res 1980; 193:505.
38. Sandberg M, Butcher S, Hagberg H. Extracellular overflow of neuroactive amino acids during severe insulin-induced hypoglycemia: in vivo dialysis of the rat hippocampus. J Neurochem 1986; 47:178.
39. Bosley T, Woodhams P, Gordon R, Balazs R. Effects of anoxia on the stimulated release of amino acid neurotransmitters in the cerebellum in vitro. J Neurochem 1983; 40:189.
40. Drejer J, Benveniste H, Diemer N, Schousboe A. Cellular origin of ischemia-induced glutamate release from brain tissue in vivo and in vitro. J Neurochem 1985; 34:145.
41. Hagberg H, Lehman A, Sandberg M, Nystrom B, Jacobson I, Hamberger A. Ischemia-induced shift of inhibitory and excitatory amino acids from intra- to extracellular compartments. J Cereb Blood Flow Metab 1985; 5:413.
42. Suzuki R, Yamaguchi T, Choh-Luh L, Klatzo I. The effects of 5-minute ischemia in Mongolian gerbils. II. Changes of spontaneous neuronal activity in cerebral cortex and CA1 sector of hippocampus. Acta Neuropathol (Ber) 1983; 60:217.
43. Schiff S, Somjen G Hyperexcitability following moderate hypoxia in hippocampal tissue slices. Brain Res 1985; 337:377.
44. Madison D, Niedermeyer E. Epileptic seizures resulting from acute cerebral anoxia. J Neurol Neurosurg Psychiatry 1970; 33:381.
45. Watanabe K, Hara K, Miyazaki S, Hakamada S. The role of perinatal brain injury in the genesis of childhood epilepsy. Folia Psychiatr Neurol Jpn 1980; 34:227.
46. Simon R, Swan J, Griffiths T, Meldrum B. Blockade of N-methyl-d-aspartate receptors may protect against ischemic damage in brain. Science 1984; 226:850.
47. Lodge D, O'Shaughnessy C, Zeman S. Reduction of ischemia-induced brain damage and of glutamate-induced calcium uptake by subanesthetic concentrations of ketamine. Neurosci Lett Suppl., 1986; 24:535.
48. Wieloch T. Hypoglycemia-induced neuronal damage prevented by an N-methyl-D-aspartate antagonist. Science 1985; 230:681.
49. Wieloch T, Engelsen G, Westerberg E, Auer R. Lesions of the glutamatergic cortico-striatal projections in the rat ameliorate hypoglycemic brain damage in the striatum. Neurosci Lett 1985; 58:25.
50. Rothman S. Synaptic release of excitatory amino acid neurotransmitter mediates anoxic neuronal death. J Neurosci 1984; 4:1884.
51. Rothman S, Thurston J, Hauhart R. Delayed neurotoxicity of excitatory amino acids in vitro. Neuroscience 1987; 22:471.
52. Choi D, Koh J, Peters S. Pharmacology of glutamate neurotoxicity in cortical cell culture: attenuation by NMDA antagonists. J Neurosci 1988; 8:185.

53. Swan J, Evans M, Meldrum B. Long-term development of selective neuronal loss and the mechanism of protection by 2-amino-7-phosphonoheptanoate in a rat model of incomplete forebrain ischaemia. J Cereb Blood Flow Metab 1988; 8:64.

54. Armanini M, Hutchins, C, Stein, B, Sapolsky R. Glucocorticoid endangerment of hippocampal neurons is NMDA-receptor dependent. Brain Research 1990; in press.

55. Nowak L, Bregestowski P, Ascher P. Magnesium gates glutamate-activated channels in mouse central neurons. Nature 1984; 307:462.

56. MacDermott A, Dale N. Receptors, ion channels and synaptic potentials underlying the integrative actions of excitatory amino acids. Trends Neurosci 1987; 10:280.

57. McBurney R, Neering I. Neuronal calcium homeostasis. Trends Neurosci 1987; 10:164.

58. Ozawa S, Makamura T, Yuzaki M. Cation permeability change caused by L-glutamate in cultured rat hippocampal neurons. Brain Res 1988; 443:85.

59. Hamon B, Heinemann U. Effects of GABA and bicuculline on NMDA and quisqualate-induced reductions in extracellular free calcium in area CA1 of the hippocampal slice. Exp Brain 1986; 64:27.

60. Ashton D, Reid K, Willems R, Wauquier A. NMDA and hypoxia induced calcium-changes in the CA1 region of the hippocampal slice. Brain Res 1986; 385:185.

61. Lazarewicz J, Lehmann A, Hagberg H, Hamberger A. Effects of kainic acid on brain calcium fluxes studied in vivo and in vitro. J Neurochem 1986; 46:494.

62. Crowder J, Croucher M, Bradford H, Collins F. Excitatory amino acid receptors and depolarization-induced calcium influx into hippocampal slices. J Neurochem 1987; 48:1917.

63. Carpenter C, Marks S, Watson D, Greenberg D. Dextromethorphan and dextrorphan as calcium channel antagonists. Brain Res 1988; 439:372.

64. Choi D. Glutamate neurotoxicity in cortical cell culture is calcium dependent. Neurosci Lett 1985; 58:293.

65. Goldberg W, Kadingo R, Barrett J. Effects of ischemia-like conditions on cultured neurons: Protection by low sodium, low calcium solutions. J Neurosci 1986; 6:3144.

66. Hori N, French-Mullen J, Carpenter D. Kainic acid responses and toxicity show pronounced calcium dependence. Brain Res 1985; 358:380.

67. Garthwaite G, Garthwaite J. Neurotoxicity of excitatory amino acid receptor agonists in rat cerebellar slices: dependence on calcium concentration. Neurosci Letts 1986; 66:193.

68. Deshpande J, Siesjo B, Wieloch T. Calcium accumulation and neuronal damage in the rat hippocampus following cerebral ischemia. J Cereb Blood Flow Metab 1987; 7:89.

69. Simon R, Griffith T, Evans M, Swan J, Meldrum B. Calcium overload in selectively vulnerable neurons of the hippocampus during and after ischemia: an electron microscopic study in the rat. J Cereb Blood Flow Metab 1984; 4:350.

70. Yanagihara T, McCall J. Ionic shifts in cerebral ischemia. Life Sci 1982; 30, 1921.
71. Dienel G. Regional accumulation of calcium in post-ischemic rat brain. J Neurochem 1984; 43:913.
72. Mabe H, Nagai H, Takagi T Effect of nimodipine on cerebral functional and metabolic recovery following ischemia in the rat brain. Stroke 1986; 17:501.
73. Cheung J, Bonventre J, Malis C, Leaf A. Calcium and ischemic injury. N Engl J Med 1986; 26:1670.
74. McCord J. Oxygen-derived free radicals in post-ischemic tissue injury. N Engl J Med 1985; 312:159.
75. Szerb J. Changes in the relative amounts of aspartate and glutamate released and retained in hippocampal slices during stimulation. J Neurochem 1988; 50:219.
76. Novelli A, Reilly J, Lysko P, Henneberry R. Glutamate becomes neurotoxic via the NMDA receptor when intracellular energy levels are reduced. Brain Res 1988; 451:205.
77. Szerb J, O'Regan P. Increase in the stimulation-induced overflow of excitatory amino acids from hippocampal slices: interaction between low glucose concentration and fluoroacetate. Neurosci Letts 1988; 86:207.
78. Nicholls D, Sihra T. Synaptosomes possess an exocytotic pool of glutamate. Nature 1986; 321:772.
79. Sanchez-Prieto J, Gonzalez P. Occurrence of a large calcium-independent release of glutamate during anoxia in isolated nerve terminals (synaptosomes). J Neurochem 1988; 50:1322.
80. Hertz L, Kvamme E, McGreer E, Schousboe E. Glutamine, glutamate and GABA in the central nervous system. New York: Alan R. Liss, 1983.
81. Kohler C, Schwarcz R. Monosodium glutamate: increased neurotoxicity after removal of neuronal re-uptake sites. Brain Res 1981; 211:485.
82. McBeen G, Roberts P. Neurotoxicity of L-glutamate and DL-threo-3-hydroxyaspartate in the rat striatum. J Neurochem 1985, 44:247.
83. Choi D. Glutamate neurotoxicity in cortical cell culture. J Neurosci 1987; 7:357.
84. Dagani F, Erecinsak M. Relationship among ATP synthesis, potassium gradients, and neurotransmitter amino acid levels in isolated rat brain synaptosomes. J Neurochem 1987; 49:1229.
85. Kauppienen R, Enkvist K, Holopainen I, Akerman K. Glucose deprivation depolarizes plasma membrane of cultured astrocytes and collapses transmembrane potasskium and glutamate gradiants. Neuroscience 1988; 26:283.
86. Barbour B, Brew H, Attwell D. Electrogenic glutamate uptake in glial cells is activated by intracellular potassium. Nature 1988; 335:433.
87. Schousboe A, Larsson O, Drejer J, Krogsgaard-Larsen P, Hertz L. Uptake and release processes for glutamine, glutamate, and GABA incultured neurons and astocytes. In Hertz L, Kvamme E, McGreer E, Schousboe A, eds. Glutamine, glutamate and GABA in the central nervous system. New York: Alan R. Liss, 1983: 297.

88. Vibulsreth S, Hefti F, Ginsberg M, Dietrich W, Busto R. Astrocytes protect cultured neurons from degeneration induced by anoxia. Brain Res 1987;422:303.

89. Garthwaite G, Garthwaite J. Receptor-linked ionic channels mediate NMDA neurotoxicity in rat cerebeller slices. Neurosci Lett 1987; 83:241.

90. Evans M, Meldrum B. Regional brain glucose metabolism in chemically-induced seizures in the rat. Brain Res 1984; 297:235.

91. Blennow G, Nilsson B, Siesjo B. Influence of reduced oxygen availability on cerebral metabolic changes during bicucullin-induced seizures in rats. J Cereb Blood Flow Metab 1985; 5:439.

92. Kreisman N, Rosenthal M, Lamanna J, Sick T. Cerebral oxygenation during recurrent seizures. Adv Neurol 1982; 34:231.

93. Sapolsky R, Stein B. Status epilepticus-induced hippocampal damage is modulated by glucose availability. Neurosi Lett 1989; 97:157.

94. Horner H, Munck A, Lienhard G. Dexamethasone causes translocation of glucose transporters from the plasma membrane to an intracellular site in human fibroblasts. J Biol Chem 1987; 262:17696.

95. Kadekaro M, Ito M, Gross P. Local cerebral glucose utilization is increased in acutely adrenalectomized rats. Neuroendocrinology 1988; 47:329.

96. Landgraf R, Mitro A, Hess J. Regional net uptake of 14C-glucose by rat brain under the influence of corticosterone. Endocrinol Exp (Bratisl) 1978; 12:119.

97. Bryan R, King J. Glucocorticoids modulate the effect of plasma epinephrine on regional cerebral glucose utilization (rCMRgl). Soc Neurosci Abst. 1988; 399.11.

98. Horner H, Packan, D, Sapolsky, R. Glucocorticoids inhibit glucose transport in hippocampal neurons and glia. Neuroendocrinolgy 1990, in press.

99. Rao V, Subba V, Gupta M. Effect of heat and cold stress on brain glutamic acid. Fed Proc 1966; 25:1185.

100. Rindi G, Ventura V. Influence of adrenalectomy, adrenal cortex hormones, and of cold on the GABA and glutamic acid content of the rat brain. Ital J Biochem 1961; 10:135.

101. Sutherland V, Rikimaru M. The regional effects of adrenalectomy and ethanol on cerebral amino acids in the rat. Int J Neuropharmacol 1964; 3:135.

102. Halpain S, McEwen B. Corticosterone decreases 3H-glutamate binding in rat hippocampal formation. Neuroendocrinology 1988; 48:235.

102a. Elliott E, Sapolsky R. Soc Neurosci Abst 1990; in press.

103. Sze P. Effects of corticosterone on calcium uptake by rat brain synaptosomes. Neurochem Abst 1985; 264.

104. Landfield P, Pitler T. Prolonged calcium-dependent afterhyperpolarizations in hippocampal neurons of aged rats. Science 1984; 226:1089.

105. Giovannelli L, Pepeu G. Cytosolic calcium concentrations in cortical synaptosomes of aging rats. Soc Neurosci Abst 1988; 509.4.

106. Kerr D, Landfield P. A corticosteroid-sensitive component of the hippocampal calcium-dependent afterhyperpolarization increases with aging. Soc Neurosci Abst 1988; 509.17.

107. Monyer H, Goldberg M, Choi D. Glucose-deprivation cortical neuronal injury is strongly influenced by the availability of extracellular amino acids. Soc Neurosci Abst 1988; 299.2.

108. Rothstein J, Tabakoff B. Alteration of striatal glutamate release after glutamine synthetase inhibition. J Neurochem 1984; 43:1438.

109. Holbrook N, Grasso R, Hackney J. Glucocorticoid receptor properties and glucocorticoid regulation of glutamine synthetase activity in sensitive C6 and resistant C6H glial cells. J Neurosci Res 1981; 6:75.

110. Juurlink B, Schousboe A, Jorgensen O, Hertz L. Induction by hydrocortisone of glutamine synthetase in mouse primary astrocyte cultures. J Neurochem 1987; 36:136.

111. Kumar S, Weingarten D, Callagan J, Schar K, De Vellis J. Regulation of mRNAs for three enzymes in the glial cell model C6 cell line. J Neurochem 1984; 43:1455.

112. Martinez-Hernandez A, Bell K, Norenberg M. Glutamine synthetase glial localization in brain. Science 1977; 195:1356.

113. Patel A, Hunt A. Observations on cell growth and regulation of glutamine synthetase by dexamethasone in primary cultures of forebrain and cerebellar astrocytes. Dev Brain Res 1985; 18:175.

114. Pishak M, Phillips A. Glucocorticoid stimulation of glutamine synthetase production in cultured rat glioma cells. J Neurochem 1980; 34:866.

114a. Tombaugh G, Sapolsky R. Hippocampal glutamine synthetase: insensitivity to glucocorticoids and stress. Am J Physiol 199; in press.

115. Cupps T, Fauci A. Corticosteroid-mediated immunoregulation in man. Immunol Rev 1982; 65:133.

116. Compton M, Cidlowski J. Rapid in vivo effects of glucocorticoids on the integrity of rat lymphocyte genomic deoxyribonucleic acid. Endocrinology 1986; 118:38.

117. Wielckens K, Delfs T. Glucocorticoid-induced cell death and poly[adenosine diphosphate (ADP)-ribosylation: increased toxicity of dexamethasone on mouse S49.1 lymphoma cells with the poly(ADP-ribosyl)ation inhibitor benzamide. Endocrinology 1986; 119:2383.

117a. Mastus J, Finch C, Sapolsky R. Glucocorticoid endangerment of hippocampal neurons does not involve DNA cleavage. Endocrinology 1989; 124:3083.

118. Stein B, Sapolsky R. Chemical adrenalectomy reduces hippocampal damage induced by kainic acid seizures. Brain Res 1988; 175.

119. Lane L, Chrousos G, Lorioux D, et al. The antiglucocorticoid and antiprogestin steroid RU 486 suppresses the adrenocorticotropin response to ovine corticotropin releasing hormone in man. J Clin Endocrinol Metab 1988; 66:290.

120. Kalimo H, Rehncrona S, Soderfeldt B, Olsson Y, Siesjo B. Brain lactic acidosis and ischemic cell damage: II. Histopathology. J Cereb Blood Flow Metab 1981; 1:313.

121. Pulsinelli W, Waldman S, Rawlinson D, Plum F. Moderate hyperglycemia augments ischemic brain damage: a neuropathologic study in the rat. Neurology 1982; 32:1239.

122. Thuggesen P, Hermann K, Willanger R. Concentration camp survivors in Denmark: persecution, disease, disability, compensation. Dan Med Bull 1970; 17:65.

123. Jensen T, Genefke I, Hyldebrandt N. Cerebral atrophy in young torture victims. N Engl J Med 1982; 307:1341.

124. Corsellis J. Mental illness and the ageing brain. Oxford: Oxford University Press, 1962.

125. Uno H, Tarara R, Else J, Suleman M, Sapolsky R. Hippocampal damage associated with prolonged and fatal stress in primates. J Neurosci 1988; 9:1705.

126. Trethowan W, Cobb S. Neuropsychiatric aspects of Cushing's syndrome. Arch Neurol Psychiatry 1952; 67:283.

127. Uno H, Thieme C, Kemnitz J, Farrell P. Effect of dexamethasone on the cerebral cortical development of the rhesus monkey. Neuroscience 1983; 320:3.

128. Sapolsky R, Uno H, Rebert C, Finch C. Hippocampal damage associated with prolonged glucocorticoid exposure in primates. J Neurosci 1990; in press.

16

SUBORDINATE ANIMALS
Behavioral and Physiological Adaptations and Opioid Tolerance

**Klaus A. Miczek, Michael L. Thompson, and
Walter Tornatzky**

Tufts University, Medford, Massachusetts

The concept of stress may be applied to events that occur in a social context. High-intensity interactions such as confrontations with a threatening or aggressive opponent include physiological and behavioral responses of a "stressful" nature. If social challenges are extended over time, even at a noncontact, physically noninjurious level, profound costs in behavior and physiology are incurred, in the extreme with life-threatening consequences. Activation of the hypothalamic–pituitary–adrenal axis generalizes to a large variety of social, sexual, maternal, aggressive, and submissive behavior patterns. More specific neurochemical events are important in the initiation of behavior in situations of social conflict and are also altered as a consequence of specific social experiences. While the short- and long-term adaptations to socially relevant events have been well documented at the behavioral level and have begun to be delineated in the cardiovascular and renal systems, our knowledge about such stress-related changes in the central nervous system (CNS) remains preliminary. We will survey briefly the behavior adaptations and maladaptations of individuals exposed to a range of social "stresses," and will then consider important physiological responses to social "stresses." We focus last on selected events in the CNS. In concert with biogenic amines and steroids, several peptides, particularly opioid peptides and their receptors, are important for behavior in a social context.

BEHAVIORAL CHARACTERISTICS OF
SUBORDINATE ANIMALS

The determinants of dispersal and aggregation of a wide range of animal orders, including mammals, have been studied mainly from an ecological and sociobiological viewpoint (e.g., 1). Games-theoretical analyses concern themselves with the long-term adaptive consequences of social conflict in a probabilistic fashion that is typical for the whole population, and less with the moment-to-moment changes in behavior in a given individual. In general, engaging in social conflict exposes individuals to the risk of injury and predatory attack, diverts precious energies from reproductive activities and feeding opportunities, and may enhance vulnerability to disease and shorten the lifespan. According to games theory, these costs are weighed, in the long term, against the potential benefits for the dominant individual of ready access to fit mating partners with high reproductive success, preferred diets, and protected niches (e.g., 2-4). This calculation applies equally to males and females of a given species.

In commonly studied mammalian species, each individual is capable of engaging in submissive as well as aggressive behavior, two types of agonistic behavior that are not poles on a continuum but rather separate dimensions of behavior. Detailed behavioral analyses of postures, movements, and facial expressions in cats, for example, illustrate the potential mixtures of offensive, defensive, and submissive patterns of body posture, facial displays, and movements in a given individual (5).

In behavioral terms, social conflict is characterized by the display of visual, olfactory, and auditory signals, acts, movements, postures, and gestures in at least two opponents. In the field as well as under laboratory conditions, these agonistic behavior patterns occur in predictable sequences in distinctive temporal episodes or bursts. The salient elements of the repertoire of agonistic behavior may be seen under various conditions that serve distinctive functions, such as in confrontations between a territorial resident and an intruder, in the formation or maintenance of groups, or in the defense of offspring by a lactating female. Like morphological characteristics, the typical elements of agonistic behavior differ between even closely related species. For example, when flight is barred, upright, supine, and crouch postures are typical for subordinate rodents, with defeated mice assuming an upright posture with the head angled upward, ears retracted, and forepaws limp, whereas the supine posture with limp extremities is characteristic of submissive rats (6-8). These behaviors have been interpreted to be adaptations of the loser to the stress of being threatened and attacked, because they may terminate or prevent attack by the opponent, either by providing a mechanism for escape or by signalling surrender to the victor (1,9,10). Animals seem to learn when to be submissive (11,12) and surrender more readily in successive encounters (13-15).

The behavioral consequences of a consistent display of submissive behavior in situations of social conflict are apparent outside of the relatively rare confrontations with an actively threatening and attacking opponent. Activity budgets reveal that most mammals engage in agonistic behavior less than 5% of their waking time, and yet the remainder of their behavioral repertoire may be greatly differentiated depending on whether or not they are subordinate or dominant in situations of social conflict (Fig. 1). In general, the subordinate animal is characterized by a restricted, impoverished behavioral repertoire, with prolonged inactive periods spent in a cowering, crouching position. Socially intolerant species such as tree shrews illustrate how a subordinate animal living in the presence of a dominant animal engages in a profoundly disrupted pattern of feeding, grooming, and sleeping, often leading to the death of the subordinate (17). Even in species with a pattern of life-long coexistence of dominant and subordinate animals, such as in various social primates, behavioral and physiological functions are profoundly compromised in subordinate members of the group. Basic

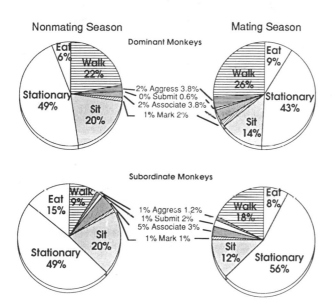

FIGURE 1   Resource allocation budgets represent the proportion of time spent walking, sitting, in stationary posture, feeding, marking, sending aggressive behaviors, associative behaviors and submissive behaviors in squirrel monkeys that are maintained as long-term social groups. The data from the nonmating season (left) and mating season (right) represent the means of four 60 min observations each for four dominant (top) and four (bottom) subordinate monkeys (from ref. 16).

survival behaviors such as feeding and drinking, sleeping, reproduction, bodily care, and defense often become opportunistic as, for example, in subordinate talapoin monkeys (18). Sapolsky (19) finds low-ranking male baboons to be subject to the highest frequency of social stressors. Their sexual consorts are frequently harassed and disrupted: sex for these subordinate individuals consists mainly of masturbation. They are the ones most frequently supplanted from food and resting sites and from bouts of social grooming. Even though these low-ranking males avoid entering into aggressive interactions, they are often attacked without having provided any discernible provocations.

One of the most prominent views of subordinate animals is that such animals have less access to mating partners and consequently leave fewer offspring than do dominant animals, an idea that was advanced by Zuckerman (20) and Maslow (21) and recently reviewed by Dewsbury (22). For example, in well-established groups of talapoin monkeys (*Miopithecus talapoin*), subordinate males fail to engage in copulatory behavior even when the dominant males are removed (18). Several studies under laboratory conditions have shown that females, when given a choice, tend to associate and mate with dominant males (lemmings, 23; rats, 24; bank voles, 25,26; vervet monkeys, 27; hamsters, 28).

The following four examples will illustrate the above generalities and their limitations. Mice and rats are selected because of their widespread and long-standing use in preclinical stress research, and squirrel monkeys as well as rhesus monkeys are chosen to highlight often-studied primates, from both the New and Old World.

Mice (*Mus musculus*)

The social behavior of mice varies greatly among *Mus, Peromyscus,* and *Onychomys* genuses. In the laboratory, *Mus musculus* is most often studied; this species is characterized by a social organization as *Grossfamilie*, with the adult male excluding other reproductively active males from his territory (29). Coexistence of adult males in the same locale is rare, and may only be seen when escape and dispersion are not readily possible (30,31). Once a male can no longer defend his own territory, he is displaced by another, usually younger, more vigorous male (32,33).

The behavioral repertoire of mice in situations of conflict has been described and catalogued in detail over the past decades (e.g., 6,14,34–36). A reproductively active adult male defends his territory by pursuits, threatening movements, and attack bites. Similarly, a maternal female defends her nest by threatening and attacking an intruder (37,38). The reactions to pursuits, threats, and attacks may initially include retaliatory attacks, eventually followed by retreat and flight. If escape is not possible, elongated alert, defensive upright, and sideways postures may be seen in an attacked mouse. Sometimes an intruder mouse may engage in nonprovoked flight responses (39) and exhibit a pronounced immobility response, even upon nonaggressive physical contact by an opponent (40). Ultimately, a defeated or submissive mouse, as illustrated in Figure 2, is characterized by an upright posture, with retracted ears, limp forepaws, squealing, even before physical contact, and failure to orient toward the threatening and attacking opponent (8,14). Mice that are submissive in these situations typically show less exploratory behavior (41). Defeated mice fail to react to painful stimuli, but develop tolerance to this analgesia (8).

At the simplest level of analysis, dominance–subordination relationships within groups of mice were defined by an assessment of wounds on the rumps, backs, and flanks of males. Dominant males were considered to be those that show little or no wound patterns, while submissive or subordinate males are those that show extensive wounding. Subordinate males often have lower body

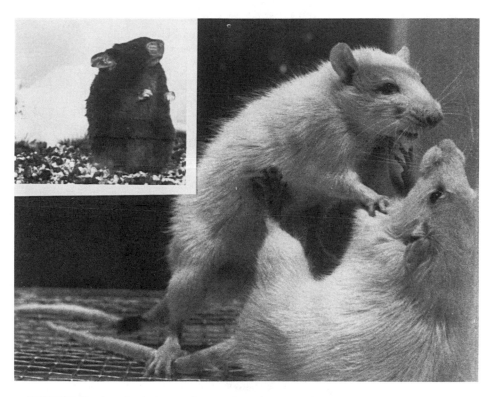

FIGURE 2 A submissive-supine posture by a rat in response to an aggressive posture by an opponent (Miczek, unpublished data, 1973). (Inset) The defeated mouse in characteristic posture (from Ref. 8).

weights and show evidence of testicular regression and adrenal hypertrophy. These physiological correlates of subordination were assumed to indicate the degree of stress associated with social rank (42,43). Weight of the pheromone-producing preputial gland is lower in subordinate males (84–86% less) than in dominants (44,45). Dominant mice tend to distribute their urine in small amounts evenly throughout their territory, whereas subordinates tend to deposit their urine in large pools at the edge of the test arena (46,47). Subordinates also show reduced activity levels in areas that have been marked with the urine of dominant mice (46). Dominant males copulate more frequently than subordinates and sire more offspring (48,49), perhaps because subordinate males that do copulate often ejaculate with fewer intromissions.

Rats (*Rattus norvegicus*)

As colonial species, rats display a spectrum of submissive postures, acts, and movements, and emit characteristic ultrasounds and odors (e.g., 50,51). The elements of agonistic behavior in wild rats can be reproduced under appropriately controlled laboratory conditions (52–56). Offensive behavior is characterized by pursuits, sideways threats, and attack bites that may be preceded by naso- and anogenital investigation and grooming of the neck region ("allogrooming"); on occasion, both opponents may rear up on their hind legs facing each other, referred to as mutual upright posture. This latter behavior is the prevalent response of two rats when exposed to electric shock pulses to their feet (57).

When threatened or attacked, a rat may retaliate or evade; however, the most prominent defensive and submissive behavioral elements are an upright posture with extended forepaws and head angled upward, a supine posture, and a crouch posture. Frequent and intense attacks are reacted to by a supine posture with reduced muscle tone, particularly in the extremities. Bites evoke audible squeals, whereas ultrasounds in the 20–30 kHz range may be recorded in a submissive rat, particularly while being threatened and after being attacked (58). Like mice, defeated rats show profound alterations in opioid-mediated pain responses (e.g., Miczek and Fier, 1990 unpublished observations).

Severely defeated wild rats that are intruding into a colony are inactive, impaired in feeding and body care, and ultimately may die if escape is barred. Death is, however, not due to wounding. Barnett and co-workers (59) showed that 34% of the intruders introduced in a homecage of three other longhaired rats (*Rattus villosissimus*) died or collapsed under attack, although unwounded.

Some intruder rats, however, do adapt to defeat and survive in the colony (50). Spencer and Cameron (60) have shown that dominance status is associated with habitat selection in the hispid cotton rat. Subordinate males are forced to occupy less desirable habitats, in this case patchy areas that are devoid of shrub cover to protect against predators. In laboratory testing, subordinate cotton

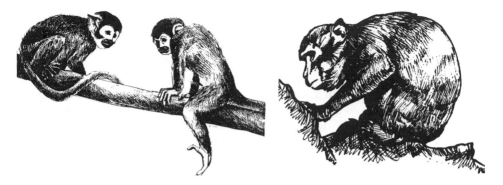

FIGURE 3 A. A crouching posture by a squirrel monkey in response to a genital display by an adult male (from Miczek and Krsiak. In: Thompson T, Dews PB, eds. Advances in behavioral pharmacology, vol. 2, 1978, Academic Press, New York drawing by Bonnie Dann). B. Crouching by a subordinate rhesus monkey (from R. A. Hinde RA. Biological bases of human social behaviour, drawing by Priscilla Barrett, McGraw-Hill, Inc., 1974).

rats explore less in a novel environment. This decreased activity might be advantageous in reducing encounters with dominant individuals (61).

Squirrel Monkeys (*Saimiri sciureus*)

The most outstanding behavior of squirrel monkeys in situations of conflict is the genital display, which consists of spreading one thigh with the knee bent and pointing the erected penis toward the opponent, who most often crouches (62, Fig. 3). When the conflict escalates, fighting may culminate, although rarely, in injurious biting at the extremities and head, but most severely at the neck. The acts, postures, movements, and displays of squirrel monkeys who are engaged in agonistic behavior have been described, catalogued, and illustrated (63,64).

More than other New World primates, squirrel monkeys engage in a relatively large amount of hostile interactions with frequent chases and retreats, possibly due to the high population density of their troops (65). The incidence of agonistic behavior is greatly increased during the breeding season when the alpha male of the subgroup shows the "fatted male syndrome," most conspicuous by the large increase in adipose tissue and testicular size (66). Subordinate males are displaced from preferred perching sites, exposed to chin thrusts, ear flaps, and bared teeth, grasped at the ears and other extremities, pulled, pushed, jumped on, restrained around the waist, mounted from behind, and, occasionally, bitten.

The behavioral consequences of engaging consistently in submissive behavior are most apparent during situations of conflict and reproduction, but also in the remainder of the behavioral repertoire of the individual. An analysis of the various types of behavior displayed during the course of the day clearly differentiates between the activity "budgets" of dominant and subordinate group members (see Fig. 1). At the motoric level, it is apparent that subordinate monkeys are less active, particularly during the mating season. Subordinates orient toward the dominant male when initiating social interactions. While it has often been noted that the introduction of an adult male into an established group of squirrel monkeys may have fatal consequences, this species appears more tolerant of strangers than, for example, Old World monkeys.

Rhesus Monkeys (*Macaca mulatta*)

Collective or "gang" aggression toward an intruder, often injurious, is seen in rhesus monkeys as well as in squirrel monkeys (e.g., 67,68). Intruder-provoked aggression is, however, relatively rare. The intensity of intragroup conflict is substantially higher in rhesus monkeys than in squirrel monkeys (69), although the actual percentage of time devoted to aggressive behavior in the entire behavioral repertoire is similarly small in both species (e.g., 2-3%, cf. Fig. 1; 70). There appear to be multiple functions of aggression within groups of rhesus monkeys, and the frequent display of submissive signals may avoid escalation to high-intensity, injurious agonism (e.g., 71). In the field, for example, the incidence of female-initiated aggression is far higher than that of males, due to the larger number of females in the troop, whereas males show higher individual aggression rates than females (70).

Submissive reactions of rhesus monkeys to threat begin by them yielding to, moving away from, and avoiding eye contact with a threatening animal. Characteristic submissive behaviors in response to attack and chase include presenting, grimaces, crouches (Fig. 4) and flight, accompanied by shrieking vocalizations (e.g., 72-74); sometimes these behavioral elements are lumped together as an index of submissiveness (e.g., 75). Mounting and presenting in rhesus monkeys, like genital displays in squirrel monkeys, may often represent a socially cohesive behavior rather than a dominance–subordination interaction (76).

CORRELATES AND CONSEQUENCES OF SOCIAL STRESS IN PERIPHERAL PHYSIOLOGY

Immediate responses to a social challenge may serve as functional adaptations that afford the subordinate individual some degree of control. Being forced to live in a subordinate role in a social group for a long time can have profound physiological consequences, which may eventually lead to pathological conditions or death.

Pituitary-Adrenal System

Rodents

Following Selye's focus on the pituitary-adrenal axis, Welch and Klopfer (77) suggested that the adrenal medullae and cortices of subordinate mice differ from those of dominants. Variability in the weight of the adrenal glands between individuals was larger with increasing group size. Welch argued that this increased variability may reflect differential autonomic stimulation in individuals of different social positions within the group. The stress of defeat in an aggressive encounter was reported to be correlated with increases in adrenocorticotropic hormone (ACTH)/glucocorticoids and decreases in circulating androgens (78–80). Wild rats that were introduced as intruders into established colonies frequently died; they had high adrenal weights and the adrenal cortex was depleted of lipid (81). They also showed low liver glycogen levels and hyperglycemia, suggesting depletion of adrenocortical hormones (82). Other studies have reported elevated corticosterone levels following fighting in both the eventual winners and losers, but found that recovery to prefight levels is more rapid in winners than in the losers (44,83,84).

Adrenal medullary response to social stress may also be related to the outcome of agonistic encounters. Dominant mice respond to social interaction with a predominantly sympathetic adrenal medullary pattern, whereas subordinates respond with a pituitary adrenocortical pattern (85). After 3 weeks of fighting experiences, defeated mice showed significantly increased adrenal epinephrine content, but no difference in norepinephrine content; by contrast, victorious mice showed the opposite pattern: increased norepinephrine content with no difference in epinephrine content (86,87).

Adrenal secretions do not only correlate with subordination or dominance but also can influence the form of agonistic behavior displayed by the individual in subsequent encounters (88). Defeat leads first to an increase in corticosterone levels, which may facilitate submission in subsequent encounters. Corticosterone replacement in adrenalectomized mice shows that the larger the replacement dose, the more readily the animal engages in submissive behavior.

The apparent correlation between glucocorticoids and submissiveness may be a direct effect of ACTH on behavior. For example, hypophysectomized mice cannot show the normal ACTH increase and testosterone decrease in response to defeat. When maintained on fixed-dose ACTH replacement therapy, these mice became submissive later in the encounter than did intact animals (15). Brain (83) reported that ACTH stimulated social aggression in mice, when acutely injected, but suppressed aggression when given over several weeks. Although injections of ACTH do increase submissiveness, they do so only in mice that are able to respond to the ACTH with increases in corticosterone levels. The submissiveness of adrenalectomized mice treated with a fixed replacement dose of corticosterone was not affected by ACTH (89,90).

In general, subordination in rodents is associated with elevated glucocorticoid levels. These increases may have the functional value of increasing the display of submissive behaviors in future agonistic encounters, thereby reducing the amount of aggression received. Sustained elevation of glucocorticoids may, however, cause downregulation of corticosterone receptors in the hippocampus (91).

Primates

In contrast to the acute stress studies in rodents, the research strategy in primates often relies on correlative studies of adrenal–pituitary responsiveness and established social rank. Leshner and Candland (92) characterized dominant and subordinate squirrel monkeys in terms of urinary 17-hydroxycorticosteroids total catecholamine, and 17-ketosteroid levels, In contrast to mice, the results with squirrel monkeys suggested that high levels of adrenal output were correlated with dominant rather than submissive behaviors. Similar differentiation in glucocorticoids can be seen in dyads or triads of squirrel monkeys (93). It should be noted, however, that these measurements were obtained in the absence of specific environmental or social challenges, and thus are not strictly comparable to the rodent studies. When challenged with one of three types of stress (a live snake, ether anesthesia, or physical restraint), dominant male squirrel monkeys had lower unstressed plasma cortisol levels than subordinates, but always showed the largest adrenal reactivity to stress (94). In a subsequent study reported by Coe et al. (93) male squirrel monkeys that lived with females in groups and that were subject to frequent environmental disturbances were examined. Under these conditions the endocrine rank correlation was shifted such that subordinates showed higher basal levels of cortisol.

Dominant male olive baboons living in the East African savannah showed lower resting levels of cortisol, but responded relatively faster and more strongly following anesthesia stress (95; similar to the findings of Manogue et al., 94). Subordinate *Macaca fascicularis* and tree shrews had heavier adrenal glands than dominants (17,96). However, McGuire et al. (97) failed to detect a clear relation between cortisol levels and dominance status in established colonies of vervet monkeys, but did find a rise in cortisol levels in all males during competition for dominance.

Interpretations of glucocorticoid measurements depend on whether the dominant or subordinate animal had to cope actively with an environmental or social challenge. Moreover, these indices of adrenal activity are subject to diurnal and seasonal rhythms. However, most results with primates suggest that the prolonged stress of subordination leads to an impairment or alteration in the normal endocrine response to stress. Subordinate individuals have higher basal levels of cortisol, but then show a blunted response to subsequent stressful events.

Gonadal

Rodents

The relationship between testosterone and subordinate status has been investigated less thoroughly than its role in aggressive behavior. Generally, androgen production -is curtailed in subordinates (98,99). However, androgens, although obviously crucial for rodent aggression, do not seem to be important to the propensity to avoid attack since castration has no effect on submissive behavior (7,100-102). Instead, the decline in androgen production alters the stimulus characteristics that elicit attack. Subordinate animals produce less androgen-dependent preputial pheromone, as evidenced by decreases in preputial weight (84-86% less) compared to dominants (44,45). That these phermones serve as aggression-provoking stimuli is demonstrated by the increased attacks toward castrates that have been marked with urine from intact males, and by the fact that males with surgically removed preputial glands are attacked less than intact males (103). The decline in androgen does apparently play a role in the stabilization of group hierarchies.

Primates

Subordinate status has been reported to be associated with lowered testosterone levels in squirrel monkeys (104), rhesus monkeys (105), and talapoins (106). In baboons, Sapolsky (95) has reported that resting testosterone levels are not related to social status. However, in response to the stress of being captured and having blood sampled, dominant males showed increased testosterone levels in response to stress, whereas subordinates showed a decline.

While most studies have focused on the male's opportunity for copulatory behavior, several studies have also shown that subordinate status can have an impact on the reproductive status of females. Abbott et al. (107) studied dominant and subordinate female marmosets in 10 well-established peer groups. The latter never ovulated, had a reduced luteinizing hormone (LH) response to LH-releasing hormone (LHRH) and showed no positive feedback LH surge after estrogen administration. Impaired ovarian function has also been reported in subordinate female cynomolgous macaques. Socially subordinate females had fewer ovulatory menstrual cycles and more cycles with deficient luteal phase plasma progesterone concentrations than did the dominant females (108,109). These hormonal alterations may decrease the attractiveness of subordinate females to males, and thus reduce their chance of being attacked by higher-ranking females. It is not clear, however, whether these changes in subordinate females result from the stress of subordinate status or the reduced exposure to male cues needed to induce normal hormonal secretions.

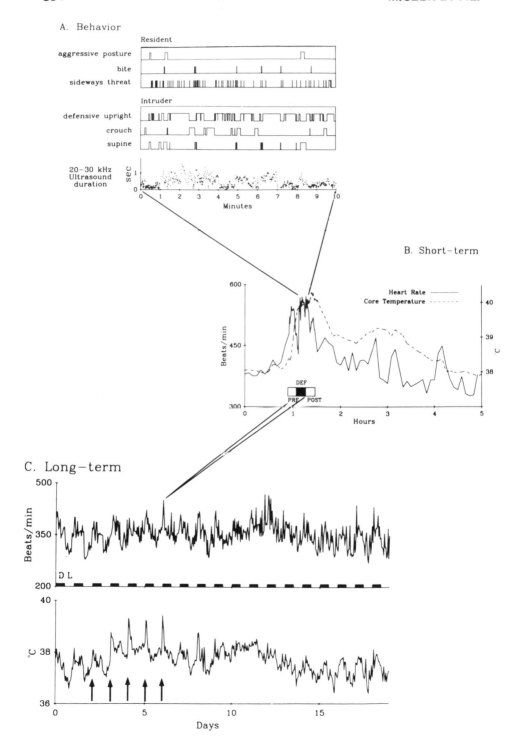

A. Behavior

Resident
- aggressive posture
- bite
- sideways threat

Intruder
- defensive upright
- crouch
- supine

20–30 kHz Ultrasound duration

Minutes

B. Short-term

Heart Rate
Core Temperature

Beats/min

°C

DEF
PRE POST

Hours

C. Long-term

Beats/min

D L

°C

Days

Renal

Henry and colleagues (110–113) found a high incidence of interstitial nephritis in colonies of inbred CBA mice housed in population cages that prompted a high level of conflict. The blood urea nitrogen level of these animals was shown to be inversely proportional to social status as measured by behavior and the appearance of fur. Urination by subordinates was suppressed when they were in the presence of dominants and hence they suffered from overfilled bladders. Henry et al. argued that the fatal tubulointerstitial involvement may originate with repeated episodes of urinary reflux.

In tree shrews (*Tupaia belangeri*), many intruders into the home range of a resident showed altered kidney function after about 6 days (17). Their serum urea nitrogen and creatine levels were elevated more than 10-fold, and many died from uremia.

The physiological mechanism of altered renal function has not been established. Because urination is often used by dominant males to mark territorial boundaries, impaired renal function most likely results from dominants suppressing such behavior in subordinates. Subordinates' access to food and water is often limited as well, which may also compromise kidney function.

Cardiovascular Correlates

Both the hypothalamic–pituitary–adrenal axis, with its effects on cardiovascular physiology, and the neural connections between CNS and the heart (114) are

---

FIGURE 4 A. Elements of aggressive behavior by a resident rat threatening and attacking an intruder are identified as upward deflections from a time line (in minutes). Three behavioral elements of the resident are selected: aggressive posture, bite, and sideways threat. The salient elements of the intruder behavior are shown similarly: defensive upright, crouch, and supine posture. Underneath, concurrently recorded ultrasounds in the 20–30 kHz range are portrayed as a time/duration scatter plot. B. Short-term effects of being attacked and threatened on the intruder's heart rate (solid line) and core temperature (dashed line) before, during, and after defeat (in hours) as obtained via Mini-Mitter Dataquest III system. PRE, intruder in the resident's home cage, separated by an opaque divider for 10 min; DEF, physical interactions leading to defeat, maximally for 10 min or until intruder has been attacked 20 times; POST, 10 min of intruder activity in the resident's cage after the defeat with the resident removed; thereafter, the intruder was placed into his own home cage (dark period, 8:00–20:00); heart rate and temperature were sampled every 20 s during resident–intruder encounters and in the home cage every 5 min. C. Long-term effects of five consecutive defeats on the magnitude and rhythmicity of heart rate and core temperature as mean values per hour (sampling rate every 5 min). Black horizontal bars denote dark periods; arrows point to the intruder's defeats. Resident–intruder encounters occurred within 1 h after the onset of the dark period.

interacting regulatory systems. They not only modulate the momentary adjustment of blood and oxygen supply to active effector organs but also prepare the metabolism of the organism for challenges by complex environmental stimuli. In the long term these systems are also important in the reestablishment of the homeostatic equilibrium of the individual. Thus, heart rate (HR) and blood pressure (BP) are often evaluated as physiological responses to emotional and stressful situations (115-118).

Rodents

Short-lived increases in blood pressure may occur in subordinate rats in response to brief dyadic behavioral interactions (119). Catheterized rats that were attacked by an experienced aggressive rat showed transient blood pressure changes that could be related to ongoing behavioral and hormonal responses. For example, the catecholamine ratios (norepinephrine/epinephrine [NE/E]) and corticosterone levels (120) were positively correlated with blood pressure responses.

More recent studies of short-term cardiovascular response in socially challenging situations have used telemetry sampling techniques to avoid restraint and handling. Moment-to-moment monitoring over long periods of time is possible, even during vigorous fighting. We have recently applied this technology to studies of the behavior and homeostasis of a subordinate male rat intruding in the home cage of a resident male. First, the behavioral adaptations of the intruder in response to the resident are characterized; concurrently, we analyzed the short-term (i.e., minutes and hours) time course in telemetered HR and body core temperature of the intruder in reaction to the behavioral event, as well as the long-term (i.e., days and weeks) effects of repeated acute defeat experiences. Defeat occurs during 10 min physical exposures to a resident 1 h after the start of the dark period. This experimental protocol permits a direct assessment of the effects of defeat on the diurnal periodicity of the cardiovascular and temperature regulatory systems. Figure 4 illustrates data recorded during one experiment from one rat before, during, and after the fifth defeat experience.

Exposure to the resident's cage is sufficient to increase HR and core temperature, which are further increased when the resident attacks and threatens the intruder. In the course of 2-4 h after the 10 min encounter, HR and core temperature recover to baseline levels. This pattern of dramatic increases and prolonged recovery is repeated during defeats on consecutive days. In severely defeated animals the circadian rhythmicity of HR and temperature is disturbed, and the basal levels of these parameters remain elevated throughout the day-night cycle. After 7-9 days normal rhythmicity returns.

Most previous information on this topic has come from studies of cardiovascular changes or adaptations in individuals who have coexisted as subordinates in colonies for a prolonged period of time. For example, Fokkema and

Koolhaas (121) assessed blood pressure in rats of varying social status that had lived in large colonies for 2 months. Mean resting blood pressure showed a significant positive correlation with a compound measure of threatening and fleeing. The subordinate rats that interacted most with the dominant while in the colony had the highest resting BP.

Cardiovascular problems such as separation of myocardial fibers, fragmentation and fibrosis, small infarcts, cardiac hypertrophy, and eventually hypertension have also been reported in long-term subordinate mice housed in population cages (122). Elevated systolic blood pressures of 145 mmHg (normal, 125) were found in the unchallenged dominant mice in these colonies, while the highest mean values (165 mmHg) were reached by subordinates. Subordinate mice showed increased erythropoiesis and splenomegaly, as well as increased reticulocyte counts (123).

Primates

Similar studies of both short- and long-term cardiovascular responses to stress have been conducted in primates. For example, Stoehr (124) monitored HR in dominant tree shrews by telemetry and found no change in the day/night variation after the second day of social confrontation. In contrast, the HR of the "actively coping" subordinate animals remained elevated for many days (17). Rather than becoming totally subordinate, these individuals instead maintain an active coping response for long periods of time, continue to interact with the dominant, and occasionally fight back. In contrast to the other subordinates, these "actively coping" tree shrews were capable of living in the dominant's cage for weeks, albeit with a reduced sphere of action. These subordinate animals showed increased sympathetic activity, characterized by a high tyrosine hydroxylase activity and elevated adrenal NE content (17,125). The behavioral, histological, and hormonal profile of the "actively coping" tree shrew meets Folkow's (126) criteria for a defense reaction: the brainstem homeostatic mechanisms are overridden and the cardiovascular system anticipates and prepares for environmental challenges that may involve vigorous physical activity. It is possible that heightened sympathetic activity, if forced to be sustained, can lead to pathological changes of the cardiovascular system and eventual heart failure (127).

An example of cardiovascular adaptation following prolonged periods of subordination is the case of the socially wild male baboons living in their natural habitat in East Africa. When compared to dominants, subordinates exhibit significant reductions in high-density lipoprotein cholesterol (HDL–C) and apolipoprotein A-I concentrations (128). These differences were not correlated with differences in age, sex hormone concentrations, rank-related diet, or body weight, but were correlated with the elevated basal cortisol concentrations associated with subordinate status. Elevated serum low-density lipoprotein cholesterol (LDL-C) levels can promote atherosclerosis and coronary heart disease, while both are retarded by increased HDL-C levels.

Hamm et al. (129) have also implicated social stress as a determining factor in coronary artery disease. Subordinate cynomolgus macaques fed a diet containing a moderate amount of cholesterol (0.56 mg/cal) for 16 months had more extensive coronary artery stenosis than did their dominant, highly competitive counterparts. A similar pattern was observed in the thoracic and abdominal portions of the aorta with respect to competitiveness but not gender. In contrast, however, Shively and Kaplan (96) found that dominant males (*Macaca fasicularis*) had higher blood pressure and worsened atherosclerosis than subordinates under some conditions.

These studies indicate that the prolonged social stress of subordination may eventually have health-impairing consequences when the effects extend to the cardiovascular system. As with the sympathetic response to stress, cardiovascular responses that are adaptive during acute stress can result in eventual pathological conditions such as hypertension and atherosclerosis when activated in a repeated or prolonged fashion. Such stress-related pathological conditions are evident even in primate species in which overt fighting and injury are infrequent in the maintenance of dominance–subordination hierarchies.

CORRELATES AND CONSEQUENCES OF SOCIAL STRESS IN CNS

The evidence for potential CNS mechanisms in social stress responses is very limited and mostly focused on the aggressive individual, but only rarely on the subject of aggression. Brain monoamines and, more recently, neuropeptides as well as their receptors have been explored.

Catecholamines

One of the proposed functions of dopamine (DA) utilization and release from terminals in frontal cortex is a role in stress reactions (e.g., 130,131). Whether or not frontal cortex DA is of critical significance in social stress has not been studied systematically. However, DA levels and DA metabolites have been measured in whole brain as well as discrete brain regions in animals that had differential experience with attack and defeat behavior.

Most relevant to the present discussion are increases in mesolimbic, but not striatal, DA metabolism in rats that were attacked by an opponent for 10 min (132). Levels of the DA metabolites DOPAC and HVA were significantly elevated in the olfactory tubercle of rats in the presence of a potential opponent as well as when physically attacked. Earlier studies of monoamine brain levels suggested that defeat by an aggressive opponent produced a time-dependent pattern of increases and decreases in cortical, hypothalamic, and amygdaloid 5-HT and NE in C57BL/6J mice (133). Amygdaloid and hypothalamic 5-HT levels declined after 2 daily defeat experiences, but increases in 5-HT in these brain regions as well as in frontal cortex were seen after 4, 8, and 16 days of defeat, whereas NE showed the opposite changes, as estimated by fluorometric methods. Group-housed mice that are scarred and wounded, presumably due to attacks by a group despot, show an increase in the number of reuptake sites for cortical NE and concurrently a decrease for affinity of reuptake for NE (134). Similar changes are reported after electroconvulsive shock or after attack experience (135). Undifferentiated defensive, submissive, or aggressive behavior in ICR mice may also change aspects of DA activity in cortical and striatal structures (e.g., 136,137). Decreases in NE and in NE turnover in olfactory bulb and in substantia nigra are also seen after the display of attack behavior in Swiss-Webster mice (138).

Marked changes in level, turnover, and reuptake of catecholamines occur in animals that are involved in aggressive behavior; yet increases as well as decreases are reported. It is apparent that the duration and precise nature of the experience are critical determinants in detecting alterations in catecholamine activity. The perplexing pattern of changes in dopamine and norepinephrine levels, turnover, and reuptake also suggests important species and situational differences; so far, evidence for selective changes in animals that exhibit submissive or defensive behavior patterns remains elusive.

We recently confirmed the increases in dopamine turnover, in n. accumbens and olfactory tubercle of adult mice that engaged in an initial resident–intruder confrontation (139). Using the micropunch technique, samples of n. accumbens, but not of striatum or amygdala, from attacking as well as defeated mice showed large elevations in DOPAC after a single behavioral experience. By contrast, DOPAC and DA levels in n. accumbens of attacking residents as well as defeated intruders with extensive fighting experience (i.e., 1 encounter per day for 10 days) were closely similar to those measured in animals without a history of aggressive, defensive, or defeat behavior, thus pointing to parallel neurochemical and behavioral adaptations.

Defeat as well as aggressive behavior may result in marked changes in cortical and limbic catecholamine systems; the direction and nature of these changes appear to depend on the specific species, agonistic behavior, and situation. A significant finding is that long-term adaptations to disturbances in catecholamine systems during repeated social confrontations appear to develop.

Serotonin

The link between heightened aggressive behavior and lowered brain 5-HT activity, originally postulated more than three decades ago, has been repeatedly investigated, albeit with varying results (e.g., 140,141). Even less clear evidence for a distinctive role of any of the brain serotonin systems specific to submissive or defeat behavior exists. Defensive reactions in tree shrews (*Tupaia*) may be correlated with marked changes in raphe cell activity, and defensive responses in rats may be facilitated by selected manipulations that impair 5-HT neurotransmission. The rate of single unit activity of dorsal raphe neurons increases three to four times when the tree shrew displays an immobile defensive posture in the presence of a dominant conspecific or when approached by a human handler (142).

In rats, defensive reactions to electric foot shock may be increased by inhibiting tryptophan hydroxylase, by electrolytic or neurotroxic lesions of 5-HT-containing neurons, and, more consistently, by chronic administration of monoamine (MAO) reuptake blockers and MAO inhibitors (see reviews in 140,143-145). No comparable data exist for submissive or defeat responses. In mice, micropunched samples of the amygdaloid complex showed approximately three-fold elevations in 5-HIAA in the resident attacker and a smaller increase in the defeated intruder after their first encounter (139). When resident and intruder mice confronted each other daily for 10 days, no significant changes in 5-HIAA or 5-HT were detectable in striatum, n. accumbens, or amygdala, pointing again to parallel behavioral and neurochemical adaptations.

Opioid Peptides

When defeated in a social confrontation for the first time, mice become analgesic (8). This analgesia is reversible by opioid receptor antagonists that act at sites in the CNS (146,147) and is associated with changes in levels of opioid peptides in brain areas associated with pain processes (148,149). These results were confirmed in other strains of mice (150-152). With repeated exposure to the "social stress" of an attacking and threatening opponent and with passage of time, the defeated animal adapts behaviorally, physiologically, and neurochemically. It is possible to correlate the behavioral adaptations that resemble the development of tolerance with alterations in indices of endogenous opioid activity, such as levels of opioid peptides in various brain regions or changes in opiate receptor binding. In mice that were sacrificed after the first defeat, in vivo [3H] diprenorphine binding relative to nondefeated mice decreased significantly in medulla pons, cortex, and diencephalon, but after additional days with defeat experiences this large decrease was not observed. Following seven defeat experiences, significantly increased binding was evident in two of the three regions (13-21%) compared to control mice not exposed to defeat. (149). This experience-dependent inversion in binding characteristic suggests that in defeat-experienced or "tolerant" mice, further "social stress" does not trigger the large opiate response, or perhaps the system was incapable of responding in day 1 fashion.

However, there was a significant increase in the amount of [^{3}H] diprenorphine labeling of receptors by day 7, which suggested a compensatory increase in the number of receptors (Fig. 5).

This finding correlates well with our results from binding studies conducted in vitro on brains from mice subjected to repeated defeat. Scatchard analyses of in vitro whole brain [^{3}H] dihydromorphine binding also revealed increased binding in defeat-tolerant mice relative to controls. These data suggested that the increase was due to an apparent significant increase in the number of binding sites (30%) and not to a significant change in affinity of the receptors for the ligand. Because [^{3}H] dihydromorphine demonstrates mainly μ activity, this suggests that chronic defeat stress upregulates the number of μ receptors in various regions of the brain.

These results might be due to chronic depletion of endogenous ligands and/or lack of their defeat-induced release in competitive amounts on day 7 following the defeat experience. [^{3}H] Diprenorphine binding in a group of mice defeated for 6 days, but not stressed on the seventh day, was similar to that seen in mice subjected to defeat on the seventh day, thus suggesting that defeat stress was no longer resulted in a large release of endogenous opioids. Furthermore, we have recently found that β-endorphin and met-enkephalin levels, as determined by radioimmunoassay, are significantly elevated in several brain regions relative to controls when measured immediately after an acute defeat, but in tolerant mice before or after defeat on the seventh day levels of these peptides are not significantly different from control values. However, the fact that binding was similar whether or not mice were exposed to defeat on the seventh day was again indicative that receptor number had been upregulated. This may represent the first report of receptor upregulation in response to behaviorally induced opioid peptide activity over time.

Benzodiazepine/GABA/Chloride Ionophore–Receptor Complex

Aside from modulating endogenous opioid systems and monoaminergic systems, social defeat stress also apparently alters benzodiazepine receptor systems in the CNS. The benzodiazepine/GABA receptor/chloride ionophore complex has been shown to be subject to regulation by the environment and to have a relevant role in mediating responses to environmental stress (153,154). File and Tucker (155) had previously reported that male hooded Lister rats treated postnatally with lorazepam showed increased submissiveness when intruding into another animal's territory. In collaboration with L. G. Miller and D. J. Greenblatt, we investigated the effect of acute defeat stress on the binding of benzodiazepine agonists and antagonists at the benzodiazepine receptor (156). Recent evidence had implicated these sites in the generation and modulation of stress. Using an

Brain dissection scheme:

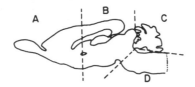

$[^3H]$ Diprenorphine binding (in vivo)

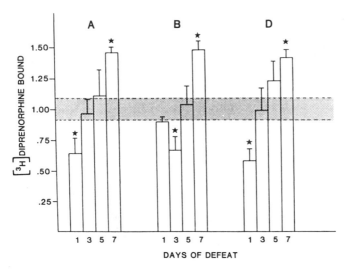

FIGURE 5 In vivo $[^3H]$ diprenorphine binding in B6AF$_1$/J mice after 1, 3, 5, or 7 days of social stress. Upper panel: Brains were rapidly removed after defeat and divided into four regions as shown (171). Lower panel: Binding in regions A, B, and D expressed as a ratio of binding determined in control mice that were not exposed to social stress. $[^3H]$ diprenorphine (4 MCi, 2 mg/kg subcutaneously) was injected immediately after defeat, and mice were sacrificed 20 min after injection. Stereospecific in vivo labeling of receptors was determined using a rapid filtration method (172). Values are means ± SEM; n = at least 7 for each group). Asterisk indicates a significant (p <0.05) difference from the naive controls.

in vivo binding procedure, we found that mice subjected to acute defeat show increased binding of benzodiazepine (BDZ) receptor ligand. Specific binding was increased approximately 80% after a single defeat experience compared to controls. This effect was maximal when injection of ligand took place immediately after stress, but binding remained elevated even when injections of the radioactive label were delayed until 30 min after stress. Greatest increases were observed in the hypothalamus, cortex, and cerebellum. Furthermore, the increases were only observed in the defeated intruder mice and not in the resident attacking mice. These results reinforce our previous suggestions that the biological function of the "stress" determines the physiological effects observed. Further analyses suggested the alterations to be due to increased receptor number and not due to alterations in affinity. These alterations were not observed in adrenalectomized mice, thus suggesting that adrenal steroids are necessary for the stress-induced increase in receptors. Since BDZs prevent the stress-induced increases in corticosterone, most likely via a central, receptor-mediated mechanism, BDZs may therefore modulate the stress response by indirectly altering circulating concentrations of adrenal steroids or by indirectly altering the number of available BDZ receptors.

NEUROPHARMACOLOGICAL CHALLENGES IN SOCIALLY STRESSED ANIMALS

During the past two decades it has been repeatedly demonstrated that many behavioral effects of all major classes of CNS drugs are profoundly affected by the social status of the individual (e.g., 55,157–159). Such socially differentiated drug effects reflect alterations in the neurochemical substrate for drug action that are brought about by the accumulated social experiences of an individual. For example, amphetamine increases locomotor activity of subordinate squirrel monkeys, but causes hypoactivity in dominant group members (159). The mechanisms by which these social experiences feed back to the brain and alter the substrates of drug action remain largely unknown.

The impact of distinctive social experiences on brain opioid peptides and their receptors as well as on opioid receptor-mediated pharmacological effects has been a particular focus of research. Distress calls due to social separation are profoundly intensified by opioid receptor blockade and attenuated by opioid receptor ligands (e.g., 160). Alterations in opioid peptides and receptors while the individual adapts to "social stress" with accruing experience over time can be revealed by appropriate pharmacological challenges. In a series of experiments, we have used this strategy of challenging the acutely defeated as well as the defeat-adapted individual with agonists and antagonists at different opioid receptor subtypes.

During the very first exposure to an attacking and threatening opponent, CF-1 mice show a potentiated analgesic response to morphine challenges (161). We recently demonstrated potentiation of morphine analgesia in rats that were briefly attacked by a resident. When the physical contact between the resident attacker and the intruder is limited to 3-5 min, it is insufficient in severity to alter the basal pain response. However, a marked potentiation of morphine analgesia is evident in the intruder as long as the threat of a potential attack persists (Miczek and Fier, 1990 unpublished observations, Fig. 6). This potentiation of opiate analgesia in animals subjected to acute social stress confirms observations with other types of physical stress in other species (e.g., 162-165). In view of the earlier discussed elevations in hypothalamic and mesencephalic met-enkephalin and β-endorphin levels and occupation of opioid receptors in acutely defeated mice, it appears that the potentiation of morphine analgesia is due to increased release of endogenous opioid peptides.

Within 24 h after the initial display of submissive behavior toward the attacking and threatening resident, a complete inversion in sensitivity to morphine's analgesic effects occurs. This tolerance to morphine's analgesic effects was first discovered in our initial studies of mice that confronted a resident attacker once a day for 8-10 min for 14 days; on day 15, the defeat-adapted mice were insensitive to an analgesic dose of morphine (8). In a further experiment, we challenged mice with the opioid antagonist naloxone after a 7 day sequence of daily exposures to an attacking opponent. Again the mice exhibited a large analgesic response after the very first defeat experience, but by day 7 their response to pain had returned to baseline levels, indicating the development of tolerance (147,166). The magnitude of the initial analgesic response and the subsequent tolerance-like decline in analgesia followed a time course closely similar to that seen in mice injected daily with morphine. On the subsequent day, all mice were challenged with naloxone, and withdrawal responses were seen in the drug-naive, defeat-adapted as well as morphine-tolerant mice. This observation, in conjunction with the earlier discussed in vivo and in vitro opioid receptor binding data, suggests that the tolerance-like change in analgesia with accruing defeat experiences may be based on changes in sensitivity or regulation of opioid receptors.

Direct pharmacological evidence for tolerance to the analgesic effects of opiate agonists that are specific to the μ receptor was developed in a series of studies examining the magnitude of opiate effects on several physiological and behavioral functions and on its long-lasting nature (147,167,168). In comparison to our earlier studies, we explored the minimal conditions under which exposure to an attacking and threatening opponent may alter opioid-mediated functions. A single exposure to a resident attacker rendered mice tolerant to morphine analgesia when challenged 3, 5, or 7 days after the defeat experience, with the largest tolerance occurring on the seventh day (147). The systematic increment in the magnitude to tolerance to morphine analgesia after a single defeat experience parallels directly the time course of increased receptor occupation by [³H]-diprenorphine, discussed earlier.

Systematic shifts to the right in dose-effect curves are the most cogent demonstrations of tolerance (169). Comparisons of morphine dose-effect curves before and after a single or five defeat experiences in mice confronting a resident attacker demonstrated large shifts to the right after defeat: four- to eight-fold higher morphine doses were required to produce analgesia in a defeat-experienced animal (167). This tolerance, however, was limited to the analgesic effects of morphine and did not extend to morphine's effects on operant behavior, providing the first indication for a functionally specific opiate tolerance development after defeat. In the course of these experiments, it became obvious that opiate tolerance was very long-lasting; to produce full morphine dose-effect curves, with each morphine dose being injected in weekly intervals, 6-8 weeks had to have elapsed since the original defeat experience.

To assess the long-lasting nature of opiate tolerance after defeat, a cumulative dosing protocol is suitably informative since it affords the opportunity to obtain dose-effect curves at specific times (e.g., 170). At the same time, we were interested in comparing μ and κ opiate receptor agonists to learn which opioid receptor subtypes may be modulated by the defeat experience. A sequence of 5 defeat experiences in mice produced tolerance to μ receptor agonists that lasted for at least 3 months (168). This tolerance was functionally selective but not specific to μ or κ opioid receptor subtypes, since only the morphine and ethylketocyclazocine dose-effect curves for analgesia shifted to the right after defeat but not the concurrently obtained dose-effect curves for hypothermia and suppression of operant behavior.

Functionally selective tolerance to the analgesic properties of morphine after defeat experiences was confirmed in separate experiments in rats that were trained in a drug discrimination paradigm (Miczek, 1990 unpublished observations). After discriminating a low morphine dose from saline with better than 95% accuracy, rats displayed submissive reactions to an attacking opponent during five brief encounters. Subsequent to these defeat experiences, half of the rats became more sensitive to the "cue" or discriminative stimulus properties of morphine, but all rats became tolerant to the analgesic effects of the drug (i.e., required four to six times higher morphine doses to produce analgesia). At the same time, the behaviorally suppressant effects of morphine as assessed by the rate of operant responding remained unaltered in defeat-experienced animals.

Even a single display of submissive behavior in laboratory rats is sufficient to produce large and long-lasting tolerance to the analgesic effects of morphine. An experimental protocol was developed that included a brief (3-5 min) confrontation between an intruder rat with a resident resulting in the unambiguous

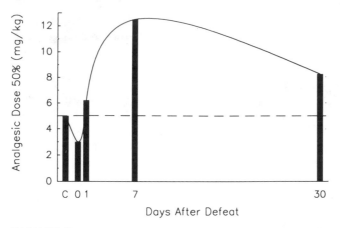

FIGURE 6 The dosage of morphine that elevated tail flick latencies to half of the maximum possible level (AD_{50}) in intruder rats that have displayed submissive behavior once during a 2–5 min encounter with an aggressive resident. Morphine doses were administered cumulatively over 1 h, either during the confrontation with the resident (0) or 1, 7, or 30 days after the single confrontation. The dotted line indicates the AD_{50} for undefeated control animals (C) (Miczek and Fier, 1990 unpublished observations, 113).

display of a submissive-supine or crouch posture and the emission of 20–30 KHz ultrasounds in reaction to the attacks by the resident (Miczek and Fier, 1990 unpublished observations, Fig. 6). After this brief period of contact aggression, the intruders remained in the presence of the threatening resident for 1 h, but were protected by a wire mesh cage. Under these conditions, no changes in pain responsiveness are detectable. However, when challenged, 1, 7, or 30 days after the single display of submissive behavior with a sequence of cumulative morphine doses, an incremental shift in dose–effect curve to the right demonstrates large and long-lasting tolerance to the analgesic effects of the drug.

Opioid-mediated analgesia serves as a sensitive and rapidly assessed index of the time-dependent bidirectional changes in certain opioid peptides and their receptors in response to the specific "stress" of defeat in a social confrontation. So far, the evidence favors the interpretation that during an initial defeat experience the large potentiation in opiate analgesia is due to enhanced release of endogenous opioid peptides in limbic and mesencephalic regions. However, if defeat experiences accrue or if time passes since the defeat, a completely inverted sensitivity to opiate challenge is detectable; within 24 h, but most prominently 1 week after as little as a single defeat experience, tolerance to opiate analgesia has developed that is parallel in time course and possibly due to upregulation in opioid receptors. It is also clear that alterations in brain opioid peptides after defeat may be seen in mice as well as in rats. These changes are functionally specific to the analgesic properties of μ opioid agonists and do not extend to the discriminative "cue," behaviorally suppressive, or hypothermic effects of these drugs.

It is unclear specifically which of the opioid peptides is critically important in the profound alteration in opiate analgesia after defeat. It will also be important to identify the critical neural "pool" of opioid peptide-containing neurons and opioid receptor populations that is most affected by defeat experiences. When one is considering the behavioral, autonomic, and endocrine facets of submissive responses, it is likely that opioid peptides in limbic, diencephalic, mesencephalic regions, as well as spinal cord are differentially activated in mediating pain, aversion, and coping responses. A more detailed exploration of the types of pain or aversion responses that are most prominently affected during and after defeat will reveal important differentiations in the reflexive versus affective components in these responses.

CONCLUSIONS

Being exposed to a threatening or aggressive opponent engenders species-specific behavioral and physiological responses that involve peptidergic and monoaminergic brain mechanisms. These CNS processes are only recently being appreciated as modulating endocrine, cardiovascular, and immune systems. Our focus on opioid peptides and their receptors as well as on the benzodiazepine/GABA/ chloride ionophore complex identifies two important brain systems that are altered by acute exposure to a specific social stress. Even more noteworthy may, however, be the long-lasting nature of the changes in sensitivity of opioid receptors that parallel the behavioral and physiological adaptations and maladaptations. The physical severity of social "stressors," although significant, may be less important than the behavioral and physiological constraints that these events impose. We have also been impressed by the varying ability of individuals to cope, behaviorally and physiologically, with specific social "stressors." Subordinate animals display an elaborate pattern of behavioral signals and adjust physiologically to rare physical assaults and the persistent threat of such assaults. The feedback relationship between specific social experiences to brain monoamines and neuropeptides, if extended from the laboratory situation, implies important mechanisms for behavioral and physiological pathological conditions and for clinical interventions.

ACKNOWLEDGMENTS

Preparation of this chapter and our own experimental work was supported by USPHS research grants AA 05122 and DA 02632.

REFERENCES

1. Wilson EO. Sociobiology. Cambridge: Harvard University Press, 1975.
2. Huntingford FA, Turner AK. Animal conflict. London/New York: Chapman and Hall 1987.
3. Maynard Smith J, Price GR. The logic of animal conflict. Nature 1973; 246:15-18.
4. Richert SE. The energetic costs of fighting. Am Zool 1988; 28:877-884.
5. Leyhausen P. Verhaltensstudien an Katzen, 2nd ed. Berlin: Paul Parey, 1960.
6. Grant EC, MacKintosh JH. A comparison of the social postures of some common laboratory rodents. Behaviour 1963; 21:246-259.
7. Leshner AI, Moyer JA. Androgens and agonistic behavior in mice: relevance to aggression and irrelevance to avoidance-of-attack. Physiol Behav 1975; 15:695-699.
8. Miczek KA, Thompson ML, Shuster L. Opioid-like analgesia in defeated mice. Science 1982; 215:1520-1522.
9. Blanchard DC, Blanchard RJ. Ethoexperimental approaches to the biology of aggression. Annu Rev Psychol 1988; 39:43-68.
10. Eibl-Eibesfeldt I B Ausdrucksformen der Saeugetiere. Handbuch Zool 1957; 8:1-26.
11. Külling P, Frischknecht HR, Pasi A, Waser PG, Siegfried B. Effects of repeated as compared to single aggressive confrontation on nociception and defense behavior in C57BL/6 and DBA/2 mice. Physiol Behav 1987; 39:01-07.
12. Siegfried B, Frischnecht H-R, Waser PG. A new learning model for submissive behavior in mice: effects of naloxone. Aggress Behav 1982; 8:112-115.
13. Scott JP, Marston MV. Nonadaptive behavior resulting from a series of defeats in fighting mice. J Abnorm Soc Psychol 1953; 48:417-428.
14. Ginsburg B, Allee WC. Some effects of conditioning on social dominance and subordination in inbred strains of mice. Physiol Zool 1942; 15:485-506.
15. Nock BL, Leshner AI. Hormonal mediation of the effects of defeat on agonistic responding in mice. Physiol Behav 1976; 17:111-119.
16. Winslow JT, Miczek KA. Naltrexone blocks amphetamine-induced hyperactivity, but not disruption of social and agonistic behavior in mice and squirrel monkeys. Psychopharmacology 1988; 96:493-499.
17. Von Holst D. Coping behaviour and stress physiology in male tree shrews. In: Hoelldobler B, Lindauer M, eds. Experimental behavioral ecology and sociobiology. Stuttgart: Gustav Fischer, 1985: 461-470.
18. Eberhart JA, Yodyingyuad U, Keverne EB. Subordination in male talapoin monkeys lowers sexual behaviour in the absence of dominants. Physiol Behav 1985; 35:673-677.
19. Sapolsky RM. Stress-induced elevation of testosterone concentrations in high ranking baboons: role of catecholamines. Endocrinology 1986; 118: 1630-1635.

20. Zuckerman S. The social life of monkeys and apes. New York: Harcourt, Brace, 1932.
21. Maslow AH. The role of dominance in the social and sexual behavior of infra-human primates: III. A theory of sexual behavior of infra-human primates. J Genet Psychol 1936; 48:310–338.
22. Dewsbury DA. Dominance rank, copulatory behavior, and differential reproduction. Q Rev Biol 1982; 57:135–159.
23. Huck UW, Banks EM. Male dominance status, female choice and mating success in the brown lemming, *Lemmus trimucronatus*. Animal Behav 1982; 30:665–675.
24. Carr WJ, Kimmel KR, Anthony SL, Schlocker DE. Female rats prefer to mate with dominant rather than subordinate males. Bull Psychonom 1982; 20(2):89–91.
25. Hoffmeyer I. Responses of female bank voles (*Clethrionomys glareolus*) to dominant vs subordinate conspecific males and to urine odors from dominant vs subordinate males. Behav Neural Biol 1982; 36:178–188.
26. Shapiro LE, Dewsbury DA. Male dominance, female choice and male copulatory in two species of voles (*Microtus ochrogaster* and *Microtus montanus*). Behav Ecol Sociobiol 1986; 18:267–274.
27. Keddy AC. Female mate choice in vervet monkeys (*Cercopithecus aethiops sabaeus*). Am J Primatol 1986; 10:125–134.
28. White PJ. Female discrimination of male dominance by urine odor cues in hamsters. Physiol Behav 1986; 37:273–277.
29. Archer J. Animals under stress. Baltimore: University Park Press, 1969.
30. Benton D, Dalrymple-Alford JC, Brain PF. Comparisons of measures of dominance in the laboratory mouse. Anim Behav 1980; 28:1274–1279.
31. Crowcroft P. Mice all over. Foulis, London: 1966.
32. Crowcroft P, Rowe FP. Social organization and territorial behaviour in the wild house mouse. Proc Zool Soc London 1963; 140:517–531.
33. Mackintosh JH. Territory formation by laboratory mice. Anim Behav 1970; 18:177–183.
34. Banks EM. A time and motion study of prefighting behavior in mice. J Genet Psychol 1962; 101:165–183.
35. Brain PF. Differentiating types of attack and defense in rodents. In: Brain PF, Benton D, eds. Multidisciplinary approaches to aggression research. Amsterdam: Elsevier, 1981: 53–78.
36. Scott JP, Fredericson E. The causes of fighting in mice and rats. Physiol Zool 1951; 24:273–309.
37. Haney M, DeBold JF, Miczek KA. Maternal aggression in mice and rats towards male and female conspecifics. Aggress Behav 1989; 15:443–453.
38. Noirot E, Goyens J, Buhot M-C. Aggressive behavior of pregnant mice towards males. Horm Behav 1975; 6:9–17.
39. Krsiak M. Timid singly-housed mice: Their value in prediction of psychtropic activity of drugs. Br J Pharmacol 1975; 55:141–150.
40. Cairns RB, Scholz SD. Fighting in mice: dyadic escalation and what is learned. J Comp Physiol Psychol 1973; 85:540–550.

41. Montgomery WI, Woods S. The effects of food deprivation in dyadic encounters in Apodemus sylvaticus. Ethology 1986; 72(4):299–310.
42. Davis DE, Christian JJ. Relation of adrenal weight to social rank of mice. Proc. Soc Exp Biol Med 1957; 94:728–731.
43. Louch CD, Higginbotham M. The relationship between social rank and plasma corticosterone levels in mice. Gen Comp Endocrinol 1967; 8:441–444.
44. Bronson FH. Establishment of social rank among grouped male mice: relative effects on circulating FSH, LH, and corticosterone. Physiol Behav 1973; 10:947–951.
45. Bronson FH, Marsden HM. The preputial gland as an indicator of social dominance in male mice. Behav Biol 1973; 9:625–628.
46. Bishop MJ, Chevins PF. Urine odours and marking patterns in territorial laboratory mice (Mus musculus). Behav Proc 1987; 15:223–248.
47. Desjardins C, Maruniak JA, Bronson FH. Social rank in house mice: differentiations revealed by ultraviolet visualization of urinary marking patterns. Science 1973; 182:939–941.
48. Dewsbury DA. Aggression copulation, and differential reproduction of deer mice (*Peromyscus maniculatus*) in a semi-natural enclosure. Behaviour 1984; 91:1–23.
49. Dewsbury DA. Kinship, familiarity, aggression, and dominance in deer mice (*Peromyscus maniculatus*) in seminatural enclosures. J Comp Psychol 1988; 102:124–128.
50. Barnett SA. The rat. A study in behavior. Chicago: University of Chicago Press, 1975.
51. Telle H-J. Beitrag zur Kenntnis der Verhaltensweise von Ratten, vergleichend dargestellt bei Rattus norvegicus und Rattus rattus. Z Angew Zool 1966; 53:129–196.
52. Blanchard RJ, Blanchard CD. Aggressive behavior in the rat. Behav Biol 1977; 21:197–224.
53. Chance MRA. An interpretation of some agonistic postures: the role of "cut-off" acts and postures. Symp Zool Soc London 1962; 8:71–89.
54. Luciano D, Lore R. Aggression and social experience in domesticated rats. J Comp Physiol Psychol 1975; 88:917–923.
55. Miczek KA. Intraspecies aggression in rats: effects of *d*-amphetamine and chlordiazepoxide. Psychopharmacologia 1974; 39:275–301.
56. Miczek KA. A new test for aggression in rats without aversive stimulation: Differential effects of *d*-amphetamine and cocaine. Psychopharmacology 1979; 60:253–259.
57. Ulrich RE, Azrin NH. Reflexive fighting in response to aversive stimulation. J Exp Anal Behav 1962; 5:511–520.
58. Sales GD, Sewell N. Ultrasound and aggressive behaviour in rats and other small mammals. Animal Behav 1972; 20:88–100.
59. Barnett SA, Hocking WE, Munro KMH, Walker KZ. Socially induced renal pathology of captive wild rats. Aggress Behav 1975; 1:123–133.

60. Spencer SR, Cameron GN. Behavioral dominance and its relationship to habitat patch utilization by the hispid cotton rat (*Sigmodon hispidus*). Behav Ecol Sociobiol 1983; 13:27-36.
61. Summerlin CT, Wolfe JL. Social influences on exploratory behavior in the cotton rat. Commun Behav Biol 1971; 6:105-109.
62. Ploog DW, MacLean PD. On the function of the mamillary bodies in the squirrel monkey. Exp Neurol 1963; 7:76-85.
63. Hopf S, Hartmann-Wiesner E, Kuhlmorgen B, Mayer S. The behavioral repertoire of the squirrel monkey (*Saimiri*). Folia Primatol 1974; 21:225-249.
64. Maurus M, Kuhlmorgen B, Hartmann-Wiesner E, Pruscha H. An approach to the interpretation of the communicative meaning of visual signals in agonistic behavior of squirrel monkeys. Folia Primatol 1975; 23:208-226.
65. Moynihan M. The New World primates: adaptive radiation and the evolution of social behavior, languages, and intelligence. Princeton: Princeton University Press, 1976.
66. Coe CL, Smith ER, Levine S. The endocrine system of the squirrel monkey. In: Rosenblum LA, Coe CL. Handbook of squirrel monkey research. New York: Plenum Press, 1985: 191-218.
67. Castell R. Communication during initial contact: a comparison of squirrel and rhesus monkeys. Folia Primatol 1969; 11:206-214.
68. Bernstein IS. The integration of Rhesus monkeys introduced to a group. Folia Primatol 1964; 2:50-63.
69. Southwick CH. Aggressive behavior of rhesus monkeys in natural and captive groups. In: Garattini S, Sigg EB. Aggressive Behavior. Amsterdam: Excerpta Medica, 1969: 32-43.
70. Teas J, Feldman HA, Richie TH, Taylor HG, Southwick CH. Aggressive behavior in free-ranging rhesus monkeys of Kathmandu, Nepal. Aggress Behav 1982; 8:63-77.
71. Bernstein IS, Ehardt CL. Intragroup agonistic behavior in rhesus monkeys (Macaca mulatta). Int J Primatol 1985; 6:209-226.
72. Altmann SA. A field study of the sociobiology of rhesus monkeys. Ann NY Acad Sci 1962; 102:338-435.
73. Hinde RA, Rowell TE. Communication by postures and facial expressions in the rhesus monkey (Macaca mulatta). Proc Zool Soc (London) 1962; 138:1-21.
74. Sade DS. Determinants of dominance in a group of free-ranging Rhesus monkeys. In: Altmann SA, ed. Social communication among primates. Chicago: University of Chicago, 1967: 99-114.
75. Zumpe D, Michael RP. Dominance index: a simple measure of relative dominance status in primates. Am J Primatol 1986; 10:291-300.
76. Reinhardt V, Reinhardt A, Bercovitch FB, Goy RW. Does intermale mounting function as a dominance demonstration in Rhesus monkeys? Folia Primatol 1986; 47:55-60.

77. Welch BL, Klopfer PH. Endocrine variability as a factor in the regulation of population density. Am Naturalist 1961; 95:256–260.
78. Brain PF. Oral lithium chloride, endocrine function and isolation-induced agonistic behaviour in male albino mice. J Endocr 1972; 55:1–2.
79. Bronson FH, Eleftheriou BE. Relative effects of fighting on bound and unbound corticosterone in mice (29781). Proc Soc Exp Biol Med 1965; 118:146–149.
80. Raab A, Dantzer R, Michaud B, et al. Behavioural, physiological and immunological consequences of social status and aggression in chronically coexisting resident-intruder dyads of male rats. Physiol Behav 1986; 36: 223–228.
81. Barnett SA. Physiological effects of "social stress" in wild rats–I. J Psychosom Res 1958; 3:1–11.
82. Barnett SA, Eaton JC, McCallum HM. Physiological effects of "social stress" in wild rats- II. J Psychosom Res 1960; 4:251–260.
83. Brain PF. Adaptive aspects of hormonal correlates of attack and defence in laboratory mice: a study in ethobiology. In: McConnell PS, Boer GT, Romijn HJ, Van der Poll NE, eds. Progress in brain research: adaptive capabilities of the nervous system. Amsterdam: Elsevier North-Holland Biomedical, 1980: 391–414.
84. Schuurman T. Hormonal correlates of agonistic behavior in adult male rats. In: McConnel PS, Boer GJ, Romijn HJ, Van de Poll NE, eds. Progress in brain research, vol. 53: adaptive capabilities of the nervous system. Amsterdam: Elsevier Biomedical Press, 1980: 415–420.
85. Ely DL, Henry JP. Neuroendocrine response patterns in dominant and subordinate mice. Horm Behav 1978; 10:156–169.
86. Gamal-el-Din LA. Some aspects of adrenomedullary function in relation to agonistic behaviour in the mouse (Mus musculus). Dissertation, Polytechnic of Central London, London, 1978.
87. Hucklebridge FH, Galamal-El-Din L, Brain PF. Social status and the adrenal medulla in the house mouse (Mus musculus, L.). Behav Neural Biol 1981; 33:345–363.
88. Leshner AI. The interaction of experience and neuroendocrine factors in determining behavioral adaptations to aggression. In: McConnell PS, Boer GJ, Romijn HJ, van der Poll NE, Progress in brain research. Adaptive capabilities of the nervous system. Amsterdam: Elsevier/North Holland Biomedical Press, 1980; 427–438.
89. Leshner AI, Moyer JA, Walker WA. Pituitary-adrenocortical activity and avoidance-of-attack in mice. Physiol Behav 1975; 15:689–693.
90. Moyer JA, Leshner AI. Pituitary–adrenal effects on avoidance-of-attack in mice: Separation of the effects of ACTH and corticosterone. Physiol Behav 1976; 17:297–301.
91. Sapolsky RM, Krey LC, McEwen BS. Stress down-regulates corticosterone receptors in a site-specific manner in the brain. Endocrinology 1984; 114: 287–292.

92. Leshner AI, Candland DK. Endocrine effects of grouping and dominance rank in squirrel monkeys. Physiol Behav 1972; 8:441-445.
93. Coe CL, Smith ER, Mendoza SP, Levine S. Varying influence of social status on hormone levels in male squirrel monkeys. In: Kling S, Steklins HD. Hormones, drugs, and social behavior. New York: Spectrum 1983: 7-32.
94. Manogue KR, Leshner AL, Candland DK. Dominance status and adrenocortical reactivity to stress in squirrel monkeys (*Samiri sciureus*). Primates 1975; 16:457-463.
95. Sapolsky RM. The endocrine stress-response and social status in the wild baboon. Horm Behav 1982; 16:279-292.
96. Shively C, Kaplan J. Effects of social factor son adrenal weight and related physiology of *Macaca fascicularis*. Physiol Behav 1984; 33:777-782.
97. McGuire MT, Brammer GL, Raleigh MJ. Resting cortisol levels and the emergence of dominant status among male vervet monkeys. Horm Behav 1986; 20:106-117.
98. Bronson FH, Stetson MH, Stiff ME. Serum FSH and LH in male mice following aggressive and nonaggressive interaction. Physiol Behav 1973; 10:369-372.
99. Sachser N, Prove E. Short-term effects of residence on the testosterone responses to fighting in alpha male guinea pigs. Aggress Behav 1984; 10: 285-292.
100. Barfield RJ, Geyer LA. Sexual behavior: ultrasonic postejaculatory song of the male rat. Science 1972; 176:1349-1350.
101. Maruniak JA, Desjardins C, Bronson FH. Dominant-subordinate relationships in castrated male mice bearing testosterone implants. Am J Physiol 1977; 233:495-499.
102. Leshner AI, Politch JA. Hormonal control of submissiveness in mice: irrelevance of the androgens and relevance of the pituitary-adrenal hormones. Physiol Behav 1979; 22:531-534.
103. Jones RB, Nowell NW. Aversive and aggression-promoting properties of urine from dominant and subordinate male mice. Animal Learning Behav 1973; 1(3):207-210.
104. Coe CL, Mendoza SP, Levine S. Social status constrains the stress response in the squirrel monkey. Physiol Behav 1979; 23:633-638.
105. Perachio AA, Alexander M, The rhesus monkey 1975; 1:382-409.
106. Eberhart JA, Keverne EB, Meller RE. Social influences on plasma testosterone levels in male talapoin monkeys. Horm Behav 1980; 14:247-266.
107. Abbott DH, McNeilly AS, Lunn SF, Hulme MJ, Burden FJ. Inhibition of ovarian function in subordinate female marmoset monkeys (Callithrix jacchus jacchus). J Reprod Fertil 1981; 63:335-345.
108. Adams MR, Kaplan JR, Koritnik DR. Psychosocial influences on ovarian endocrine and ovulatory function in Macaca fascicularis. Physiol Behav 1985; 35:935-940.

109. Kaplan JR, Adams MR, Kortnik DR, Rose JC. Adrenal responsiveness and soical status in intact and ovariectomized *Macaca fascicularis*. Am J Primatol 1986; 11:181–193.

110. Henry JP. The relation of social to biological processes in disease. Soc Sci Med 1982; 16:369–380.

111. Henry JP, Ely DL, Stephens PM. Cardiovascular disease in rodent communities suffering from chronic social disorders. Excerpta Med Int Cong Series 1971; 1477–1488.

112. Henry JP, Stephens PM, Santistebon GA. A model of psychosocial hypertension showing reversibility and progression of cardiovascular complications. Circulation Res 1975; 36:156–164.

113. Miczek KA, Krsiak M. Drug effects on agonstic behavior. In: Thompson T, Dews PB, eds. Advances in behavioral phramcology, vol. 2. Academic Press, New York, 1978.

114. Natelson BH. Neurocardiology. Arch Neurol 1985; 42:176–184.

115. Candland DK, Bryan DC, Nazar BL, Kopf KJ, Sendor M. Squirrel monkey heart rate during formation of status orders. J Comp Physiol Psychol 1970; 70:417–423.

116. Cherkovich GM, Tatoyan SK. Heart rate (radiotelemetrical registration) in macaques and baboons according to dominant-submissive rank in a group. Folia Primatol 1973; 20:265–273.

117. Adams DB, Baccelli G, Mancia G, Zanchetti A. Relation of cardiovascular changes in fighting to emotion and exercise. J Physiol 1971; 212:321–335.

118. Buttner D, Plonait H. Langfristige Messungen der maximalen, mittleren und Ruheherzfrequenzen an Laborratten mittels implantierbarer Telemetriesender. Zentralbl Veterinmcd 1980; 27:269–278.

119. Fokkema DS. Social behavior and blood-pressure (a study of rats). Dissertation, Groningen University, The Netherlands, 1985.

120. Fokkema DS, Smit K, Van der Gugten J, Koolhaas JM. A coherent pattern among social behavior, blood pressure, corticosterone and catecholamine measures in individual male rats. Physiol Behav 1988; 42:485–489.

121. Fokkema DS, Koolhaas JM. Acute and conditioned blood pressure changes in relation to social and psychosocial stimuli in rats. Physiol Behav 1985; 34:33–38.

122. Ely DL. Hypertension, social rank, and aortic arteriosclerosis in CBA/J mice. Physiol. Behav 1981; 26:655–661.

123. Turney TH, Harmsen AG. Splenomegaly and other hematological parameters in the socially dominant mouse. Physiol Behav 1984; 33:559–562.

124. Stoehr W. Longterm heartrate telemetry in small mammals: a comprehensive approach as a prerequisite for valid results. Physiol Behav 1988; 43:567–576.

125. Raab A, Oswald R. Coping with social conflict; impact on the activity of tyrosine hydroxylase in the limbic system and in the adrenals. Physiol Behav 1980:24:387–394.

126. Folkow B. Physiological aspects of primary hypertension. Physiol Rev 1982; 62:347–409.

127. Rona G. Catecholamine cardiotoxicity. J Mol Cell Cardiol 1985; 17:291–306.

128. Sapolsky RM, Mott GE. Social subordinance in wild baboons is associated with suppressed high density lipoprotein-cholesterol concentrations: the possible role of chronic social stress. Endocrinology 1987; 121:1605–1610.

129. Hamm TE Jr, Kaplan JR, Clarkson TB, Bullock BC. Effects of gender and social behavior on the development of coronary artery atherosclerosis in cynomolgus macaques. Atherosclerosis 1983; 48:221–233.

130. Lavielle S, Tassin JP, Thierry AM, et al. Blockade by benzodiazepines of the selective high increase in dopamine turnover induced by stress in mesocortical dopaminergic neurons of the rat. Brain Res 1978; 168:585–594.

131. Thierry AM, Tassin JP, Blank G, Glowinsky G. Topographic and pharmacological study of the mesocortical dopaminergic system. In: Wauquier A, Rolls ET, eds. Brain-stimulation reward. Amsterdam: North Holland, 1976.

132. Mos J, Van Valkenburg CFM. Specific effect on social stress and aggression on regional dopamine metabolism in rat brain. Neurosci Letts 1979; 15:325–327.

133. Eleftheriou BE, Church RL. Brain levels of serotonin and norepinephrine in mice after exposure to aggression and defeat. Physiol Behav 1968; 3:977–980.

134. Hendley ED, Moisset B, Welch BL. Catecholamine uptake in cerebral cortex: adaptive change induced by fighting. Science 1973; 180:1050–1052.

135. Welch B, Hendley ED, Turek I. Norepinephrine uptake into cerebral cortical synaptosomes after one fight or electroconvulsive shock. Science 1974; 183:220–221.

136. Hadfield MG, Milio C. Isolation-induced fighting in mice and regional brain monoamine utilization. Behav Brain Res 1988; 31:93–96.

137. Hadfield MG, Rigby WFC. Dopamine-adaptive uptake changes in striatal synaptosomes after 30 seconds of shock-induced fighting. Biochem Pharmacol 1976; 25:2752–2754.

138. Tizabi Y, Massari VJ, Jacobowitz DM. Isolation induced aggression and catecholamine variations in discrete brain areas of the mouse. Brain Res Bull 1980; 5:81–86.

139. Haney M, Noda K, Kream R, Miczek KA. Regional 5HT and dopamine activity: Sensitivity to amphetamine and aggressive behavior in mice. Aggress Behav 1990; in press.

140. Miczek KA, Donat P. Brain 5-HT systems and inhibitions of aggressive behavior. In: Archer T, Bevan P, Cools A, eds. The behavioural pharmacology of 5-HT. Hillsdale, NJ: Lawrence Erlbaum Associates, 1989: 117.

141. Miczek KA, Mos J, Olivier B. Brain 5-HT and inhibition of aggressive behavior in animals: 5-HIAA and receptor subtypes. Psychopharmacology Bull 1989; 25:

142. Walletschek H, Raab A. Spontaneous activity of dorsal raphe neurons during defensive and offensive encounters in the tree-shrew. Physiol Behav 1982; 28:697–705.
143. Eichelman B. Role of biogenic amines in aggressive behavior. In: Sandler M. Psychopharmacology of aggression. New York: Raven Press, 1979: 61–93.
144. Prasad V, Sheard MH. Time course of chronic desipramine on shock-elicited fighting in rats. Agressologie 1983; 24:15–17.
145. Pucilowski O, Kostowski W. Aggressive behaviour and the central serotonergic systems. Behav Brain Res 1983; 9:33–48.
146. Miczek KA, Thompson ML. Shuster L. Naloxone injections into periaqueductal grey area and arcuate nucleus block analgesia in defeated mice. Psychopharmacology 1985; 87:39–42.
147. Miczek KA, Thompson ML, Shuster L. Analgesia following defeat in an aggressive encounter: development of tolerance and changes in opioid receptors. Ann NY Acad Sci 1986; 467:14–29.
148. Külling P, Frischknecht H-R,Pasi A, Waser PG, Siegfried B. Social conflict-induced changes in nociception and β-endorphin-like immunoreactivity in pituitary and discrete brain areas of C57BL/6 and DBA/2 mice. Brain Res 1988; 450:237–246.
149. Thompson ML, Brunner E, Hoefler H, et al. Changes in opioid receptor binding and levels of opioid peptides in the brain following acute and chronic defeat in mice. Soc Neurosci Abstr 1986; 12:411.
150. Teskey GC, Kavaliers M, Hirst M. Social conflict activates opioid analgesic and ingestive behaviors in male mice. Life Sci 1984; 35:303–315.
151. Siegried B, Frischknecht H-R, Waser PG. Defeat, learned submissiveness, and analgesia in mice: effect of genotype. Behav Neural Biol 1984; 42:91–97.
152. Rodgers RJ, Randall JI. Social conflict analgesia: studies on naloxone antagonism and morphine cross-tolerance in male DBA/2 mice. Pharmacol Biochem Behav 1985; 23:883–887.
153. Trullas R, Havoundjian H, Zamir N, Paul S, Skolnick P. Environmentally-induced modification of the benzodiazepine/GABA receptor coupled chloride ionophore. Psychopharmacology 1987; 91:384–390.
154. Havoundjian H, Paul SM, Skolnick R. Rapid, stress-induced modifications of the benzodiazepine receptor-coupled chloride ionophore. Brain Res 1986; 375:401–408.
155. File SE, Tucker JC. Lorazepam treatment in the neonatal rat alters submissive behavior in adulthood. Neurobehav Toxicol Teratol 1983; 5:280–294.
156. Miller LG, Thompson ML, Greenblatt DJ, Deutsch SI, Shader RI, Paul SM. Rapid increase in brain benzodiazepine receptor binding following defeat stress in mice. Brain Res 1987; 414:395–400.
157. Miczek KA, Barry H III. Effects of alcohol on attack and defensive-submissive reactions in rats. Psychopharmacology 1977; 52:231–237.

158. Miczek KA, O'Donnell JM. Intruder-evoked aggression in isolated and nonisolated mice: effects of psychomotor stimulants and l-dopa. Psychopharmacology 1978; 57:47–55.

159. Miczek KA, Gold LH. d-Amphetamine in squirrel monkeys of different social status: effects on social and agonistic behavior, locomotion, and stereotypies. Psychopharmacology 1983; 81:183–190.

160. Panksepp J. Brain opioids—a neurochemical substrate for narcotic and social dependence. In: Cooper SJ, ed. Theory in psychopharmacology. London, Academic Press, 1981: 149–175.

161. Donat P, Miczek KA. Time dependent hyper- and hyposensitivity to morphine analgesia after defeat in mice. Psychopharmacology 1988; 96:S17 (abstr).

162. Appelbaum BD, Holtzman SG. Characterization of stress-induced potentiation of opioid effects in the rat. J Pharmacol Exp Ther 1984; 231:555–565.

163. Appelbaum BD, Holtzman SG. Restraint stress enhances morphine-induced analgesia in the rat without changing apparent affinity of receptor. Life Sci 1985; 36:1069–1074.

164. Appelbaum BD, Holtzman SG. Stress-induced changes in the analgesic and thermic effects of opioid peptides in the rat. Brain Res. 1986; 377:330–336.

165. Adams JU, Andrews JS, Hiller JM, Simon EJ, Holtzman SG. Effects of stress and β-funaltrexamine pretreatment on morphine analgesia and opioid binding in rats. Life Sci 1987; 41:2835–2844.

166. Miczek KA, Thompson ML. Analgesia resulting from defeat in a social confrontation: the role of endogenous opioids in brain. In: Bandler R, ed. Modulation of sensorimotor activity during altered behavioural states. New York: Alan R. Liss, 1984: 431–456.

167. Miczek KA, Winslow JT. Analgesia and decrement in operant performance in socially defeated mice: selective cross-tolerance to morphine and antagonism by naltrexone. Psychopharmacology 1987; 92:444–451.

168. Miczek KA. Long-lasting functionally specific tolerance to μ and κ opioid agonists after brief social defeat: analgesia, hypothermia and suppression of operant performance. Psychopharmacology

169. Kalant H, LeBlanc AE, Gibbins RJ. Tolerance to, and dependence on, some non-opiate psychotropic drugs. Pharmacol Rev 1971; 23:135–191.

170. Wenger GR. Cumulative dose-response curves in behavioral pharmacology. Pharmacol Biochem Behav 1980; 13:647–651.

171. Glowinski J, Iversen LL. Regional studies of catecholamines in the rat brain. I. The disposition of [^{3}H]norepinephrine, [^{3}H]dopamine, and [^{3}H]DOPA in various regions of the brain. J Neurochem 1966; 13:655–669.

172. Pert CB, Snyder SH. Identification of opiate receptor binding in intact animals. Life Sci 1975; 16:1623–1634.

17

DEFENSIVE BEHAVIOR IN NONHUMAN PRIMATES

Ned H. Kalin

William S. Middleton Memorial VA Hospital, Madison, Wisconsin

Defensive behaviors are motivated by fear and they protect organisms from dangerous situations. These behaviors have been well characterized in numerous species. Their expression depends on the specific elements of the threatening situation. Activation of these behaviors is almost always associated with autonomic and endocrinological changes that provide metabolic support for the organism during the period of stress.

To survive, primates must detect potentially dangerous situations and then activate the appropriate protective behaviors. Studying primates' defensive behaviors leads to an understanding of both adaptive and maladaptive responses to stressful situations. Intense fearfulness or activation of defensive behaviors inappropriate to the environmental context can result in behavioral, social, and physiological dysfunction, and therefore may have particular relevance to understanding the development of neuropsychiatric illnesses.

This chapter will focus on the expression and regulation of defensive behaviors in the Rhesus monkey. The Rhesus monkey is of interest because, like humans, it is a highly social primate and its survival depends on other members of its group. Disruption of important relationships or separation from the group is frequently associated with fearfulness and distress, and may make a primate more vulnerable to predators.

RESPONSE TO BRIEF SEPARATION

Infant Rhesus monkeys briefly separated from their mothers undergo a dramatic behavioral and physiological response characterized by autonomic and pituitary-adrenal activation, increased vocalizations, and behavioral agitation (1-4). The "coo" is the most frequent vocalization emitted by infant Rhesus monkeys after maternal separation. A coo is produced by rounding and pursing the lips and is characterized by an increase followed by a decrease in pitch and intensity (Fig. 1). This vocalization probably alerts the mother to the separated infant, facilitating its retrieval. Increases in plasma concentrations of adrenocorticotropic hormone (ACTH) and cortisol, but not prolactin, accompany the behavioral activation (Fig. 2; 4).

We initially examined the effects of opiate (4), benzodiazepine (5), and a-2 and β-adrenergic (6) agents on the response of infants to brief maternal separation. In these studies, infants living in dyads with their mothers were removed from their mothers and placed in a cage in another room for 60 min. Behavioral testing was performed by trained observers sitting in the room with the infants. The results demonstrated that opiate systems play a major role in mediating the species-typical coos emitted by the infant monkey when it is separated from its mother. As seen in Figure 3, morphine administered to infants before maternal separation causes a marked reduction in the level of cooing during a 60 min separation. This effect was observed using morphine dosages (0.1 mg/kg) that did not alter other behaviors, including the infants' amount of locomotor behavior. This indicates that the effect of morphine was not due to sedation.

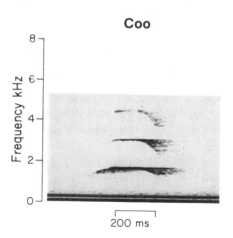

FIGURE 1 Sonogram of a typical coo emitted by an infant Rhesus monkey separated from its mother.

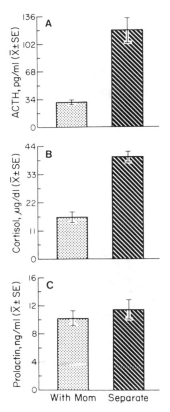

FIGURE 2 Plasma concentrations of (A) ACTH, (B) cortisol, and (C) prolactin in eight Rhesus monkeys with their mothers (stippled bars) and separated from their mothers for 60-75 min (striped bars). *p <0.005 (reprinted from ref. 4 with permission from the publisher).

Naloxone had the opposite effect. Naloxone (1.0 mg/kg) increased the number of coos emitted by separated infants. Lower dosages of naloxone administered alone were without effect. Figure 4 supports the contention that the coo-reducing effects of morphine are mediated through opiate receptors, since dosages of naloxone (0.1 mg/kg) that did not have intrinsic effects blocked the effect of morphine (4).

Benzodiazepine and α-2 and β-adrenergic agents also affected the infants' level of distress vocalizations. However, these effects do not appear to be mediated by specific receptor systems. For example, diazepam reduced infants' level of distress vocalizations, but this effect was not blocked by pretreating the

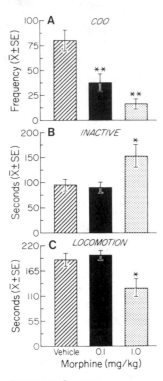

FIGURE 3 Effects of morphine on separation-induced behaviors in eight infant Rhesus monkcys. *p <0.05; **p <0.01 (reprinted from ref. 4 with permission of the publisher).

infants with the benzodiazepine antagonist Ro-15788. The same dosage of Ro-15788 did block the diazepam-induced increase in activity levels (5).

Corticotropin-releasing hormone (CRH) (0.5–10 μg) administered either peripherally or ICV was without significant effect on the infants' level of cooing. ICV dosages less than 10 μg were without any behavioral effect. However, 10 μg inhibited behavior while increasing plasma concentrations of ACTH and cortisol. The behavioral inhibition did not appear to be secondary to nonspecific sedation and might be related to increased fearfulness (7).

In summary, separation-induced cooing is an adaptive response in infant Rhesus monkeys separated from their mothers. In the wild, it is likely that the infant's cooing signals its location, facilitating retrieval by its mother. Our findings demonstrate that the expression of this response is regulated by brain opiate systems. Studies have been performed in other species and are consistent with our results (8,9). MacLean (10) has hypothesized that in mammals the anterior cingulate cortex mediates behaviors associated with attachment and parenting. It is therefore of interest that this region has a high density of μ-opiate receptors (11). Studies examining the function of the anterior cingulate cortex in nonhuman primates show that electrical stimulation of this area selectively elicits coo vocalizations (12). Primates with anterior cingulate lesions are unable to coo but are capable of producing other types of vocalizations (13,14).

RESPONSE TO THREAT

To study other types of defensive behaviors, we capitalized on observations made during our first brief separation studies. In these early experiments we noticed that the behavior of infants tested in the absence of their mothers was affected by the presence of the observers. Some observers had a greater effect than others; what appeared to be important was whether the observer spent time staring directly at the infant. This is of interest because in primates eyes are extremely important in conveying and receiving nonverbal social signals. For example, intense eye contact is frequently associated with aggression and, depending on the situation, may either predict or prevent an attack.

We therefore designed an experiment to characterize the effect of a human "intruder" on the infants' response (15). In these studies, the trained observer did not sit in the room with the infants. Instead, behavior was recorded on videotape for rating at a later time. Infant monkeys were tested twice, with 1

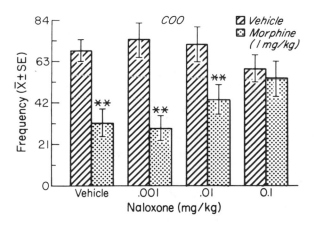

FIGURE 4 Effects of naloxone administered before morphine on separation-induced coos in eight infant monkeys. **Indicates significant difference ($p <$ 0.01) between morphine treatment and vehicle at the same dosage of naloxone (reprinted from ref. 4 with permission of the publisher).

week between tests. During the first test the infant was separated from its mother and placed in a cage in a different room. The infant remained alone (A1) for 10 min, after which a human entered the room and stood 2.5 m from the cage, presenting the profile of his face to the infant while gazing at the wall. This "no eye contact" (NEC) period lasted 10 min. It was followed by another 10 min during which the infant remained alone (A2). A similar test was conducted 1 week later, but during this test when the human entered the room he faced the monkey and stared at it continuously (ST). The infant's behavior during the 10 min exposure to each test condition was videotaped and scored from the videotape in 3 min epochs by expert observers.

The human intruder had dramatic effects on the infants' behavior, and these clearly depended on the direction of the human's gaze (Fig. 5). When the infants were alone they emitted numerous coos and were very active. In the ST condition the infants vocalized even more, with "barking" and an increased frequency of coos. Barks are brief, low-pitched, rasping vocalizations produced with the mouth slightly open while the abdominal musculature forces air through the vocal cords (Fig. 6). Barks are frequently assoociated with threat or used as a warning (16). They are of particular interest because they rarely occurred in the A and NEC conditions. This result confirmed our undocumented impressions of the effects our behavioral raters produced when they stared at the monkeys.

The behaviors observed during the NEC period were unexpected. In this condition we found that the infants became behaviorally inhibited to the extent of actually "freezing" in one position. There was considerable variability in how long each animal froze; some animals remained motionless for the entire 10 min period. After freezing, the animal remained crouched in the same position. Finally it would begin to move using a slow and deliberate gait, its face constantly oriented to the intruder. It eventually resumed its normal gait, moved freely about the cage, and began to coo.

These effects could have been due to an idiosyncratic response to the particular male intruder we used. We therefore repeated the experiment with a female intruder. The results were identical (unpublished data). We also used videotape presentations of profile and frontal views of a human face and obtained results similar to those elicited by actual presence of the intruder (unpublished data). These findings demonstrated that the salient cue is the direction of the human's gaze, and the effects are not due to affective interactions between the human and the infant monkey.

Thus the infant Rhesus monkey changes its pattern of defensive behavior according to its perception of the environment. When alone, the adaptive response is to call for its mother. However, when the infant is separated from its mother and a threat is perceived, it responds differently. The characteristic behavior elicited by NEC was freezing. This is a common response to threatening conditions. and in an animal's natural environment it may reduce the likelihood of detection and/or attack by a predator (17,18). Barking is frequently

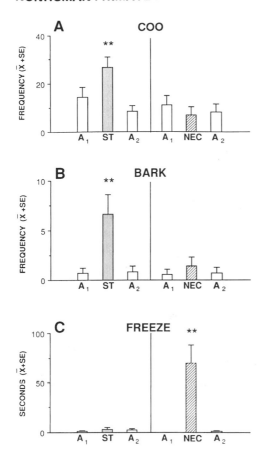

FIGURE 5 Behavioral response (mean ± SD of three 3 min epochs) of 11 infant Rhesus monkeys 6–11 months old to (A1 and A2) brief separation from their mothers, (ST) a human entering and staring at the infant, and (NEC) a human entering and avoiding eye contact with the infant. **p <0.01 (reprinted from ref. 15 with permission of the publisher).

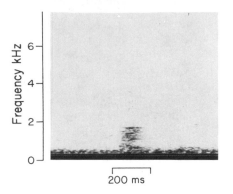

FIGURE 6 Sonogram of a typical bark emitted by an infant Rhesus monkey during brief maternal separation.

associated with aggression and was specific to the ST condition. In many species, aggressive displays occur when retreat is impossible, and such behavior frequently discourages the attacker.

NEUROBIOLOGICAL MECHANISMS UNDERLYING BEHAVIORS INDUCED BY THREAT

We performed neuropharmacological experiments to establish which neurobiological systems regulate the expression of these defensive behaviors. As before, infant monkeys were separated from their mothers and their behavior was videotaped in the A1, NEC, ST, and A2 conditions. This time, however, various pharmacological agents were administered and their effects were compared to the effects of vehicle in the same animals. As in our earlier study, CRH did not affect the frequency of coos. Compared to vehicle, ICV-administered CRH (7 μg) reduced locomotion on both test days; when the infants were exposed to the NEC condition, ICV CRH significantly increased the time spent freezing (with vehicle, 34.2 ± 7.7 s; with CRH, 53.3 ± 12.0 s; p <.03). It is important that CRH did not induce freezing on the day the monkeys were exposed to the ST condition.

a-Helical CRH (9–41) is a specific antagonist that binds to the CRH receptor. We tested the CRH antagonist to see if it would attenuate the freezing induced by the NEC condition. However, it had only weak and inconsistent effects (unpublished data). This could be due in part to the relatively low doses we used, because a-helical CRH (9–41) is not very potent.

To study the involvement of the opiate and benzodiazepine systems, we modified the test paradigm so that the monkeys were exposed to ST and NEC conditions on the same day (15). Infants were separated from their mothers and left alone for 10 min (A1). This was followed by successive 10 min exposures to NEC, ST, and alone (A2). The intruder induced the same effects as in the earlier studies, except that now we were able to observe the infants rapidly changing their defensive responses as the environmental stimuli changed. Morphine (0.1 mg/kg) selectively reduced the frequency of coos without affecting the frequency of ST-induced barking or the duration of NEC-induced freezing. Naloxone (1 mg/kg) increased coos, but like morphine, it had no effect on the other behaviors (Fig. 7).

The effects of diazepam (1.0 mg/kg) were quite different from those of morphine. Diazepam did not significantly reduce cooing but markedly decreased the infants' amount of barking during the ST condition. It also attenuated the effects of NEC, reducing the amount of time spent freezing and crouching (Fig. 8).

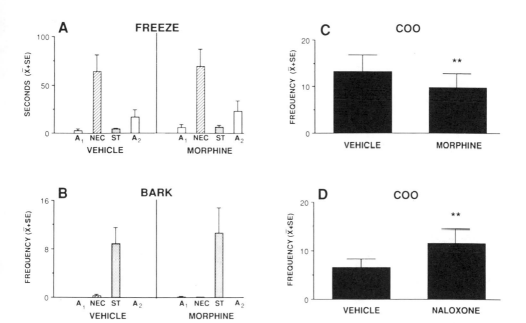

FIGURE 7 Effects of opiate system alterations on defensive behaviors in 12 infant rhesus monkeys. A, B. Effects of the NEC conditions on freezing and the ST condition on barking (mean ± SE). Neither morphine (0.2 mg/kg) nor naloxone (1.0 mg/kg) significantly affected these behaviors. C, D. Main effects of one drug or the other on the frequency of coos (mean ± SE) emitted across all test conditions. Morphine reduced the frequency of coos, whereas naloxone increased their frequency. Mean ± SE; **p <0.01 (reprinted from ref. 15 with permission of the publisher).

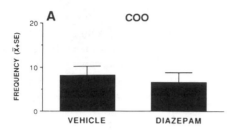

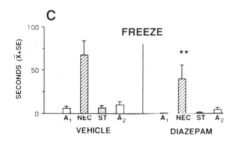

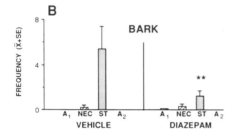

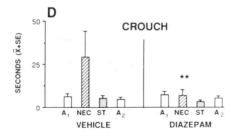

FIGURE 8   Effects of diazepam (1 mg/kg) on defensive behaviors. The effects of diazepam were quite different from those of morphine and naloxone. Diazepam had no statistically significant effect on (A) coos but significantly reduced the frequency of (B) barks under ST conditions. Diazepam also significantly reduced behaviors elicited by the NEC condition: (C) freezing and (D) crouching. Mean ± SE; **p <0.01 (reprinted from ref. 15 with permission of the publisher).

These studies demonstrate that different defensive behaviors are controlled by different neurotransmitter systems and that it is not merely the animal's level of arousal that is important in mediating these responses. If manipulations of the opiate system produced their effects simply by changing the level of arousal, barking and freezing would decrease with morphine and increase with naloxone. The selective effects seen with CRH and diazepam would also not be expected.

ONTOGENY OF THE PRIMATE'S DEFENSIVE BEHAVIORS AND RELATIONSHIP TO PSYCHOPATHOLOGY

Fear-related behaviors are expressed early in life and are adaptive in the appropriate context. For example, human and other primate infants have a period when they are excessively fearful, exhibiting behavioral inhibition associated with physiological arousal when exposed to strangers (1,5). The ontogeny and expression of these behaviors appear to be controlled genetically (19). Through development, the circumstances that elicit this response become more specific as the infant acquires a refined and more accurate understanding of what constitutes danger. The emergence of fear-related behaviors in Rhesus monkey and human infants is linked to development of the affectional system between infant and mother. Harlow (20) described developmental stages in the Rhesus infant that, although they appear at an earlier age, are similar for human infants. Other studies suggest that very young Rhesus infants have innate undifferentiated fear responses that peak between the ages of 2 and 4 months (21). However, these studies were performed in only a few animals, the infants had had prior experience with fearful stimuli, and the investigators did not consider whether the infants were capable of activating the behavioral repertoire best suited to the threat.

We have recently completed a study of the development of the infant monkey's responses to a human intruder. We compared the responses of infants 0-2 weeks old with those of infants 9-12 weeks old. Each infant remained with its mother until the study was performed, and thus had no prior experience with the paradigm. At the appropriate age, infants were separated from their mothers and tested in the A1, NEC, ST, A2 sequence described above. Immediately after separation, during the A1 period, the younger infants emitted significantly more coos than the older infants. The animal's age, however, did not seem to influence the number of barks it emitted. Younger monkeys engaged in very little freezing under the NEC condition. In contrast, the 9-12-week-old infants responded to NEC by freezing for long period of time (unpublished data).

We also examined whether a Rhesus infant's tendency to freeze is a stable characteristic (15). We tested 12 infants 5-7 months old twice in the NEC condition, with 1 month between tests. There was a strong linear relation between the amount of freezing in the two tests (slope ± SE = 1.06 ± 0.11) (Fig. 9). We continued to evaluate eight of these animals and found that the relation pesisted 5.5 months later, even after eight intervening experiences with the paradigm (slope ± SE = 0.91 ± 0.22).

Individual differences in fear-related behavior (e.g., shyness or behavioral inhibition) in 2-year-old humans are highly correlated with fear-related behavior at 7 years of age and are associated with a child's level of autonomic arousal and pituitary-adrenal activation (22). Human infants rated as extremely behaviorally inhibited become, at 7 years of age, children with pathological fears. Suomi has reported similar findings in the behavioral development of Rhesus monkeys (2). Furthermore, children of parents with panic disorder and agoraphobia exhibit significantly more behavioral inhibition when exposed to novelty than do age-matched controls (23). Our observations in the rhesus infant are consistent with our understanding of human development. The marked increase in freezing at 9–12 weeks may be analagous to the onset of "stranger anxiety" in human infants that occurs between 7 and 9 months. This suggests that in primates fearfulness is a stable trait that originates early in life and may predispose to, or be a marker for, psychopathological conditions in adult life.

SUMMARY

We have characterized defensive behaviors in Rhesus monkeys and investigated environmental factors that elicit them. These behaviors are induced by stressful

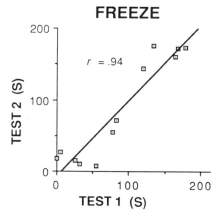

FIGURE 9 Relation between amounts of freezing elicited by identical conditions in two tests performed 1 month apart (y = –5.7 + 1.05x; SE of the slope = 0.11). Twelve rhesus monkeys 5–7 months old were exposed to a human who maintained a constant distance from them, keeping his gaze averted to avoid eye contact (reprinted from ref. 15 with permission of the publisher).

situations, are accompanied by hypothalamic–pituitary–adrenal activation, and serve to reduce the potential negative consequences of the stress. It is interesting that eye contact is an important cue for the Rhesus monkey in directing its type of defensive response. Because of the social importance of eye contact in humans, it is likely that the meaning of intense eye contact is similar for the two species. The effects of lack of eye contact were unexpected. Lack of eye contact resulted in freezing, a response that appears similar to the behavioral inhibition observed in children exposed to threatening situations. As in humans, the onset of behavioral inhibition in the infant Rhesus follows a developmental time course: by the time they are 12 weeks old the infants selectively respond to the NEC condition by freezing. While freezing is induced by the NEC condition (a state-related change), we have also shown that each animal's tendency to freeze remains stable over time. Our neuropharmacological studies suggest that the different defensive behaviors displayed by the Rhesus infant are under the control of different neurotransmitters. The opiate system is very much involved in behaviors motivated by disruption of attachment bonds, whereas CRH and benzodiazepine systems regulate those behaviors induced by threat.

Studies of the neurobiological changes underlying the emergence of fearfulness in infant Rhesus monkeys can provide important insights into the striking individual differences in this trait that occur in all primates, human and nonhuman. These differences may be mediated by opiate, CRH, and benzodiazepine systems and may contribute to the development of psychopathological conditions characterized by excessive or inappropriate fear responses.

ACKNOWLEDGMENT

This work was supported by the Medical Research Service, Department of Veterans Affairs, and grant No. AM-35641 from the National Institutes of Health. The author acknowledges the technical assistance of S. Shelton, H. Van Valkenberger, and K. Renk and the editorial assitance of C. Stcinhart.

REFERENCES

1. Harlow HF, Zimmermann RR Affectional responses in the infant monkey. Science 1959; 130:421–432.
2. Suomi SJ. Genetic and maternal contributions to individual differences in rhesus monkey biobehavioral development. In: Krasnegor N, Blass E, Hofer M, Smotherman W, eds. Perinatal development: a psychobiological perspective. Orlando, FL: Academic Press, 1987: 397–420.
3. Reite M, Short RA. Nocturnal sleep in separated monkey infants. Arch Gen Psychiatry 1978; 35:1247–1253.
4. Kalin NH, Shelton SE, Barksdale CM. Opiate modulation of separation-induced distress in non-human primates. Brain Res 1988; 440:285–292.

5. Kalin NH, Shelton SE, Barksdale CM. Separation distress in infant rhesus monkeys: effects of diazepam and Ro 15-1788. Brain Res 1987; 408:192–198.

6. Kalin NH, Shelton SE. Effects of clonidine and propranolol on separation-induced distress in infant rhesus monkeys. Dev Brain Res 1988; 42:289–195.

7. Kalin NH, Shelton SE, Barksdale CM. Behavioral and physiological effects of CRH administered to infant primates undergoing maternal separation. Neuropsychopharmacology 1989; 2:97–104.

8. Panksepp J, Herman B, Conner R, Bishop P, Scott JP. The biology of social attachments: opiates alleviate separation distress. Biol Psychiatry 1976; 13:607–618.

9. Blass EM, Kehoe P. Behavioral characteristics of emerging opioid systems in newborn rats. In: Krasnegor N, Blass E, Hofer M, Smotherman W, eds. Perinatal development: a psychobiological perspective. Academic Press: Orlando, FL, 1987: 61–84.

10. MacLean PD. Culminating developments in the evolution of the limbic system: the thalamocingulate division. In: Doane BK, Livingston KE, eds. The limbic system: functional organization and clinical disorders. New York: Raven Press, 1986; 1–29.

11. Wise SP, Herkenham M. Opiate receptor distribution in the cerebral cortex of the rhesus monkey. Science 1982; 218:387–389.

12. Robinson BW. Vocalization evoked from forebrain in *Macaca mulatta*. Physiol Behav 1967; 2:345–354.

13. Sutton D, Larson C, Lindeman RC. Neocortical and limbic lesion effects on primate phonation. Brain Res 1974; 71:61–75.

14. MacLean PD, Newman JD. Role of frontolimbic cortex in production of the isolation call of squirrel monkeys. Brain Res 1988; 450: 111–123.

15. Kalin NH, Shelton SE. Defensive behaviors in infant rhesus monkeys; environmental cues and neurochemical regulation. Science 1989; 243: 1718–1721.

16. Rowell TE, Hinde RA. Vocal communication by the rhesus monkey (*Macaca mulatta*). Proc Zool Soc London 1962; 138:279–294.

17. Bolles RC. Species-specific defense reactions and avoidance learning. Psychol Rev 1970; 77:32–48.

18. Gallup GG Jr, Suares SD. An ethological analysis of open-field behavior in chickens. Anim Behav 1980; 28:368–378.

19. Plomin R, Rowe DC. Genetic and environmental etiology of social behavior in infancy. Dev Psychol 1979; 15:62–72.

20. Harlow HF. Development of affection in primates. In: Bliss EL, ed. Roots of behavior. New York: Harper, 1962: 157–166.

21. Sackett GP. Monkeys reared in isolation with pictures as visual input: evidence of an innate releasing mechanism. Science 1966; 154:1468–1473.

22. Kagan J, Reznick JS, Snidman S. Biological bases of childhood shyness. Science 1988; 240:167–171.

23. Rosenbaum JF, Biderman J, Gersten M, et al. Behavioral inhibition in children of parents with panic disorder and agoraphobia. Arch Gen Psychiatry 1988; 45:463–470.

18

STRESS-ASSOCIATED PSYCHIATRIC DISORDERS
Focus on the Role of Neuropeptides

James C. Pryor
Vanderbilt University School of Medicine, Nashville, Tennessee

Charles B. Nemeroff
Duke University Medical Center, Durham, North Carolina

The depressive temperament is characterized by a permanent gloomy emotional stress in all the experiences of life.

Emil Kraeplin

INTRODUCTION AND BACKGROUND

Since the early days of disease description, observers have tried to correlate a person's mood state with a disruption in body chemistry. The term *melancholia*, for example, contributed to the notions of black bile, and early physicians prescribed the letting of this substance for melancholic patients with the idea that an overabundance of black bile caused their dark, depressed moods. Today, the term *melancholia* is still used to describe one severe form of affective disorder, although we know bile has little to do with the pathogenesis of depression. Yet an overabundance or deficiency of a substance or substances in the brain may well be related to certain psychiatric disorders. As the title of this volume suggests, the experience of stress by an organism has measurable and reproducible effects on the chemistry of the brain, especially the neuroendocrine system. Since clinical and experimental evidence has shown reproducible alterations in neuroendocrine systems in affective disorders, and because many of these same systems are altered by stress, this chapter will discuss the relationship between stress, neuropeptides, and neuroendocrine alterations and psychiatric disorders.

In the past 30 years a number of neurotransmitters have been identified in the mammalian central nervous system. Much attention has been focused on the monoamine transmitters norepinephrine, dopamine, and serotonin, and their relevance to the present subject matter is discussed in the chapter by Veith in this volume. Increasing attention has recently been paid to the neuropeptide neurotransmitters such as somatostatin (SRIF), corticotropin-releasing factor (CRF), and thyrotropin-releasing hormone (TRH). There is considerable evidence that neurons containing these peptidergic neurotransmitters are altered in patients with neuropsychiatric disorders including depression. This is the subject matter of this review. It should be recognized, however, that there is much interaction between peptidergic and monoaminergic neurons, including documented examples of colocalization within the same neuron and peptidergic innervation of monoamine neurons as well as the converse.

The neuropeptides CRF, TRH, and SRIF were all discovered within the past 20 years. They were first described as hypothalamic hypophysiotrophic hormones, that is, modulators of anterior pituitary hormone release. Thus CRF stimulates the synthesis and secretion of adrenocorticotropin (ACTH), TRH has similar effects on thyroid-stimulating hormones (TSH), and SRIF inhibits the release of growth hormone and a variety of other adenohypophysial hormones. However, these peptides were quickly found to have a wide distribution in brain regions that apparently had little to do with anterior pituitary function. This neuroanatomical evidence led to a study of their roles as neuromodulators and neurotransmitters in higher central nervous system (CNS) centers.

We will begin with a discussion of CRF and its relation to stress and psychiatric disease. This will be followed by a description of TRH and somatostatin in relation to affective disorder and we shall finish with a discussion of the possible interactions of these chemical messengers in human disease states.

CRF

Introduction to the Hypothalamic–Pituitary–Adrenal Axis and CRF

The cephalic representation of the hypothalamic–pituitary–adrenal (HPA) axis is CRF by virtue of its role as the hypothalamic releasing factor controlling ACTH secretion. CRF neurons appear to make up one of the major systems that mediate an organism's response to stress. The HPA axis is one of the major transducers between one's perception of a stressful event and the body's physiological response to it (1,2). In rodents and primates, stress is well known to be associated with a rise in circulating plasma concentrations of glucocorticoids produced in the adrenal cortex. These hormones (corticosterone in rats, cortisol in primates) then produce physiological changes that help prepare the body for acute emergencies (i.e., the flight or fight response). However, since these are catabolic hormones, prolonged exposure is detrimental, resulting in multisystem pathological conditions in chronically stressed animals (3).

Glucocorticoid secretion is, of course, primarily stimulated by circulating ACTH, a hormone released from anterior pituitary corticotrophs. ACTH release from these cells is stimulated by CRF (4), which is found in highest concentration in nerve terminals in the median eminence (ME) where they secrete directly into the hypothalamopituitary portal system (5–7).

CRF Identification and Localization

Other substances have been shown to increase ACTH secretion including vasopressin, endorphins, vasoactive-intestinal peptide (VIP), angiotensin II, and norepinephrine (8–10). The presence of these "CRFs" rendered the purification of CRF difficult, as did problems with the ACTH radioimmunoassay. It was not until 1981, 25 years after physiological activity was discovered by Saffran and Schally (11), that Vale and his colleagues (12) reported on the elucidation of the structure of CRF isolated from an extract of 490,000 sheep hypothalami. In addition to its presence in the hypothalamus, CRF has been demonstrated in several extrahypothalamic regions of the rodent and primate brain. CRF is a 41 amino acid polypeptide found in all species studied thus far; its amino acid sequence is highly conserved between species, with substitutions being clearly homologous (4). Antibodies to CRF have been raised in animals, thus providing a powerful tool to localize CRF accurately in the nervous system through immunohistochemical techniques. As expected, there is a large concentration of these cells in the parvocellular division of the paraventricular nucleus (PVN) of the hypothalamus that projects to the median eminence (5–7,13,14); these are believed to mediate the hypophysiotrophic action of the peptide. Another group of CRF-positive-staining cells is found in the central and medial nuclei of the amygdala, which project to the hypothalamus, bed nucleus of the stria terminalis, and the parabrachial nuclei (15,16). There are also wider projections to the cerebral cortex, and also to the locus ceruleus (LC) (7), which is the site of the A_6 norepinephrine-containing cell bodies that project to the forebrain (17).

Using a specific and sensitive radioimmunoassay (RIA) for CRF coupled with the micropunch dissection technique of Palkovits, our group (18) measured the concentration of CRF in 32 different brain nuclei of the rat. As would be predicted, the highest concentrations of the peptide were found in the ME. Measurable amounts of CRF were found in all areas studied, however. These included the substantia nigra (site of the A_9 dopamine cell bodies), the raphe nuclei (site of the origin of a major serotonergic pathway), and the locus ceruleus. Thus it appears that CRF is linked to the major monoamine perikarya in the CNS.

Other experimental work consistent with the view that CRF is a neurotransmitter in the CNS has documented its calcium-dependent release from brain slices by depolarizing concentrations of potassium (19), potent effects on the firing rate of CNS neurons (e.g., LC neurons) (20); preferential synaptosomal localization after density gradient centrifugation (4); and high-affinity binding sites for CRF that are heterogeneously distributed throughout the brain (21).

CRF and Stress: Experimental Studies

The demonstration that hypothalamic CRF is secreted when mammals are exposed to stress has been reported in a number of studies. For example, Vale and colleagues (22) reported that the loss of 15% of total blood volume (hemorrhage stress) in the rat caused a 10-fold rise in plasma ACTH concentration. At the same time, CRF concentrations in pituitary portal blood doubled compared to nonstressed conditions. Others have noted that immunoneutralization of CRF can block the rise in rat plasma ACTH concentrations in response to stressful stimuli (23).

To delineate further the stress-associated change in CRF neurons in the rat brain, our group (18) measured the concentration of the peptide in 36 different brain nuclei using the Palkovits micropunch technique after rats were exposed to either acute or chronic unpredictable stress. The acute stress (3 h of cold immobilization) decreased the concentration of CRF in the median eminence/arcuate nucleus (ME/ARC) by 52%. This decrease was associated with an increase in both plasma ACTH and corticosterone concentrations. This finding is consistent with the sequence of release of prepackaged CRF from the nerve terminals of the ME to the pituitary portal capillary system; vascular transport to the anterior pituitary corticotrophs, with subsequent release of ACTH; transport of ACTH in the general circulation to the adrenal cortex with release of glucocorticosteroids. A consistent decrease in CRF concentrations after acute stress was also noted in the median preoptic nucleus, an area that has been found both to contain a high density of CRF cell bodies (24) and to be implicated in the stress response (25). A perhaps more intriguing and surprising observation was the marked increase in CRF concentrations in the locus ceruleus after acute stress (a finding recently confirmed by Kalin [personal communication 1988]). As noted above, this area is the origin of a major noradrenergic (A_6) cell group that contributes 70% of the norepinephrine to the forebrain. As discussed elsewhere in this volume, this nucleus has also been implicated in the stress response and in the pathophysiology of affective and anxiety disorders.

The chronic stress paradigm (13 days of daily, unpredictable stress) produced increases in adrenal weight, plasma corticosterone concentrations, and a return of plasma ACTH concentrations to normal levels. Corticosterone concentrations most likely remained elevated despite normal plasma ACTH concentrations because of increased adrenal size so that for each pulse of ACTH, a greater than normal corticosterone response occurred. There were changes in CNS CRF concentrations as well. As with the acute stress group, CRF concentration was also noted in the dorsal vagal complex, consistent with a role for CRF in autonomic nervous system regulation. A dramatic and consistent increase in CRF concentrations was also noted in the LC after chronic stress, again implicating this region in the neurochemical response to stress.

Our group recently (26) reported that the acute administration of two agents effective in the treatment of generalized anxiety disorder, panic disorders, and perhaps depression, adinazolam and alprazolam, but not the tricyclic antidepressant imipramine, produced a decrease in the LC concentration of CRF as well as an increase in hypothalamic CRF concentrations. These effects are the opposite to those of stress. It is tempting to speculate that the LC is a major integration site between peptide and monoamine transmitter systems affected by stress.

Behavioral and Physiological Studies with CRF

When administered directly into the CNS of laboratory animals, CRF produces a number of physiological and behavioral changes similar to the physiological alterations observed in stress and not dissimilar to many of the signs and symptoms of depression and anxiety disorders. When injected intracerebroventricularly (ICV), CRF increases mean arterial pressure, heart rate, oxygen consumption, plasma glucose levels, and catecholamine concentrations (27-30). This collection of responses is similar to the fight or flight response of autonomic arousal, as well as spontaneous (31) or lactate-induced panic attacks (32). ICV administered CRF also produces alterations in locomotor activity (33), a decrease in sexual activity in rats (34,35), reduced food consumption (36,37), increased "emotionality" (33), and sleep disturbances (38).

A review of the *Diagnostic and Statistical Manual*, 3rd edition (revised) (DSM-III-R; 39) reveals that decreased appetite with weight loss, decreased libido, disrupted sleep, and psychomotor activity changes are all diagnostic criteria for major depression. It is difficult to make direct correlations between findings in animal experiments and clinical observations, nevertheless, these preclinical studies do provide evidence that clinical studies of CRF in humans with affective and anxiety disorders are warranted.

CRF and the HPA Axis: Clinical Studies

It is now well established that patients with major depression, especially those with melancholic or psychotic features, demonstrate dysregulation of the HPA axis. Beginning with early observations of a high rate of depression in patients with Cushing's disease (an overproduction of cortisol by the adrenal cortex) (40), depressed patients free of medical disorders were noted to display changes in cortisol secretion (41). These include findings of hypercortisolemia and increased urinary free cortisol excretion (42), a shift or loss of the diurnal variation in plasma cortisol concentrations (43,44), and the finding that approximately 60% of patients hospitalized for treatment of major depression do not display the normal suppression of plasma cortisol secretion after the administration of the long-acting synthetic glucocorticoid dexamethasone, commonly referred to as the dexamethasone suppression test (DST) (45,46). Since glucocorticoids normally act at the pituitary and hypothalamus to regulate their own secretion (through negative feedback loops), this "escape" from the suppression of dexamethasone indicates a dysregulation of the HPA axis. This defect appears primarily to be of central rather than pituitary or adrenal origin (47), although nonsuppression of ACTH after dexamethasone has been observed in depressed patients and there are now several reports of increased adrenocortical sensitivity to ACTH in depressed patients (47-54).

To investigate directly the hypothesis that CRF hypersecretion occurs in depressed patients, our group, in association with Widerlov in Sweden (48), measured CRF concentrations in the cerebrospinal fluid (CSF) of drug-free patients with depression, schizophrenia, or dementia, and in normal controls. A significant elevation in the CSF CRF concentration was found only in the depressed group. There was, however, no correlation between CSF CRF concentrations and baseline or postdexamethasone plasma cortisol concentrations. In a second study with a large group of sex- and age-matched neurological controls, in collaboration with Banki and Arato in Hungary (49), we observed an almost twofold elevation in CSF CRF concentrations in depressed patients compared to controls. In a third study (50), we obtained CSF from suicide victims, depressed patients who died of other means, and sudden death controls. We were able to assay samples of CSF from both cisternal and lumbar regions for CRF concentrations and noted a rostral–caudal gradient for CRF, indicating a supraspinal souce for the peptide. As a group, the depressed patients had marked elevations of CSF CRF concentrations. In a recent study conducted in collaboration with Fink, we demonstrated that the elevation in CSF CRF concentrations is state-dependent. After patients received treatment with electroconvulsive therapy and experienced concomitant clinical recovery, CSF CRF concentrations returned to normal (101).

Another well-documented property of neurotransmitters and hormones is the ability of their cell surface receptors to adjust to a long-term relative abundance or deficiency in the concentration of their ligands. This is the basis for the well-documented phenomenon of receptor up- and downregulation. Thus, if we hypothesize CRF hypersecretion in depression, there should be demonstrable CRF receptor downregulation in depressed patients. Gold and his colleagues (47,51) as well as Holsboer et al. (52,53) have administered CRF intravenously to depressed patients and controls and measured plasma ACTH and adrenocortical response. As a group, the patients with major depression display a blunted

ACTH response to CRF when compared to controls. This indicates either negative feedback on ACTH release due to the hypercortisolemia present in these depressed patients or a CRF receptor downregulation at the corticotroph in response to chronic CRF hypersecretion. Our group has replicated these findings in a group of depressed DST nonsuppressors (Nemeroff, Krishnan, and Carroll, unpublished observations 1988), as well as in patients with posttraumatic stress disorder (54).

To obtain further evidence of CRF hypersecretion in depression, we measured CRF receptor binding in postmortem brain samples from suicide victims and sudden death controls (55). While the binding affinity for CRF was similar for both groups, there was a marked decrease in the number of CRF binding sites in the frontal cortices of suicide victims compared to age- and sex-matched controls (see Figure 1).

Another potential measure of CRF hypersecretion would be to quantify CRF mRNA levels in the postmortem brain tissue of depressed patients and appropriate controls. As yet no data are available in this area.

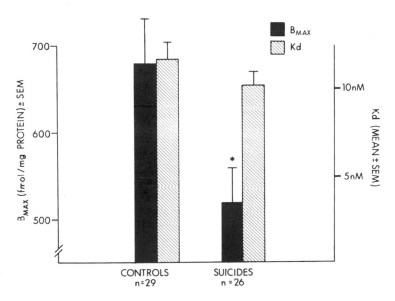

FIGURE 1 Bmax (maxium binding) and K_d (binding affinity) of $[^{125}I]$ Try^0-ovine corticotropin-releasing factor binding sites from frontal cortex of suicide victims and age- and sex-matched sudden death victims. Postmortem interval was 16.4 ± 8.0 h for the suicide group and 16.9 ± 6.3 h for the control group. Binding data were analyzed by Scatchard plots. There was no difference in binding affinity between groups. There was a 23% reduction in Bmax in the suicide group compared to control (* p=0.020 vs. control by Student's t test) (from ref. 100 in the public domain.)

This concatenation of findings supports the hypothesis of CRF hypersecretion during depressive episodes in a subgroup of depressed patients. If we refer back to the chronic stress studies, which noted elevated plasma cortisol levels, an increase in adrenal weight, but normal plasma ACTH concentrations, this may indicate an increased sensitivity of the adrenal cortex to ACTH. Gold and Chrousos (47) described a state of "late" depression due to endogenous CRF hypersecretion that would produce these same findings in humans. In a recent study (56), the adrenal weights from a group of violent suicide victims was compared to that of other sudden death victims. There was significant adrenal hypertrophy in the suicide group compared to the other group. Since 40–60% of suicide victims suffer from depression, it can be argued that a majority of the suicide group was indeed depressed and that the state of depression may have affected the adrenal weights through HPA axis overactivity. Similar conclusions were reached by Amsterdam et al. (57) in a study using computerized tomography to assess adrenal size, and we have made similar observations (Nemeroff, Krishnan, and Dunnik, unpublished observations 1988).

Much experimental work has tried to link stressful life events with depression (58). The above findings in both experimental stress as well as in depressed patients indicate that the HPA axis disruption observed in stress and depression may have some commonalities.

HYPOTHALAMIC–PITUITARY–THYROID AXIS

It is well known that one of the medical disorders associated with major depression is primary hypothyroidism (40,59,60). An interesting corollary to this is the finding of dysregulation of the hypothalamic–pituitary–thyroid (HPT) axis in some patients with affective disorder (59–62). Furthermore, thyroid hormones have been used as adjunctive treatments with tricyclic antidepressants in affective disorder (62).

In contrast, elevation in the circulating concentrations of thyroid hormones (hyperthyroidism) may be associated with many anxiety symptoms (40). The HPT axis is organized in a hierarchical fashion with TRH being secreted from the hypothalamic median eminence and transported to the anterior pituitary where it binds to thyrotrophs that secrete thyrotropin (TSH); TSH in turn is transported to the thyroid gland where it stimulates the secretion of thyroid hormones. Several feedback loops in the system contribute to the regulation of target gland hormone release (63,64).

TRH Stimulation Tests and Clinical Observations

In parallel to ACTH blunting in major depression, a subpopulation (approximately 25%) of depressed patients display a blunted TSH response after intravenous (i.v.) TRH challenge. This finding was first reported by Prange and colleagues (65), who also reported normal baseline plasma TSH and thyroid hormone concentrations in these patients. These findings have been replicated many times and have been reviewed by Loosen (61). It is interesting that approximately 15% of depressed patients exhibit a markedly enhanced response to TRH.

What are the mechanisms that cause TSH blunting in depressed patients? It is not the normal feedback regulation of T_3 and T_4 on the pituitary thyrotroph, because circulating thyroid hormone levels in depressed patients are normal. Somatostatin inhibits TSH release and its elevation could be responsible for the TSH blunting; however, CSF SRIF concentrations are decreased in depressed populations (see below) (66,67). Overall, patients with TSH blunting do not necessarily have abnormal DST results nor blunted ACTH responses to CRF (61). One possible mechanism for TSH blunting would be hypersecretion of TRH analogous to CRF overproduction in depression, resulting in TRH receptor downregulation at the thryotrope. To test this hypothesis, in collaboration with Banki and colleagues (68) we measured the CSF concentrations of TRH in a group of drug-free depressed patients without evidence of thyroid disease and in controls. Eleven of the 14 depressed group had higher CSF concentrations of TRH than the highest control value. Even after comparison for demographic variables (age, sex, height, and weight), the group differences persisted. No correlation was found between CRF TRH concentration and TSH blunting, or result of a dexamethasone suppression test. Since more than 70% of the brain TRH is extrahypothalamic, this increase in TRH secretion in depression may not always be associated with disruption of the HPT axis.

TRH and Stress: Experimental Observations

Are CNS TRH neurons altered in association with stress? As yet, this question remains unanswered in the experimental setting. However, it is known that in animals TRH produces increased arousal, increased locomotor activity, and a reversal of the sedation caused by CNS depressants such as barbiturates and ethanol (69). TRH has been described as an "endogenous ergotropic substance" (70), and as such a decrease in its secretion in the patients described above may contribute to the anergy and lack of motivation observed in many depressed patients.

SOMATOSTATIN

The identity of the growth hormone release-inhibiting factor somatostatin (SRIF) was established in 1972 during a search for the long-elusive growth hormone releasing factor (71,72). As with CRF and TRH, SRIF was identified in extrahypothalamic brain areas including the hippocampus, striatum, and cerebral cortex and has been shown to be involved in a large number of brain functions

(73-75). Putative SRIF receptors have been identified in the CNS (76,77), and the peptide is released by depolarizing concentrations of potassium (78). In addition, it is preferentially localized to synaptosomes after density gradient centrifugation (79). SRIF therefore fulfills many of the requisite neurotransmitter criteria.

Somatostatin neurons are present throughout the CNS, in both long pathways and short interneurons (72). Parikarya containing SRIF in the periventricular hypothalamic nucleus project both rostrally and caudally to other nuclei, including the LC. A pathway from the amygdala to the solitary tract nucleus (80) indicates that SRIF may be involved in regulation of the cardiovascular and autonomic responses.

In addition to its actions on growth hormone secretion, SRIF inhibits the release of TSH and prolactin from the anterior pituitary and has been termed paninhibin. Of particular relevance to the present discussion is the observation that stress causes a profound inhibition of growth hormone secretion mediated by increased SRIF release (82).

Experimental Studies

Behavioral studies involving the injections of SRIF directly into the brains of experimental animals have revealed a number of effects of SRIF. In both intact and hypophysectomized animals (81), ICV SRIF produces marked excitation associated with reductions in both slow-wave and rapid eye movement (REM) sleep. There appear to be dose-dependent effects of SRIF injections; for example, low doses of SRIF (1 μg) increase, while higher doses (5 μg) decrease, the rate of electrical self-stimulation in the lateral hypothalamus of the rat (83). SRIF also appears to alter learning and memory; ICV SRIF inhibits extinction of active avoidance behavior in the rat (84,85). Cysteamine is an agent that has been reported to deplete SRIF in brain tissue, but there are several problems associated with its use (86).

Somatostatin: Clinical Studies

Two neuropsychiatric disorders most frequently associated with alterations in SRIF neurons are major depression (66,67) and Alzheimer's disease (AD) (87-89). Alzheimer's disease is characterized clinically by a profound loss of higher cognitive function including associative learning and memory, and pathologically by the presence of senile plaques and neurofibrillary tangles. Patients with major depression often complain of short-term memory deficits, and elderly depressed patients may display a pseudodementia that resembles AD but reverses with appropriate somatic treatments. In the postmortem brains of AD patients, marked reductions of SRIF concentrations were initially observed in the hippocampus, frontal cortex, parietal cortex, and superior temporal gyrus (87). Our group confirmed these findings in the frontal and temporal cortex and hypothalamus (90). Normal SRIF concentrations were found in other CNS regions, indicating that the presumed loss of SRIF neurons is not widespread throughout the brain.

The CSF concentration of SRIF has been measured in several neuropsychiatric disorders. Several investigators have shown a marked decrease in the CSF concentration of SRIF in AD patients compared to control subjects (67,91,92). To assess the effect of environment on the concentration of SRIF in the CSF of AD patients, our group in association with Karlsson and colleagues (93) measured CSF SRIF in two groups of AD patients exposed to different environmental conditions. In the group in traditional custodial care a small decrease or no change in CSF SRIF concentration was found. The group exposed to intense stimulation displayed an increase in the concentration of SRIF in the CSF. This work, taken together with preclinical findings, indicates that SRIF is associated with cognitive processes and the clinical data described below support this view.

Several groups have measured SRIF concentrations in CSF in patients with major depression. Gerner and Yamada (94) were the first to report the decrease of SRIF concentrations in the CSF of patients with major depression. Rubinow and colleagues (66) confirmed and extended these results to include bipolar depressed patients. They also noted a correlation between DST nonsuppression and the reduction in CSF SRIF concentrations. Our group (67) reported decreased CSF SRIF concentrations in patients with major depression and in AD patients. However, we were unable to find a correlation between HPA axis activity and SRIF concentrations. In a later study of older depressed patients, AD patients, and age-matched controls, the NIMH group (95) reported that while there was no correlation between Hamilton Depression Scale ratings and CSF SRIF concentrations, there was an overall group correlation between SRIF content and results on Weschler Memory Quotient tests. This supports the role of SRIF in cognitive processes. In an earlier study, Rubinow et al. (66) also reported that SRIF concentrations were negatively correlated with CSF norepinephrine levels and positively correlated with 2-methoxy-4-hydroxyphenyl glycol and 5-hydroxyindole acetic acid levels in CSF. Although this finding has not yet been replicated, because both norepinephrine and serotonin alter SRIF secretion in the CNS, a relative change in these monoamines could account for changes in CSF SRIF concentrations in depression.

CONCLUSIONS

Modern medicine has often identified conditions due to an absolute or relative deficiency on the one hand or overabundance on the other. Endocrinology is replete with such examples including hyper- and hypothyroidism, Cushing's and Addison's diseases, and type I diabetes mellitus. Major affective disorder has also been conceptualized as a relative lack of synaptic availability of cate-cholamines or indoleamines in certain brain areas (96–98). However, as our understanding of this illness has progressed, the findings do not support such a view. Siever and Davis (99) suggest that major depression more closely resembles type II diabetes, in which there is an alteration in hormone (transmitter) secre-tion and receptor sensitivity. They suggest six criteria for a dysregulated neuro-transmitter system in psychiatric disease: (1) a dysregulated neurotransmitter system is impaired in one or more regulatory or homeostatic mechanisms; (2) basal output of a dysregulated neurotransmitter system is more erratic; (3) normal periodicities, including circadian rhythmicities, of a dysregulated neuro-transmitter system are disrupted; (4) A dysregulated neurotransmitter system is less selectively responsive to environmental stimuli; (5) a dysregulated neuro-transmitter system returns more slowly to basal activity following a perturba-tion; and (6) clinically efficacious pharmacological agents restore efficient regula-tion of the dysregulated neurotransmitter system (99). CRF and the HPA axis in depression appear to fit this schema. As noted above, there is a blunting of CRF-induced ACTH release in depressed patients (criterion 1). Serum cortisol levels in depressed patients do not show the normal circadian pattern of secretion (criter-ion 3). Many depressed patients exhibit DST nonsuppression (criterion 2). The DST, ACTH blunting, and perhaps CSF CRF concentrations return to baseline after effective treatment for major depression (criterion 6). Criterion number 4 has not been clearly tested in relation to the HPA axis. The work of Sapolsky (3), discussed elsewhere in this volume, may well speak to criteria 5. His work has shown that increased cortisol secretion in response to stress in aged rats may persist up to 24 h after the stressful event. It may well be that a series of per-ceived stressful events may disrupt the control of the HPA axis severely enough to result in a change in regional brain CRF concentrations. The resultant CRF hypersecretion in susceptible individuals and dysregulation of the HPA axis may then contribute to the signs and symptoms of major depression.

Dysregulation of both the HPT axis and somatostatin neurons in the CNS in neuropsychiatric diseases are not as well established as the disturbances of the HPA axis. Both systems are clearly disrupted in subgroups of depressed patients. Study of the HPT axis with a focus on identifying patients with subclinical hypothyroidism and autoimmune thyroiditis appears to be a fruitful area of research. It is evident that decreases in CSF SRIF are associated with a disrup-tion of cognitive processes as found in Alzheimer's disease, multiple sclerosis, and depression.

As discussed elsewhere in this volume, the monoamine neurotransmitter sys-tems are also stress-responsive. Since all three neuromodulators we have dis-cussed are both colocalized and have synaptic connections with monoaminergic neurons, there must be a great deal of interaction of these systems during stress-ful events and possibly in disease states such as major depression. As novel tools become available, such as the ability to measure neuropeptide turnover and biosynthesis as well as neuropeptide receptor signal transduction, novel information about peptidergic involvement in stress and stress-related psychiatric disorders will become available.

ACKNOWLEDGMENTS

This research was supported by NIMH MH-42088, MH-39415, and MH-40159.

REFERENCES

1. Owens MJ, Nemeroff CB. The neurobiology of corticotropin-releasing factor: implications for affective disorders. In: Schatzberg, AF Nemeroff CB, eds. The hypothalamic–pituitary–adrenal axis: physiology, pathophysiology, and psychiatric implications. New York: Raven Press, 1988:1–36.
2. Reisine TD. Cellular mechanisms regulating adrenocorticotropin release. J Recept Res 1984; 4:291–300.
3. Sapolsky R, Armanini MS, Packan D, Tombaugh G. Stress and glucocorticoids in aging. Endocrinol Metab Clin North Am 1987; 16:965–980.
4. Rivier CL, Plotsky PM. Mediation by corticotropin-releasing factor of adenohypophysial hormone secretion. Annu Rev Physiol 1986; 48:475–494.
5. Bloom FE, Battenberg EL, Rivier J, Vale W. Corticotropin-releasing factor (CRF): immunoreactive neurons and fibers in the rat hypothalamus. Regul Pept 1982; 4:43–48.
6. Swanson LW, Sawchenko PE, Rivier J, Vale WW. Organization of ovine corticotropin-releasing factor immunoreactive cells and fibers in the rat brain: an immunohistochemical study. Neuroendocrinology 1982; 36:165–186.
7. Sawchencko PE, Swanson LW. Localization, colocalization, and plasticity of corticotropin-releasing factor immunoreactivity in the rat brain. Fed Proc 1985; 44:221–227.
8. Aguilera G, Harwood JP, Wilson JX, Morell J, Brown JH, Catt KJ. Mechanisms of action of corticotropin-releasing factor and other regulators of corticotropin release in rat pituitary cells. J Biol Chem 1983; 258:8039–8045.
9. Antoni FH. Hypothalamic control of adrenocorticotropin secretion: advances since the discovery of 41-residue corticotropin-releasing factor. Neuroendocrinology 1986; 43:79–88.
10. Vale W, Vaughn J, Smith M, Yamamoto G, Rivier J, Rivier C. Effects of synthetic ovine corticotropin-releasing factor, glucocorticoids, catecholamines, neurohypophysial peptides, and other substances on cultured corticotropin cells. Endocrinology 1983; 113:1121–1131.
11. Saffran M, Schally AV. Release of corticotropin by anterior pituitary tissue in vitro. Can J Biochem Physiol 1955; 33:408–415.

12. Vale W, Speiss C, Rivier C, Rivier J. Characterization of a 41-residue ovine hypothalamic peptide that stimulates secretion of corticotropin and β-endorphin. Science 1981; 213:1394–1397.
13. Antoni FA, Palkovits M, Makara GB, Linton EA, Lowery PJ, Kiss JZ. Immunoreactive corticotropin-releasing hormone in the hypothalamo-infudibular tract. Neuroendocrinology 1983; 36:415–423.
14. Sawchenko PE, Swanson LW, Vale WW. Co-expression of corticotropin-releasing factor and vasopressin immunoreactivity in parvocellular neurosecretory neurons of the adrenalectomized rat. Proc Natl Acad Sci USA 1984; 81:1883–1887.
15. Fellmann D, Bugnon C, Gouget A. Immunocytochemical demonstration of corticoliberin-like immunoreactivity (CLI) in neurons of the rat amygdala central nucleus (ACN). Neurosci Lett 1982; 34:253–258.
16. Moga MM, Gray TS. Evidence for corticotropin-releasing factor, neurotensin, and somatostatin in the neural pathway from the central nucleus of the amygdala to the parabrachial nucleus. J Comp Neurol 1985; 241:275–284.
17. Foote SL, Bloom FE, Aston-Jones G. Nucleus locus ceruleus: new evidence of anatomical and physiological specificity. Physiol Rev 1983; 63:844–914.
18. Chappell PB, Smith MA, Kilts CD, et al. Alterations in corticotropin-releasing factor-like immunoreactivity in discrete rat brain regions after acute and chronic stress. J Neurosci 1986; 6:2908–2914.
19. Smith MA, Bissette G, Slotkin TA, Knight DL, Nemeroff CB. Release of corticotropin-releasing factor from rat brain regions in vitro. Endocrinology 1986; 118:1997–2001.
20. Valentino RJ, Foote, SL, Aston-Jones G. Corticotropin-releasing factor acitivates noradrenergic neurons of the locus coeruleus. Brain Res 1983; 270:363–367.
21. DeSouza EB, Insel TR, Perrin MH, Rivier J, Vale WW, Kuhar MJ. Corticotropin-releasing factor receptors are widely distributed within the rat central nervous system: an autoradiographic study. J Neurosci 1985; 5:3189–3203.
22. Plotsky PM, Vale W. Hemorrhage-induced secretion of corticotropin-releasing factor-like immunoreactivity into the rat hypophysial-portal circulation and its inhibition by glucocorticoids. Endocrinology 1984; 114:164–169.
23. Linton EA, Tilders FJH, Hodgkinson S, Berkenbosch F, Vermes I, Lowry PJ. Stress-induced secretion of adrenocorticotropin in rats is inhibited by administration of antisera to ovine corticotropin-releasing factor and vasopressin. Endocrinology 1985; 116:966–969.
24. Petrusz P, Merchenthaler I, Maderdrut JL, Heitz PU. Central and peripheral distribution of corticotropin-releasing factor. Fed Proc 1985; 44:229–235.
25. Saavedra JM. Changes in dopamine, noradrenaline, and adrenaline in specific septal and preoptic nuclei after acute immobilization stress. Neuroendocrinology 1982; 35:396–401.
26. Owens MJ, Bissette G, Lundberg D, Nemeroff CB. Acute effects of antidepressant and anxiolytic drugs on CRF–LI in microdissected rat brain

regions. Proceedings, 26th Annual Meeting of the American College of Neuropsychopharmacology, 1987: 167.

27. Brown MR, Fisher LA, Spiess J, Rivier J, Rivier C, Vale W. Corticotropin-releasing factor: effects on the sympathetic nervous system and oxygen consumption. Life Sci 1982; 30:207–210.

28. Brown MR, Fisher LA, Spiess J, Rivier C, Rivier J, Vale W. Corticotropin-releasing factor: actions on the sympathetic nervous system and metabolism. Endocrinology 1982; 111:928–931.

29. Brown MR, Fisher LA. Central nervous system effects of corticotropin-releasing factor in the dog. Brain Res 1983; 280:75–79.

30. Fisher LA, Brown MR. Corticotropin-releasing factor and angiotensin II: comparison of CNS actions to influence neuroendocrine and cardiovascular function. Brain Res 1984; 296:41–47.

31. Breier A, Charney DS, Henniger GR. Agoraphobia with panic attacks: development, diagnostic stability, and course of illness. Arch Gen. Psychiatry 1986; 43:1029–1036.

32. Liebowitz MR, Gorman JM, Fryer A, Dillon D, Levitt M, Klein DF. Possible mechanisms for lactate's induction of panic. Am J Psychiatry 1987; 143:495–502.

33. Koob GF, Bloom FE. Corticotropin-releasing factor and behaviour. Fed Proc 1985; 44:259–263.

34. Sirinathsinghji DJS, Rees LH, Rivier J, Vale W. Corticotropin-releasing factor is a potent inhibitor of sexual receptivity in the female rat. Nature 1983; 305:232–235.

35. Sirinathsinghji DJS. Regulation of lordosis behaviour in the female rat by corticotropin-releasing factor, beta-endorphin/corticotropin, and lutenizing hormone-releasing hormone neuronal systems in the medial preoptic area. Brain Res 1986; 375:49–56.

36. Morley JE, Levine AS, Rowland NE. Stress-induced eating. Life Sci 1983; 32:2169–2182.

37. Morley JE, Levine AS. Corticotropin-releasing factor, grooming, and ingestive behavior. Life Sci 1982; 31:1459–1464.

38. Ehlers C, Henriksen S, Wang M, Rivier J, Vale W, Bloom F. Corticotropin-releasing factor produces increases in brain excitability and convulsive seizures in rats. Brain Res 1983; 278:332–336.

39. Diagnostic and statistical manual of mental disorders, 3rd ed, rev. Washington, D.C.: American Psychiatric Association 1987: 228–230.

40. Leigh H, Kramer SI. The psychiatric manifestations of endocrine disease. Adv Intern Med 1984; 29:413–445.

41. Schlesser MA. Neuroendocrine abnormalities in affective disorders. In: Rush AJ, Altshuler KZ, eds. Depression: basic mechanisms, diagnosis, and treatment. New York: Guilford Press, 1986: 45–71.

42. Carroll BJ, Curtis GC, Davies BM, Mendels J, Sugerman AA. Urinary free cortisol excretion in depression. Psychol Med 1976; 6:43–50.

43. Carroll BJ, Curtis GC, Mendels J. Neuroendocrine regulation in depression: I. Limbic system adrenocortical dysfunction. Arch Gen Psychiatry 1976; 33:1039–1044.

44. Sachar EJ, Hellman L, Roffwarg HP, Halpern FS, Fukushima DK, Gallagher TF. Disrupted 24-hour patterns of cortisol secretions in psychotic depression. Arch Gen Psychiatry 1973; 28:19–24.
45. Carroll BJ, Feinberg M, Greden JF, et al. A specific laboratory test for the diagnosis of melancholia. Arch Gen Psychiatry 1981; 38:15–22.
46. Carroll BJ. The dexamethasone suppression test for melancholia. Br J Psychiatry 1982; 140:292–304.
47. Gold PW, Chrousos GP. Clinical studies with corticotropin-releasing factor: implications for the diagnosis and pathophysiology of depression, Cushing's disease, and adrenal insufficiency. Psychoneuroendocrinology 1985; 10: 401–419.
48. Nemeroff CB, Widerlov E, Bissette G, et al. Elevated concentrations of CSF corticotropin-releasing factor-like immunoreactivity in depressed patients. Science 1984; 226:1342–1344.
49. Banki CM, Bissette G, Arato M, O'Connor L, Nemeroff CB. Cerebrospinal fluid CRF-LI in depression and schizophrenia. Am J Psychiatry 1987; 144: 873–877.
50. Arato M, Banki CM, Bissette G, Nemeroff CB. Elevated CSF CRF in suicide victims. Biol Psychiatry 1989; 25:355–359.
51. Gold PW, Chrousos GP, Kellner C, et al. Psychiatric implications of basic and clinical studies with corticotropin-releasing factor. Am J Psychiatry 1984; 141:619–627.
52. Holsboer F, Gerken A, Stalla GK, Muller OA. Blunted aldosterone and ACTH release after human CRF administration in depressed patients. Am J Psychiatry 1987; 144:229–231.
53. Holsboer F, Bardeleben UV, Green A, Stalla GK, Muller OA. Blunted corticotropin and normal cortisol response to human corticotropin-releasing factor in depression. N Engl J Med 1985; 311:1127.
54. Smith MA, Davidson J, Ritchie JC, et al. The corticotropin-releasing hormone test in post-traumatic stress disorder. Biol Psychiatry 1989; 26: 349–355.
55. Nemeroff CB, Owens MJ, Bissette G, Andorn AC, Stanley M. Reduced corticotropin-releasing factor binding sites in the frontal cortex of suicide victims. Arch Gen Psychiatry 1988; 45:577–580.
56. Dorovini-Zis K, Zis AP. Increased adrenal weight in victims of violent suicide. Am J Psychiatry 1987; 144:1214–1215.
57. Amsterdam JD, Marinelli DL, Arger P, Winokur A. Assessment of adrenal gland volume by computed tomography in depressed patients and healthy volunteers: a pilot study. Psychiatry Res 1987; 21:189–197.
58. Anisman H, Zacharko RM. Depression: the predisposing influence of stress. Behav Brain Sci 1982; 5:89–137.
59. Bauer MS, Dobra M, Shybrow PC. Disorders of the thyroid and parathyroid. In Nemeroff CB, Loosen PT, eds. Handbook of clinical psychoneuroendocrinology. New York: Guilford Press 1987: 41–70.
60. Gold MS, Pottash A, Extein I. Hypothyroidism and depression. Evidence from complete thyroid function evaluation. JAMA 1981; 245:1919–1921.

61. Loosen PT. The TRH-induced TSH response in psychiatric patients: a possible neuroendocrine marker. Psychoneuroendocrinology. (1985) 10: 237–260.

62. Nemeroff CB, Evans DL. Thyrotropin-releasing hormone (TRH), the thyroid axis and affective disorder. Ann NY Acad Sci 1989; 553:304–310.

63. Griffiths EC. Thyrotropin-releasing hormone: endocrine and central effects. Psychoneuroendocrinology 1985; 10:225–235.

64. Morley JE. Neuroendocrine control of thyrotropin secretion. Endocr Rev 1981; 2:396–436.

65. Prange AJ Jr, Wilson IC, Lara PP, Alltop LB, Breese GR. Effects of thyrotropin-releasing hormone in depression. Lancet 1972; 2:999–1002.

66. Rubinow DR, Gold PW, Post RM, et al. CSF somatostatin in affective illness. Arch Gen Psychiatry 1983; 40:409–412.

67. Bissette G, Widerlov E, Walleus H, et al. Alterations in cerebrospinal fluid concentrations of somatostatin-like immunoreactivity in neuropsychiatric disorders. Arch Gen Psychiatry 1986; 43:1148–1154.

68. Banki CM, Bissette G, Arato M, Nemeroff CB. Elevation of immunoreactive CSF TRH in depressed patients. Am J Psychiatry 1989; 145:1526–1531.

69. Nemeroff CB, Kalivas PW, Golden RN, Prange AJ. Behavioral effects of hypothalamic hypophysiotrophic hormones, neurotensin, substance P, and other neuropeptides. Pharmacol Ther 1984; 24:1–56.

70. Metcalf G, Dettmar PW. Is thyrotropin-releasing hormone an endogenous ergotropic substance in the brain? Lancet 1981; 1:586–589.

71. Brazeau P, Vale W, Burgus R, et al. Hypothalamic polypeptide that inhibits the secretion of immunoreactive pituitary growth hormone. Science 1972; 129:77–79.

72. Epelbaum J. Somatostatin in the central nervous system: physiology and pathological modifications. Prog Neurobio 1986; 27:63–100.

73. Brownstein M, Arimava A, Sato H, Schally AV, Kizer JS. The regional distribution of somatostatin in rat brain. Endocrinology 1975; 96:1456–1461.

74. Geola FL, Yamada T, Warwick RJ, Tourtelotte WW, Hershman JM. Regional distribution of somatostatin-like immunoreactivity in the human brain. Brain Res 1981; 229:35–42.

75. Nemeroff CB, Walsh TJ, Bissette G. Somatostatin and behavior: preclinical and clinical studies. In Reichlin S, ed. Somatostatin. New York: Plenum Press, 1987; 157–167.

76. Reubi JC, Rivier J, Perrin M, Brown M, Vale W. High affinity binding sites for a somatostatin-28 analog in rat brain. Life Sci 1981; 28:1049–1053.

77. Segal DS, Mandell AJ. Differential behavioral effects of hypothalamic polypeptides. In Prange AJ Jr, ed. The thyroid, drugs, and behavior. New York: Raven Press, 1974; 129–133.

78. Iversen LL, Iversen SD, Bloom F, Douglas C, Brown M, Vale W. Calcium-dependent release of somatostatin and neurotensin from rat brain in vitro. Nature 1978; 273:161–163.

79. Epelbaum J, Brazeau P, Tsang D, Brawer J, Martin JB. Subcellular distribution of radioimmunoassayable somatostatin in rat brain. Brain Res 1977; 126:309–323.
80. Higgins GA, Schwaber JS. Somatostatinergic projections from the central nucleus of the amygdala to the vagal nuclei. Peptides 1983; 4:663–668.
81. Halicek V, Rezek M, Friesen H. Somatostatin and thyrotropin-releasing hormone: cental effect on sleep and motor systems. Pharmacol Biochem Behav 1976; 5:73–77.
82. Terry LC, Willoughby JO, Brazeau P, Martin JB, Patel Y. Antiserum to somatostatin prevents stress-induced inhibition of growth hormone secretion in the rat. Science 1976; 192:565–566.
83. Vecsei L, Schwarzberg H, Telegdy G. The effect of somatostatin on the self-stimulation of rats. Neuroendocr Lett 1982; 4:37–41.
84. Vecsei L, Bollok L, Telegdy G. Intracerebroventricular somatostatin attenuates electroconvulsive shock-induced amnesia in rats. Peptides 1983; 4:293–295.
85. Vecsei L, Bollok L, Penke B, Telegdy G. Somatostatin and (D–Trp8, D–Cys14)-somatostatin delay extinction and reverse electroconvulsive shock-induced amnesia in rats. Psychoneuroendocrinology 1986; 11:111–115.
86. Cook LL, Bissette G, Dole K, Nemeroff CB. A critical evaluation of cysteamine as a tool to deplete somatostatin in the rat central nervous system. Endocrinology 1989; 124:855–861.
87. Davies P, Katzman R, Terry RD. Reduced somatostatin-like immunoreactivity in cerebral cortex from cases of Alzheimer's disease and Alzheimer senile dementia. Nature 1980; 288:279–280.
88. Nemeroff CB, Bissette G. Neuropeptides in psychiatric disorders. In: Berger PA, Brodie HKH, eds. American handbook of psychiatry, vol. VIII. New York: Basic Books, 1986: 64–110.
89. Cain ST, Nemeroff CB. Neuropeptides and neurotransmitters in Alzheimer's disease. In: Maddox GL, Busse EW, eds. Aging: the universal human experience. New York: Springer, 1987: 63–80.
90. Nemeroff CB, Bissette G, Busby WH Jr, et al. Regional concentrations of neurotensin, thyrotropin-releasing hormone and somatostatin in Alzheimer's disease. Soc Neurosci Abstr 1983; 9:1052.
91. Wood PL, Etienne P, Lal S, Gauthier S, Cajal S, Nair NPV. Reduced lumbar CSF somatostatin levels in Alzheimer's senile dementia. Life Sci 1982; 31:2073–2079.
92. Oram JJ, Edwardson J, Millard PH. Investigation of cerebrospinal fluid neuropeptides in idiopathic senile dementia. Gerontology 1981; 27:216–223.
93. Karlsson J, Widerlov E, Melin EV, et al. Changes of CSF neuropeptides after environmental stimulation in dementia. Nord Psykiatr Tidsskr 1985; 39(suppl. 11):75–81.
94. Gerner RH, Yamada T. Altered neuropeptide concentrations in cerebrospinal fluid of psychiatric patients. Brain Res 1982; 238:298–302.

95. Sunderland T, Rubinow DR, Tariot PN, et al. CSF somatostatin in patients with Alzheimer's disease, older depressed patients, and age-matched control subjects. Am J Psychiatry 1987; 144:1313–1316.

96. Schildkrault JJ. The catecholamine hypothesis of depression: a review of supporting evidence. Am J Psychiatry 1965; 122:509–522.

97. Schildkrault JJ, Kety SS. Biogenic amines and emotion. Science 1967; 156:21–30.

98. Jesberger JA, Richardson JS. Neurochemical aspects of depression: the past and the future? Int J Neuroscience 1985; 27:19–47.

99. Siever LJ, Davis KL. Overview: toward a dysregulation hypothesis of depression. Am J Psychiatry 1985; 142:1017–1031.

100. Owens MJ, Nemeroff CB. Preclinical and clinical studies with corticotropin-releasing factor: implications for affective disorders. Psychopharmacology Bull 1988; 24:355–359.

101. Nemeroff CB, Bissette G, Akil H, Fink M. Cerebrospinal neuropeptides in depressed patients treated with ECT: corticotropin-releasing factor, β-endorphin, and somatostatin. Br J Psychiatry 1990 (in press).

19

SYMPATHETIC NERVOUS SYSTEM FUNCTION IN DEPRESSION AND PANIC DISORDER

Richard C. Veith

*Seattle/American Lake Veterans Administration Medical
Centers and University of Washington School of Medicine
Seattle, Washington*

Pathological states of depression and anxiety have been observed since antiquity. Similar states or their analogs are also often observed in nonhumans and, although the subjective emotional experience may be difficult to discern or absent in less developed organisms, there is frequently no mistaking the behavioral and physiological manifestations of these states. Humans are unique, however, in their ability to communicate intellectually the occasionally overwhelming character of these conditions, which in their full intensity are pervasive and life-threatening. It might be expected, therefore, that these emotional states, which in more recent times have been systematically scrutinized, categorized, and glorified with diagnostic status, should elicit in their subjects evidence that psychological, behavioral, and physiological coping responses have been appropriately mobilized in defense of the perceived threat to homeostasis (1-3). One of the paramount physiological resources available in such an adaptive confrontation is activation of the cardiovascular, hemodynamic, and metabolic defenses of the sympathetic nervous system (SNS). The fundamental historical, neuro-anatomical and physiological aspects of autonomic responses to stress are well described elsewhere in this volume. Thus, the principal focus of this chapter is to review evidence from human studies for SNS disturbances in major depressive illness and panic disorder.

SYMPATHETIC NERVOUS SYSTEM FUNCTION IN MAJOR DEPRESSIVE ILLNESS

Diagnosis and Epidemiology

Affective disturbances span a spectrum of severity from transient alterations in mood to pervasive periods of melancholia or episodes of acute mania. Although highly familiar and casually employed clinically, "depression" is a troublesome term that can be applied to an array of conditions that include a normal fluctuation in mood state, demoralization, an episode of bereavement, a transient psychological reaction to injury or loss, or the neurovegetative syndrome characterized in the recently revised *Diagnostic and Statistical Manual* (DSM-III-R) (4) of the American Psychiatric Association as a major depressive episode (Table 1). The heterogeneity of depressive states and ambiguity of the term "depression" are sources of potential confusion in clinical research. For the purpose of this review, we will consider "depression" to represent the diagnosis of those patients who fulfill DSM-III-R criteria for major depressive episode with or without melancholia (Table 2).

Recent studies using DSM-III criteria for major depressive episode indicate that 2-4% of the population fulfill criteria for major depression (5). Rates for depression among individuals enrolled in outpatient medical clinics and on inpatient medical services typically range between 20 and 30% (6,7). Rates for institutionalized elderly patients suggest that depression is especially prevalent (8), but methodological and diagnostic difficulties are more problematic in this setting.

The consequences of major depression represent a serious public health problem. The lifetime risk for suicide among individuals suffering from depression is approximately 15% (9) and suicide rates are particularly high among the elderly (10). Studies in younger individuals indicate that, in addition to the risk of suicide, inadequately treated depression is associated with increased mortality from cardiovascular causes (11). Thus, depression represents an important, potentially preventable cause of mortality and morbidity.

Measurement of SNS Activity in Humans

It has long been recognized that activation of the SNS plays an important role in the physiological response of the organism to stress. However, that SNS activity is increased in some depressed and, possibly, anxious patients has been recognized only recently. This is somewhat surprising, particularly for depression, because the suspicion that a disturbance involving CNS norepinephrine (NE) is causative in this disorder has been popular since the 1960s (12, 13). Progress in this research area has been hindered, in part, because sensitive

TABLE 1   DSM–III–R Diagnostic Criteria for Major Depressive Episode

---

A. At least five of the following symptoms have been present during the same 2 week period and represent a change from previous functioning; at least one of the symptoms is either depressed mood or loss of interest or pleasure.

Depressed mood most of the day, nearly every day, as indicated either by subjective account or observation by others

Markedly diminished interest or pleasure in all, or almost all, activities most of the day, nearly every day (as indicated either by subjective account or observation by others of apathy most of the time)

Significant weight loss or weight gain when not dieting (e.g., more than 5% of body weight in a month), or decrease or increase in appetite nearly every day

Insomnia or hypersomnia nearly every day

Psychomotor agitation or retardation nearly every day (observable by others, not merely subjective feelings of restlessness or being slowed down)

Fatigue or loss of energy nearly every day

Feelings of worthlessness or excessive or inappropriate guilt (which may be delusional) nearly every day (not merely self-reproach or guilt about being sick)

Diminished ability to think or concentrate, or indecisiveness, nearly every day (either by subjective account or as observed by others)

Recurrent thoughts of death (not just fear of dying), recurrent suicidal ideation without a specific plan, or a suicide attempt or a specific plan for committing suicide.

B. It cannot be established that an organic factor initiated and maintained the disturbance

The disturbance is not a normal reaction to the death of a loved one (uncomplicated bereavement)

C. At no time during the disturbance have there been delusions or hallucinations for as long as 2 weeks in the absence of prominent mood symptoms (i e., before the mood symptoms developed or after they have remitted)

D. Not superimposed on schizophrenia, schizophreniform disorder, or delusional disorder

---

TABLE 2   DSM–III– Diagnostic Criteria for Major Depressive Episode,
Melancholic Type

A. Meets criteria for major depressive episode
B. The presence of at least five of the following:
   Loss of interest or pleasure in all, or almost all, activities
   Lack of reactivity to usually pleasurable stimuli (does not feel much better,
      even temporarily, when something good happens)
   Depression regularly worse in the morning
   Early morning awakening (at least 2 h before usual time of awakening)
   Psychomotor retardation or agitation (not merely subjective complaints)
   Significant anorexia or weight loss (e.g., more than 5% of body weight in a
      month)
   No significant personality disturbance before first major depressive episode
   One or more previous major depressive episodes followed by complete, or
      nearly complete, recovery
   Previous good response to specific and adequate somatic antidepressant
      therapy: tricyclics, electroconvulsive therapy, MAOI, lithium

---

measures of SNS activity in humans have only recently become available. In
addition, however, biological psychiatry has traditionally adopted pharmacological or biochemical models of the pathogenesis of depression and anxiety,
and has tended to conceptualize emerging evidence for disturbances of SNS
function in these disorders as alterations of "noradrenergic function" rather than
incorporating these observations in more physiological models. Moreover, the
field has been slow to adopt new methodological and technical advances that
have been more quickly applied to human investigation in endocrinology and
cardiovascular physiology.

For the purposes of examining studies in humans, the peripheral SNS can be
organized into two major components: SNS nerves regulating cardiovascular
function and those to the adrenal medulla (14). Postganglionic SNS nerves innervating the heart, major organs, skeletal muscles, and vasculature make up the
cardiovascular component of the SNS, which is principally involved in regulating
blood pressure and mediating hemodynamic adaptations to stress. Accordingly,
such "stressors" as hypotension, the assumption of upright posture, and exercise
are potent stimuli for activating this component of the SNS. This is reflected by
increased firing of pre- and postganglionic SNS nerves and the release of NE into
the circulation (14). The adrenomedullary component of the SNS, comprised
of cholinergic preganglionic SNS nerves directly innervating the adrenal medulla,
serves important homeostatic and adaptive functions primarily involving glucose
regulation and metabolism (14). This component of the SNS is preferentially

activated in response to such simuli as hypoglycemia, which results in a prompt release of epinephrine (EPI) into the circulation (14).

Although SNS activation has traditionally been viewed as an "all or none" system (2,3), and this is generally true for severe stressors such as hypovolemic shock, profound hypoglycemia, or maximal exercise (14), it is increasingly recognized that the SNS is capable of differential activation (15,16) and that this capacity for specificity in SNS responses is orchestrated within the CNS (16,17). For example, direct microneurographic measurements in humans reveal that resting SNS activity in sympathetic nerves to skeletal muscle is regulated by baroreceptor activity (16,18) whereas SNS activity in cutaneous sympathetic nerves is not entrained to the cardiac cycle (16). Moreover, muscle SNS activity increases during the Valsalva maneuver but cutaneous SNS activity is unaffected (16). Cooling of the skin, however, increases SNS discharge in cutaneous SNS nerves but does not influence muscle SNS nerve activity (16). Differential responses in cardiac and skeletal muscle SNS nerve activity have also been observed. Victor and associates (19) have shown that the cold pressor test evokes an immediate elevation in heart rate, thought to be sympathetically mediated because it is abolished by beta-adrenergic blockade, but activity in muscle SNS nerves does not increase until approximately 30 s later.

The remarkable specificity and regional selectivity of SNS responses are evident in recent studies in dogs from our laboratories, which demonstrated that the SNS nerves to the pancreas were stimulated by CNS neuroglucopenia induced by 2-deoxyglucose but not by profound hypotension or hypoxemia. This was despite the fact that all three stressors produced similar elevations of systemic NE, presumably reflecting equivalent activation of the cardiovascular component of the SNS (20). Finally, as described by Folkow (15) and by Hilton (21), the adaptive nature of differential SNS activation is particularly evident during the "defense reaction" when cardiac, splanchnic, renal, and cutaneous SNS activity is increased but sympathetic vasoconstrictor fibers to skeletal muscle are inhibited. Coupled with reduced vagal tone, this pattern of SNS response increases cardiac output and blood pressure and increases neurogenic constriction of capacitance and most resistance vessels, except to the heart, skeletal muscle, and brain, where blood flow increases. Such hemodynamic adjustments optimally prepare the organism for "fight or flight." It is important to point out, however, that qualitatively similar responses have been demonstrated in humans in less threatening circumstances simply requiring attention, vigilance, and concentration such as mental arithmetic or other cognitive challenges (15,22,23).

The availability within the last 10–15 years of sensitive and specific assays for catecholamines and the direct measurement of peripheral SNS nerve activity using microneurographic techniques have allowed a more accurate assessment of SNS activity in humans than had previously been possible by reliance on heart rate or blood pressure. The microneurographic technique, developed by Wallin and associates (16,18), has been particularly useful in demonstrating the intra-individual stability of SNS "tone" over extended periods of time and has been successfully used to assess responses to a number of physiological stimuli that activate the SNS (16,18,19,24). To our knowledge, this approach has not been used to assess SNS function in depressed or anxious patients. Plasma NE levels rise in response to acute stressful illness, surgery, exercise, and assumption of upright posture and fall with blockade of SNS outflow by spinal anesthesia, thus providing a potentially useful index of the cardiovascular component of peripheral SNS activity (14,25-28). In similar fashion, plasma EPI has been shown to be a sensitive index of adrenomedullary SNS activity (14). However, it is important to recognize that the circulating levels of NE and EPI in plasma do not necessarily reflect release from postganglionic neurons and the adrenal medulla, respectively, because the plasma concentration is also determined by the clearance of catecholamines from plasma (29-31). Furthermore, only a small portion of the NE released at postganglionic SNS synapses escapes reuptake or local metabolism and spills over into the circulation where it can be measured (32). These potential limitations have been mitigated by the development by Esler and associates of isotope dilution tracer methods to measure NE and EPI kinetics (29,30). This technique allows determination of both the plasma appearance rate and clearance of catecholamines, has proven useful in examining differences in plasma catecholamines among clinical populations and in response to physiological or pharmacological perturbations of the SNS (23,29,33-35), and has more recently been used to measure organ-specific NE kinetics in humans (29). In addition, Linares and associates (36) have recently developed a two-compartment mathematical model to analyze plasma NE kinetics, which provides estimates of several parameters of peripheral NE function not amenable to direct experimental measurement or not estimated by the original one-compartment NE kinetic model (30).

The site of plasma catecholamine sampling deserves emphasis as an important factor in the use of plasma catecholamine determinations as indices of SNS activity. The majority of clinical studies utilizing plasma catecholamine measurements for this purpose have relied on antecubital venous measurements, which have been shown to have several limitations (22,23,31). Several recent studies have demonstrated that sampling from arterial or arterialized venous blood provides a more accurate measure of systemic SNS activity than catecholamine sampling from antecubital venous blood (22,23,31,35). This is due, in part, to the 40-50% fractional extraction of circulating catecholamines that occurs as they traverse the forearm tissues and are subjected to neuronal uptake at SNS synapses. Furthermore, the forearm is a site of net NE production, resulting in higher NE levels in antecubital venous blood than in simultaneously obtained arterial or arterialized venous (35,37) measurements (obtained by heating the hand in a warming box or heating pad). Thus, antecubital venous NE levels are greatly influenced by the local production and release of NE from forearm tissues and provide an index largely of skeletal muscle, not total body, SNS activity. Because circulating EPI is derived exclusively from the adrenal medulla, the fractional extraction of EPI by the forearm results in an approximate 50% fall in plasma EPI in venous compared to arterial sampling and basal values often fall below the sensitivity of many assay techniques.

These sampling issues become particularly important if SNS activity or regional blood flow, which affects clearance, differs in skeletal muscle compared to the rest of the body. In fact, precisely these factors may require revision of the traditional view that mental or cognitive stress preferentially activates the adrenomedullary component of the SNS, as suggested by several studies that have observed that such stimuli produce a greater elevation of plasma EPI than NE when sampled in venous blood (22,38,39). Hjemdahl and associates (22) used the Stroop Color Word test to induce mental stress in normal subjects and demonstrated an increase in heart rate, blood pressure, and cardiac output. These effects were associated with an increase in both NE and EPI measured in arterial blood. Although venous EPI levels increased, there was no change in antecubital venous NE levels. These findings were recently confirmed and extended by Goldstein and associates (23), who investigated SNS responses to a somewhat less noxious "stress": a video challenge task. They observed an increase in heart rate, blood pressure, and cardiac output that was associated with a significant increase in forearm blood flow. Arterial NE, but not antecubital venous NE, was increased without a significant change in arterial or venous EPI. Using a tritiated NE kinetic technique, Goldstein and associates (23) observed a significant increase in total body NE appearance rate, which was closely correlated with cardiac output. Although the study by Hjemdahl and associates (22) suggested that a decrease in skeletal muscle SNS activity accounted for their arterial–venous NE findings, Goldstein and associates found a modest increase in forearm NE appearance rate in response to their challenge, but a greater relative increase in forearm blood flow resulted in no change in the antecubital NE level.

Both studies are compatible with a hemodynamic response similar to a "defense reaction" (15,21) with marked cardiac stimulation and peripheral vasodilatation. Had these studies, like several earlier investigations, relied on venous catecholamine measurements alone, the Hjemdahl study would have been interpreted as indicating a preferential effect of mental stress on adrenomedullary SNS activity and plasma EPI, and both studies would have overlooked the important effect of these challenges on the cardiovascular component of the SNS. It is important to consider these sampling issues in appraising the clinical studies of SNS function in depression and anxiety disorders because the majority have utilized venous catecholamine measurements.

Clinical Studies of Sympathetic Nervous System Activity
in Depression

Growing evidence indicates that peripheral SNS activity is increased in patients with major depression (40-54). For example, the average venous plasma NE level is approximately 75% higher in depressed patients than basal values in controls (41,43,45,48-53) and the urinary NE excretion is also increased (44,54). Maas and associates (44) analyzed the relative urinary excretion rates of NE, EPI, and their metabolites and estimated that the systemic synthesis and release of EPI, as well as NE, are increased in depression. These elevations appear to be largely attributable to patients with unipolar disease (depressed patients without a history of mania) who fulfill criteria for melancholia (Table 2). Melancholia is a subclassification of major depressive episode applied to patients with marked anhedonia (diminished ability to experience pleasure) and prominent neuro-vegetative symptoms who are typically also among the more severely depressed (45,55). Although increased urinary excretion of EPI has been noted (45,54), to our knowledge there has been no report of increased plasma EPI in depressed patients diagnosed by DMS-III criteria, which suggests the absence of generalized SNS activation in this disorder.

There appears to be a relationship between increased SNS activity in depression and hyperactivity of the hypothalamic–pituitary–adrenal (HPA) axis, as reflected by nonsuppression of plasma cortisol in response to dexamethasone feedback inhibition (dexamethasone suppression test, DST) (56,57). For example, studies from our laboratory indicate that supine and standing venous NE and EPI levels are higher in depressed patients who are dexamathasone nonsuppressors than in suppressors (40). This has also been reported by Roy and associates (45) and by Rubin and associates (58), who found increased supine plasma NE levels in depressed patients resistant to dexamethasone suppression than in suppressors. In our depressed patients as a group, the overall higher plasma NE levels can be largely attributed to the DST nonsuppressors (53). Additional evidence for a relationship between SNS activity and HPA function in depression is the observation that plasma and urinary NE are correlated with postdexamethasone cortisol values in depressed patients (49,51,59). It was interesting that plasma and urinary levels of NE and its major metabolite, 3-methoxy-4-hydroxyphenylglycol (MHPG), tend to be low in depressed patients with bipolar disease (patients with a history of both depression and mania) compared both to controls and to depressed patients without a history of mania (45,46,60), but this is not a consistent finding (54).

Although evidence now convincingly indicates that basal activity of the cardiovascular component of the SNS is increased in some populations of depressed patients, few studies have explored whether depressed patients exhibit heightened SNS responses to provocative stimuli thought to activate the SNS

However, limited data suggest increased SNS responsiveness, at least in some patients. As noted above, we have shown greater plasma NE responses to the assumption of upright posture in DST nonsuppressors than in suppressors (40). Three studies comparing depressed patients and controls have demonstrated greater absolute (43,45) or percentage (46) increments in plasma NE with orthostasis, despite equivalent blood pressure responses. It is interesting that the exaggerated NE response to standing is present in depressed patients with bipolar disease as well, despite lower basal plasma NE levels in this subgroup (45,46). Roy and associates (50) found that depressed patients also had higher absolute plasma NE levels basally and during a cold pressor test, but as in an earlier study by Ackenheil and associates (61), the percentage increase in plasma NE in response to the cold challenge was not greater in patients than in controls.

The trend toward higher plasma NE levels in patients with unipolar disease is compatible with increased SNS activity, unless plasma NE clearance is reduced. The latter is an important consideration because glucocorticoids antagonize nonneuronal NE uptake (62-64) and, as noted above, the 24 h plasma cortisol production is increased in some depressed patients. To examine this possibility, we have measured plasma appearance rate and clearance in depressed patients in ongoing studies using a tritiated NE isotope dilution technique (53). Preliminary findings suggest that NE appearance rate is increased in the DST nonsuppressors compared to suppressors and controls but that plasma NE clearance is similar (53). These findings are compatible with increased SNS outflow as the cause of elevated plasma NE in major depression, which, in our patients, is found most often in patients with HPA hyperactivity. These findings are in general agreement with the report of Esler and associates (41), who documented increased NE appearance rates in five depressed patients with "endogenous" features.

Several additional lines of evidence are also compatible with increased SNS activity in depression. The adenylate cyclase response of the lymphocyte beta-adrenergic receptor to agonist stimultion is reduced, and a shift of these beta-adrenergic receptors to the low-affinity state has been reported in depressed patients (65-68). These findings are likely to represent the development of subsensitivity of these beta-receptors in response to higher circulating plasma NE levels in depression. Elevated plasma NE levels might also be expected to produce subsensitivity of the peripheral alpha-1 and postsynaptic alpha-2 adrenergic receptors that mediate vasoconstriction of peripheral blood vessels (69). In the subsensitive state, a greater NE stimulus might be required to produce a given blood pressure response. It is intriguing to speculate that such a mechanism might account for the fact that resting blood pressure is not increased in depressed patients and for the observation (43,45,46) that the assumption of upright posture elicits a greater plasma NE rise despite an equal blood pressure response in depressed patients compared to controls. However, such a model does not explain why exaggerated NE responses to standing also occur in patients with bipolar disease, who tend to have low plasma NE levels.

Taken together, these findings indicate that major depression is associated with increased outflow to the cardiovascular component of the SNS and possibly with increased SNS responsiveness to upright posture. Increased SNS activity is most pronounced in those patients who exhibit symptoms of melancholia, HPA axis hyperactivity, and DST nonsuppression, who tend to be the more severely depressed patients.

CNS Regulation of SNS Outflow

Because it is presumed that a disturbance of CNS function in genetically vulnerable individuals underlies the clinical syndrome of depression, attempts to interpret pathophysiologically the finding of increased SNS activity in depressed patients requires an understanding of the CNS regulation of SNS outflow. This topic is more fully developed elsewhere in this volume, but several aspects will be highlighted here because of their importance in several models that can be advanced to account for the apparent increase in SNS activity in patients with depression and, possibly, panic disorder.

Recent studies have demonstrated the prominent role of the rostral ventrolateral medulla (RVLM) in integrating peripheral somatic and baroreceptor afferents with brainstem, hypothalamic, forebrain, and cortical efferents that collectively determine SNS activity. Several groups have shown that RVLM neurons tonically stimulate the preganglionic SNS neurons of the intermediolateral spinal cord (70-72). RVLM neurons are themselves inhibited by nucleus tractus solitarius neurons (NTS), which relay baroreceptor input from the periphery, and these RVLM neurons are phasically synchronized with the cardiac cycle (70, 72). The importance of this region of the brainstem for the maintenance of SNS tone is illustrated by the observation that discrete lesions in this region result in SNS collapse and prevent SNS responses to stimulation from higher brain regions known to activate the SNS (70). RVLM cells project rostrally to the pontine locus ceruleus, the site of origin of the majority of forebraine NE neurons (70, 73-76). This pathway is probably responsible for the integration of CNS noradrenergic and peripheral SNS nerves that can be demonstrated by the similar activity profiles of these nerves in some circumstances (77,78). Evidence for this interaction in humans derives from the close correlation that exists between plasma and cerebrospinal fluid (CSF) NE levels (49,79) and, as noted by recent studies in our laboratory, from the parallel responses of plasma and CSF NE to alpha-2 adrenergic stimulation and inhibition in young subjects (80).

Although the specific neurotransmitters involved in the baroreceptor-NTS-RVLM-SNS reflex loop have not been determined definitively (70,81-83), several candidates deserve note in this context. Neuropharmacological evidence suggests that RVLM neurons are tonically inhibited by gamma-aminobutyric acid (GABA)ergic mechanisms and that local GABA neurons provide the principal input to the RVLM from the NTS (70). Noradrenergic input to this area, possibly derived from more caudally situated cells, inhibits the RVLM cells via alpha-2 receptors and possibly a non-alpha-2 imidazole receptor (70,81). The RVLM area also contains muscarinic cholinergic receptors and acetylcholine is an excitatory neurotransmitter in this area (70). In addition, the excitatory neurotransmitter L-glutamate activates the SNS when applied to the RVLM, but a source for L-glutamate input to this region is unknown (70). The RVLM cells are distinguished by the presence of the epinephrine synthesizing enzyme phenylethanolamine N-methyltransferase (PNMT) and are presumed to produce EPI. However, EPI inhibits rather than stimulates preganglionic SNS cells (70). Reis and associates (70) suggest that the corelease of other neurotransmitters, possibly L-glutamate, neuropeptide Y, or substance P (83), might mediate excitatory, descending RVLM input to SNS preganglionic nerve cells.

The RVLM receives descending inputs from several brain areas thought to be involved in neuroendocrine dysregulation in depression. Prominent among these is the paraventricular nucleus of the hypothalamus, which sends projections directly to the RVLM as well as providing monosynaptic inputs to the preganglionic SNS neurons of the thoracic and lumbar intermediolateral spinal nuclei (84). Fibers in these pathways contain CRF, somatostatin, vasopressin, and several other peptides thought to serve as neuropeptide transmitters that functionally integrate SNS and hypothalamic neuroendocrine activity (85,86).

Increased SNS Activity in Depression: Possible CNS Mechanisms

Increased CRF Activity in the CNS

Because of the difficulties inherent in gaining direct access to the CNS in humans, the clinical investigation of the neurobiology of depression has relied heavily on inferences from neuroendocrine studies. As described by Pryor and Nemeroff in Chapter 18, one of the most robust neuroendocrine disturbances in depression is hyperactivity of the HPA axis. This is exhibited by elevated 24 h plasma cortisol concentrations and feedback resistance to suppression of cortisol production by the synthetic glucocorticoid, dexamethasone (56,57). Nonsuppression on the DST occurs in approximately 50% of patients sufficiently depressed to require hospitalization (56,57). As reported by Nemeroff and associates, depression is also associated with increased corticotropin-releasing factor (CRF) in the CSF (87-89). In addition, adrenocorticotropic hormone (ACTH) responses to exogenous CRF administration are blunted (90). These findings suggest that a disturbance involving increased CRF activity at or above the hypothalamus accounts for HPA hyperactivity in depressed patients (90). Consistent with this interpretation, Bissette and associates (91) have reported decreased CRF-receptor binding in the frontal cortex of suicide victims, which suggests increased CRF input to this region.

CRF injected into the brains of laboratory animals not only stimulates the HPA axis but also produces behavioral and neuroendocrine responses compatible with SNS activation (92,93). CRF-induced activation of the CNS is likely to be mediated by CRF pathways that project from the paraventricular nucleus of the hypothalamus to brainstem centers regulating SNS outflow and to the preganglionic SNS nerves of the intermediolateral spinal cord (84-86). CRF pathways also project from the paraventricular nucleus to the median eminence, regulating release of ACTH (84-86). Thus, neuroanatomical mechanisms are present in the CNS that could be invoked to explain the apparent association between HPA and SNS hyperactivity in depression and that implicate increased CRF activity in the CNS as a plausible mediator of these neuroendocrine findings.

Diminished CNS Somatostatin Activity

CSF levels of somatostatin are reduced in patients with depression (88,95,96) and several lines of evidence suggest mechanisms involving reduced CNS somatostatin activity that could explain increased SNS activity in depression. Neuronal cell bodies containing somatostatin-like immunoreactivity are anatomically distributed in a variety of brain regions involved in the physiological control of pituitary hormone secretion and autonomic regulation (84). Prominent among these are the paraventricular preoptic nuclei, amygdala, hippocampus, locus ceruleus, and septal nuclei (84,96). In addition, somatostatin-like immunoreactivity is also present in descending projections from the paraventricular nucleus to the RVLM and to the preganglionic SNS cells of the intermediolateral spinal cord (96). These pathways may be responsible for the suppression of plasma catecholamines produced by somatostatin when administered centrally in dogs (97).

Several studies suggest an inhibitory effect of somatostatin on CRF activity in the CNS. Brown and associates (17,98) have shown that somatostatin analogs antagonize CRF-induced elevations of plasma epinephrine when given centrally. Somatostatin also antagonizes CRF-stimulated ACTH secretion from isolated pituitary cells (99). Doran and associates (100) have observed an inverse relationship between CSF somatostatin levels and maximum postdexamethasone cortisol values in depressed patients, providing evidence for an inhibitory influence of CNS somatostatin pathways, possibly via CRF, on HPA axis functioning in humans. However, this finding was not confirmed in a recent study by Widerlov and associates (88). Nevertheless, this research area deserves further study because, taken together, these findings suggest that reduced CNS somatostatin activity could increase SNS outflow directly by a reduction in the inhibitory restraint by somatostatin on SNS outflow or indirectly by enhancing CRF activity. It must be noted, however, that the predominant effect of somatostatin analogs on the SNS is to antagonize stress-induced adrenomedullary EPI release with minimal effect on baroreceptor-dependent EPI or NE stimulation (17,98). In depressed patients SNS hyperactivity primarily, if not exclusively, involves the noradrenergic SNS outflow; this argues against a causative role for somatostatin in the SNS hyperactivity present in this disorder.

CNS NE Deficiency or Alpha-2 Noradrenergic Defect

The advent in the late 1950s and early 1960s of effective pharmacological treatment for depression led to clinical and in vitro observations that produced theories regarding possible disturbances in CNS neurochemical function that might underlie depression. Prominent among these was the hypothesis proposed by Schildkraut et al. (13) and Bunney and Davis (12) that depression might result from a CNS deficiency of NE and/or serotonin. The original NE deficiency model of depression derived from the clinical observation that reserpine, which depletes the CNS of NE and several other monoamines, causes depression in some individuals (12,13). In addition, several compounds capable of at least temporarily elevating mood (e.g., amphetamine, monoamine oxidase [MAO] inhibitors, and tricyclic antidepressants) exhibited in vitro properties suggesting the ability to enhance synaptic concentrations of such CNS neurotransmitters as NE. In addition to the historical precedent for considering the possible role of NE CNS mechanisms in the pathogenesis of depression, it is also appropriate to consider that disturbances of NE might explain increased SNS activity in depression because CNS NE pathways are important in the brainstem regulation of SNS outflow.

Early human studies undertaken in the 1970s that attempted to validate the theory that depression might result from a defect or deficiency in CNS NE activity relied upon measurements of urinary or plasma MHPG, the major metabolite of brain NE metabolism in primates, as an index of CNS NE metabolism (32). At that time it was generally accepted that as much as 60% of peripherally measured MHPG originated in the CNS (101). However, this belief was subsequently challenged by evidence indicating that the majority of MHPG in plasma and urine is of peripheral, not CNS, origin (32,102-104). Furthermore, most clinical studies demonstrated that plasma or urinary MHPG levels were either normal (54,60) or increased (42) in depressed patients and not low, as might have been predicted by the original NE depletion model of depression. Although not universally accepted, elevations of plasma and urinary MHPG levels observed in subgroups of depressed patients most likely represent increased peripheral SNS activity.

In a somewhat more direct approach to exploring possible CNS NE disturbances in major depression, later studies measured NE or its metabolites in CSF to gain closer access to the CNS (42,49,54,105-110). The assumption that CSF

NE is a valid measure of brain noradrenergic activity is based upon several factors. Noradrenergic cell bodies in the locus ceruleus, the major nucleus of CNS NE neurons, richly innervate brain areas close to the cerebroventricular surface (111). Norepinephrine injected into CSF is taken up by catecholaminergic neurons of central origin (112). In addition, and in contrast to MHPG (32, 103), an effective blood–brain barrier for NE has been well documented (113). Studies from our laboratory have further validated CSF NE as an index of CNS noradrenergic activity by demonstrating the lack of an effect of extensive peripheral sympathectomy on CSF NE levels in rats (114).

CSF studies have not provided consistent evidence indicating a difference in NE concentration in depressed patients, although levels tend to be higher in depressed patients with prominent anxiety or dexamethasone nonsuppression and in manic patients compared to controls (49,108,109). Studies of CSF MHPG are conflicting (108). In apparent contradiction to the original NE depletion model, CSF MHPG levels have been reported in several recent studies to be *higher* in depressed patients with increased anxiety, postmenopausal status, or hyperactivity of the HPA axis compared to normal subjects (49,54,109,110). Because MHPG passes freely from the plasma compartment to the CSF (32), it is difficult to exclude the possibility that higher CSF MHPG levels in some depressed groups of patients are not the result of increased motor activity or increased peripheral SNS activity. Christensen and co-workers have reported reduced CSF EPI but normal NE levels in two studies of depressed patients (105, 106). The physiological significance of this finding and the role of EPI as a CNS neurotransmitter are unclear but this observation is interesting since iontophoretically applied EPI appears to inhibit preganglionic SNS neurons (70).

Recent studies exploring possible CNS neurochemical disturbances in depressive illness have also examined postmortem CSF samples and brain tissue from suicide victims and depressed patients who died of other causes. Low levels of NE have been reported in the putamen of suicide victims (115), but levels were not reduced in the hypothalamus or caudate nucleus (115,116). An inverse relationship between CSF levels of MHPG and the violence of the suicide attempt has also been reported (117). Mann and co-workers (118) recently found a 73% increase in frontal cortex beta-adrenergic receptor binding in brain tissue from suicide victims who were largely drug-free. These investigators suggested that *low* NE concentrations in the vicinity of these receptors might account for an increase in beta-adrenergic receptor sensitivity in the frontal cortex. These latter findings provide, albeit indirectly, the most compelling evidence for diminished CNS NE activity in major depression and are particularly intriguing because most pharmacologically effective antidepressant agents, as well as electroconvulsive treatment, produce subsensitivity of brain beta-adrenergic receptors in animal studies (119). The potential influence, if any, of CNS beta-adrenergic receptor mechanisms on SNS activity is presently unknown. It is important to consider also that possible changes in presynaptic NE availability and/or postsynaptic receptor binding might represent compensatory responses to a primary defect in postreceptor mechanisms.

A major regulator of SNS outflow is an NE-mediated CNS pathway that inhibits SNS outflow in the medullary brainstem and spinal cord by alpha-2 adrenergic mechanisms (70,84,119–121). Accordingly, local administration in animals of NE or other alpha-adrenergic agonists exerts a profound sympathoinhibitory response (120). We have shown similarly that oral clonidine, a centrally active alpha-2 agonist, produces a dose-related suppression of plasma NE appearance rate in humans (35), indicating a marked reduction of SNS outflow. Furthermore, we have shown that oral clonidine and yohimbine produce parallel decreases and increases, respectively, in both plasma and CSF NE in young normal subjects (80,122). These findings suggest that similar mechanisms involving alpha-2 adrenergic receptors regulate peripheral SNS outflow and CSF NE release.

In view of the inhibitory effect of NE on brainstem mechanisms regulating SNS outflow, it is possible that *decreased* CNS or brainstem NE activity, as proposed in the original NE depletion model of depression, could result in *increased* SNS outflow. Reduced CNS NE activity might also be expected to produce upregulation of CNS beta-adrenergic receptors and, thereby, possibly account for increased brain beta-adrenergic receptor binding observed in the postmortem studies of Mann and associates (118). However, such an NE-depletion model should also lead to upregulation of the CNS postsynaptic alpha-2 adrenergic receptors regulating blood pressure and SNS outflow. However, blood pressure (123–125), plasma NE (125), and plasma NE appearance rate (Veith et. al., unpublished findings) responses to the alpha-2 agonist clonidine or the alpha-2 antagonist yohimbine (124,126) are not increased in depressed patients, as might be expected if the sensitivity of brainstem alpha-2 receptors were increased. These findings argue against a primary CNS NE-depletion model, at least at the level of the brainstem. It is important to consider, however, that studies from our laboratory demonstrating in elderly volunteers a clonidine-induced fall in plasma NE without a corresponding reduction in CSF NE (80) raise uncertainty regarding the use of peripheral SNS or cardiovascular responses to centrally acting alpha-2 agents as means to assess CNS alpha-2 adrenergic receptor function.

The apparent lack of altered sensitivity of alpha-2 adrenergic mechanisms regulating SNS outflow in depression contrasts with neuroendocrine challenge studies examining alpha-2 adrenergic regulation of the HPA axis. Although controversy exists (127), alpha-2 adrenergic input is thought to inhibit CRF release and HPA axis activity (128,129), which suggests that increased HPA activity in depression might reflect diminished CNS NE input to the hypothalamus or pituitary.

Consistent with this model, plasma cortisol elevations in response to alpha-2 adrenergic antagonist yohimbine (124) are enhanced and plasma cortisol reductions following the alpha-2 agonist clonidine (130) are larger in depressed patients than in controls. This might be interpreted as upregulation of CNS alpha-2 receptor pathways that inhibit the HPA axis in response to low NE levels in this region. The demonstration of an inverse relationship between CSF NE levels and 4 p.m. plasma cortisol in a small sample of depressed patients (107) is also consistent with this model. In apparent contradiction, Roy and co-workers (131) found a trend for a positive correlation between NE and CRF levels in the CSF of depressed patients.

Alpha-2 adrenergic agonists stimulate growth hormone release in humans (132,133) and many studies examining growth hormone responses to test the integrity of CNS alpha-2 adrenergic receptor function have found blunted responses in depressed patients (123,134–136). These blunted clonidine-induced growth hormone responses have been interpreted as evidence for either a defect in or subsensitivity of CNS postsynaptic alpha-2 adrenergic receptors regulating growth hormone release. However, as noted above, this is difficult to reconcile with the absence of comparable effects on SNS outflow (123,124), which is also regulated by postsynaptic alpha-2 receptors. Furthermore, it is difficult to argue for the presence of subsensitivity of the postsynaptic alpha-2 adrenergic receptors regulating growth hormone release when the most parsimonious interpretation of the available CNS NE data is a reduction in CNS NE activity, which should upregulate these receptors. Finally, it is possible that the blunted growth hormone responses to clonidine result from increased 24 h growth hormone release (137), which would be expected to blunt growth hormone response to stimulation.

As an alternative approach to assessing alpha-2 receptor function in patients with depression, numerous studies have used the blood platelet alpha-2 receptor as a possible marker of CNS alpha-2 adrenergic receptor function because platelet receptors closely resemble those on CNS neurons (138). Although highly variable, the majority of these studies have reported *increased* platelet alpha-2 adrenergic receptor binding in platelets from depressed patients and reduced platelet alpha-2 receptor responsiveness, as indicated by diminished platelet aggregation, in response to adrenergic agonists (67,125,138–140). These findings have fueled speculation that depression might be associated with a generalized defect in CNS alpha-2 adrenergic receptor function. However, as noted in the careful review by Kafka and Paul (138), the interpretation of binding studies is complex. It is also important to acknowledge that the ability of the platelet alpha-2 adrenergic receptor to regulate normally in the physiological range of plasma NE concentrations has been questioned (141).

Increased CNS Acetylcholine Activity

Janowsky and associates (142) have hypothesized that depression might be a consequence of increased CNS acetylcholine activity and such a mechanism could also be invoked to account for elevated SNS activity in depressed patients. Both animal and human studies suggest that CNS acetylcholine mechanisms can stimulate the SNS through direct effects on descending cholinergic fibers regulating SNS outflow (143-145) or by releasing CRF, which also stimulates SNS outflow (92). Increased cholinergic activity could also account for HPA hyperactivity in depression because hypothalamic CRF and the pituitary release of ACTH appear to be stimulated by CNS cholinergic pathways in humans (146). Also consistent with this interpretation, plasma beta endorphin, which is coreleased with ACTH from the anterior pituitary, is elevated (147,148) and there is diminished feedback suppression of beta endorphin and ACTH by dexamethasone in these patients (146). In addition, plasma ACTH and beta endorphin responses to the centrally acting acetylcholinesterase inhibitor physotigmine are increased in patients with depression (149). Thus, increased acetylcholine activity in the CNS of depressed patients might result in dual activation of both the HPA axis and the SNS.

Reduced CNS Serotonin Activity

Many effective antidepressant agents affect serotonin metabolism in vitro (119, 150). Furthermore, chronic antidepressant treatment reduces maximal binding of serotonin receptors in vivo in animals (151), possibly reflecting an increase in the synaptic concentration of serotonin. These findings have led to considerable interest in the potential role of CNS serotonergic systems in affective illness.

Numerous studies in depressed patients have employed measurements of serotonin or its major metabolite, 5-hydroxyindole acetic acid (5-HIAA) in brain tissue or CSF (108,116,117,152-154), serotonin receptor binding in postmortem brain tissue (118,155,156), platelet serotonin uptake and the closely related tritiated-imipramine binding (157-159), and neuroendocrine challenge strategies (160,161) to assess presumed CNS serotonin function in depression. As recently reviewed (162), these studies generally suggest decreased CNS serotonin activity in patients with depression. The demonstration of a reduction in tritiated imipramine binding sites in the frontal cortex of suicide victims (155), thought to indicate fewer presynaptic serotonin neurons, supports this interpretation. Maximal binding of serotonin$_2$ receptor is increased in the cortex of suicide victims and this is compatible with upregulation of postsynaptic serotonin receptors in response to low concentrations of serotonin in the vicinity of these receptors (118,156). In addition, an important interrelationship appears to exist between CNS serotonin and NE neuronal systems that is relevant to the observation that beta-adrenergic receptor binding is increased in postmortem brains of suicide victims and to the mechanism of action of some antidepressant medications (118,119,151,163). Lesions of ascending CNS serotonin pathways result in up-regulation of both postsynaptic serotonin and beta-adrenergic receptor maximal binding (164). Moreover, an intact CNS serotonin system appears to be necessary for the development of antidepressant-induced beta-adrenergic receptor downregulation (163).

In addition to these findings suggesting a role for serotonin in the causes of depression and the mechanism of action of some antidepressant treatments, neuroanatomical evidence suggests that serotonin pathways might be involved in autonomic regulation in the brainstem (82,83). However, the specific role, if any, of CNS serotonin systems in the physiological regulation of SNS outflow is poorly defined. Although a minority of locus ceruleus afferents appear to be serotonergic (74), nerve fibers staining with serotonin-like immunoreactivity are closely associated with baroreceptor-inhibited RVLM neurons that project to the intermediolateral cell column of spinal cord (72). In addition, descending serotonin neurons are closely approximated to preganglionic SNS nerves in the rat, but their function is unknown (82,83). Finally, neither intravenous nor oral administration of serotonin precursors or agonists affects blood pressure, heart rate, or plasma MHPG or NE in humans (165-167). Thus, it is presently difficult to ascribe a role for CNS serotonin systems in the observed increase in SNS activity in depressed patients.

SYMPATHETIC NERVOUS SYSTEM FUNCTION IN PANIC DISORDER

Diagnosis and Epidemiology

Although often unrecognized in the primary care setting (168), anxiety disorders affect approximately 7% of the U.S. population (5,169). Phenomenological, genetic, and treatment outcome studies of patients with anxiety have been conducted in the past two decades and have resulted in the definition of several clinical syndromes characterized by DSM-III-R criteria. The most striking of these conditions is panic disorder (Table 3), which has a prevalence rate of 0.5% of the population (5). This form of anxiety has received the most scrutiny from clinical investigators attempting to identify a biological cause for anxiety disorders.

Individuals with panic disorder experience repeated, sudden attacks of acute anxiety associated with an array of symptoms suggestive of autonomic arousal (Table 3). In an attempt to avoid circumstances that become associated with the onset of symptoms or are considered likely to provoke anxiety attacks, patients

TABLE 3   DSM–III–R Diagnostic Criteria for Panic Disorder

A. At some time during the disturbance, one or more panic attacks (discrete periods of intense fear or discomfort) have occurred that were unexpected (i.e., did not occur immediately before or on exposure to a situation that almost always caused anxiety) and not triggered by situations in which the person was the focus of others' attention.
B. Either four attacks, as defined in criterion A, have occurred within a 4 week period, or one or more attacks have been followed by a period of at least 1 month of persistent fear of having another attack.
C. At least four of the following symptoms developed during at least one of the attacks:
   Shortness of breath (dyspnea) or smothering sensations
   Dizziness, unsteady feelings, or faintness
   Palpitations or accelerated heart rate (tachycardia)
   Trembling or shaking
   Sweating
   Choking
   Nausea or abdominal distress
   Depersonalization or derealization
   Numbness or tingling sensations (paresthesias)
   Flushes (hot flashes) or chills
   Chest pain or discomfort
   Fear of dying
   Fear of going crazy or of doing something uncontrolled
D. During at least some of the attacks, at least four of the symptoms in C developed suddenly and increased in intensity within 10 min of the beginning of the first symptom noticed in the attack.
E. It cannot be established that an organic factor initiated and maintained the the disturbance (e.g., amphetamine or caffeine intoxication, hyperthyroidism).

Panic Disorder with Agoraphobia

A. Meets the criteria for panic disorder;
B. Agoraphobia: Fear of being in places or situations from which escape might be difficult (or embarrassing) or in which help might not be available in the event of a panic attack. As a result of this fear, the person either restricts travel or needs a companion when away from home, or else endures agoraphobic situations despite intense anxiety. Common agoraphobic situations include being outside the home alone, being in a crowd or standing in a line, being on a bridge, and traveling in a bus, train, or car.

---

with panic disorder often develop agoraphobia (Table 3): a progressive restriction of their social functioning or a fear of public settings where attacks might be restricted, such as bridges or elevators. In addition to the obvious psychosocial morbidity caused by such symptoms, epidemiological evidence indicates that patients with panic disorder are at increased risk for cardiovascular death, from causes that remain obscure (170).

Clinical Studies of SNS Function in Panic Disorder

Disturbances of SNS function have been implicated in the pathogenesis of anxiety disorders since the Civil War era, when Jacob Mendes Da Costa hypothesized heightened SNS activity as the cause for cardiac symptoms in patients suffering from what he termed "irritable heart syndrome" (171). Recent studies exploring SNS activity in patients with anxiety disorders offer modest support for this hypothesis.

Several studies have reported an elevated resting heart rate in patients with various anxiety states (172-174) but this has not been a consistent finding (175-179). Likewise, modest elevations of resting blood pressure have been reported (172,180). Increased plasma catecholamine (unfractionated NE and EPI) levels were first reported in a group of patients with mixed anxiety and depression in the early 1970s (48). This early report has been confirmed by several recent studies using rigorous diagnostic criteria and more sensitive catecholamine assays. These studies have revealed that some patients with panic disorder or agoraphobia have significantly elevated EPI levels during the resting, nonpanic state (176,181-183). The majority of other studies have found trends toward higher EPI levels (173,179,184,185). Plasma EPI values typically average 75% higher in patients with panic disorder. Corresponding elevations of plasma NE levels in panic patients have been less frequently observed (182,183) although, when combined with occasional elevations of plasma MHPG (187), these reports suggest modest increases in cardiovascular SNS activity in some patients. Nesse and associates (188) noted decreased heart rate responses to isoproterenol, and two studies have shown diminished cyclic AMP responses to isoproterenol in lymphocytes in patients with panic disorder (189,190). These finidngs are compatible with reduced peripheral beta-adrenergic function, which could be attributable to increased circulating catecholamine levels in patients with panic disorder. The recent report by Castellani and associates (174) describing exaggerated plasma EPI responses to TRH infusions in panic patients compared to controls suggests increased adrenomedullary responsiveness in these patients.

It is important to note that the majority of the studies reporting plasma catecholamines in patients with panic disorder have relied on venous measurements. Villacres and associates (178) from our laboratory found no difference in arterialized plasma NE or NE appearance rate, but did find significantly elevated plasma EPI in 10 panic disorder patients compared to controls. Moreover, there was a close correlation between arterialized EPI levels and severity ratings of anxiety. Papp and associates (191) measured arterial plasma catecholamines in patients with panic disorder and controls and found no differences.

It has not yet been confirmed by plasma EPI kinetic studies that elevated plasma EPI levels in patients with panic disorder reflect increased adrenomedullary EPI release and not diminished clearance from plasma. However, studies from our laboratory (176) have found no difference between patients and controls in the clearance of NE from plasma, which is thought to be mediated in a manner similar to EPI clearance. Although recent evidence (192) suggests that EPI and NE are not necessarily cleared from plasma by identical mechanisms, it appears most likely that increased plasma EPI levels in patients with panic disorder represents increased resting adrenomedullary tone. It is important to note, however, that the plasma EPI elevations in patients with panic disorder are modest, have not yet been confirmed in large patient samples, and are not present in all patients, although inconsistencies in the literature might partly reflect methodological differences among studies (176).

If panic disorder is associated with a disturbance in resting autonomic function, specifically an increase in adrenomedullary activity, it might be expected that this would be most evident during a panic attack, especially if it is additionally assumed that SNS activation is somehow related to the cause or accounts for the symptoms of a panic attack. However, evidence to support this hypothesis is limited.

It is possible to induce panic attacks experimentally in predisposed patients by infusions of sodium lactate. Numerous studies have examined hemodynamic, ventilatory, and neuroendocrine measures in response to this provocative stimulus in an attempt to identify physiological or biochemical clues to the pathogenesis of panic disorder (173,179,181,185). In general, such studies reveal that sodium lactate more often induces a panic attack in patients than controls and reliably elevates heart rate, systolic blood pressure, and cardiac output. However, cardiovascular, ventilatory, or metabolic responses are not exaggerated in patients compared to controls despite the fact that patients experience these physiological changes with accentuated self-ratings of anxiety on rating scales. Moreover, lactate-induced panic is not associated with elevations of plasma catecholamine levels.

It has been suggested (179) that the absence of a rise in plasma norepinephrine level in response to lactate-induced panic is the result of the large volume load delivered during the lactate infusion protocol, which would be expected to activate baroreceptor reflexes to suppress SNS outflow. The increase in cardiac output associated with lactate infusions (179) might also be expected to offset an elevation in plasma NE levels or actually promote a fall in catecholamine levels, by enhancing their clearance from plasma. Thus, it is difficult to interpret plasma catecholamine responses to lactate infusion.

An alternative approach that avoids this confounding aspect of lactate-induced panic yet reliably induces panic attacks in a substantial portion of patients is the inhalation of carbon dioxide (172,193). In contrast to findings in lactate-induced panic, Gorman and associates (172) recently reported that carbon dioxide inhalation caused an overall increase in plasma NE and EPI as well as pulse and blood pressure in a group of patients with panic disorder or other anxiety disorders and controls. The diastolic blood pressure and NE elevations responses were greater in patients who panicked than in nonpanickers and controls. It was interesting, however, that carbon dioxide-induced panic was not associated with a greater increase in plasma EPI. The interpretation of the catecholamine data is unfortunately complicated by the fact that the reported values were obtained from either arterial or venous samplings, which were pooled for the analysis. Nevertheless, the exaggerated plasma NE and diastolic responses to carbon-dioxide-induced panic suggest participation of at least the cardiovascular component of the SNS in carbon-dioxide-induced panic.

Several investigators have successfully measured cardiovascular and catecholamine responses in panic patients during either spontaneous or situationally induced panic attacks (175,179,194–196). Ko and associates (194) reported a significant plasma MHPG elevation in phobic patients who panicked in response to phobic exposure. Cameron and associates (195) found no increase in MHPG but did observe increases in heart rate and NE, but not EPI, in four patients who experienced "spontaneous" panic attacks during hospitalization on a research ward. Woods and associates (175) reported increases in heart rate but an absence of blood pressure elevations in patients who developed spontaneous panic attacks. The above studies revealed marked variability of responses among individuals, despite the presence of observed and subjectively identified panic attacks. This variability conforms with evidence that fewer than 50% of spontaneous panic attacks are associated with increases in heart rate or ventricular arrhythmias measured by continuous ambulatory monitoring (177,178,197).

Sellew and associates (196) recently reported pilot data providing the most compelling evidence to date for SNS activation during panic. Spontaneous and imagery-induced panic attacks were observed in four patients during continuous venous sampling using a pump that allows for plasma catecholamine measurement at 1 min intervals, thereby avoiding the potential problem of missing plasma catecholamine elevations due to the short half-life of catecholamines in plasma. Panic was associated with seven-to ninefold plasma NE elevations from baseline, to values exceeding 1000 pg/ml for two subjects. Plasma EPI elevations were more variable, but ranged from slightly increased above basal to a sixfold elevation to 238 pg/ml in one patient (A.P. Sellew, personal communication, 1988). Plasma NE values obtained during panic attacks exceeded those obtained earlier during bicycle exercise, which is a potent stimulus for SNS activation. Although preliminary, these promising findings suggest that a robust activation of the SNS occurs in some patients during panic attacks.

Pharmacological challenge strategies have also been used to assess behavioral and neuroendocrine function in patients with panic disorder and other anxiety states (187,198,199). As is true for the lactate and carbon dioxide studies, panic patients experience greater self-rated anxiety and a higher frequency of panic attacks in response to caffeine infusions, but this is not associated with significant differences from controls in objective physiological variables (199). In contrast, however, Charney and associates (187) demonstrated that 54% of their panic patients developed panic attacks in response to infusions of the alpha-2 antagonist yohimbine compared to 5% of controls. As a group, the patients reported significantly greater sensitivity to yohimbine on anxiety ratings, largely due to the patients who panicked. In addition, yohimbine produced greater overall increases in blood pressure, heart rate, and plasma cortisol in patients than controls. The yohimbine-induced elevation in plasma MHPG was not greater in patients than controls but was greater in patients who panicked compared both to those who did not and to controls. However, it is possible that the exaggerated MHPG responses in patients who panicked reflected basal differences, because patients who panicked had the highest baseline levels and there was evidence suggesting a relationship between basal levels and peak MHPG responses to yohimbine among patients and controls. Using a similar approach, Nutt (198) found that clonidine produced greater reductions in blood pressure and heart rate in panic patients compared to controls, despite comparable baseline values. This apparent increased sensitivity to alpha-2 adrenergic suppression of sympathetic outflow is in agreement with the increased sensitivity to the alpha-2 antagonist yohimbine described by Charney and associates (187).

In summary, several lines of evidence suggest that panic disorder is associated with a modest increase in resting adrenomedullary activity and possibly increased adrenomedullary responsiveness (174). Panic attacks that occur spontaneously or in response to imagery, carbon dioxide, or yohimbine are occasionally, but not invariably, associated with signs of SNS activation. It is unlikely that the concentrations of circulating catecholamines occurring at rest or during panic directly account for anxiety symptoms in these patients. Consistent with this view, Papp and associates (200) elicited observable anxiety in only 1 of 11 patients with social phobia (i.e., irrational fear of specific activity such as public speaking, etc.) in whom mean plasma EPI values of 928 pg/ml were obtained during exogenous EPI infusions. In addition, subjective anxiety is not a prominent feature in patients with pheochromocytoma, who have extreme elevations of plasma catecholamines (201). Finally it is clear that the heightened behavioral sensitivity of panic patients to anxiogenic stimuli can occur in the absence of correspondingly notable cardiovascular or neuroendocrine responses.

It must be emphasized that few studies have been performed using measurements of arterial or arterialized plasma catecholamines and plasma catecholamine kinetics, and to our knowledge none have used direct measurement of peripheral SNS activity by microneurographic techniques. Because some panic attacks are likely to be associated with an increase in cardiac output (179) that would be expected to increase catecholamine clearance, it is likely that plasma catecholamine levels in venous plasma will underestimate actual SNS activity during panic attacks. It is also important to consider that spontaneous and experimentally induced panic attacks may not be identical physiologically. Finally, caution must be exercised in assuming a causative role of any neuroendocrine or metabolic disturbance in these patients who, as suggested by Liebowitz and associates (173) and emphasized by Gaffney and associates (179), might be conditioned to overrespond emotionally to the physiological changes produced by a variety of nonspecific stimuli.

SNS Mechanisms Implicated in the Pathogenesis of Panic Disorder: Role of the Locus Ceruleus

A substantial body of research in animal studies indicates an important relationship between locus ceruleus activity and the behavioral and physiological manifestations of anxiety (73,76,202). Not surprisingly, theoretical and experimental efforts to explore the pathogenesis of anxiety disorders in humans have focused upon efforts to assess presumed CNS noradrenergic functioning in patients. However, the recognition that panic disorder represents a distinct clinical entity and the investigation of its pathogenesis are recent developments, particularly compared to the 20–30 year exploration of the neurobiology of depression. As a consequence, efforts to identify specific CNS mechanisms that might predispose patients or account for the profound symptoms of panic disorder are in the preliminary stages of development. As is true for the investigation of other psychiatric conditions, progress in this area is additionally hindered by limited access to the CNS in living humans.

The clinical investigation of the pathogenesis of panic disorder has relied upon neuroendocrine or pharmacological challenge strategies in an effort to identify differential cardiovascular or endocrine responses in patients and controls that might allow us to make inferences regarding CNS functioning. For example, the yohimbine studies of Charney and associates (187) have yielded the most specific hypothesis to date and have been interpreted as evidence for hyperresponsiveness of the locus ceruleus noradrenergic system in panic disorder. However, as Charney and associates readily acknowledge (187), such conclusions must be made cautiously considering the complex neurotransmitter input to this important brain region; the possibility that alpha-2 antagonism is modulating alternative neurotransmitter systems to evoke the observed neuroendocrine and cardiovascular responses in their patients; the possibility that yohimbine is acting peripherally; and that yohimbine might be acting nonspecifically to produce symptoms that themselves trigger a panic attack or are interpreted as panic symptoms by susceptible patients.

Future Studies

Although efforts to determine the physiological substrate for panic disorder have only recently been initiated and the modest findings to date must be considered preliminary, suggestive leads emerging from recent studies offer several intriguing avenues for speculation and future investigation.

Adrenomedullary Hyperactivity

As noted herein, several studies suggest the presence of heightened basal adrenomedullary activity in some patients with panic disorder. If this is confirmed by larger study populations using appropriate sampling and kinetic methods, future studies should explore mechanisms not only that underlie SNS regulation by the CNS but also specifically those that preferentially stimulate the adrenal medulla.

It would be interesting to assess, for example, if enhanced adrenomedullary responsiveness to stimulation is present in panic disorder. Is the plasma EPI response to such provocative stimuli as relative hypoglycemia (203) increased? Alternatively, plasma EPI responses to the centrally acting anticholinesterase, physostigmine, could be assessed. Physostigmine is a pharmacologic stimulus that reliably activates the adrenal medulla (143–145). This approach to assessing adrenomedullary responsiveness in panic disorder might also have CNS implications because physostigmine is thought to stimulate the adrenal medulla through activation of central nervous system cholinergic pathways (143–145). The recent report by Castellani and associates (174) demonstrating that panic patients exhibit heightened EPI responses to thyrotropin-releasing hormone (TRH) provides an additional rationale for exploring CNS cholinergic function in panic disorder, because TRH-mediated pressor and catecholamine responses (204,205) are thought to be mediated in the CNS (205–208) by mechanisms involving cholinergic pathways (209,210).

CNS Peptidergic Systems

The studies by Brown and Fisher and their associates (17,92,98,205) implicate CNS peptidergic mechanisms in the differential activation of the adrenomedullary and cardiovascular components of the SNS and suggest several possible avenues for future research if adrenomedullary hyperactivity is confirmed in panic disorder. They have shown in animals, for example, that centrally administered bombesin preferentially elevates plasma EPI levels, whereas administration of CRF produces a greater effect on plasma NE (17). CRF acts in the CNS to increase heart rate and blood pressure, but bombesin decreases heart rate and blood pressure. Evidence that somatostatin analogs act centrally to antagonize the plasma EPI rise associated with several stress paradigms but have no effect on the plasma NE responses to these stimuli (98) is additional support for the hypothesis proposed by Brown and Fisher (17) that mechanisms controlling adrenomedullary sympathetic outflow might be entirely independent from the baroreceptor-dependent mechanisms controlling cardiovascular SNS outflow.

The possibility that CNS peptidergic mechanisms might underlie the modest, but possibly selective, elevation of plasma EPI in some patients with panic disorder has not been explored. However, HPA axis function has been assessed in this disorder and these data allow for speculative inferences regarding the activity of CRF systems in the CNS (211,212). Roy-Byrne and associates (213) have shown that the ACTH and cortisol response to intravenously infused CRF are attenuated in patients with panic disorder despite normal baseline cortisol levels. Because hypercortisolemia and DST nonsuppression are also occasionally reported in patients with panic disorder (211), it has been proposed that this condition is associated with episodic bursts of HPA activity rather than the persistent elevation seen in depression. These findings, coupled with the evidence from most studies that basal plasma NE levels in panic disorder are not significantly elevated, argue against persistently increased CRF activity in the CNS as a primary neuroendocrine disturbance in panic disorder. To our knowledge, altered CSF levels of CRF, bombesin, or somatostatin have not been reported in panic disorder but the above findings emphasize the value of exploring further the potential contribution of CNS peptidergic mechanisms in the neuroendocrine disturbances present in some patients.

CNS Benzodiazepine Receptor Mechanisms

Recent studies have identified specific receptors for benzodiazepines in the brain and have shown that they are functionally linked to GABA, the major inhibitory neurotransmitter in the CNS (214). Animal and human studies using specific benzodiazepine receptor inverse agonists demonstrate that these agents produce the behavioral and physiological manifestations of anxiety, thus suggesting that the benzodiazepine/GABA receptor complex may mediate aspects of the anxiety state (214). Evidence that the specific benzodiazepine antagonist RO15-1788 blocks the behavioral, cognitive, neuroendocrine, and saccadic eye movement effects of intravenous diazepam suggests that these measures are influenced by pathways involving benzodiazepine receptors (214,215). These findings are relevant in the present context because it has also been shown that GABA is a potent inhibitor of SNS outflow when applied to the RVLM (70). The GABA antagonist bicuculline causes a marked elevation of blood pressure and heart rate, suggesting that GABAergic mechanisms are tonically active (70). These effects are thought to occur at local GABAergic neurons intrinsic to the brainstem nucleus tractus solitarii and RVLM region (70).

Observations from our laboratory indicate that diazepam suppresses SNS outflow in humans, as reflected in a reduction in the rate of plasma NE appearance (216). This lends clinical support to the concept that CNS benzodiazepine/ GABA mechanisms participate in SNS regulation. Moreover, Roy-Byrne and associates (217) have recently shown that this response is blunted in patients with panic disorder. Thus, future studies are required to examine further the potential role of CNS benzodiazepine receptor function in panic disorder.

SUMMARY AND CONCLUSION

Based on the extensive clinical research reviewed herein, it is reasonable to conclude that major depressive illness is associated with hyperactivity of the cardiovascular component of the SNS and that this is compatible with findings suggesting increased CRF activity in the CNS in depression. Research evidence for a disturbance of SNS function in panic disorder points more to increased basal adrenomedullary than to generalized SNS activation, but this impression must be considered preliminary.

The potential importance of these observations hinges on the assumption that the demonstration of SNS, or other physiological, disturbances in psychiatric disorders will provide opportunities to derive specific inferences regarding brain function that will have causative or therapeutic significance. In many respects, this review reflects this prevailing tenet in clinical biological psychiatry, because highly specific CNS models are promoted to explain the emerging clinical evidence for SNS disturbances in depression and panic disorder. Although intended to be provocative, it must be emphasized that these unitary models are speculative and unrealistically simplistic, considering the redundancy of CNS mechanisms regulating the neuroendocrine systems reviewed. There has been a tendency in biological psychiatry to adopt uncritically such unitary models and to employ clinical measurements with insufficient attention to their physiological determinants, and it is not the intent of this chapter to promote such approaches.

Indeed, perhaps the most striking observation to be derived from this review is that the degree of SNS activation present in these disorders is quantitatively modest and does not exceed levels of activation that might be entirely commensurate with nonspecific stress associated with a serious illness. The preliminary findings of Sellew and associates (196) are a notable exception. Although the approximately 75% average increase in basal NE in depression and EPI in panic disorder is modest, this is roughly equivalent to the response of the SNS to orthostasis, which is not inconsequential. However, in view of the occasionally profound clinical intensity of these disorders, the absence of more impressive SNS activation is a compelling argument for exercising caution in adopting causative inferences related to SNS disturbances and the pathogenesis of these disorders. Nevertheless, these suggestive findings deserve further research exploration. We hope that such efforts, combined with the anticipated technical developments in molecular genetics (218) and brain imaging, will promote progress in the understanding and treatment of these disorders.

ACKNOWLEDGMENT

This work was supported by the Medical Research Service of the Veterans Administration. Maxine Cormier provided excellent secretarial support.

REFERENCES

1. Selye H. Stress. Montreal, Acta Inc., Med. Publ.; 1950.
2. Cannon W B. Bodily changes in pain, hunger, fear and rage.New York: D. Appeton, 1929.
3. Cannon W B. The wisdom of the body. New York: W. W. Norton, 1939.
4. Diagnostic and statistical manual of mental disorders, 3rd ed, revised. Washington, D.C.: American Psychiatric Association, 1987.
5. Regier D A, Boyd J H, Burke J D Jr, et al. One-month prevalence of mental disorders in the United States. Based on five epidemiologic catchment area sites. Arch Gen Psychiatry 1988; 45:977–986.
6. Borson S, Barnes R A, Kukull W A, et al. Symptomatic depression in elderly medical outpatients. J Am Geriatr Soc 1986; 34:341–347.
7. Okimoto JT, Barnes R F, Veith R C, Raskind M A, Inui T S, Carter W B. Screening for depression in geriatric medical patients. Am J Psychiatry 1962; 139: 699.
8. Blazer DB. Depression in late life. St. Louis: C.V. Mosby, 1982: 105–117.
9. Guze S F, Robins E. Suicide and primary affective disorders. Br J Psychiatry 1970; 117:437–438.
10. Matnon K G, Blazer D G, Woodbury M A. Suicide in middle age and later life: sex and race specific life table and cohort analyses. J Gerontol 1987; 42(2):219–227.
11. Avery D, Winokur G. Mortality in depressed patients treated with electroconvulsive therapy and antidepressants. Arch Gen Psychiatry 1976; 33: 1029–1037.
12. Bunney W E Jr, Davis J M. Norepinephrine and depressive reactions: a review. Arch Gen Psychiatry 1965; 13:483–494.
13. Schildkraut J J. The catecholamine hypothesis of affective disorders: a review of supporting evidence. Am J Psychiatry 1965; 122:509–522.
14. Cryer P E. Physiology and pathophysiology of the human sympathoadrenal system. N Engl J Med 1980; 303:436–444.
15. Folkow B. Physiological aspects of primary hypertension. Physiol Rev 1982; 62(2):347–504.

16. Vallbo A B, Hagbarth K-E, Torebjök H E, Wallin B G. Somatosensory, proprioceptive, and sympathetic activity in human peripheral nerves. Physiol Rev 1979; 59(4): 919–957.

17. Brown M R, Fisher L A. Brain peptide regulation of adrenal epinephrine secretion. Am J Physiol 1984; 247:E41–E46.

18. Wallin B G. Muscle sympathetic activity and plasma concentrations of noradrenaline. Acta Physiol Scand 1984; 527: 25–29.

19. Victor R G, Leimbach W N Jr, Seals D R, Wallin B G, Mark A L. Effects of the cold pressor test on muscle sympathetic nerve activity in humans. Hypertension 1987; 9: 429–436.

20. Havel P J, Veith R C, Dunning B E, Taborsky G J Jr. Pancreatic noradrenergic nerves are activated by neuroglucopenia but not by hypotension or hypoxia in the dog. J Clin Invest 1988; 82:1538–1545.

21. Hilton S M. The defence-arousal system and its relevance for circulatory and respiratory control. J Exp Biol 1982; 100:159–174.

22. Hjemdahl P, Freyschuss U, Juhlin-Dannfelt A, Linde B. Differential sympathetic activation during neutral stress evoked by the Stroop test. Acta Physiol Scand 1984; 527(Suppl):25–29.

23. Goldstein D S, Eisenhofer G, Sax F L, Keiser H R, Kopin I J. Plasma norepinephrine pharmacokinetics during mental challenge. Psychosom Med 1987; 49:591–605.

24. Victor R G, Seals D R, Mark A L. Differential control of heart rate and sympathetic nerve activity during dynamic exercise. J Clin Invest 1987; 79: 508–516.

25. Christensen N J, Brandsburg O. The relationship between plasma catecholamine concentration and pulse rate during exercise and standing. Eur J Clin Invest 1973; 3; 399–406.

26. Goldstein D S, McCarty R, Polinsky R J, Kopin I J. Relationship between plasma norepinephrine and sympathetic neural activity. Hypertension 1983; 5:552–559.

27. Halter J B, Pflug A E, Porte D Jr. Mechanism of plasma catecholamine increases during surgical stress in man. J Clin Endocrinol Metab 1977; 45: 930–944.

28. Pflug A E, Halter J B. Effect of spinal anesthesia on adrenergic tone and the neuroendocrine responses to surgical stress in man. Anesthesiology 1981; 55:120–126.

29. Esler M, Jennings G, Korner P, et al. Assessment of human sympathetic nervous system activity from measurements of norepinephrine turnover. Hypertension 1988; 11(1): 3–20.

30. Esler M, Jackman G, Bobik A, et al. Determination of norepinephrine apparent release rate and clearance in humans. Life Sci 1979; 25:1461–1470.

31. Best J D, Halter J B. Release and clearance rates of epinephrine in man: importance of arterial measurements. J Clin Endocrinol Metab 1982; 55: 263–268.

32. Kopin I J. Catecholamine metabolism: basic aspects and clinical significance. Pharmacol Rev 1985; 37(4):333–364.

33. Schwartz R S, Jaeger L F, Veith R C. The importance of body composition to the increase in plasma norepinephrine appearance rate in elderly men. J Gerontol 1987; 42: 546–551.

34. Veith R C, Featherstone J A, Linares O A, Halter J B. Age differences in plasma norepinephrine kinetics in humans. J Gerontol 1986; 41:319–324.

35. Veith R C, Best J D, Halter J B. Dose-dependent suppression of norepinephrine appearance rate in plasma by clonidine in man. J Clin Endocrinol Metab 1984; 59: 151–1155.

36. Linares O A, Jacquez J A, Zech L A, et al. Norepinephrine metabolism in humans. Kinetic analysis and model. J Clin Invest 1987; 80:1332–1341.

37. Abumrad N N, Rabin D, Diamond M P, Lacy W W. Use of a heated superficial hand vein as an alternative site for the measurement of amino acid concentrations and for the study of glucose and alanine kinetics in man. Metabolism 1981; 30:936–940.

38. Barnes R F, Raskind M A, Gumbrecht G, Halter J B. The effects of age on the plasma catecholamine response to mental stress in man. J Clin Endocrinol Metab 1982; 54:64–69.

39. Dimsdale J E, Moss J. Short term catecholamine response to psychological stress. Psychosom Med 1980; 62:347–504.

40. Barnes R F, Veith R C, Borson S, Verhey J, Raskind M A, Halter J B. High levels of plasma catecholamines in dexamethasone-resistant depressed patients. Am J Psychiatry 1983; 140:1623–1625.

41. Esler M, Turbott J, Schwarz R, et al. The peripheral kinetics of norepinephrine in depressive illness. Arch Gen Psychiatry 1982; 39:295–300.

42. Jimerson D C, Insel T R, Reus V I, Kopin I W. Increased plasma MHPG in dexamethasone-resistant depressed patients. Arch Gen Psychiatry 1983; 40: 173–176.

43. Lake C R, Pickar D, Ziegler M G, Lipper S, Slater S, Murphy D L. High plasma norepinephrine levels in patients with major affective disorder. Am J Psychiatry 1982; 139:1315–1318.

44. Maas J W, Koslow S H, Davis J, et al. Catecholamine metabolism and disposition in healthy and depressed subjects. Arch Gen Psychiatry 1987; 44: 337–344.

45. Roy A, Pickar D, Linnoila M, Potter W Z. Plasma norepinephrine level in affective disorders. Relationship to melancholia. Arch Gen Psychiatry 1985; 42:1181–1185.

46. Rudorfer M V, Ross R J, Linnoila M, Sherer M A, Potter W Z. Exaggerated orthostatic responsivity of plasma norepinephrine in depression. Arch Gen Psychiatry 1985; 42:1186–1192.

47. Siever L J, Pickar D, Lake R, Cohen R M, Uhde T W, Murphy D L. Extreme elevations in plasma norepinephrine associated with decreased alpha-adrenergic responsivity in major depressive disorder: two case reports. J Clin Psychopharmacol 1983; 3(1):39–41.

48. Wyatt R J, Portnoy B, Kupfer D J, Snyder F, Engelman K. Resting plasma catecholamine concentrations in patients with depression and anxiety. Arch Gen Psychiatry 1971; 24:65-70.

49. Roy A, Pickar D, De Jong J, Karoum F, Linnoila M. Norepinephrine and its metabolites in cerebrospinal fluid, plasma, and urine. Arch Gen Psychiatry 1988; 45:849-857.

50. Roy A, Guthrie S, Pickar D, Linnoila M. Plasma norepinephrine responses to cold challenge in depressed patients and normal controls. Psychiatry Res 1987; 21:161-168.

51. de Villiers A S, Russell V A, Carstens M E, et al. Noradrenergic function and hypothalamic-pituitary-adrenal axis activity in primary unipolar major depressive disorder. Psychiatry Res 1987; 22:127-140.

52. Louis W J, Doyle A E, Anavekar S N. Plasma noradrenaline concentration and blood pressure in essential hypertension, phaeochromocytoma and depression. Clin Sci Mol Med 1975; 48:239s-242s.

53. Veith R C, Barnes R F, Villacres E C, et al. Plasma catecholamines and norepinephrine kinetics in depression and panic disorder. In: Belmaker R, ed. Catecholamines: clinical aspects. New York: Alan R. Liss. 1988.

54. Koslow S H, Maas J W, Bowden C L, Davis J M, Hanin I, Javaid J. CSF and urinary biogenic amines and metabolites in depression and mania. A controlled, univariate analysis. Arch Gen Psychiatry 1983; 40:999-1010.

55. Kumar A, Alcser K, Grunhaus L, Greden J F. Relationships of the dexamethasone suppression test to clinical severity and degree of melancholia. Biol Psychiatry 1986; 21:436-444.

56. Carroll B J, Feinberg M, Greden J F, et al. A specific laboratory test for the diagnosis of melancholia: Standardization, validation, and clinical utility. Arch Gen Psychiatry 1981; 38:15-22.

57. Arana G W, Baldessarini R J, Ornsteen M. The dexamethasone suppression test for diagnosis and prognosis in psychiatry. Arch Gen Psychiatry 1985; 42:1193-1204.

58. Rubin L, Price L, Charney D, Heninger G. Noradrenergic function and the cortisol response to dexamethasone in depression. Psychiatry Res 1985; 15: 5-15.

59. Rosenbaum A, Schatzberg M T, Orsulak P, Jiang N, Cole J, Schildkraut J. Towards a biochemical classification of depressive disorders: VII. Urinary-free cortisol and urinary MHPG in depression. Am J Psychiatry 1983; 140: 314-317.

60. Muscettola G, Potter W Z, Pickar D, Goodwin F K. Urinary 3-methoxy-4-hydroxyphenylglycol and major affective disorders. Arch Gen Psychiatry 1984; 41:337-342.

61. Ackenheil M, Albus M, Muller F, et al. Catecholamine response to short-time stress in schizophrenic and depressive patients. In: Usdin E, Kopin IJ, Barchas J, eds. Catecholamines: basic and clinical frontiers. New York: Pergamon Press, 1979.

62. Paton D. The mechanisms of neuronal and extraneuronal transport of catecholamines. New York: Raven Press, 1976: 95-153, 325, 354.

63. Trendelenburg U. A kinetic analysis of the extraneuronal uptake and metabolism of catecholamines. Rev Physiol Biochem Pharmacol 1980; 87: 33-115.

64. Iversen L, Salt P. Inhibition of catecholamine uptake$_2$ by steroids in the isolated rat heart. Br J Pharmacol 1970; 40:528-530.

65. Carstens M E, Engelbrecht A H, Russell V A, et al. Beta-adrenoceptors on lymphocytes of patients with major depressive disorder. Psychiatry Res. 1987; 20:239-248.

66. Mann J J, Brown R P, Halper J R, et al. Reduced sensitivity of lymphocyte beta- adrenergic receptors in patients with endogenous depression and psychomotor agitation. N Engl J Med 1985; 313:715-720.

67. Wood K, Whiting K, Coppen A. Lymphocyte beta-adrenergic receptor density of patients with recurrent affective illness. J Affect Dis 10:3-8.

68. halper J P, Brown R P, Sweeney J A, Kocsis J H, Peters A, Mann J J. Blunted beta-adrenergic responsivity of peripheral blood mononuclear cells in endogenous depression. Arch Gen Psychiatry 1988; 45:241-244.

69. Matthews W D, Jim K F, Hieble J P, DeMarinis R M. Postsynaptic alpha adrenoceptors on vascular smooth muscle. Fed Proc 1984; 43:2923-2928.

70. Reis D J, Morrison S, Ruggiero D A. The C1 area of the brainstem in tonic and reflex control of blood pressure. State of the art lecture. Hypertension 1988; 11(Suppl I): I8-I13.

71. Morrison S F, Milner T A, Reis D J. Reticulospinal vasomotor neurons of the rat rostral ventrolateral medulla: relationship to sympathetic nerve activity and the C1 adrenergic cell group. J Neurosci 1988; 8(4):1286-1301.

72. Brown D L, Guyenet P G. Cardiovascular neurons of brain stem with projections to spinal cord. Am Physiol Soc 1984; 247:R-1009-R1016.

73. Aston-Jones G, Ennis M, Pieribone V A, Nicell W T, Shipley M T. The brain nucleus locus coeruleus: restricted afferent control of a broad efferent network. Science 1986; 234:734-737.

74. Pieribone V A, Aston-Jones G, Bohn M C. Adrenergic and noradrenergic neurons in the C1 and C3 areas project to locus coeruleus: a fluorescent double labeling study. Neurosci Lett 1988; 85:297-303.

75. Ennis M, Aston-Jones G. Two physiologically distinct populations of neurons in the ventrolateral medulla innervate the locus coeruleus. Brain Res 1987; 425:275-282.

76. Foote S L, Bloom F E, Aston-Jones G. Nucleus locus ceruleus: new evidence of anatomical and physiological specificity. Physiol Rev 1983; 63: 844-914.

77. Elam M, Yao T, Thoren P, Svennson T H. Hypercapnia and hypoxia: chemoreceptor-mediated control of locus coeruleus neurons and splanchnic sympathetic nerves. Brain Res 1981; 222:373-381.

78. Elam M, Yao T, Svennson T H, Thoren P. Regulation of locus coeruleus neurons and splanchnic sympathetic nerves by cardiovascular efferents. Brain Res 1984; 290:281-287.

79. Raskind M, Peskind E, Halter J, Jimerson D. Norepinephrine and MHPG levels in CSF and plasma in Alzheimer's disease. Arch Gen Psychiatry 1984; 42:343-346.

80. Raskind M A, Peskind E R, Veith R C, Beard J C, Gumbrecht G, Halter J B. Increased plasma and cerebrospinal fluid norepinephrine in older men: differential suppression by clonidine. J Clin Endocrinol Metab 66:438-443.

81. Meeley M P, Ernsberger P R, Granata A R, Reis D J. An endogenous clonidine-displacing substance from bovine brain: receptor binding and hypotensive actions in the ventrolateral medulla. Life Sci 1986; 38:1119-1126.

82. Loewy A D, McKellar S. Serotonergic projections from the ventral medulla to the intermediolateral cell column in the rat. Brain Res 1981; 211:146-152.

83. Appel N M, Wessendorf M W, Elde R P. Coexistence of serotonin- and substance P-like immunoreactivity in nerve fibers apposing identified sympathoadrenal preganglionic neurons in rat intermediolateral cell column. Neurosci Lett 1986; 65:241-246.

84. Swanson L W. Organization of mammalian neuroendocrine system. In: Mountcastle V B, Bloom F E, Geiger S R, eds. Handbook of physiology, vol. 4, intrinsic regulatory systems of the brain. Baltimore: Waverly Press, 1986; 317-363.

85. Swanson L W, Sawchenko P E. Paraventricular nucleus: a site for the integration of neuroendocrine and autonomic mechanisms. Neuroendocrinology 1980; 31;410-417.

86. Sawchenko P E, Swanson L W. Immunohistochemical identification of neurons in the paraventricular nucleus of the hypothalamus that project to the medulla or to the spinal cord in the rat. J Comp Neurol 1982; 205:260-272.

87. Nemeroff C B, Widerlöv E, Bissette G, et al. Elevated concentrations of CSF corticotropin-releasing factor-like immunoreactivity in depressed patients. Science 1984; 226:1342-1343.

88. Widerlöv E, Bissette G, Nemeroff C B. Monoamine metabolites, corticotropin releasing factor and somatostatin as CSF markers in depressed patients. J Affect Dis 1988; 14:99-107.

89. Banki C M, Bissette G, Arato M, O'Connor L, Nemeroff C B. Cerebrospinal fluid corticotropin releasing factor-like immunoreactivity in depression and schizophrenia. Am J Psychiatry 1987; 145:1526-1531.

90. Gold P W, Loriaux D L, Roy A, et al. Responses to corticotropin-releasing hormone in the hypercortisolism of depression and Cushing's disease. Pathophysiologic and diagnostic implications. N Engl J Med 1986; 314:1329-1335.

91. Nemeroff C B, Owens M J, Bissette G, Andorn A C, Stanley M. Reduced corticotropin releasing factor binding sites in the frontal cortex of suicide victims. Arch Gen Psychiatry 1988; 45:577-579.

93. Koob G F, Bloom F E. Corticotropin-releasing factor and behavior. Fed Proc 1985; 44:259–263.
94. Rubinow D R. Cerebrospinal fluid somatostatin and psychiatric illness. Biol Psychiatry 1986; 21:341–365.
95. Bissette G, Widerlöv E, Walleus H, et al. Alterations in cerebrospinal concentrations of somatostatin-like immunoreactivity in neuropsychiatric disorders. Arch Gen Psychiatry 1986; 43:1148–1151.
96. Gold P W, Rubinow D R. Neuropeptide function in affective illness: corticotropin-releasing hormone and somatostatin as model systems. In: Meltzer HY, ed. Psychopharmacology: the third generation of progress. New York: Raven Press, 1987: 617–627.
97. Weitzmann R E, Firemark H, Riviczky A, Nelson J C. Hypotension following intraventricular somatostatin (SRIF) is mediated by lowering of plasma catecholamines. Endocrinology 104:292 (abstract).
98. Fisher D A, Brown M R. Somatostatin analog: plasma catecholamine suppression mediated by the central nervous system. Endocrinology 1980; 107:714–718.
99. Heisler S, Reisine T D, Hook V Y H, Axelrod J. Somatostatin inhibits multireceptor stimulation of cyclic AMP formation and corticotropin secretion in mouse pituitary tumor cells. Proc Natl Acad Sci 1982; 79: 6502–6506.
100. Doran A R, Rubinow D R, Roy A, Pickar D. CSF somatostatin and abnormal response to dexamethasone administration in schizophrenic and depressed patients. Arch Gen Psychiatry 1986; 43:365–369.
101. Maas J W, Hattox S E, Green N M, Lanois D S. MHPG production by human brain in vivo. Science 1979; 205: 1025–1027.
102. Blombery P A, Kopin I J, Gordon E K, Mackey S R, Ebert M H. Conversion of MHPG to vanillylmandelic acid. Arch Gen Psychiatry 1980; 37: 1095–1098.
103. Kopin I J, Polinsky R J, Oliver J A, Oddershede I R, Ebert M H. Urinary catecholamine metabolites distinguish different types of sympathetic neuronal dysfunction in patients with orthostatic hypotension. J Clin Endocrinol Metab 1983; 57:632–637.
104. Mardh G, Sjoqvist B, Anggard E. Norepinephrine metabolism in man using deuterium labeling: the conversion of 4-hydroxy-3-methoxy-phenylglycol to 4-hydroxy-3-methyoxymandelic acid. J Neurochem 1981; 36:1181–1185.
105. Christensen N J, Vestergaard P, Sorensen T, Rafaelsen D J. Cerebrospinal fluid adrenaline and noradrenaline in depressed patients. Acta Psychiatr Scand 1980; 61:178–182.
106. Gjerris A, Rafaelsen O J, Christensen N J. CSF-adrenaline—low in "somatizing depression." Acta Psychiatr Scand 1987; 75:516–520.
107. Lu R-B, Ho S-L, Ho B T, Leu S-Y, Shian L-R, Chen W-L. Correlation between plasma cortisol and CSF catecholamines in endogenous depressed dexamethasone nonsuppressors. J Affect Dis 10:177–184.

108. Post R M, Ballenger J C, Goodwin F K. Cerebrospinal fluid studies of neurotransmitter function in manic and depressive illness. In: Post RN, Ballenger JC, eds. Neurobiology of mood disorders. Baltimore: Williams & Wilkins, 1984: 685–717.

109. Redmond D E, Katz M M, Maas J W, Swann A, Casper R, David J M. Cerebrospinal fluid amine metabolites. Arch Gen Psychiatry 1986; 43: 939–947.

110. Roy A, Pickar D, Linnoila M, Doran A R, Ninan P, Paul S M. Cerebrospinal fluid monoamine and monoamine metabolite concentrations in melancholia. Psychiatry Res 1985; 15:281–292.

111. Moore R Y. Central catecholamine neuron systems: anatomy and physiology of the norepinephrine and epinephrine systems. Annu Rev Neurosci 1979; 2:113–168.

112. Fuxe K, Ungerstedt U. Localization of catecholamine uptake in rat brain after intraventricular injection. Life Sci 1966; 5:1817–1824.

113. Ziegler M D, Lake C R, Wood J H, Ebert M H. Norepinephrine in cerebrospinal fluid: basic studies, effects of drugs and disease. In: Wood JH, ed. Neurobiology of cerebrospinal fluid. New York: Plenum Press, 1980: 141–152.

114. Peskind E R, Raskind M A, Wilkinson C W, Flatness D E, Halter J B. Peripheral sympathectomy and adrenal medullectomy do not alter cerebrospinal fluid norepinephrine. Brain Res 1986; 367:258–264.

115. Beskow J, Gottfries C G, Roos B E, Winblad B. Determination of monoamine and monoamine metabolites in the human brain: postmortem studies in a group of suicides and in a control group. Acta Psychiatr Scand 1976; 53:7–20.

116. Pare C M B, Young D P H, Price K, Stacey R S. 5-hydroxytryptamine, noradrenaline, and dopamine in brain stem, hypothalamus, and caudate nucleus of controls and patients committing suicide by coal-gas poisoning. Lancet 1969; 2:113–135.

117. Agren H. Symptom patterns in unipolar and bipolar depression correlating with monoamine metabolites in the cerebrospinal fluid. II. Suicide. Psychiatry Res 1980; 3:225–236.

118. Mann J J, Stanley M, McBride A, McEwen B S. Increased serotonin$_2$ and beta-adrenergic receptor binding in the frontal cortices of suicide victims. Arch Gen Psychiatry 1986; 43:954–959.

119. Sulser F. Serotonin–norepinephrine receptor interactions in the brain: implications for the pharmacology and pathophysiology of affective disorders. J Clin Psychiatry 1987; 48:3(Suppl):12–18.

120. Kobinger W. Alpha-adrenoceptors in cardiovascular regulation. In: Ziegler M G, Lake C R, eds. Norepinephrine. Baltimore: Williams & Wilkins, 1984:307–326.

121. Reis D J, Granata A R, Joh T H, Ross C A, Ruggiero D A, Park D H. Brain stem catecholamine mechanisms in tonic and reflex control of blood pressure. Hypertension 1984; 6(Suppl II):7–15).

122. Peskind E R, Veith R C, Dorsa D M, Gumbrecht G, Raskind M A. Yohimbine increases CSF and plasma norepinephrine but not arginine vasopressin in humans. Neuroendocrinology 1989; 50:286-291.

123. Charney D S, Heninger G R, Sternberg D E, Hafstad K M, Giddings S, Landis H. Adrenergic receptor sensitivity in depression. Arch Gen Psychiatry 1982; 39: 290-294.

124. Price L H, Charney D S, Rubin L, Heninger G R. Alpha-2 adrenergic receptor function in depression. Arch Gen Psychiatry 1986; 43:849-858.

125. Siever L J, Kafka M S, Targum S, Lake C R. Platelet alpha-adrenergic binding and biochemical responsiveness in depressed patients and controls. Psychiatry Res 1984; 11:287-302.

126. Heninger G R, Charney D S, Price L H. Alpha$_2$-adrenergic receptor sensitivity in depression. The plasma MHPG, behavioral, and cardiovascular responses to yohimbine. Arch Gen Psychiatry 1988; 45:718-726.

127. Calogero A E, Gallucci W T, Chrousos G P, Gold P W. Catecholamine effects upon rat hypothalamic corticotropin-releasing hormone secretion in vitro. J Clin Invest 1988; 82:839-846.

128. Ganong W F. Neurotransmitters and pituitary function regulation of ACTH secretion. Fed Proc 1980; 39:2912-2930.

129. Lancranajan I, Ohnaus E, Girard J. The alpha-adrenoreceptor control of adrenocorticotropin secretion in man. J Clin Endocrinol Metab 1979; 49: 227-230.

130. Siever L J, Uhde T W, Jimerson D C, Post R M, Lake R, Murphy D L. Plasma cortisol responses to clonidine in depressed patients and controls. Arch Gen Psychiatry 1984; 41:63-68.

131. Roy A D, Pickar M, Linnoila M, Chrousos G P, Gold P W. Cerebrospinal fluid corticotropin-releasing hormone in depression: relationship to noradrenergic function. Psychiatry Res 1986; 20:229-237.

132. Lal S, Tolis G, Martin J B N, Brown G M, Guyda H. Effect of clonidine on growth hormone, prolactin, luteinizing hormone, follicle stimulating hormone, and thyroid stimulating hormone in the serum of normal men. J Clin Endocrinol Metab 1975; 41:827.

133. Lancranjan I, Marbach P. New evidence for growth hormone modulation by the alpha-adrenergic system in man. Metabolism 1977; 26:1225.

134. Checkley S A, Slade A P, Shur E. Growth hormone and other responses to clonidine in patients with endogenous depression. Br J Psychiatry 1981; 138:51-55.

135. Matussek N, Ackenheil M, Hippis H, et al. Effect of clonidine on growth hormone release in psychiatric patients and controls. Psychiatry Res 1980; 2:25-36.

136. Siever L J, Uhde T W, Silberman E K, et al. Growth hormone response to clonidine as a probe of noradrenergic receptor responsiveness in affective disorder patients and controls. Psychiatry Res 1982; 6:171-183.

137. Mendlewich J, Linkowski P, Kerkhofs M, et al. Diurnal hypersecretion of growth hormone in depression. J Clin Endocrinol Metab 1985; 60:505-512.

138. Kafka M S, Paul S W. Platelet alpha $_2$-adrenergic receptors in depression. Arch Gen Psychiatry 1986; 43:91–95.

139. Mitrius J C, Micuni M, Arora R C, Meltzer H Y, U'Prichard D C. Responsiveness of alpha-2-adrenergic receptors is decreased in platelets from depressed patients. Soc Neurosci Abstr 1983; 9:990.

140. Piletz J E, Schubert D S P, Halaris A. Evaluation of studies on platelet alpha$_2$ receptors in depressive illness. LifeSci 1986; 39:1589–1616.

141. Pfeifer M A, Ward K, Malpass T, et al. Variations in circulating catecholamines fail to alter human platelet alpha-2-adrenergic receptor number or affinity for [^{3}H] yohimbine or [^{3}H] dihydroergocryptine. J Clin Invest 1984; 74:1063–1072.

142. Janowsky D S, El-Yousef M K, Davis J M, Sekerke H J. A cholinergic-adrenergic hypothesis of mania and depression. Lancet 1972; 2:632–635.

143. Brezenoff H E. Cardiovascular regulation by brain acteylcholine. Fed Proc 1984; 43:17–20.

144. Kennedy B. Janowsky D S, Risch S C, Ziegler M G. Central cholinergic stimulation causes adrenal epinephrine release. J Clin Invest 1984; 74: 972–975.

145. Risch S C, Janowsky D S, Mott M A, et al. Central and peripheral cholinesterase inhibition: effects on anterior pituitary and sympathomimetic function. Psychoneuroendocrinology 1986; 11(2):221–230.

146. Risch S C, Kalin N H, Janowsky D L, Cohen R M, Pickar D, Murphy D L. Co-release of ACTH and beta-endorphin immunoreactivity in human subjects in response to cnetral cholinergic stimulation. Science 1983; 222:77.

147. Norman T R, Piperoglou M, McIntyre I M, Lynch C, Burrows G D. Plasma immunoreactive beta-endorphin in dexamethasone suppressors and nonsuppressors of cortisol. J Affect Dis 1987; 12:233–239.

148. Risch S C. Beta-endorphin hypersecretion in depression: possible cholinergic mechanisms. Biol Psychiatry 1982; 17:1071–1079.

149. Risch S C, Janowsky D S, Gillin J C. Muscarinic supersensitivity of anterior pituitary ACTH and beta-endorphin release in major depressive illness. Peptides 1983; 4:789–792.

150. Segawa T, Midzuta T, Nomura Y. Modifications of central 5-hydroxytryptamine binding sites in synaptic membranes from rat brain after long-term administration of tricyclic antidepressants. Eur J Pharmacol 1979; 58:75–83.

151. Wamsley J K, Byerley W F, McCabe R T, McConnell E J, Dawson T M, Grosser B I. Receptor alterations associated with sertonergic agents: an autoradiographic analysis. J Clin Psychiatry 1987; 48(3):19–25.

152. Asberg M, Traskman L, Thoren P. 5-H1AA in the cerebrospinal fluid: a biochemical suicide predictor? Arch Gen Psychiatry 1976; 38:1193–1197.

153. Banki C M, Arato M. Amine metabolites and neuroendocrine responses related to depression and suicide. J Affect Dis 1983; 5:223–232.

154. Roy-Byrne P, Post R M, Rubinow D R, Linnoila M, Savard R, Davis D. CSF 5HIAA and personal and family history of suicide in affectively ill patients: a negative study. Psychiatry Res 1983; 10:263–274.

155. Stanley M, Birgilio J, Gershon S. Tritiated imipramine binding sites are decreased in frontal cortex of suicides. Science 1982; 216:1337–1339.

156. Owen F, Cross A J, Crow T J, et al. Brain 5-HT$_2$ receptors and suicide. Lancet 1983; 1:1256.

157. Roy A, Everett D, Pickar D, Paul S M. Platelet tritiated imipramine binding and serotonin uptake in depressed patients and controls. Relationship to plasma cortisol levels before and after dexamethasone administration. Arc Gen Psychiatry 1987; 44:320–327.

158. Meltzer H Y, Arora R C, Baber R, Tricou B J. Serotonin uptake in blood platelets of psychiatric patients. Arch Gen Psychiatry 1981; 38:1322–1326.

159. Tuomisto J, Takiainen E, Alfors U G. Decreased uptake of 5-hydroxytryptamine in blood platelets from patients with endogenous depression. Psychopharmacology 1979; 65: 141–147.

160. Meltzer H Y Umberkoman-Wiita B, Robertson A, Tricou B J, Lowy M, Perline R. Effect of 5-hydroxytryptophan on serum cortisol levels in major affective disorders. Arch Gen Psychiatry 1984; 41:366–374.

161. Koyama T, Lowy M T, Meltzer H Y. 5-hydroxytryptophan-induced cortisol response and CSF 5-HIAA in depressed patients. Am J Psychiatry 1987; 144:334–337.

162. Veith R C, Raskind M A. The neurobiology of aging: does it predispose to depression. Neurobiol Aging 1987; 9:101–117.

163. Brunello N, Barbaccia M L, Chuang D-M, Costa E. Down-regulation of beta-adrenergic receptors following repeated injections of desmethylimipramine: permissive role of serotonergic axons. Neuropharmacology 1982; 21:1145–1149.

164. Stockmeier C A, Martino A M, Kellar K J. A strong influence of serotonin axons on beta-adrenergic receptors in rat brain. Science 1985; 230:323–325.

165. Mueller E A, Murphy D L, Sunderland T. Neuroendocrine effects of M-chlorophenylpiperazine, a serotonin agonist, in humans. J Clin Endocrinol Metab 1985; 61(6):1179–1184.

166. Mashchak C A, Kletzky O A, Spencer C, Artal R. Transient effect of L-5-hydroxytryptophan on pituitary function in men and women. J Clin Endocrinol Metab 1983; 56:170–176.

167. de la Vega C E, Slater S, Ziegler M G, Lake C R, Murphy D L. Reduction in plasma norepinephrine during fenfluramine treatment. Clin Pharmacol Ther 1977; 21(2):216–221.

168. Katon W, Vialiano P P, Russo J, Cormier L, Anderson K, Jones M. Panic disorder: epidemiology in primary care. J Fam Practice 1986; 23(3):233–239.

169. Weissman M M, Merikangas K R. The epidemiology of anxiety and panic disorders: an update. J Clin Psychiatry 1986; 47 (Suppl 6): 11–17.

170. Coryell W, Noyes R, Clancy J. Excess mortality in panic disorder. A comparison with primary unipolar depression. Arch Gen Psychiatry 1982; 39: 701–703.

171. DaCosta J M. On irritable heart: a clinical study of a form of functional cardiac disorder and its consequences. Am J Med Sci 1871; 61:17-21.

172. Gorman J M, Fyer M R, Goetz R, et al. Ventilatory physiology of patients with panic disorder. Arch Gen Psychiatry 1988; 45:31-39.

173. Liebowitz M R, Gorman J M, Fyer A J, et al. Lactate provocation of panic attacks: II. Biochemical and physiological findings. Arch Gen Psychiatry 1985; 42:709-719.

174. Castellani S, Quillen M A, Vaughan D A, et al. TSH and catecholamine response to TRH in panic disorder. Biol Psychiatry 1988; 24:87-90.

175. Woods S W, Charney D S, McPherson C A, Gradman A H, Heninger G R. Situational panic attacks. Behavioral, physiologic, and biochemical characterization. Arch Gen Psychiatry 1987; 44:365-375.

176. Villacres E C, Hollifield M, Katon W J, Wilkinson C W, Veith R C. Sympathetic nervous system activity in panic disorder. Psychiatry Res 1987; 21: 313-321.

177. Shear M K, Kligfield P, Harshfield G, et al. Cardiac rate and rhythm in panic patients. Am J Psychiatry 1987; 144:633-637.

178. Freedman R R, Ianni P, Ettedgui E, Puthezhath N. Ambulatory monitoring of panic disorder. Arch Gen Psychiatry 1985; 42:244-248.

179. Gaffney F A, Fenton B J, Lane L D, Lake C R. Hemodynamic, ventilatory and biochemical responses of panic patients and normal controls with sodium lactate infusion and spontaneous panic attacks. Arch Gen Psychiatry 1988; 45:53-60.

180. Nesse R M, Curtis G C, Thyer B A, McCann D S, Huber-Smith B A, Knoff R F. Endocrine and cardiovascular responses during phobic anxiety. Psychosom Med 1985; 47:320-332.

181. Appleby I L, Klein D F, Sachar E J, Levitt M. Biochemical indices of lactate-induced panic; a preliminary report. In: Klein DF, Rabkin J, eds. Anxiety: new research and changing concepts. New York: Raven Press, 1981: 411-423.

182. Nesse R M, Cameron O G, Curtis G C, McCann D S, Huber-Smith M J. Adrenergic function in patients with panic anxiety. Arch Gen Psychiatry 1984; 41:771-776.

183. Ballenger J C, Peterson G A, Laraia M, et al. A study of plasma catecholamines in agoraphobia and the relationship of serum tricyclic levels to treatment response. In: Ballenger JC, ed. Biology of agoraphobia. Washington, D. C.: American Psychiatric Press, 1984: 28-63.

184. Cameron O G, Smith C B, Hollingsworth P J, Nesse R M, Curtis G C. Platelet alpha$_2$-adrenergic receptor binding and plasma catecholamines: before and during imipramine treatment in patients with panic anxiety. Arch Gen Psychiatry 1984; 41:1144-1148.

185. Carr D B, Sheehan D V, Surman O S, et al. Neuroendocrine correlates of lactate-induced anxiety and their response to chronic alprazolam therapy. Am J Psychiatry 1986; 143:483-493.

186. Matthew R J, Ho B T, Francis D J, Weinman M L. Catecholamines and anxiety. Acta Psychiatr Scand 1982; 65:142-147.

187. Charney D S, Woods S W, Goodman W K, Heninger G R. Neurobiological mechanisms of panic anxiety: biochemical and behavioral correlates of yohimbine-induced panic attacks. Am J Psychiatry 1987; 144:1030–1036.

188. Mathew R J, Ho B T, Kralik P, et al. Catechol-O-methyl transferase and catecholamines in anxiety and relaxation. Psychiatry Res 1980; 3:85–91.

189. Lima D R, Turner P. Propranolol increases reduced beta-receptor function in severely anxious patients. Lancet 1983; 2:1505.

190. Mann J J, Shear K D, Halper J P, et al. Beta adrenergic receptor subsensitivity in anxiety disorders. Proceedings of the Society for Biological Psychiatry, Dallas, Texas, May, 1985.

191. Papp L A, Martinez J, Gorman J M. Arterial epinephrine levels in panic disorder. Psychiatry Res 1988; 25:111–112.

192. Morrow L A, Linares O A, Hill T J, et al. Age differences in the plasma clearance mechanisms for epinephrine and norepinephrine in humans. J Clin Endocrinol Metab 1987; 65:508–511.

193. Woods S W, Charney D S, Goodman W K, Heninger G R. Carbon dioxide-induced anxiety. Behavioral, physiologic, and biochemical effects of carbon dioxide in patients with panic disorders and healthy subjects. Arch Gen Psychiatry 1988; 45:43–52.

194. Ko G N, Elsworth J D, Roth R H, Rifkin B G, Leigh H, Redmond E Jr. Panic-induced elevation of plasma MHPG levels in phobic-anxious patients. Effects of clonidine and imipramine. Arch Gen Psychiatry 1983; 40:425–430.

195. Cameron O G, Lee M A, Curtis G C, McCann D S. Endocrine and physiological changes during "spontaneous" panic attacks. Psychoneuroendocrinology 1987; 12:321–331.

196. Sellew A P, Low J A, Shear M K, Mann J J, James G. Norepinephrine increase during panic attacks (abstr). Proceedings of the American Psychiatric Association annual meeting, 1987: 232.

197. Taylor C B, Sheikh J, Agras S, et al. Ambulatory heart rate changes in patients with panic attacks. Am J Psychiatry 1986; 143:478–482.

198. Nutt D J. Increased central alpha$_2$-adrenoceptor sensitivity in panic disorder. Psychopharmacology 1986; 90:268–269.

199. Charney D S, Heninger G R, Jatlow P I. Increased anxiogenic effects of caffeine in panic disorders. Arch Gen Psychiatry 1985; 42:233–243.

200. Papp L A, Gorman J M, Liebowitz M R, Fyer A J, Cohen B, Klein D F. Epinephrine infusions in patients with social phobia. Am J Psychiatry 1988; 145:733–736.

201. Starkman M N, Zelnik T C, Nesse R M, et al. Anxiety in patients with pheochromocytomas. Arch Intern Med 1985; 145:248–252.

202. Redmond D E Jr. Studies of the nucleus locus coeruleus in monkeys and hypotheses for neuropsychopharmacology. In: Meltzer HY, ed. The third generation of progress. New York: Raven Press, 1987.

203. Schwartz N S, Clutter W E, Shah S D, Cryer P E. Glycemic thresholds for activation of glucose counterregulatory systems are higher than the threshold for symptoms. J Clin Invest 1987; 79:777–781.

204. Morley J E, Tuck M L, Mayes D M, Rosenblatt S, Hershman J M. Thyrotropin-releasing hormone increases plasma norephinephrine in man. Hormone Res 1981; 14:18–23.

205. Brown M R. Thyrotropin releasing factor: a putative CNS regulator of the autonomic nervous system. Life Sci 1981; 28:1789–1795.

206. Horita A, Carino M A, Lai H, LaHann T R. Behavioral and autonomic effects of TRH in animals. In: Collu, ed. Central nervous system effects of hypothalamic hormones and other peptides. New York: Raven Press, 1979: 65–74.

207. Okuda C, Tanaka H, Miyazaki M. Cardiovascular effect of intravenously administered thyrotropin-releasing hormone and its concentration in push–pull perfusion of the fourth ventricle in conscious and pentobarbital-anesthetized rats. Life Sci 1988; 42:1181–1188.

208. Feuerstein G, Hassen A H, Faden A I. TRH: cardiovascular and sympathetic modulation in brain nuclei of the rat. Peptides 1983; 4:617–620.

209. Okkuda C, Mizobe T, Miyazaki M. The involvement of central cholinergic mechanisms in cardiovascular responses to intracerebroventricular and intravenous administration of thyrotropin-releasing hormone. Life Sci 1987; 40:1293–1299.

210. Yarbrough G G. Thyrotropin releasing hormone and CNS cholinergic neurons. Life Sci 1983; 33:111–118.

211. Cameron O G, Nesse R M. Systemic hormonal and physiological abnormalities in anxiety disorders. Psychoneuroendocrinology 1988; 13(4): 287–307.

212. Mason J W. A review of the psychoneuroendocrine research on the pituitary-adrenal cortical system. Psychosom Med 1968; 30:576–607.

213. Roy-Byrne P P, Uhde T W, Post R M, Gallucci W, Chrousos G P, Gold P W. The corticotropin-releasing hormone stimulation test in patients with panic disorder. Am J Psychiatry 1986; 143:896–899.

214. Hommer D W, Skolnick P, Paul S M. The benzodiazepine/GABA receptor complex and anxiety. In: Meltzer HY, ed. Psychopharmacology: The third generation of progess. New York: Raven Press, 1987; pp 977-984.

215. Hommer D W, Matsuo V, Wokowitz O, et al. Benzodiazepine sensitivity in normal human subjects. Arch Gen Psychiatry 1986; 43:542–551.

216. Roy-Byrne P P, Lewis N, Villacres E, Greenblatt D J, Shader R I, Veith R C. Suppression of norepinephrine appearance rate in plasma by diazepam in humans. Life Sci 1988; 43:1615–1623.

217. Roy-Byrne P P, Lewis N, Villacres E, et al. Preliminary evidence of benzodiazepine subsensitivity in panic disorder. Biol Psychiatry 1989; 26: 744.

218. Egeland J A, Gerhard D S, Pauls D L, et al. Bipolar affective disorders linked to DNA markers on chromosome 11. Nature 1987; 325:783–787.

20

STRESS, SLEEP, AND VULNERABILITY TO VENTRICULAR FIBRILLATION

Richard L. Verrier
Georgetown University Medical Center, Washington, D.C.

Experimental study of the influence of behavioral states such as sleep and wakefulness on susceptibility to cardiac arrhythmias constitutes an area in which notable advances have been made. This has been largely due to the development of well-defined behavioral models and to the evolution of quantitative methods for assessing myocardial electrical stability. The advent of improved pharmacological probes to factor out the effects of the various components of the nervous system and the refinement of selective denervation procedures have contributed further to the elucidation of mechanisms.

The main objective of this chapter is to review progress that has been made in defining the influence of a broad spectrum of behavioral states, ranging from sleep to anger, on susceptibility to cardiac arrhythmias. Ventricular fibrillation is the focus of attention, because it is the primary rhythm disturbance responsible for sudden cardiac death (1). Some of the fundamental insights that have been derived are illustrated and directions for future research discussed.

ASSESSMENT OF VENTRICULAR ELECTRICAL STABILITY

Approximately 10 years ago we developed a method for quantifying the effects of alterations in levels of behavioral arousal on vulnerability to ventricular fibrillation (1-3). The technique involves using the repetitive extrasystole threshold as an index of susceptibility to fibrillation. A bipolar catheter is positioned fluoroscopically in the right ventricular apex via a jugular vein (1-4). Cardiac electrical testing is carried out by scanning the vulnerable period that coincides with the first half of the T-wave of the surface electrocardiogram. By increasing the test current in a stepwise fashion, the minimum intensity required to provoke a repetitive extrasystole is determined. This end point parallels the ventricular fibrillation threshold and thus provides a quantitative measure of the propensity for fibrillation under diverse conditions of changing autonomic tone (1-4). Because animals do not perceive the test stimuli, the repetitive extrasystole threshold method permits detailed study of the effects of behavioral state on the vulnerable period threshold.

BEHAVIORAL STRESS AND VENTRICULAR VULNERABILITY

Experimental Models

Aversive Conditioning

Our early attempts at behavioral modeling involved a passive aversive shock conditioning paradigm (1,2). Dogs were placed alternately in a sling where they received a mild chest shock and in a nonstressful cage environment where they were left undisturbed. This sequence was repeated for 3 consecutive days after which time no further shocks were administered. The only behavioral input was the recollection of the previous noxious experience. In the sling environment, the animals exhibited somatic tremor and salivated excessively, and their heart rate and arterial blood pressure were markedly elevated. Most remarkable, however, was the pattern of neurohumoral release. The predominant catecholamine in the plasma was epinephrine rather than norepinephrine (5). In fact, the norepinephrine to epinephrine ratio decreased from a resting level of 1.35 to a stress value of 0.6. This pattern of catecholamine release is in sharp contrast to that observed in response to anger, in which there is a major increase in plasma norepinephrine with little or no increase in epinephrine (6).

The aversive conditioning paradigm proved to be a valuable biological model. It led to the demonstration that stress was not only capable of lowering the vulnerable period threshold but could also precipitate ventricular tachycardias during myocardial infarction (7) and ventricular fibrillation during acute ischemia (8,9) (Fig. 1). It was also demonstrated that adrenergic factors play a key role, since beta-adrenergic blockade and stellectomy prevented stress-induced vulnerability (8,10). Another discovery was that spontaneous vagal tone was capable of annulling the adverse effects of enhanced adrenergic activity associated with behavioral stress (11,12). This finding provided essential verification of the fact that the mechanism of accentuated antagonism of adrenergic inputs by the vagus nerve (13) operates both in the conscious (11,12,14,15) and anesthetized state (1,16-18).

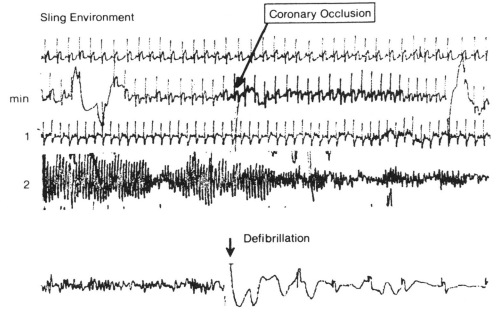

FIGURE 1 Coronary occlusion while the animal was in a sling environment resulted within 2 min in ventricular fibrillation. Note the instability of the baseline related to restlessness when the animal was merely standing quietly. When coronary occlusion was carried out while the animal was in the nonaversive cage environment, ventricular fibrillation did not occur (106).

Anger Paradigm

A few years ago we undertook to develop an experimental counterpart to anger (19). This was prompted by clinical reports linking this emotional state with cardiovascular disorders, including angina pectoris and cardiac arrhythmias (20–24). The experimental paradigm consisted of inducing an angerlike state in dogs by denying them access to food. After an overnight fast, the instrumented dog was brought to the experimental laboratory and allowed to acclimate for 20–30 min. While secured by a leash, the animal was presented with a dish of food. At this point, the food was moved just out of reach and a second leashed dog was permitted to consume the food. Upon observing this, the first dog almost invariably exhibited an angerlike behavioral state as evidenced by growling and exposing its teeth. At no time were the animals allowed to come into contact. The anger response persisted as long as the animals remained within sight of each other. The behavioral response was associated with consistent increases in heart rate, mean arterial blood pressure, and plasma catecholamine levels and a significant decrease in the repetitive extrasystole threshold. The latter effect indicates that induction of anger is capable of substantially decreasing the electrical stability of even the normal myocardium. It is reasonable to assume, although it has not yet been established, that in the damaged myocardium major arrhythmias would be precipitated.

Fear Paradigm

A crucial remaining question was whether a fearlike state can be induced without the need for delivering noxious stimuli. Recently obtained data suggest an affirmative answer to this question (25). The paradigm is as follows. First, the animals are screened and those that fail to exhibit an angerlike state (anger-negative dogs) are selected. Next the animals are suspended in a pavlovian sling with their feet 3–4 inches above the floor. At this point, a leashed anger-positive dog is brought into the room. The dog in the sling immediately exhibits a fear-like state because it is unable to escape. No contact is allowed between the animals. There are major reproducible changes in heart rate, systemic blood pressure, and coronary arterial flow. Most notable, however, is the rise in epinephrine as well as norepinephrine levels. Thus, during the same confrontation situation, the dog exhibiting an angerlike state releases predominantly norepinephrine with little change in epinephrine, whereas in the dog expressing fear, levels of both catecholamines are significantly elevated (Fig. 2).

In the future we plan to address the following questions: What are the neurochemical and cardiovascular consequences of inducing the fearlike state? Is there habituation with repeated exposure? Can the changes in plasma constituents be related to the observed alterations in coronary hemodynamic and cardiac electrophysiological function? How do these relationships differ from those discovered using the anger paradigm? Thus, the overall objective of these experiments is to obtain a relatively comprehensive understanding of the impact of a continuum of behavioral states. Since the same animals can be used in the different paradigms, the analytical power of the experimental designs is enhanced.

Central Nervous System Pathways Involved in Behaviorally Induced Arrhythmias

Skinner and Reed (26) have characterized some of the neural tracts that mediate the arrhythmogenic effect of behavioral stress by implanting probes into selected regions in the brain of the pig. They demonstrated that cryogenic blockade of the thalamic gating system or its output from the frontal cortex to the brainstem delayed or prevented the occurrence of ventricular fibrillation during stress. Cooling of adjacent structures in a separate group of animals had no effect on susceptibility to ventricular fibrillation. Thus distinct pathways within the central nervous system appear to mediate the influence of stress on heart rhythm. The topic of central nervous system regulation of cardiovascular function has been discussed in detail by Smith and DeVito (27).

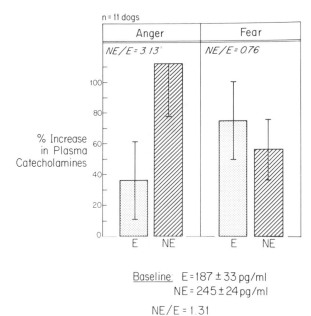

Baseline: E = 187 ± 33 pg/ml
NE = 245 ± 24 pg/ml

NE/E = 1.31

FIGURE 2 Contrasting effects of inducing anger or fear on plasma catccholamine levels in 11 dogs. Provocation of anger elicits a predominant increase in norepinephrine (NE/E = 3.13). By comparison, elicitation of fear produces a predominant increase in epinephrine (NE/E = 0.76). This differing pattern of neurochemical response occurred despite comparable changes in heart rate and arterial blood pressure induced by the behavioral states of anger and fear (105).

Role of the Sympathetic Nervous System

There is cogent evidence that adrenergic factors play a primary role in the provocation of arrhythmias (7,28-32). In particular, several investigations indicate that pharmacological (10,33) or surgical sympathectomy (10) is effective in decreasing the profibrillatory effects of various types of stress. It has been found that beta-adrenergic blockade with propranolol or the cardioselective drugs tolamolol or metoprolol completely abolishes the effects of aversive conditioning or induction of anger on vulnerability to ventricular fibrillation (10,33) (Fig. 3). It is significant that unilateral or bilateral stellectomy is only partially effective in blocking fibrillation (10). Thus, adrenergic inputs in addition to those provided by the stellate ganglia affect ventricular vulnerability during behavioral stress. Most likely these adrenergic influences arise from other thoracic ganglia and from adrenal medullary catecholamines.

The neural mechanisms responsible for behaviorally induced arrhythmias during myocardial ischemia and infarction are not well understood. Pigs adapted

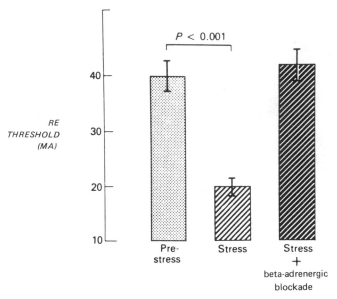

FIGURE 3 Effect of behavioral stress and beta-adrenergic blockade (tolamolol, 4 mg/kg) on the repetitive extrasystole threshold. Stress induces a significant decrease in threshold that is prevented by beta-blockade (107).

to a laboratory environment have a reduced and delayed onset of ventricular fibrillation during coronary artery obstruction, but beta-adrenergic blockade with propranolol does not afford any protection against the development of ventricular fibrillation in unadapted animals (34). It remains to be clarified whether the failure of propranolol to protect against ventricular fibrillation in the pig model resulted from inadequate blockade of adrenergic inputs to the heart or from the involvement of extra-adrenergic factors in the antifibrillatory effect possibly associated with the behavioral habituation paradigm (34).

This suggestion is in accord with the report that beta-adrenergic blockade protected against malignant ventricular arrhythmias shown to be associated with acute coronary artery occlusion in dogs exposed to behavioral stresses (35). The animals were instrumented for long-term recording of electrograms from ischemic and normal regions of the myocardium and were subjected to several forms of stress. These experimental stresses included introduction of the animal to a novel environment in which stressful stimuli, such as a light followed by a sudden noise or a noise followed by a subcutaneous electrical shock, were presented. Shock significantly decreased the latency and increased the severity of ventricular arrhythmias. Beta-adrenergic blockade with the cardioselective agent tolamolol significantly ameliorated the adverse effects of stress on cardiac rhythm. Moreover it was demonstrated that the quaternary analog of propranolol, UM 272, which lacks beta-adrenergic blocking properties but exerts direct local anesthetic effects on the myocardium, did not result in a protective action. Thus the salutary influence of tolamolol appears to result from its antiadrenergic action rather than from a nonspecific effect on myocardial tissue. These investigators also found an antiarrhythmic effect of the antianxiety drug diazepam.

Precise characterization of the influence of alpha-adrenergic receptors on ventricular electrical stability has been difficult. This has been due in part to the complexity of their influences, which include both direct actions on myocardial excitable properties (36,37) and indirect effects on insulin secretion (38), platelet aggregability (39), and coronary hemodynamic function (40,41). The latter consideration may be of particular importance in view of evidence implicating coronary vasospasm as a factor in the genesis of lethal arrhythmias (42).

In the normal heart, alpha-adrenergic stimulation or blockade does not appear to alter ventricular electrical stability (43,44). This is based on several lines of evidence. In particular, intravenous administration of the alpha-adrenergic agonists phenylephrine (44) or methoxamine (43) has been found to be without effect on the vulnerable period threshold when the pressor response is controlled to prevent the reflex changes in autonomic tone. It has also been shown that beta-adrenergic receptor blockade completely abolishes the reduction in the ventricular fibrillation threshold produced by posterior hypothalamic or stellate ganglion stimulation (8,45). If alpha-adrenergic receptors were involved in the regulation of vulnerability in the normal heart, some component of the effect of sympathetic stimulation would have remained after beta-adrenergic blockade.

In the ischemic heart, alpha-adrenergic receptor kinetic properties (36) may be altered by sustained ischemia, and this may in turn alter their role in cardiac arrhythmogenesis. Corr and colleagues (46) have demonstrated that the idioventricular rate is enhanced during reflow by localized infusion of methoxamine, an alpha-agonist, into the reperfused zone. This finding is in contrast to the effects mediated by beta-adrenergic receptors on idioventricular rate in nonischemic animals. Thus it appears that $alpha_1$-adrenergic stimulation may result in electrophysiological derangements peculiar to ischemia and reperfusion and not evident in normal tissue. Recent work using x-ray microprobe analysis also suggests that alpha-adrenergic mechanisms may mediate a large portion of the increase in intracellular calcium during reperfusion (47).

Sympathetic–Parasympathetic Interactions and Myocardial Electrical Stability

Several studies indicate that vagal activity modulates myocardial electrical stability in response to changes in behavioral state. It has been demonstrated that the deleterious effects of aversive conditioning on vulnerability can be decreased by accentuating vagal tone (14). When dogs were exposed to a stress-ful environment after pretreatment with morphine sulfate, the decrease in vul-nerable period threshold was abolished. Blockade of vagal efferent influences by intravenous injection of atropine cancelled a major component of morphine's antifibrillatory effect. When morphine was administered in the nonaversive environment, where adrenergic activation was absent or decreased as indicated by low circulating catecholamine levels (5,14), drug-induced vagotonia did not alter ventricular vulnerability. Thus, the protective action of morphine during exposure to experimentally imposed stressors appeared to result partly from vagal antagonism of the fibrillatory influence of enhanced adrenergic stimulation of the heart and partly from the drug's sedative action. It is of particular interest that the opioid agonist fentanyl exerts its antifibrillatory effect in the context of hemorrhage by stimulating reflex withdrawal of cardiac sympathetic tone (Fig. 4). By contrast, in the setting of myocardial ischemia, fentanyl acts primarily by increasing vagal drive to the heart, thus reducing susceptibility to fibrillation (48, 49).

It remained to be determined whether spontaneous vagal tone in the stressed animal was sufficient to modulate myocardial electrical stability. To examine

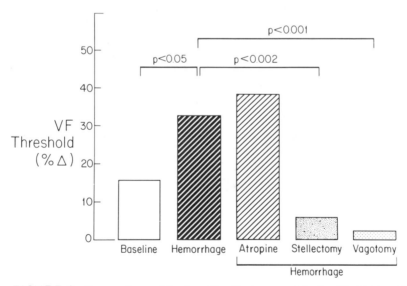

FIGURE 4 Comparison of fentanyl's effect on ventricular fibrillation threshold during different autonomic interventions. Hemorrhage significantly increased fentanyl's antifibrillatory effect. Muscarinic blockade with atropine did not alter the drug's action whereas stellectomy significantly reduced it. Bilateral cervical vagotomy abolished fentanyl's effect completely. Values are percentage changes in ventricular fibrillation threshold after administration of fentanyl (48).

this question, low dosages of atropine (0.05 mg/kg) were given to block selectively vagal efferent activity to the myocardium (12). In the aversive sling setting, vagal efferent blockade produced a significant decrease in the vulnerable period threshold. The inference is that in the stressed animal the level of vagal tone partly offset the deleterious effects of aversive conditioning. In the cage, where adrenergic input was reduced, vagal blockade was without influence on the threshold.

The diminution of adrenergic effects by muscarinic agents has been characterized at the receptor level. Muscarinic agents inhibit the release of norepinephrine from sympathetic nerve endings (13,50,51) and blunt the response to norepinephrine at receptor sites by cyclic nucleotide interactions (52,53). The effects of vagus nerve activation on the ischemic heart during behavioral stress have not been adequately defined. Clarification of this issue will require careful delineation of the role of heart rate and sympathetic–parasympathetic interactions as discussed in relation to the normal heart. It will also be important to consider the impact of ischemic injury on the nerve supply to the myocardium. The net effect of neural activation on heart rhythm during infarction may be further complicated by necrotic changes in afferent and efferent sympathetic and vagal pathways within the ventricles (54). A particularly relevant observation in terms of cardiac arrhythmogenesis is that myocardial infarction can produce functionally denervated areas within the ventricle. Zipes and co-workers (55-58) have shown that zones apical to the infarction fail to exhibit afferent reflexes in response to bradykinin or nicotine. Moreover, refractoriness of the affected areas is not altered by vagus nerve or stellate ganglion stimulation. There is a significant reduction in norepinephrine levels in myocardial tissue. The affected zone exhibits supersensitivity to infused norepinephrine or isoproterenol (59). Thus these investigators suggest that selective myocardial damage to the epicardium or endocardium may preferentially interrupt one or the other limb of the autonomic nervous system, and this in turn may predispose to the genesis of some ventricular arrhythmias.

The current view of the influence of vagus nerve activity on cardiac arrhythmogenesis is summarized in Table 1.

Poststress State and Delayed Myocardial Ischemia

Using the anger model, we made a serendipitous observation regarding the effects of the poststress state on myocardial perfusion (19). We specifically observed that after induction of the angerlike state, there is a progressive increase in coronary vascular resistance that ensues within 2-3 min and persists for 10-15 min after the anger episode (Fig. 5). The vasoconstrictor state lasts well after heart rate and arterial blood pressure have returned to control levels, indicating primary coronary vasoconstriction. In some animals the response is so

TABLE 1   Sympathetic–Parasympathetic Interactions and Cardiac Arrhythmogenesis

---

Vagal tone increases myocardial electrical stability and protects against ventricular fibrillation during myocardial ischemia. This effect is indirect and results
from antagonism of adrenergic influences.
The bases for parasympathetic–sympathetic interactions are inhibition of
norepinephrine release from nerve endings, and attenuation of response to
catecholamines at receptor sites.
Beneficial effects of vagal activity may be annulled if profound bradycardia and
hypotension ensue.
Myocardial infarction may alter autonomic influences by damaging neural pathways.

Source: Ref. 103.

intense as to obstruct flow in the affected vessel completely. The presence of
myocardial ischemia is indicated by significant ST segment changes. Although
this phenomenon, which we termed *delayed myocardial ischemia*, is not fully
understood, some important insights have emerged from recent studies. Specifically, it appears that activation of the sympathetic nervous system is a critical
factor. This is based on two lines of evidence. The first is that the phenomenon
can be induced by direct electrical stimulation of the left stellate ganglion and
that the vasoconstrictor response can be averted by alpha-adrenergic blockade
with prazosin (60). The second line of evidence is based on the recent observation that bilateral stellectomy prevents delayed ischemia induced by anger (6).

The basis for the delayed nature of the response remained a puzzle. A clue
was provided by the finding that there is a close temporal association between
the onset of ischemia and the return of coronary arterial blood pressure to the
control level following anger or sympathetic stimulation (19,60). Experimental
interventions were carried out to define the role of pressure in delayed ischemia
(61). The first involved preventing the hypertensive response to stellate stimulation by controlled exsanguination. When this procedure was carried out, the
coronary vasoconstrictor response was not delayed but occurred during stimulation. A series of interventions designed to raise arterial blood pressure was performed next. These entailed stimulating the left stellate ganglion without blood
pressure regulation and allowing the delayed coronary vasoconstriction to occur.
Thereafter, systemic blood pressure was raised to the stimulation level by occluding the aorta with a snare. Increasing arterial blood pressure in this manner
consistently returned coronary arterial flow and intracoronary pressure to the
control values. By contrast, elevating systemic pressure by restimulating the
stellate ganglion failed to restore flow through the coronary artery.

Our working hypothesis is that delayed myocardial ischemia results from an interplay between adrenergic and hemodynamic factors and that this interaction is the likely basis for the delayed nature of the ischemic response. The following hypothesis is proposed to account for the available data (6,19,60,61). During activation of the sympathetic nervous system, arterial blood pressure increases in response to either behavioral stress or direct excitation of the stellate ganglia, thereby opposing the vasoconstrictor influence of alpha-adrenergic receptor stimulation on vascular smooth muscle. The net result is that coronary vascular resistance remains unaltered. However, during the postexcitation phase, systemic pressure returns abruptly to the control level, thereby lessening distending pressure within the coronary vessel. We hypothesize that the dissipation of catecholamines is delayed and thus the active adrenergic vasoconstrictor influence predominates over the passive distending force. The imbalance leads to a decrease

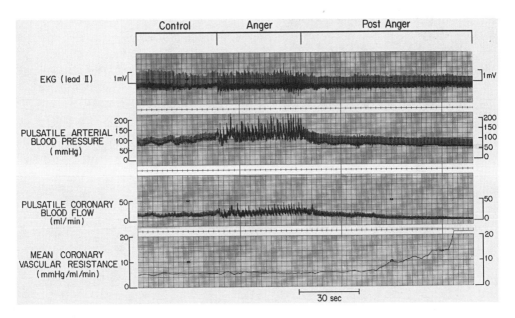

FIGURE 5 Effects of inducing an angerlike state on coronary hemodynamic function in a dog with coronary artery stenosis. During the stress state, coronary arterial blood flow increased substantially and coronary vascular resistance decreased (panels 1 and 2). However, during the poststress recovery phase (panels 3 and 4) a pronounced coronary vasoconstriction was evidenced by a fall in coronary arterial blood flow and an increase in coronary vascular resistance. These changes occurred when heart rate and arterial blood pressure returned to the prestress levels, suggesting primary coronary vasoconstriction. Published by permission of the American Heart Association from *Circulation* 75:251, 1987 (19).

in coronary diameter and to an increase in vascular resistance. This formulation is analogous to that proposed by Masuda and Levy (62) to account for a delayed recovery of heart rate and contractility following cessation of sympathetic nerve stimulation. Our findings are summarized in Table 2.

Clinical Implications of Poststress Ischemia

These findings indicate that several characteristics of the poststress state are conducive to myocardial ischemia and arrhythmias. They include relatively elevated catecholamine levels and reduced coronary distending pressure in the face of lingering neurohumorally mediated vasoconstrictor drive. These factors may be responsible for the delayed onset of ischemia following cessation of exercise or intense emotional arousal. This hazardous coexistence of enhanced neurogenic activity and inadequate coronary distending pressure may also occur under conditions such as heart failure or hemorrhage. Schwartz et al. (63) have postulated that the markedly elevated sympathetic tone and concomitantly low coronary distending pressure may be responsible for the occurrence of coronary insufficiency and myocardial ischemia during hemorrhage (64). Finally, a highly relevant case has been reported by McLaughlin and co-workers of a 34-year-old patient who experienced severe myocardial ischemia within 3–4 min following coitus (65) (Fig. 6). Lahiri and others have reported five cases of protracted exercise stress-induced myocardial ischemia (66).

SLEEP AND CARDIAC DISORDERS

Arrhythmias

Clinical studies indicate that sleep suppresses ventricular arrhythmias (46,67–74). Lown et al. (69) found that 45 of 54 subjects undergoing 24 h ambulatory

TABLE 2 Mechanisms Responsible for Delayed Myocardial Ischemia

---

The ischemic state ensues 2–3 min following provocation of stress.

Delayed ischemia can be prevented by stellectomy and induced by sympathetic stimulation. The latter effect can be blocked by alpha$_1$-adrenergic blockade.

The interaction between coronary distending pressure and adrenergic factors appears to be responsible for the delayed nature of the response.

These findings carry important clinical implications: they may help to explain the occurrence of myocardial ischemia in response to hemorrhage and heart failure. Under such conditions, the neurally induced rise in intravascular pressure may not be sufficient to offset the coronary vasoconstrictor influence.

Source: Ref. 104.

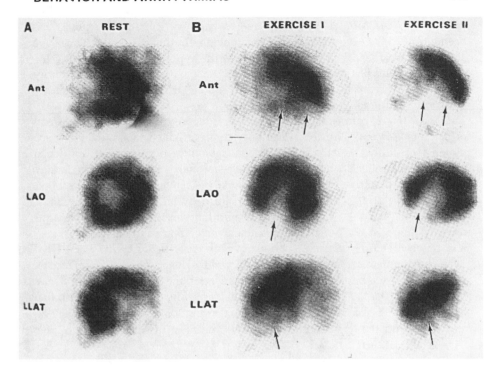

FIGURE 6 Thallium 201 images at rest (A) and during chest pain (B) 4 min after each of two maximal exercise tests (exercise I and II). Arrows indicate the perfusion defect in the inferior segment of the heart, as seen in the anterior (Ant), left anterior oblique (LAO), and left lateral (LLAT) views of the two postexercise studies (65).

monitoring exhibited significant reduction in ventricular ectopic activity during sleep. When sleep stages were monitored, these investigators noted reduction of ventricular premature beats during all stages except rapid eye movement (REM) sleep (68). The most marked lessening of arrhythmias was recorded during slow-wave sleep (stages 3 and 4). The change in ventricular ectopic activity was not correlated with changes in heart rate because heart rate remained relatively stable during the various sleep stages. The frequency of ventricular premature beats was similar during the awake and REM periods. Pickering et al. (71,72) and others (67,74) reported results comparable to those of Lown et al. (68,69). A beneficial effect of sleep on myocardial electrical stability is also suggested by the infrequency of sudden cardiac death during sleep, although it occupies about one-third of the diurnal cycle (75,76). Ventricular tachycardia and fibrillation, however, have been noted to occur in association with violent or frightening dreams (77,78). Arousal from sleep due to auditory stimuli in particular has been linked to the occurrence of life-threatening arrhythmias (79,80). Topaz and co-workers have suggested the involvement of the hypothalamus and quadrigeminal bodies in this phenomenon since they are the loci of convergence of auditory pathways. Nevertheless, it remains highly inferential that when sudden death does occur nocturnally, it is during REM sleep.

Only a few experimental studies have been conducted to define the effects of sleep on susceptibility to cardiac arrhythmias. Skinner et al. (81) have explored specifically the influences of sleep stage on the occurrence of ventricular arrhythmias during left anterior descending coronary artery occlusion in pigs. They found that the period during the early sleep in at which transitional and slow-wave sleep alternate was accompanied by an increase in arrhythmias compared to the awake state. This was true both in the acutely infarcted and the recently infarcted pig heart. The maximum increase in ventricular arrhythmias was observed during sustained periods of slow-wave sleep. Later, when REM sleep predominated, the overall arrhythmia incidence abruptly diminished. Acute coronary artery occlusion performed after the inception of slow-wave sleep reduced the latency in onset of ventricular fibrillation compared with that observed during the awake state. Coronary occlusion during REM sleep was associated with the opposite effect, namely a delay in the development of ventricular fibrillation.

These investigators reached some unexpected conclusions: (1) slow-wave sleep, but not REM sleep, has a deleterious influence on the ischemic heart; (2) REM sleep may be beneficial because it delays the development of ventricular fibrillation during coronary artery occlusion; and (3) the heart rate changes during sleep do not correlate with the effects of slow-wave or REM sleep on cardiac rhythm.

The explanation for these changes remains unclear. It is curious that in the pigs with coronary artery occlusion, arrhythmia was reduced not only during REM sleep but also during wakefulness. These investigators cite Baust and Bohnert (82) who found in cats that reduction in sympathetic tone accounts for the slow tonic heart rates during REM sleep, whereas during slow-wave sleep bradycardia was due to increased parasympathetic tone. However, increased sympathetic tone is certainly an attribute of the awake state. Snyder et al. (83) and others (84,85) have demonstrated that heart rate and arterial blood pressure are higher during wakefulness than during sleep.

We have obtained evidence suggesting that alterations in vagal tone may modulate cardiac electrophysiological properties during sleep (86). The effects of REM and slow-wave sleep on ventricular refractoriness were studied in chronically instrumented cats. Electrodes were implanted to record electro-oculograms, electromyograms, and electroencephalograms to determine sleep stage. A right ventricular catheter was employed for cardiac electrical testing using the single-stimulus technique. Both REM and slow-wave sleep significantly increased the effective refractory period. This effect was independent of alterations in heart rate since this variable was maintained constant by pacing. These alterations were not prevented by bilateral stellectomy. However, when the muscarinic blocking agent atropine methylnitrate was administered, the sleep-induced changes were completely abolished. These results suggest that the electrophysiological changes associated with sleep are mediated through fluctuations in cardiac vagal tone.

Myocardial Ischemia

There may indeed be hemodynamic concomitants, as well as coronary artery flow changes, linked to neural alterations during sleep stages that influence the electrically unstable ischemic heart. Clinical studies indicate that phasic changes in coronary blood flow occur throughout the diurnal cycle. In particular, Deanfield et al. (87) have found during 24 h Holter monitoring in patients with stable angina that ST segments fluctuate substantially during day and night. King et al. (88) studied the effects of sleep on the occurrence of Prinzmetal's variant angina. In an individual with angiographically documented coronary artery spasm, they found that the episodes of nocturnal chest pain accompanied by ST segment elevation occurred primarily during the REM stage of sleep. The factors responsible for the episodes of nocturnal angina, however, were not defined.

In the experimental laboratory, Vatner et al. (89) noted that in the nocturnal period, when baboons were apparently asleep, coronary artery blood flow increased by as much as 100%. The periodic oscillations in blood flow were not associated with changes in heart rate or arterial blood pressure and occurred while the animals remained motionless with eyes closed. Since the baboons were not instrumented for electrographic recordings, no data were obtained regarding sleep stage, nor was the mechanism for the coronary blood flow surge defined.

We addressed the issue of sleep-induced coronary blood flow changes in a recent series of experiments carried out in chronically instrumented dogs (90). The animals were prepared for recordings of sleep stage and systemic and coronary hemodynamic function. The animals were studied during natural sleep and the cycles were divided into 1 min periods of either quiet wakefulness, slow-wave sleep, or REM sleep. The findings indicate that during slow-wave sleep there are moderate but significant reductions in heart rate and coronary blood flow and increases in coronary vascular resistance. In REM, the coronary blood flow baseline is moderately elevated compared to slow-wave sleep and there are striking, episodic surges in flow. Coronary vascular resistance is reduced correspondingly. Heart rate but not mean arterial pressure is elevated during the flow surges, indicating that an increase in cardiac metabolic activity may be the basis for the coronary vasodilation (Figure 7). Since bilateral stellectomy

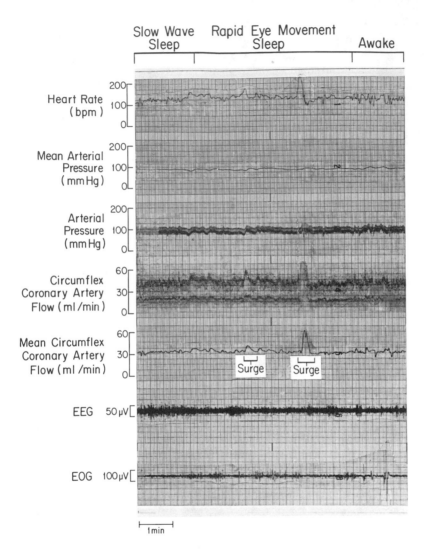

FIGURE 7 Effects of slow-wave (SW) sleep, rapid eye movement (REM) sleep, and quiet wakefulness on heart rate, phasic and mean arterial blood pressure, phasic and mean left coronary artery flow, electroencephalogram, electrocardiogram, and electrooculogram in the dog. Electromyogram is not shown. Sleep spindles are evident during SW sleep, minor eye movements during REM, and grosser eye movements upon awakening. Surges in heart rate and coronary flow occur during REM sleep (90).

prevented the surges in coronary blood flow, this response does not appear to be due to nonspecific effects of somatic activity or respiratory fluctuations. Instead, the changes appear to be the direct result of enhanced adrenergic discharge. We have also examined the influence of sleep on coronary hemodynamic function during coronary stenosis. The results indicate that in the presence of coronary stenosis the phasic increases in sympathetic discharge during REM sleep result in a decrease rather than an increase in coronary arterial blood flow (91).

FUTURE DIRECTIONS

Taken collectively, these studies point to a link between neural activity, behavioral stress, and the initiation of cardiac arrhythmias. It is likely that in the next few years major progress will be made both experimentally and clinically in defining this relationship further. The development of highly relevant biological models, in conjunction with an increased understanding of the neurochemistry of stress, will contribute significantly to this end. Ultimately, this should result in a better comprehension of the influence of brain states on myocardial electrical stability and lead to innovative approaches to the management of coronary vasospastic disease and life-threatening arrhythmias. Research should therefore proceed along several levels, drawing upon the advances in the fields of neuroscience and cardiovascular physiology.

From the standpoint of the cardiovascular system, it is important to explore the role of myocardial perfusion as an intermediary mechanism in the genesis of arrhythmias during behavioral stress. The significance of this consideration is highlighted by growing clinical evidence that mental activity is capable of eliciting significant perfusion deficits in patients with coronary artery disease (92,93). (See chapter 23 by Rozanski in this volume.)

In the field of cardiac electrophysiology, sophisticated mapping techniques have been evolved that could be applied for more detailed study of the impact of behavior on the stability of heart rhythm (94-97). The relationship of anatomically inhomogeneous sympathetic and parasympathetic innervation to electrophysiological inhomogeneity has yet to be explored and will necessitate three-dimensional mapping techniques. We anticipate that such studies will shed new light on the electrophysiological mechanisms of sympathetic-parasympathetic interactions. Finally, the intriguing frontier of chaos research could help to provide a fresh approach to our understanding of stress-induced perturbations in heart rhythm (98).

In the domains of neuroscience and behavior, the role of various brainstem nuclei in integrating the cardiovascular adaptation to behavioral stress needs to be studied. For example, experiments using the selective ablation of the nucleus tractus solitarius have yielded valuable insights into the role of baro-reflex integration in the development of behaviorally induced hypertension (99,100). Application of such techniques to the study of behaviorally induced arrhythmias is warranted. Localized neuroinjection techniques need to be adapted to the freely moving, conscious animal. This would allow the experimental study of specific neurotransmitter systems at specific brain sites and might open new avenues for the pharmacotherapy of arrhythmias.

The neurohumoral component of brain–heart interactions remains largely unexplored. Pituitary secretion of beta-endorphin as well as the other hormones may play a role in longer-term fluctuations in cardiac electrophysiological properties. The recent discoveries of circulating peptides with significant cardiovascular effects (atrial natriuretic factor, gamma-MSH, enkephalins) (101,102) add other promising dimensions to the study of brain–heart relationships.

An overall research strategy is outlined in Table 3.

TABLE 3 Future Directions for Study of Neurocardiac Interactions

Research focus	Research approaches
Behavior	Modeling of relevant states such as anxiety, panic, and depression
Central nervous system mapping	Application of lesioning and neuro-chemical techniques to delineate arrhythmogenic centers in the brain. Also, pharmacological study of the role of neurotransmitters in behaviorally induced arrhythmias
Myocardial perfusion	Use of advanced imaging methods to determine mechanisms involved in stress-induced coronary artery spasm. Also, application of platelet antibodies to characterize the role of platelets in the observed perfusion deficits
Cardiac electrophysiological mechanisms	Use of mapping techniques and application of chaos theory to define electrophysiological mechanisms responsible for behaviorally induced arrhythmias

Source: Ref. 105.

ACKNOWLEDGMENT

This work was supported by grants HL-32905, HL-33567, and HL-35138 from the National Institutes of Health, Bethesda, Maryland.

REFERENCES

1. Lown B, Verrier RL. Neural activity and ventricular fibrillation. N Engl J Med 1976; 294:1165–1170.
2. Lown B, Verrier RL, Corbalan R. Psychologic stress and threshold for repetitive ventricular response. Science 1973; 182:834–836.
3. Matta RJ, Verrier RL, Lown B. Repetitive extrasystole as an index of vulnerability to ventricular fibrillation. Am J Physiol 1976; 230:1469–1473.
4. Saini V, Verrier RL. The experimental study of behaviorally induced arrhythmias. In: Schneiderman N, Weiss SM, Kaufmann P, eds. Handbook of methods and measurement in cardiovascular behavioral medicine. New York: Plenum Press, 1989; 51–67.
5. Liang B, Verrier RL, Melman J, Lown B. Correlation between circulating catecholamine levels and ventricular vulnerability during psychological stress in conscious dogs. Proc Soc Exp Biol Med 1979; 161: 266–269.
6. Verrier RL, Kirby DA, Papageorgiou P. Plasma catecholamines and anger-induced delayed myocardial ischemia [abstract]. Circulation 1988; 78: II555.
7. Corbalan R, Verrier RL, Lown B. Psychological stress and ventricular arrhythmias during myocardial infarction in the conscious dog. Am J Cardiol 1974; 34:692–696.
8. Verrier RL, Lown B. Influence of neural activity on ventricular electrical stability during acute myocardial ischemia and infarction. In: Sandoe E, Julian DG, Bell JW, eds. Management of ventricular tachycardia: role of mexiletine. Amsterdam: Excerpta Medica, 1978: 133–150.
9. Verrier RL, Lown B. Influence of psychologic stress on susceptibility to spontaneous ventricular fibrillation during acute myocardial ischemia and reperfusion [abstract]. Clin Res 1979; 27:570A.
10. Verrier RL, Lown B. Effects of left stellectomy on enhanced cardiac vulnerability induced by psychologic stress [abstract]. Circulation 1977; 55/56: III80.
11. Verrier RL, Lown B. Behavioral stress and cardiac arrhythmias. Annu. Rev. Physiol. 1984; 46:155–176.
12. Verrier RL, Lown B. Vagal tone and ventricular vulnerability during psychological stress [abstract]. Circulation 1980; 62:II176.
13. Levy MN. Sympathetic-parasympathetic interactions in the heart. Circ Res 1971; 29: 437–445.
14. DeSilva RA, Verrier RL, Lown B. The effects of psychological stress and vagal stimulation with morphine on vulnerability to ventricular fibrillation (VF) in the conscious dog. Am Heart J 1978; 95:197–203.

15. De Ferrari GM, Vanoli E, Stramba-Badiale M, Foreman RD, Schwartz PJ. Vagal stimulation and sudden death in conscious dogs with a healed myocardial infarction [abstract]. Circulation 1987; 76:IV107.

16. Kolman BS, Verrier RL, Lown B. The effect of vagus nerve stimulation upon vulnerability of the canine ventricle: role of sympathetic–parasympathetic interactions. Circulation 1975; 52:578–585.

17. Zuanetti G, De Ferrari GM, Priori SG, Schwartz PJ. Protective effect of vagal stimulation on reperfusion arrhythmias in cats. Circ Res 1987; 61: 429–435.

18. Rabinowitz SH, Verrier RL, Lown B. Muscarinic effects of vagosympathetic trunk stimulation on the repetitive extrasystole (RE) threshold. Circulation 1976; 53:622–627.

19. Verrier RL, Hagestad EL, Lown B. Delayed myocardial ischemia induced by anger. Circulation 1987; 75:249–254.

20. Reich P, DeSilva RA, Lown B, Murawski BJ. Acute psychological disturbances preceding life-threatening ventricular arrhythmias. JAMA 1981; 246:233–235.

21. Schwartz GE, Weinberger DA, Singer JA. Cardiovascular differentiation of happiness, sadness, anger, and fear following imagery and exercise. Psychosom Med 1981; 43: 343–364.

22. Heberden W. Some account of a disorder of the breast. Read at the College, July 21, 1768. Med Trans Coll Physicians London 1772;2:59.

23. Kligfield P. John Hunter, angina pectoris and medical education. Am J Cardiol 1980; 45:367–369.

24. Kobayashi T, Ishikawa H, Tawara I. Psychosomatic aspects of angina pectoris. Scand J Rehab Med 1970; 2:87–91.

25. Verrier RL, Moya-Huff FA. Fear-induced changes in plasma catecholamines and coronary hemodynamic function [abstract]. Soc Neurosci Abstr 1988; 14:617.

26. Skinner JE, Reed JC. Blockade of frontocortical-brain stem pathway prevents ventricular fibrillation of ischemic heart. Am J Physiol 1981; 240: H156–H163.

27. Smith OA, DeVito JL. Central neural integration for the control of autonomic responses associated with emotion. Annu Rev Neurosci 1984; 7: 43–65.

28. Natelson BH. Stress, predisposition and the onset of serious disease: implications about psychosomatic etiology. Neurosci Biobehav Rev 1983; 7: 511–527.

29. Randall DC, Hasson DM. Cardiac arrhythmias in the monkey during classically conditioned fear and excitement. Pavlov J Biol Sci 1981; 16:97–107.

30. Verrier RL, Lown B. Myocardial perfusion and neurally induced cardiac arrhythmias. Ann NY Acad Sci 1984; 427:171–186.

31. Schwartz PJ, Randall WC, Anderson EA, et al. Task force on sudden cardiac death. Non-pharmacologic interventions. Circulation 1987; 76: I215–I219.

32. Schwartz PJ, Vanoli E, Zaza A, Zuanetti G. The effect of antiarrhythmic drugs on life-threatening arrhythmias induced by the interaction between acute myocardial ischemia and sympathetic hyperactivity. Am Heart J 1985; 109:937–948.
33. Matta RJ, Lawler JE, Lown B. Ventricular electrical instability in the conscious dog. Effects of psychologic stress and beta adrenergic blockade. Am J Cardiol 1976; 38:594–598.
34. Skinner JE, Lie JT, Entman ML. Modification of ventricular fibrillation latency following coronary artery occlusion in the conscious pig. The effects of psychological stress and beta-adrenergic blockade. Circulation 1975; 51:656–667.
35. Rosenfeld J, Rosen MR, Hoffman BF. Pharmacologic and behavioral effects on arrhythmias that immediately follow abrupt coronary occlusion: a canine model of sudden coronary death. Am J Cardiol 1978; 41:1075–1082.
36. Corr PB, Yamada KA, Witkowski FX. Mechanisms controlling cardiac autonomic function and their relation to arrhythmogenesis. In: Fozzard HA, ed. The heart and cardiovascular system. New York: Raven Press, 1986: 1343–1403.
37. Rosen MR, Danilo P Jr, Robinson RB, Shah A, Steinberg SF. Sympathetic neural and alpha-adrenergic modulation of arrhythmias. Ann NY Acad Sci 1988; 533:200–209.
38. Majid PA, Saxton C, Dykes JRW, Galvin MC, Taylor SH. Autonomic control of insulin secretion and the treatment of heart failure. Br Med J 1970; 4:328–334.
39. Pfister B, Imhof PR. Inhibition of adrenaline-induced platelet aggregation by the orally administered alpha-adrenergic receptor blocker phentolamine (Regitine). Eur J Clin Pharmacol 1977; 11:7–10.
40. Mohrman DE, Feigl EO. Competition between sympathetic vasoconstriction and metabolic vasodilation in the canine coronary circulation. Circ Res 1978; 42:79–86.
41. Schwartz PJ, Stone HL. Tonic influence of the sympathetic nervous system on myocardial reactive hyperemia and on coronary blood flow distribution in dogs. Circ Res 1977; 41:51–58.
42. Maseri A, L'Abbate A, Chierchia S, et al. Significance of spasm in the pathogenesis of ischemic heart disease. Am J Cardiol 1979; 44:788–792.
43. Kowey PR, Verrier RL, Lown B. Effect of alpha-adrenergic receptor stimulation on ventricular electrical properties in the normal canine heart. Am Heart J 1983; 105:366–371.
44. Verrier RL, Calvert A, Lown B, Axelrod P. Effect of acute blood pressure elevation on the ventricular fibrillation threshold. Am J Physiol 1974; 226:893–897.
45. Smith R, Johnson L, Rothfeld D, Zir L, Tharp B. Sleep and cardiac arrhythmias. Arch Intern Med 1972; 130:751–753.

46. Sheridan DJ, Penkoske PA, Sobel BE, Corr PB. Alpha adrenergic contributions to dysrhythmia during myocardial ischemia and reperfusion in cats. J Clin Invest 1980; 65:161–171.

47. Sharma AD, Saffitz JE, Lee BI, Sobel BE, Corr PB. Alpha-adrenergic-mediated accumulation of calcium in reperfused myocardium. J Clin Invest 1983; 72:802–818.

48. Saini V, Carr DB, Hagestad EL, Lown B, Verrier RL. Antifibrillatory mechanism of the narcotic agonist fentanyl. Am Heart J 1988; 115:598–605.

49. Saini V, Carr DB, Verrier RL. Comparative effects of the opioids fentanyl and buprenorphine on ventricular vulnerability during acute coronary artery occlusion. Cardiovasc Res 1989; 1001–1006.

50. Levy MN, Blattberg B. Effect of vagal stimulation on the overflow of norepinephrine into the coronary sinus during cardiac sympathetic nerve stimulation in the dog. Circ Res 1976; 38:81–85.

51. Levy MN, Martin PJ, Stuesse SL. Neural regulation of the heart beat. Annu Rev Physiol 1981; 43:443–453.

52. Watanabe AM, Besch HR Jr. Interaction between cyclic adenosine monophosphate and cyclic guanosine monophosphate in guinea pig ventricular myocardium. Circ Res 1975; 37:309–317.

53. Watanabe AM, Lindemann JP, Jones LR, Besch HR Jr, Bailey JC. Biochemical mechanisms mediating neural control of the heart. In: Abboud FM, Fozzard HA, Gilmore JP, Reis DJ, eds. Disturbances in neurogenic control of the circulation. Bethesda, MD: American Physiological Society, 1981: 189–203.

54. Zipes DP, Barber MJ, Takahashi N, Gilmour RF Jr. Recent observations on autonomic innervation of the heart. In: Zipes DP, Jalife J, eds. Cardiac electrophysiology and arrhythmias. Orlando, FL: Grune & Stratton, 1985: 181–189.

55. Barber MJ, Mueller TM, Davies BG, Gill RM, Zipes DP. Interruption of sympathetic and vagal-mediated afferent responses by transmural myocardial infarction. Circulation 1985; 72:623–631.

56. Barber MJ, Mueller TM, Davies BG, Zipes DP. Phenol topically applied to canine left ventricular epicardium interrupts sympathetic but not vagal afferents. Circ Res 1984; 55:532–544.

57. Barber MJ, Mueller TM, Henry DP, Felten SY, Zipes DP. Transmural myocardial infarction in the dog produces sympathectomy in noninfarcted myocardium. Circulation 1983; 67:787–796.

58. Martins JB, Zipes DP. Epicardial phenol interrupts refractory period responses to sympathetic but not vagal stimulation in canine left ventricular epicardium and endocardium. Circ Res 1980; 47:33–40.

59. Inoue H, Zipes DP. Results of sympathetic denervation in the canine heart: supersensitivity that may be arrhythmogenic. Circulation 1987; 75:877–887.

60. Hagestad EL, Verrier RL. Delayed myocardial ischemia following the cessation of sympathetic stimulation. Am Heart J 1988; 115:45–53.

61. Papageorgiou P, Hagestad EL, Verrier RL. Coronary distending pressure and delayed myocardial ischemia. Am Heart J 1988; 116:59–66.

62. Masuda Y, Levy MN. Heart rate modulates the disposition of neurally released norepinephrine in cardiac tissues. Circ Res 1985; 57:19–27.

63. Schwartz JS, Carlyle PF, Cohn JN. Effect of coronary arterial pressure on coronary stenosis resistance. Circulation 1980; 61:70–76.

64. Master AM, Dack S, Horn H, Freedman BI, Field LE. Acute coronary insufficiency due to acute hemorrhage: an analysis of one hundred and three cases. Circulation 1950; 1:1302–1317.

65. McLaughlin PR, Doherty PW, Martin RP, Goris ML, Harrison DC. Myocardial imaging in a patient with reproducible variant angina. Am J Cardiol 1977; 39:126–129.

66. Lahiri A, Subramanian B, Millar-Craig M, Crawley J, Raftery EB. Exercise induced S-T segment elevation in variant angina. Am J Cardiol 1980; 45:887–894.

67. Brodsky M, Wu D, Denes P, Kanakis C, Rosen KM. Arrhythmias documented by 24 hour continuous electrocardiographic monitoring in 50 male medical students without apparent heart disease. Am J Cardiol 1977; 39:390–395.

68. DeSilva RA. Central nervous system risk factors for sudden cardiac death. Ann NY Acad Sci 1982; 382:143–161.

69. Lown B, Tykocinski M, Garfein A, Brooks P. Sleep and ventricular premature beats. Circulation 1973; 48: 691–701.

70. Monti JM, Folle LE, Peluffo C, et al. The incidence of premature contractions in coronary patients during the sleep-awake cycle. Cardiology 1975; 60:257–264.

71. Pickering TG, Goulding L, Cobern BA. Diurnal variations in ventricular ectopic beats and heart rate. Cardiovasc Med 1977; 2:1013–1022.

72. Pickering TG, Johnston J, Honour AJ. Comparison of the effects of sleep, exercise and autonomic drugs on ventricular extrasystoles, using ambulatory monitoring of electrocardiogram and electroencephalogram. Am J Med 1978; 65:575–583.

73. Rosenblatt G, Hartmann E, Zwilling GR. Cardiac irritability during sleep and dreaming. J Psychosom Res 1973; 17:129–134.

74. Winkle RA, Lopes MG, Fitzgerald JW, Goodman DJ, Schroeder JS, Harrison DC. Arrhythmias in patients with mitral valve prolapse. Circulation 1975; 52:73–81.

75. Friedman M, Manwaring JH, Rosenman RH, Donlon G, Ortega P, Grube SM. Instantaneous and sudden deaths. Clinical and pathological differentiation in coronary artery disease. JAMA 1973; 225:1319–1328.

76. Myers A, Dewar HA. Circumstances attending 100 sudden deaths from coronary artery disease with coroners' necropsies. Br Heart J 1975; 37:1133–1143.

77. Lown B, Temte JV, Reich P, Gaughan C, Regestein Q, Hai H. Basis for recurring ventricular fibrillation in the absence of coronary heart disease and its management. N Engl J Med 1976; 294:623–629.

78. Skinner JE, Verrier RL. Task force report on sudden cardiac death and arrhythmias. In: Smith OA, Galosy RA, Weiss SM, eds. Circulation, Neurobiology, and Behavior. New York: Elsevier Science, 1982: 309–316.

79. Wellens HJJ, Vermeulen A, Durrer D. Ventricular fibrillation occurring on arousal from sleep by auditory stimuli. Circulation 1972; 46:661–665.

80. Topaz O, Castellanos A, Grobman LR, Myerburg RJ. The role of arrhythmogenic auditory stimuli in sudden cardiac death. Am Heart J 1988; 116:222–226.

81. Skinner JE, Mohr DN, Kellaway P. Sleep-stage regulation of ventricular arrhythmias in the unanesthetized pig. Circ Res 1975; 37:342–349.

82. Baust W, Bohnert B. The regulation of heart rate during sleep. Exp Brain Res 1969; 7:169–180.

83. Snyder F, Hobson JA, Goldfrank F. Blood pressure changes during human sleep. Science 1963; 142:1313–1314.

84. Baccelli G, Guazzi M, Mancia G, Zanchetti A. Neural and non-neural mechanisms influencing circulation during sleep. Nature 1969; 223:184–185.

85. Coccagna G, Mantovani M, Brignani F, Manzini A, Lugaresi E. Arterial pressure changes during spontaneous sleep in man. Electroencephalogr Clin Neurophysiol 1971; 31:277–281.

86. Francis GC, Hagestad EL, Verrier RL. Influence of sleep stage on ventricular refractoriness [abstract]. Physiologist 1986; 29:163.

87. Deanfield JE, Maseri A, Selwyn AP, et al. Myocardial ischaemia during daily life in patients with stable angina: its relation to symptoms and heart rate changes. Lancet 1983; 2:753–758.

88. King MJ, Zir LM, Kaltman AJ, Fox AC. Variant angina associated with angiographically demonstrated coronary artery spasm and REM sleep. Am J Med Sci 1973; 265:419–422.

89. Vatner SF, Franklin D, Higgins CB, Patrick T, White S, Van Citters RL. Coronary dynamics in unrestrained conscious baboons. Am J Physiol 1971; 221:1396–1401.

90. Kirby DA, Verrier RL. Differential effects of sleep stage on coronary hemodynamic function. Am J Physiol 1989; 256:H1378–1383.

91. Kirby DA, Verrier RL. Differential effects of sleep stage on coronary hemodynamic function during stenosis. Physiol Behav 1989; 45:1017–1020.

92. Deanfield JE, Shea M, Kennett M, et al. Silent myocardial ischaemia due to mental stress. Lancet 1984; 2:1001–1005.

93. Rozanski A, Bairey CN, Krantz DS, et al. Mental stress and the induction of silent myocardial ischemia in patients with coronary artery disease. N Engl J Med 1988; 318:1005–1012.

94. Burgess MJ. Ventricular repolarization and electrocardiographic T wave form and arrhythmia vulnerability. In: Levy MN, Vassalle M, eds. Excitation and neural control of the heart. Bethesda, MD: American Physiological Society, 1982: 181–202.

95. Janse MJ, Wilms-Schopman F, Wilensky RJ, Tranum-Jensen J. Role of the subendocardium in arrhythmogenesis during acute ischemia. In: Zipes DP,

Jalife J, eds. Cardiac electrophysiology and arrhythmias. Orlando, FL: Grune & Stratton, 1985: 353–362.

96. Kramer JB, Saffitz JE, Witkowski FX, Corr PB. Intramural reentry as a mechanism of ventricular tachycardia during evolving canine myocardial infarction. Circ Res 1985; 56:736–754.

97. Wit AL, Josephson ME. Fractionated electrograms and continuous electrical activity: fact or artifact. In: Zipes DP, Jalife J, eds. Cardiac electrophysiology and arrhythmias. Orlando, FL: Grune & Stratton, 1985: 343–351.

98. Jalife J, Chialvo D. Non-linear dynamics and chaos in conducting, nonpacemaker cells. In: Zipes DP, Jalife J, eds. Cardiac electrophysiology: from cell to bedside. Philadelphia: WB Saunders, 1990.

99. Nathan MA, Reis DJ. Chronic labile hypertension produced by lesions of the nucleus tractus solitarii in the cat. Circ Res 1977; 40:72–81.

100. Nathan MA, Tucker LW, Severini WH, Reis DJ. Enhancement of conditioned arterial pressure responses in cats after brainstem lesions. Science 1978; 201:71–73.

101. Holtz J, Sommer O, Bassenge E. Inhibition of sympathoadrenal activity by atrial natriuretic factor in dogs. Hypertension 1987; 9:350–354.

102. Sander GE, Giles TD, Kastin AJ, Quiroz AC, Kaneish A, Coy DH. Cardiopulmonary pharmacology of enkephalins in the conscious dog. Peptides 1981; 2:403–407.

103. Verrier RL. Autonomic substrates for arrhythmias. Prog Cardiol 1988; 1: 65–85.

104. Verrier RL. Central nervous system modulation of cardiac rhythm. In: Rosen MR, Palti Y, eds. Lethal arrhythmias resulting from myocardial ischemia and infarction. Boston: Kluwer Academic, 1989: 149–164.

105. Verrier RL. Behavioral stress, myocardial ischemia, and arrhythmias. In: Zipes DP, Jalife J, eds. Cardiac electrophysiology: from cell to bedside. Philadelphia: WB Saunders, 1990.

106. Verrier RL. Neural factors and ventricular electrical instability. In: Kulbertis HE, Wellens HJJ, eds. Sudden Death. The Hague: Martinus Nijhoff, 1980: 137–155.

107. Verrier RL, Lown B. Adrenergic blockade and the prevention of behaviourally-induced cardiac arrhythmias. In: Zanchetti A, ed. Advances in beta-blocker therapy II. Amsterdam: Excerpta Medica, 1982: 130–146.

21

STRESS AND CARDIOVASCULAR
PHYSIOLOGY IN ANIMALS

Laurel A. Fisher

University of Arizona College of Medicine, Tucson, Arizona

Successful organisms adapt to their environments. The ability to thrive when confronted with adverse ambient conditions entails meeting immediate cellular requirements while temporarily suspending less essential physiological functions. Cellular viability, and thus survival itself, depends upon the delivery of adequate metabolic substrate, a function subserved by the cardiovascular system. Cardiovascular responses to environmental exigencies are therefore of utmost importance to the organism. It should be borne in mind, however, that the coordinated adjustments of multiple organ systems are required for beneficial organism–environment interactions. Thus, cardiovascular responses to a given environmental stimulus occur simultaneously with a broad spectrum of behavioral and somatic reactions; these concurrent outputs may directly or indirectly influence cardiovascular function and, hence, contribute to the expression of stress-induced circulatory responses. As such, cardiovascular changes measured during stressful events cannot be viewed independently of the whole animal's response.

A pervasive concept is that emotional stress may be an antecedent or at least an exacerbating factor in the pathogenesis of cardiovascular disease. Since nearly half of all deaths in the United States are attributed to heart and circulatory disorders, it is imperative that we understand the cardiovascular sequelae of acute and chronic stress. To this end, a variety of paradigms have been developed to investigate stress-induced cardiovascular responses. Indeed, the scientific literature is replete with studies on the cardiovascular effects of physical and psychological stressors in humans and animals. Even a cursory review of this literature is well beyond the scope of this chapter. The following discussion, therefore, is intended only to highlight some conclusions and some questions arising from animal research on stress-induced cardiovascular responses. Particular emphasis is placed on studies designed to assess the influence of psychological stressors on cardiovascular function in mammals.

COUPLING BETWEEN BLOOD FLOW AND METABOLISM

The cardiovascular system executes the critical function of providing tissues with adequate amounts of oxygen and substrates to maintain cellular metabolism. Different organs and tissues confront differential metabolic demands depending on the nature of the particular stressor. It follows that appropriate circulatory responses to different stressful stimuli are variable and may be predicted on the basis of individual tissue metabolic rates during a given condition. It is undeniable that most physical stressors are associated with blood flow changes relevant to individual tissue or whole body requirements. For example, blood flow to working skeletal muscle is dramatically increased during exercise. Deviations in ambient temperature likewise produce predictable patterns of cutaneous blood flow to promote either heat loss or heat conservation. Efficient coupling between blood flow and metabolism is indeed accepted as a hallmark of successful adaptation to environmental fluctuations.

A logical extension of the foregoing discussion to emotional or psychogenic stress is not readily obvious, especially with regard to humans. Except for acute exposures to selected visual or auditory cues (e.g., an ambulance siren), emotional distress is most often precipitated internally. In this sense, it is not the environment posing a threat to homeostasis. Instead, endogenous stimuli (i.e., one's own thoughts), elicit cardiovascular responses that are not related to meeting immediate cellular and metabolic requirements. If metabolic demand was the sole determinant of stress-induced circulatory responses, one would hypothesize that psychological stressors would, at most, elicit selective alterations of cerebral blood flow. In actuality, much more complicated patterns of cardiovascular and hemodynamic responses are measured during "mental" stress in humans (1-3) and animals (4-6). These complex adjustments cannot always be explained satisfactorily on the basis of concomitant metabolic demands. An important question is whether this uncoupling of blood flow and metabolism is necessarily maladaptive.

ANIMAL MODELS OF PSYCHOLOGICAL STRESS

Perhaps the most difficult task animal investigators are faced with is designing experimental interventions that simulate emotional distress as defined for humans. First, it is not known whether animals experience psychological phenomena comparable to human emotions. Without verbal accounts of the subject's emotional state, there is the potential for anthropomorphic biasing of experimental design and interpretation (7). In humans, moreover, emotional discomfort is highly subjective, being shaped by previous experience and socialization; hence, it is difficult for investigators to agree on a strict definition of stress (8). Attempting to replicate an ill-defined human syndrome in experimental animals engenders obvious problems related to quantifying the subject's perception of the stimulus.

Furthermore, in studies using unrestrained conscious animal models, somatomotor responses may, depending on your perspective, complicate the interpretation of simultaneous cardiovascular changes. Locomotor and other skeletomuscular activity engages local and reflex mechanisms that have an impact on cardiovascular and hemodynamic status (9). Discerning the primary versus secondary cardiovascular responses to a given stimulus is made difficult if behavioral concomitants are expressed. On the other hand, if the behavioral or somatomotor response is actually the primary constituent of the animal's stress reaction, perhaps the concurrent cardiovascular alterations may be explained entirely on the basis of supporting or subserving such behaviors (10).

A wide variety of stressful stimuli have been utilized to elicit cardiovascular responses in animals (Table 1). Most psychological stressors used to date are either known to be nociceptive (e.g., electroshock) or are considered to be

TABLE 1　Psychological Stress Models in Animals

Acute exposure to aversive/novel stimuli
Noise
Air jet
Water jet
Electroshock
Restraint
Centrifugation
Vibration
Same-species confrontation
Different-species confrontation
Classical conditioning
Aversive
Appetitive
Operant conditioning
Signalled avoidance
Unsignalled avoidance
Conflict paradigms

---

aversive based on the gross behavior of the animals during presentation of the stimulus; if unrestrained, most species attempt to escape. As in all research fields, technical limitations as well as intrinsic flaws in experimental designs often hamper meaningful analysis of the data. For example, in many experimental situations animals are subject to a combination of aversive conditions in that they are restrained, to various extents, to enable efficient delivery of the chosen stressor. Moreover, until relatively recently, simultaneous direct measurement of multiple physiological variables was not possible or at least not a standard feature of most studies. Despite these and other limitations, both overt and subtle differences have been identified in the cardiovascular and hemodynamic adjustments to various psychological stimuli.

CARDIOVASCULAR RESPONSES TO STRESSFUL STIMULI

Coordinated behavioral, somatic, and visceral responses to the environment are dependent on central nervous system integrative mechanisms. Multiple efferent avenues exist by which the central nervous system may influence cardiovascular function. While the cardiovascular system is subject to important intrinsic or local regulatory processes, stress-induced circulatory responses are, in the main, effected via extrinsic (neural and hormonal) mechanisms (Fig. 1). Rapid homeostatic adjustments of vessel diameter and cardiac rate and contractility are mediated primarily by sympathetic and parasympathetic nerves supplying the heart and vasculature. Hormonal effectors under central nervous system control include bloodborne catecholamines and glucocorticoids derived from the adrenal medulla and adrenal cortex, respectively; circulating vasopressin released from the posterior pituitary; and the renin-angiotensin-aldosterone system. Both neural and humoral regulatory mechanisms mediate stress-induced cardiovascular responses, although differences exist with regard to both the stressor and the species under study.

When relatively gross measures of cardiovascular function are assessed, two basic patterns of centrally mediated cardiovascular responses are observed in animals on exposure to aversive stimuli (Table 2). One response, termed the defense reaction, consists of elevated arterial pressure, heart rate, and cardiac output associated with mesenteric and renal vasoconstriction and skeletal muscle vasodilation; total peripheral resistance declines or changes little owing to the vasodilatory response in skeletomuscular beds. The other cardiovascular response pattern, often attending states of increased vigilance, differs mainly with regard to cardiac function and skeletal muscle blood flow. In this case, bradycardia and decreased cardiac output are associated with increased total peripheral resistance as vasoconstriction occurs in all beds, including skeletal muscle. In general, the defense reaction is presumed to subserve behavioral responses consisting of

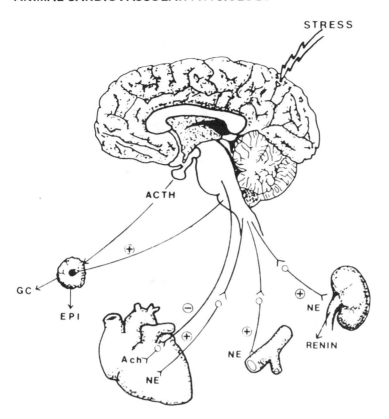

FIGURE 1 Efferent mechanisms by which the central nervous system converts stressful stimuli into cardiovascular changes.

increased motor activity (i.e., "fight or flight"), whereas the vigilance response is associated with motor behaviors such as immobility or "freezing." As discussed below, however, these divergent patterns of cardiovascular responses are not strictly related to the concomitant somatomotor responses.

Cardiovascular responses representative of the defense reaction have been reported for several species on acute exposure to aversive stimuli. In conscious unrestrained mongrel dogs, sudden presentation of a loud noise produces elevations of arterial pressure and heart rate accompanied by mesenteric and renal vasoconstriction and iliac vasodilation (11,12). Comparing noise-induced cardiovascular changes before and after various combinations of sympathetic and vagal blockade indicated that vagal withdrawal was of primary importance in eliciting the immediate tachycardic and pressor responses to this stimulus (12). Spontaneous transitions from a quiet resting state to one of alertness were associated

TABLE 2 Patterned Cardiovascular Responses to Stressful Stimuli

Variable	Defense	Vigilance
Arterial pressure	↑	↑
Heart rate	↑	↓
Cardiac output	↑	↓
Total peripheral resistance	↓	↑
Mesenteric vascular resistance	↑	↑
Renal vascular resistance	↑	↑
Iliac vascular resistance	↓	↑

with similar, although smaller, cardiovascular changes, except for the iliac vaso-dilation, which was quite robust in both situations. Although elevations in iliac blood flow often occurred in the absence of gross movements, hindlimb electro-myographic activity was not measured directly in these studies. Thus, it is not known whether the observed iliac vasodilation was related to skeletal muscle activity.

The relationship between stress-induced somatomotor and cardiovascular responses was investigated in a series of experiments conducted by Zanchetti and co-workers (13–16). Cardiovascular and hemodynamic variables were measured in unrestrained cats during various stages of arousal and fighting. When cats were confronted with an attacking cat, while the animal remained immobile, the immediate circulatory responses consisted of bradycardia and decreased cardiac output associated with mesenteric and iliac vasoconstriction. As soon as the animal engaged in fighting, the hemodynamic pattern changed to one of tachy-cardia, increased cardiac output, and marked elevation of iliac blood flow. Hind-limb electromyographic activity was positively correlated to iliac blood flow, which suggested that skeletomuscular activity was the primary determinant of vasodilation in this bed (13,14). Thus, the authors concluded that the emotional component of the cardiovascular response was a generalized vasoconstriction and that local metabolic factors, not the central nervous system, mediated the skele-tal muscle vasodilation.

This conclusion was soon modified as being restricted to the experimental situation of confrontation between two cats; subsequent studies by these workers demonstrated complete dissociation of hindlimb electromyographic activity and iliac blood flow when using different stimuli for arousal (15,16). If the cats were presented with a barking dog, a mouse, or fire, iliac blood flow responses were variable, ranging from vasoconstriction to marked vasodilation. Moreover, while iliac vasoconstriction was a consistent initial response to presen-tation of another cat, individual animals demonstrated different blood flow responses to each of the other stimuli. In all of these situations, increases and decreases in iliac blood flow occurred in the absence of hindlimb electromyographic activity, and both the vasodilatory and vasoconstrictive responses were abolished by sympathectomy. Thus, in the cat, differential activation of cholinergic versus adrenergic sympathetic nerves occurred depending on the particular psychological stimulus. The authors reasoned that the different stimuli employed possessed varying degrees of emotional significance for individual cats, perhaps related to their experiential backgrounds.

In the very least, the variable nature of the sympathetic responses indicates that the transduction of environmental signals into cardiovascular changes by the central nervous system is a dynamic process. Indeed, ample evidence exists that stress-induced cardiovascular responses are modulated by multiple factors that may or may not be related to the actual stressor. It is known, for example, that habituation or sensitization may occur such that cardiovascular responses become smaller or larger upon repeated presentations of the same stimulus (17–19). Moreover, experimental conditions may heavily influence specific components of stress-induced cardiovascular responses. For example, the direction of conditioned heart rate responses to electroshock in rats is demonstrated to depend on whether the animals are freely moving (tachycardia) or restrained (bradycardia); the conditioned heart rate responses do not necessarily correlate with motor activity as assessed by electromyographic recording (20). Other factors that may acutely modulate stress-induced cardiovascular responses include, but are not limited to, sensory information arising from chemoreceptors and baroreceptors (21–23).

In addition to the studies discussed above in which animals were presented acutely with emotional or noxious stimuli, neurally mediated cardiovascular changes have been examined in dogs trained to avoid electric shock (24–26). While they were performing the avoidance task, arterial pressure, heart rate, and cardiac output were elevated while total peripheral resistance was decreased. In contrast, while they were anticipating the avoidance task (i.e., during the preavoidance interval), reductions of heart rate and cardiac output were measured in association with elevated arterial pressure and total peripheral resistance. Propranolol treatment attenuated the avoidance-induced tachycardia but did not modify preavoidance alterations in heart rate and arterial pressure (27). Thus, in this stressful paradigm, heart rate is controlled predominantly by vagal mechanisms during preavoidance, whereas during avoidance, cardiac sympathetic tone is increased with coincident withdrawal of vagal tone. Using a similar experimental paradigm, Galosy et al. (28) demonstrated that during avoidance, sympathetically mediated cardiac changes are not limited to tachycardia. Positive ionotropic influences were measured as assessed by recording left ventricular systolic pressure and maximum rate of ventricular pressure development. In contrast to the above studies, these investigators found that during preavoidance intervals, heart rate was elevated above baseline due mainly to withdrawal of cardiac vagal tone (28).

Discrete cardiac and vascular changes are also reported for classical conditioning paradigms. In dogs (29,30) and Rhesus monkeys (31), aversively conditioned tachycardia is mediated by a combination of increased sympathetic outflow and decreased vagal activity. Appetitive conditioning using food as the unconditioned stimulus also results in conditioned tachycardia in dogs (30,32). Appetitively conditioned tachycardia differs from aversively conditioned tachycardia in that it is smaller in magnitude and mediated completely by sympathetic outflow. Sympathetic nervous activity also underlies the conditioned positive ionotropic changes evoked by both aversive and appetitive stimuli (29,30,32). Other conditioned cardiac changes in dogs mediated by sympathetic outflow include transient reductions of coronary blood flow (29) and increased atrioventricular nodal conduction fidelity (32). Conditioned emotional responses in baboons are associated with elevations in arterial pressure, heart rate, and terminal aortic blood flow and reductions of renal blood flow (33). The increased terminal aortic flow is not correlated with hind limb movements and is prevented by propranolol pretreatment, suggesting that it is mediated by circulating epinephrine versus local metabolic processes. Moreover, propranolol pretreatment prevents the stress-induced tachycardia in this paradigm.

Baroreflex function is profoundly affected by stressful stimuli. In normal settings, acute elevations of arterial pressure evoke, via the baroreflexes, slowing of heart rate and withdrawal of sympathetic outflow to selected vascular beds. As described above, stressful stimuli often elicit simultaneous elevations of arterial pressure and heart rate. Indeed, reflex sensitivity of the cardiac limb is significantly decreased in baboons during wheel turning, a conditioned behavior having an emotional component (34,35). Likewise, in cats cardiac baroreflex gain is markedly reduced during confrontation with an attacking cat (36). The primary mechanism underlying the reduction of cardiac reflex gain in these studies was demonstrated to be vagal withdrawal. It was interesting that reflex sensitivities of the cardiac versus vasomotor components are differentially influenced by various behaviors (35). Moreover, the effects of behavior on baroreflex-mediated vasomotor responses are similarly differentiated with respect to the particular vascular bed. Thus, the effects of a given stressor on reflex regulation of blood flow in a specific artery cannot be predicted from changes in cardiac baroreflex sensitivity nor from changes occurring in other vessels. These observations indicate that central nervous system processing of afferent baroreceptor information is subject to variable and highly discrete modulation by stressful stimuli.

Relatively little is known regarding stress-induced cardiovascular and hemodynamic changes in normotensive rats. This stems in part from the technical difficulties related to obtaining simultaneous direct measurements of multiple cardiovascular variables in such a small animal. A consistent finding in rat studies, however, is that the spontaneous hypertensive rat (SHR) exhibits enhanced cardiovascular responses to stressful stimuli. Compared to normotensive Wistar (37) or Wistar-Kyoto rats (19,38–40), SHRs display larger pressor and tachycardic responses to aversive stimuli such as presentations of a loud noise or a jet of air. Likewise, significantly greater elevations of arterial pressure and heart rate are observed in SHRs during immobilization (41) and footshock (42), respectively. In studies in which regional blood flows were measured (40,42), stress-induced increases in mesenteric and renal vascular resistance are accentuated in SHRs compared with Wistar-Kyoto rats. Similar observations are reported in studies utilizing aversive conditioning paradigms in which SHRs, compared to Wistar-Kyoto rats, demonstrate larger pressor responses (43–45). In several of the aforementioned studies, evidence was provided to suggest a role for enhanced sympathetic and adrenomedullary outflow in mediating the more pronounced cardiovascular responses observed in the SHR.

CONCLUSION

The aggregate results of these and other studies demonstrate clear autonomic and cardiovascular responses to stressful stimuli in a variety of species. Stress-induced cardiovascular responses are not fixed or invariant, and are subject to dynamic modulation by a variety of exogenous and endogenous factors. The central nervous system mechanisms underlying these differential responses have been studied extensively with electrical and chemical stimulation and ablation procedures. As available experimental techniques become increasingly sophisticated, our understanding of the anatomical and chemical substrates mediating stress-induced cardiovascular changes will improve further. A multidisciplinary approach will prove critical for meaningful investigation of the transduction of environmental signals into appropriate behavioral and physiological adaptations.

REFERENCES

1. Herd JA. Cardiovascular response to stress in man. Annu Rev Physiol 1984; 46: 177–185.
2. Williams RB, Lane JD, Kuhn CM, Melosh W, White AD, Schanberg SM. Type A behavior and elevated physiological and neuroendocrine responses to cognitive tasks. Science 1982; 218: 483–485.
3. Freyschuss U, Hjemdahl P, Juhlin-Dannfelt A, Linde B. Cardiovascular and sympathoadrenal responses to mental stress: influence of β-blockade. Am J Physiol 1988; 255: H1443–H1451.
4. Galosy RA, Clarke LK, Vasko MR, Crawford IL. Neurophysiology and neuropharmacology of cardiovascular regulation and stress. Neurosci Biobehav Rev 1981; 5: 137–175.

5. Cohen DH, Randall DC. Classical conditioning of cardiovascular responses. Annu Rev Physiol 1984; 46: 187–197.

6. Engel BT, Schneiderman N. Operant conditioning and the modulation of cardiovascular function. Annu Rev Physiol 1984; 46: 199–210.

7. Moberg GP. Biological response to stess: key to assessment of animal well-being? In: Moberg GP, ed. Animal stress. Bethesda, MD: American Physiological Society, 1985: 27–49.

8. Levine S. A definition of stress? In Moberg GP, ed. Animal stress. Bethesda, MD: American Physiological Society, 1985: 51–69.

9. Abboud FM, Thames MD. Interaction of cardiovascular reflexes in circulatory control. In: Shepherd JT, Abboud FM, eds. Handbook of physiology. Section 2. The cardiovascular system. Vol. III. Washington, DC: American Physiological Society, 1983: 675–753.

10. Cohen DH, Obrist PA. Interactions between behavior and the cardiovascular system. Circ Res 1975; 37: 693–706.

11. Caraffa-Braga E, Granata L, Pinotti O. Changes in blood-flow distribution during acute emotional stress in dogs. Pflugers Arch 1973; 339: 203–216.

12. Federici A, Rizzo A, Cevese A. Role of the autonomic nervous system in the control of heart rate and blood pressure in the defense reaction in conscious dogs. J Auton Nerv Syst 1985; 12: 333–345.

13. Adams DB, Baccelli G, Mancia G, Zanchetti A. Cardiovascular changes during naturally elicited fighting behavior in the cat. Am J Physiol 1969; 216: 1226–1235.

14. Adams DB, Baccelli G, Mancia G, Zanchetti A. Relation of cardiovascular changes in fighting to emotion and exercise. J Physiol 1971; 212: 321–335.

15. Baccelli G, Ellison GD, Mancia G, Zanchetti A. Opposite responses of muscle circulation to different emotional stimuli. Experientia 1971; 27: 1183–1184.

16. Mancia G, Baccelli G, Zanchetti A. Hemodynamic responses to different emotional stimuli in the cat: patterns and mechanisms. Am J Physiol 1972; 223: 925–933.

17. Martin J, Sutherland CJ, Zbrozyna AW. Habituation and conditioning of defense reactions and their cardiovascular components in cats and dogs. Pflugers Arch 1976; 365: 37–47.

18. Abrahams VC, Hilton SM, Zbrozyna AW. The role of active muscle vasodilation in the alerting stage of the defense reaction. J Physiol 1964; 171: 189–202.

19. Rettig R, Geyer MA, Printz MP. Cardiovascular concomitants of tactile and acoustic startle responses in spontaneously hypertensive and normotensive rats. Physiol Behav 1986; 36: 1123–1128.

20. Martin GK, Fitzgerald RD. Heart rate and somatomotor activity in rats during signalled escape and yoked classical conditioning. Physiol Behav 1980; 25: 519–526.

21. Baccelli G, Albertini R, Del Bo A, Mancia G, Zanchetti A. Role of sinoaortic reflexes in hemodynamic patterns of natural defense behaviors in the cat. Am J Physiol 1981; 240: H421–H429.

22. Hatton DC, Foutz SR, Fitzgerald RD. Baroreceptor involvement in classically conditioned heart rate responses of restrained rats. Physiol Behav 1984; 33: 31–35.

23. Buchholz RA, Hubbard JW, Keeton TK, Nathan MA. Cardiovascular and neuroendocrine responses to behavioral stress after central or peripheral barodenervation in rats. Brain Res 1986; 365: 360–364.

24. Anderson DE, Brady JV. Preavoidance blood pressure elevations accompanied by heart rate decreases in the dog. Science 1971; 172: 595–597.

25. Anderson DE, Tosheff JG. Cardiac output and total peripheral resistance changes during preavoidance periods in the dog. J Appl Physiol 1973; 34: 650–654.

26. Lawler JE, Obrist PA, Lawler KA. Cardiovascular function during preavoidance, avoidance and post-avoidance in dogs. Psychophysiology 1975; 12: 4–11.

27. Anderson DE, Brady JV. Cardiovascular responses to avoidance conditioning in the dog: effects of beta adrenergic blockade. Psychosom Med 1976; 38: 181–189.

28. Galosy RA, Clarke LK, Mitchell JH. Cardiac changes during behavioral stress in dogs. Am J Physiol 1979; 236: H750–H758.

29. Billman GE, Randall DC. Mechanisms mediating the coronary vascular response to behavioral stress in the dog. Circ Res 1981; 48: 214–223.

30. Randall DC, Skinner TL, Billman GE. A comparison of the autonomic nervous control of the heart during classical aversive vs appetitive conditioning in dog. J Auton Nerv Syst 1985; 13: 125–136.

31. Schoenfeld WN, Kadden RM, Tremont PJ, McCullough MR, Steele WA. Effects of pharmacological autonomic blockade upon cardiac rate and blood pressure conditioned and unconditioned responses in *Macaca mulatta*. J Auton Nerv Syst 1980; 2: 365–375.

32. Skinner TL, Randall DC. Behaviorally conditioned changes in atrioventricular transmission in awake dog. J Auton Nerv Syst 1985; 12:23–34.

33. Smith OA, Hohimer AR, Astley CA, Taylor DJ. Renal and hindlimb vascular control during acute emotion in the baboon. Am J Physiol 1979; 236: R198–R205.

34. Stephenson RB, Smith OA, Scher AM. Baroreceptor regulation of heart rate in baboons during different behavioral states. Am J Physiol 1981; 241: R277–R285.

35. Combs CA, Smith OA, Astley CA, Feigl EO. Differential effect of behavior on cardiac and vasomotor baroflex responses. Am J Physiol 1986; 251: R126–R136.

36. Schlor K-H, Stumpf H, Stock G. Baroreceptor reflex during arousal induced by electrical stimulation of the amygdala or by natural stimuli. J Auton Nerv Syst 1984; 10: 157–165.

37. Hallback M, Folkow B. Cardiovascular responses to acute mental "stress" in spontaneously hypertensive rats. Acta Physiol Scand 1974; 90: 684–698.

38. Lundin S, Thoren P. Renal function and sympathetic activity during mental stress in normotensive and spontaneously hypertensive rats. Acta Physiol Scand 1982; 115: 115–124.
39. Lundin S, Ricksten S-E, Thoren P. Interaction between "mental stress" and baroreceptor reflexes concerning effects on heart rate, mean arterial pressure and renal sympathetic activity in conscious spontaneously hypertensive rats. Acta Physiol Scand 1984; 120: 273–281.
40. Galeno TM, Van Hoesen GW, Brody MJ. Central amygdaloid nucleus lesion attenuates exaggerated hemodynamic responses to noise stress in the spontaneously hypertensive rat. Brain Res 1984; 291: 249–259.
41. Kvetnansky R, McCarty R, Thoa NB, Lake CR, Kopin IJ. Sympatho-adrenal responses of spontaneously hypertensive rats to immobilization stress. Am J Physiol 1979; 236: H457–H462.
42. Kirby RF, Callahan MF, Johnson AK. Regional vascular responses to an acute stressor in spontaneously hypertensive and Wistar-Kyoto rats. J Auton Nerv Syst 1987; 20: 185–188.
43. Hatton DC, Buchholz RA, Fitzgerald RD. Autonomic control of heart rate and blood pressure in spontaneously hypertensive rats during aversive classical conditioning. J Comp Physiol Psychol 1981; 95: 978–990.
44. Sakaguchi A, LeDoux JE, Reis DJ. Sympathetic nerves and adrenal medulla: contributions to cardiovascular-conditioned emotional responses in spontaneously hypertensive rats. Hypertension 1983; 5: 728–738.
45. LeDoux JE, Sakaguchi A, Reis DJ. Strain differences in fear between spontaneously hypertensive and normotensive rats. Brain Res 1983; 277: 137–143.

22

EFFECTS OF PSYCHOLOGICAL STRESS ON CARDIAC RATE AND RHYTHM

Michael A. Brodsky and Byron J. Allen

University of California School of Medicine, Irvine Medical Center
Orange, California

ANECDOTAL INFORMATION ON STRESS AND SUDDEN DEATH

An organism's homeostasis depends in part on the myriad connections between the nervous and cardiovascular systems. These ties include well-defined nervous and hormonal linkages. Although many of the actions and reactions between these systems have been characterized, those within the brain and especially with regard to emotions have not been clearly elucidated. The cardiovascular responses to emotional stress range from insignificant to catastrophic, and it has been suggested that psychologically stressful emotions can result in sudden cardiac death (1).

Many reports suggest a connection between psychological stress and sudden death. In the 18th century, when the first association was made between coronary artery disease and sudden death, there was a dramatic story of stress-provoked sudden death. John Hunter, an English surgeon and anatomist, was reported prone to violent rages and later in life he began to experience cardiovascular symptoms associated with his loss of temper. He realized his problem ("My life is at the mercy of any rogue who chooses to provoke me.") but could not control it. His final moments were spent engaged in a vigorous quarrel; he left the room, collapsed and died. An autopsy later documented that he had significant coronary artery disease (2).

Psychological stress is reportedly associated with sudden death in individuals without structural heart disease as well. In 1942, Walter Cannon, a physiologist, published a review on "voodoo" death (3). He collated descriptions of individuals among tribal cultures who experienced unexplained death temporally associated with spiritual phenomena. In some cases, later pathological analysis noted no readily identifiable cause of death. Cannon speculated that these deaths were due to shocking emotional stress. Medical reports from the United States armed services during World War II documented that 10% of all sudden and unexpected deaths of young soldiers occurred in the absence of any identifiable pathological findings (4). United States military reports from the Korean conflict suggested that soldiers may die due to stress rather than physical injury, as in the case of "prisoner-of-war syndrome" (5). These publications support the notion that stress-associated sudden death can occur in the absence of identifiable cardiovascular disease.

The type of stress able to provoke sudden death has also been reviewed. George Engel, an upstate New York physician, categorized the multiple precipitants of sudden death while collating 170 newspaper reports over a 6 year period (6). Sudden death could occur as a result of adverse feelings over the impact of terrible news, a threat of loss, or during a phase of mourning. On occasion, extremely positive feelings such as elation could also precipitate sudden death. He suggested that sudden death occurred because victims could not control their overwhelming emotional response. Myers and Dewar, pathologists from England, reviewed the cases of 100 male victims of sudden death in the setting of coronary artery disease (7). They showed that acute psychological stress was the most significant risk factor for the development of sudden death, while chronic psychological stress was not a related factor. Reich and others documented that acute psychological disturbances occurred the day before presentation of life-threatening ventricular arrhythmias in 21% of 117 patients (8). They suggested that a disproportionate number of patients without structural heart disease were included in the group of patients with significant antecedent psychological disturbances. Trichopoulos et al. studied the medical results from the Athens earthquake of 1981 and documented a significant increase in deaths from cardiac causes approximately 3 days after the earthquake. These investigators suggested that the psychological stress of the 3 days of tremors following the initial quake registering 6.7 on the Richter scale precipitated a marked increase in cardiovascular deaths (9). These anecdotal reports provide historical per- spective on the association between stress and sudden death. None of these reports document specific evidence, but taken together they suggest that acute psychological stress may be temporally associated with sudden unexpected death.

RISK FACTORS FOR SUDDEN DEATH AND THEIR ASSOCIATION WITH PSYCHOLOGICAL STRESS

General

The likely cause of sudden death depends on the degree of suddenness and expectation. Literature on pathology suggests that if sudden death occurs within an hour of the onset of symptoms in an otherwise unexpected situation, the likelihood of a cardiovascular cause is greater than 90% (10). This cutoff period allows for a homogeneity of diagnosis. The most common cardiac cause of sudden death is an unstable arrhythmia. Ventricular fibrillation is the most common arrhythmia noted terminally, occurring between 75 and 90% of the time. Coronary artery disease is the most common underlying cardiovascular disorder present in patients with ventricular fibrillation, but miscellaneous conditions occur in 10%, and structural heart disease is absent in 10% of victims. Therefore, sudden death is most likely cardiac in origin, occurs in the setting of coronary artery disease, and is terminally due to ventricular fibrillation.

Psychological imbalance has been implicated as a risk factor for sudden cardiac death, both by itself and as a multiplier of other factors. A University of Iowa study showed that there was an increased risk of natural sudden deaths among young female patients hospitalized for schizophrenia or depression (11). Many of these deaths occurred within the first 2 years after discharge from hospital.

Coronary Disease

Coronary artery disease is a major risk factor for sudden cardiac death. Rosenman and others have suggested that behavior patterns related to the response to psychological stress can be associated with the incidence and degree of coronary disease (12). Type A personality, also known as coronary-prone behavior, may be associated with abnormal neuroendocrine responses and may in turn provoke coronary artery disease (13). Others have shown that psychological factors have been specifically correlated to the presence and degree of coronary artery disease (14). The mechanism of these associations probably relates to some of the risk factors for coronary artery disease (hypercholesterolemia, hypertension, and tobacco use). Recent data suggest that psychological stress can precipitate coronary atherosclerosis in monkeys even when they are fed a low-fat, low-cholesterol diet (15). Hypertension can be provoked as a result of psychological-stress-induced cardiovascular reactivity (16). The mechanism of this stress-induced hypertension is multifactorial and includes changes in vascular tone, downregulation of alpha receptors, and changes in the regulation of mineral and water balance.

Psychological stress remains an important factor even after coronary artery disease has become manifest. Talbott and others showed that a history of psychiatric treatment is an important risk factor for sudden death in women with coronary disease (17,18). In men with coronary disease, significant risk factors for sudden cardiac death include a high degree of life stress, social isolation, and low education level (19). Rahe and others reported that stress-associated recent life changes were related to the incidence of sudden cardiac death in patients with coronary disease (20). In their study, the highest graded factor was death of a spouse. Bereavement has also been documented by others to be associated with an adverse outcome (21). Type A personality and the Sisyphus personality type (an effort-oriented person who strives against odds with little sense of accomplishment or satisfaction) are both associated with adverse outcomes in patients with ischemic heart disease (12,22).

Once coronary disease is present, mental stress can provoke active ischemia. Recent data document both symptomatic and asymptomatic myocardial ischemia in response to stressful activities such as mental arithmetic, public speaking, and the recall of emotionally arousing personal experiences (23-27). These episodes of ischemia have been documented by electrocardiographic changes as well as alterations in myocardial perfusion. There are multiple potential mechanisms of these changes including increased heart rate, coronary vasospasm, and platelet activation. These types of changes have been confirmed by Verrier and others (28). They showed that animals provoked with anger had significant alterations in coronary blood flow if there was preexisting coronary artery obstruction.

Cardiomyopathy

Diminished cardiac contractibility of any cause is commonly noted in individuals resuscitated from cardiac arrest. While ischemic heart disease is the usual cause of myocardial dysfunction, this disorder can also occur unrelated to coronary artery disease. This problem, also known as cardiomyopathy, has been noted to develop in response to psychological stress. Raab and others detailed primary myocardial necrosis in rats after exposure to a psychologically stressful environment for as short a time as 3 days (29). These unique findings were confirmed in swine as well (30). Rona suggests that the pathological changes in this stress cardiomyopathy were similar to experimental cardiomyopathy caused by infusion of catecholamine (31).

Ventricular Arrhythmia

Cardiac arrhythmia has been considered an important risk factor for sudden cardiac death. Lown and others suggest that fatal cardiac arrhythmias can develop given the proper conditions of a vulnerable substrate, electrical instability, and transient risk factors (32). This fragile substrate is often a diseased myocardium as a result of ischemia or other factors, but may be a structurally normal heart. Cardiac electrical instability is commonly manifest as frequent and complex ventricular arrhythmia. Transient risk factors include alterations in pH, electrolytes, oxygen, and, perhaps most importantly, psychological stress (32). The relationship between ventricular arrhythmias and psychological stress has been studied by many investigators.

Animal Studies

Lown and others reviewed various animal experiments, mostly involving canines, that tested the role of neural and psychological mechanisms in cardiac arrhythmia (32). Stimulation of the brain, especially the hypothalamus, can produce different types of arrhythmia, including ventricular fibrillation. Brain stimulation provokes arrhythmia much more readily in susceptible animals, especially those with myocardial ischemia. Manipulation of neurotransmitters of the central nervous system can alter the susceptibility to ventricular fibrillation. The peripheral parts of the nervous system are also important in arrhythmogenesis. Enhanced activity in the sympathetic branch of the autonomic nervous system is directly correlated with ventricular arrhythmia. Direct stimulation of the stellate ganglia can affect the threshold for ventricular fibrillation. Myocardial ischemia can stimulate activity in the stellate ganglia, which then predisposes the heart to ventricular fibrillation. The parasympathetic branch of the autonomic nervous system also has a role, but exerts its effect on the heart rhythm mostly through its association with adrenergic tone and not by itself. Several experiments have suggested that psychological stress has an important effect on the production of arrhythmia. A stressful environment increases the likelihood of ventricular fibrillation in both normal and ischemic hearts. Skinner and others have shown that swine are also prone to arrhythmia in response to psychological stress (33).

Human Studies

HEART RATE, VENTRICULAR ARRHYTHMIA   Although ethical considerations and inadequate models have limited investigation in humans, some studies have evaluated the effect of psychological stress on cardiac arrhythmias. Stevenson and others reported that emotions such as anxiety, fear, anger, and elation were associated with cardiac arrhythmia. Arrhythmia was noted regardless of the underlying cardiovascular status (34). Sigler detailed various changes in the electrocardiogram in patients under stress (35). In a later publication he reported that a psychologically stressful interview could provoke electrocardiographic changes. In response to the interview, patients manifested an increase in heart rate, including changes in conduction and differences in repolarization, the latter suggesting ischemia (36). Moss and Wynar showed that a significant increase in

heart rate occurred during public speaking. The magnitude of heart rate elevation was equivalent to that of moderate exercise (37). Taggart and others investigated the effects of various stressful activities on the cardiac rate and rhythm.
They noted an increase in heart rate, changes in the ST segment of the electrocardiogram, and ventricular arrhythmia in response to diverse activities such as
driving an automobile or public speaking (38,39). Lown and colleagues utilized
a psychological-stress interview in 19 patients with a history of life-threatening
cardiac arrhythmias. They documented that 11 of 19 subjects had a significant
increase in the frequency of ventricular arrhythmia during a purposely stressful
interaction. The heart rate increased significantly from a mean of 71 to 82 beats/
min with a direct correlation between increases in heart rate and arrhythmia
(40). Orth-Gomer and others evaluated the relationship between psychological
characteristics and ventricular arrhythmias in 150 men with various underlying
disorders. They concluded that depression had the most significant association
with ventricular arrhythmia. This correlation was important, however, only in
the absence of ischemic heart disease (41). Katz and others compared the
psychological profile with electrocardiograms of 102 patients and found that
arrhythmia was associated with significant psychological variables, including
hysteria, anxiety, and depression (42). Follick and others suggested that psychological distress was associated with cardiac arrhythmia in a group of patients
following myocardial infarction (43). These studies taken together suggest that
cardiac arrhythmia is related to psychological variables in a variety of different
individuals.

VENTRICULAR TACHYARRHYTHMIA   There have been many case reports
of sustained ventricular tachyarrhythmia provoked by psychologically stressful
events. Harvey and Levine detailed paroxysmal ventricular tachycardia in
response to fear. In their report physicians were able to recreate the arrhythmia
using stressful situations (44). Levine later described the sudden death of
another individual following an intense emotional upset (45). Lown and others
detailed the thorough evaluation of a patient with ventricular fibrillation associated with psychological stress (46). Vlay reported the case of a young woman
who experienced cardiac arrest with documented ventricular fibrillation on her
first day of medical school (47). Brodsky and others reported the case histories
of six patients with sustained ventricular tachyarrhythmia and no evidence of
heart disease. Five of these six patients had significant psychological stress as
their only risk factor (48). The patients in these case reports were without
evidence of significant cardiac disease, yet each experienced life-threatening
arrhythmia. The risk factor for ventricular tachyarrhythmia in these patients was
their psychological status.

Certain groups of patients have been reported to have ventricular tachyar-
rhythmias in response to psychological stress. A recent study showed that among
those patients with syncope in the setting of a prolonged QT interval (long QT

syndrome), 58% had at least one syncopal spell precipitated by intense emotions (49). Wellens and others reported the recurrent loss of consciousness and ventricular fibrillation in a young woman with QT prolongation following auditory arousal from sleep. According to her history, the patient's initial loss of consciousness occurred following a thunderclap. Medical investigation documented further prolongation of the QT interval and ventricular fibrillation following auditory arousal from loud stimuli (50). Young male Laotian and Cambodian refugees who have moved to the United States have had a disproportionately high frequency of sudden death (51). Ventricular tachyarrhythmia has been documented as the preterminal event (52). Psychological stress and "posttraumatic stress disorder" in particular have been considered important factors in the death of these refugees (51,53).

Patients with cardiac disease are occasionally tested using invasive techniques in an attempt to stratify future prognosis. Cardiac electophysiological testing can provoke arrhythmia in patients who may be prone to it. Tavazzi and others used a combination of invasive cardiac electrophysiological testing and psychological stress testing to evaluate patients following myocardial infarction. While under mental stress, as compared to baseline, patients had a significant change in myocardial electrical properties, including a shortening of the ventricular refractory period and an increase in the frequency of provocable ventricular tachyarrhythmia (54). These reports support the notion that psychological stress can provoke significant changes in the cardiac rate and rhythm, even to the degree of precipitating cardiac arrest.

MECHANISMS/TREATMENT OF ARRHYTHMIA RELATED TO PSYCHOLOGICAL STRESS

Cardiovascular Function

Life-threatening cardiac arrhythmia can develop in response to acute myocardial ischemia. Different types of stress can provoke ischemia (23-28). There are many potential mechanisms for ischemia. Treatment of patients at risk for ventricular tachyarrhythmia should focus on controlling the tendency for ischemia. Since many of these patients will also have baseline cardiac arrhythmia, antiarrhythmic medication will often be helpful.

Nervous System

Parasympathetic

Some investigators have suggested that the mechanism of stress-induced sudden death may be related to excessive parasympathetic tone (55,56). In 1957 Richter showed that rats exposed to persistent stress died from progressive bradycardia (55). The animals initially had an accelerated heart rate, but later the rate slowed. Pretreatment with atropine had a beneficial effect while para-sympathetic stimulants were associated with a more rapid death. These findings suggested that the animals died in the setting of excessive vagal tone (55). In 1967 Wolf documented how syncope occurred after increasing vagal tone and further speculated that this might be a mechanism of death. He suggested that the oxygen-conserving reflex, frequently seen during diving, may be associated with sudden cardiac death (56). Despite these considerations, there are limited therapeutic options for controlling arrhythmia as a result of this mechanism. Atropine can effectively prevent serious arrhythmias, but it is only available in a parenteral form. Even then, it has a relatively short duration of action. Also, the dosage must be greater than 0.5 mg and less than 2.0 mg or there may be a para-doxical effect. Synthetic atropine-like agents such as scopolamine are inadequate in controlling cardiac disorders.

Adrenergic Tone

In 1942 Walter Cannon suggested that sudden unexplained death in tribal cul-tures was due to persistent excessive activity of the sympathoadrenal sytstem (2). Since then, many investigators have concurred that an alteration in adrener-gic tone is the most likely explanation for stress-induced sudden death. Taggart documented that excessive catecholamine levels were generated in response to psychological stress (38,39). In a later study, Dimsdale and Moss also showed that plasma catecholamines increased in response to either psychological or physical stress (57). They documented that norepinephrine levels are predomini-nantly elevated in response to exercise, and epinephrine levels rise to a greater extent during stress-provoking public speaking. They suggested that psychologi-cal stress induced a response primarily from the adrenal medulla, as opposed to the generalized sympathetic nervous system reaction induced from exercise (57).

Since a commonly speculated mechanism of stress-associated arrhythmia is an alteration in adrenergic tone and response, many investigators have attempted therapy with beta adrenergic blocking agents. Lown and colleagues protected animals exposed to psychological stress from developing serious arrhythmia by using beta blockers (32). Skinner and others also documented the beneficial effects of beta blockers in swine, but they suggested that this therapy was only of limited value (33). Taggart showed that beta blocker therapy suppressed the electrocardiographic abnormalities (tachycardia and ectopic beats) but did not affect the catecholamine level (39). Lown and others showed that beta blockade was necessary for control of arrhythmia in their patient with stress-associated cardiac arrest (46). Vlay also used beta blocker therapy in an attempt to control arrhythmia, but it had only a partial effect (47). Brodsy and co-workers evalu-ated the adrenergic tone and responsiveness in five patients with stress-associated life-threatening cardiac arrhythmia (48). Ventricular tachyarrhythmia was pro-voked during exercise or isoprotenenol infusion in four of the five patients.

Evidence of the potential protective effect of a reduction in adrenergic tone was seen as arrhythmia suppressed during sleep in four of five patients. Solitary beta blocker therapy effectively reduced arrhythmia during recurrent testing and had a beneficial long-term effect in four of five patients.

Moss and others have reviewed the role of the sympathetic nervous system in the prolonged QT syndrome (49). Alterations in the QT interval can be achieved with manipulation of the nervous system through the stellate ganglia. The ganglia are part of the chain of neurons of the sympathetic branch of the autonomic nervous system. The prolonged QT syndrome is thought to be related to an imbalance of the innervation of the heart through these ganglia, with the left ganglion predominating. Treatment has been successfully accomplished with left ganglion excision. Alternative therapies include beta blockade. Wellens and others showed that propranolol reduced the arrhythmia in their patient with paroxysmal ventricular fibrillation, but a recurrent attack while the patient was receiving propranolol prompted a change in therapy (50).

Morady and others evaluated the role of epinephrine infusions using invasive cardiac electrophysiological testing. They tested these infusions in patients with baseline provocable sustained ventricular tachycardia that was later controllled by quinidine (58). The infusion provided a serum epinephrine level consistent with that provoked by psychological stress (57). When epinephrine was given in addition to quinidine, many of the patients were no longer protected by quinidine and had provocable ventricular tachycardia (58).

There are difficulties in assessing the efficacy of beta blocking therapy in many of these situations. First, the standard beta blockers are competitive antagonists and their effect can be overwhelmed by a strong enough stimulus. Second, there are many different agents available with different potency, and widely disparate dosages have been used in the studies. Taggart used oxprenolol 40 mg, Wellens' patient was given propranolol 80 mg per day, Lown's patient was given propranolol 160 mg per day (along with other therapy), Vlay used atenolol, and Brodsky and others used metoprolol 150–250 mg per day in 5 patients and propranolol 240 mg per day in 1 patient (39,46–48,50). To ascertain the actual potency of beta blocker therapy, one usually tests the patient with exercise or isoproterenol. Only Brodsky and others reported titrating the therapy to limit the exercise heart rate (to less than 120 beat/min) (49). It is doubtful that 80 mg of propranolol would act as effective block for the patient in the study by Wellens, and this may explain the recurrence of symptoms (50). Third, even if the patients are prescribed an adequate dosage of therapy, one cannot be sure if the therapy is taken. Compliance is limited (especially due to side effects), and blood levels of these agents are not readily available. Stellate ganglion excision is more definitive therapy, but even that cannot interrupt the important adrenergic input to the heart. The sympathetic chain of ganglia is bilateral and often diffuse. In addition, the adrenal medulla may be the area most responsible for the catecholamine surge to psychological stress, and adrenalectomy is often unreasonable and excessive treatment for this disorder.

Other Mechanisms/Treatments

Other neural–cardiac interactions reportedly have been associated with life-threatening arrhythmias. Topaz and others detailed the association between auditory stimuli, cardiac arrhythmia, and sudden cardiac death (59). They discussed the link between hearing and congenital cardiac disorders as well as the many case reports implicating auditory events and cardiac arrest. They suggested that the mechanism of arrhythmia formation (as a result of auditory stimuli) was eventually due to increased tone in the stellate ganglia and sympathetic nervous system.

Lown and others reviewed how different central nervous system actions were responsible for critical interactions between the nervous and cardiovascular systems (32). In testing these interactions, they altered the production of important neurotransmitters by intravenous administration of amino acids and, in turn, influenced the cardiac electrical state (60). These results could have far-reaching implications since dietary manipulation could change the risk of life-threatening cardiac arrhythmia.

Biobehavioral Status

Counseling

In evaluating the effect of stress on the cardiac rate and rhythm, the physician must understand each patient's biobehavioral make-up. Therapeutic options depend on the patient as well as the type and duration of stress. Counseling is frequently helpful in reducing the ramifications of psychological stress. Friedman and colleagues used behavioral counseling to reduce the intensity of type A behavior and, as a result, reduced the rate of cardiac events (61). Ragland and Brand suggested that type A personality was not even a risk factor in patients with coronary disease. However, many of the patients in this study had already undergone behavioral and personality counseling (62). Other types of counseling, including behavior modification and relaxation techniques, have been helpful. Noncultic meditation, as introduced by Benson and colleagues, has been shown to reduce cardiac arrhythmia in patients with stable ischemic heart disease and frequent baseline ventricular arrhythmia (63).

Pharmacological Therapy

Psychoactive medications are helpful in controlling many of the psychic responses to stress. Benzodiazepine agents reduce anxiety and depression and control sleep disturbances (64,65). Benzodiazepines have also been shown to blunt the catecholamine response to psychological and physical stress (66,67). Wheatley suggested that propranolol was as effective as chlordiazepoxide in control of anxiety, but less effective in combating sleep disturbances and depression (64). Mazzuero and others suggested that beta blockers controlled the cardiovascular response to stress better that benzodiazepines in patients following myocardial infarction (65).

FUTURE INVESTIGATIONS

New Directions

Psychological stress's impact on the nervous and cardiovascular systems includes altering neural traffic as well as hormonal levels. Future research will focus on defining these associations better for the purposes of positive intervention. Lane and Schwartz have recently postulated a neurophysiological mechanism for stress-induced cardiac arrhythmias (68). They have suggested that a specific area for the brain deals with emotional arousal. This area is typically lateralized. At the same time, the neural input to the heart is also typically lateralized. These investigators suggest that stress generates lateralized central nervous system activity that in turn induces a lateralized imbalance of sympathetic input to the heart. They further suggest that an overwhelming emotional experience could conceivably result in a massive sympathetic imbalance that could lead to life-threatening cardiac arrhythmia (68).

While individuals without heart disease experience some arrhythmia in response to stress, the most significant arrhythmia typically occurs in subjects with serious underlying heart disease. Psychological stress has been suggested to be an important risk factor for sudden death in many victims with significant cardiac disease. The risk for ventricular tachyarrhythmia could be calculated by assigning value to underlying disease (ischemia, myocardial dysfunction, baseline arrhythmia) as well as to the amount of stress (duration, intensity, suddenness). An equation could be designed to take these values into account in order to assign risk.

In many situations some individuals have an excessive response to catecholamines (e.g., the heart rate is excessively increased with minimal exercise). Despite the possibility of catecholamine excess (as may occur with adrenal tumor such as pheochromocytoma), many of these subjects have normal catecholamine levels. Adrenal tumors are exceedingly rare despite being commonly considered. The excessive response to catecholamines may result from an excess of beta receptors or a more dramatic response per beta stimulant. This could occur as a result of a sensitized myocardium from prolonged catecholamine exposure due to drugs such as cocaine, excessive athletic conditioning, or a hyperthyroid state. An evaluation of the quantity and characteristics of beta receptor–stimulation interaction could unlock the secret of many of these subjects' reactions.

Methods for Research

Susceptible Populations

It is important to investigate populations at greatest risk to provide the highest yield. Many animals models currently exist for ventricular tachyarrhythmia (32, 33,69). Additional animal models exist for cardiac disorders potentially predisposed to cardiac arrhythmia including coronary atherosclerosis and dilated cardiomyopathy (15,70,71). The study of these populations should help to establish the neural–cardiac linkages.

Ethical considerations have limited human research in the area of psychological stress, especially in individuals at risk for cardiac arrest. Patients need not be subjected to induction of cardiac arrest as an endpoint of research. Instead, well-described premonitory arrhythmias such as nonsustained ventricular tachycardia could be utilized as endpoints. The populations at risk would include those patients with the disorders most commonly found in patients resuscitated from cardiac arrest, which would include coronary artery disease, myocardial infarction, and cardiomyopathy. Certain exceptions to that rule would include certain populations of individuals who have been shown to be at risk for cardiac arrest in the setting of structurally normal hearts. This could include such groups as patients with prolonged QT syndrome and refugees from Laos and Cambodia.

Techniques of Evaluation

In evaluating the effects of stress on cardiac arrhythmia, many different physiological measurements are important. Indirect factors include levels of electrolytes, brain wave activity and blood pressure. Direct measurements of arrhythmia can be done invasively or noninvasively. Invasive testing may require anesthesia (thoracotomy and/or repeated ventricular fibrillation threshold testing) or not (catheter placement), but typically these interfere with the individual's psychological state. Noninvasive techniques can quantitate the cardiovascular response to a variety of stimuli and are generally less intrusive and disruptive to the underlying psychological state. These include ambulatory electrocardiographic recording (to assess the QT interval and arrhythmia) and excercise testing.

Baseline and stress psychological testing are important to assess the role of stress in susceptible subjects. Baseline psychological testing to assess personality and attitudes is helpful to understand a subject's basic behavioral make-up. This can be repeated at different stages of intervention to assess the effect of therapy. Provocative "psychological stress" testing is often complicated and must be done in a safe environment. Some of the previously utilized techniques have included mental arithmetic, auditory stimulation, public speaking, automobile driving, and the recall of emotionally sensitive issues. Since these processes are potentially very provocative, appropriate precautions must be taken to avoid serious complications.

CONCLUSION

In summary, psychological stress should be considered a risk factor for sudden cardiac death. Stress may provoke coronary disease, active ischemia, and allow for the development of cardiomyopathy. Stress affects the cardiac rate and rhythm in various degrees and may provoke a life-threatening arrhythmia even in the absence of heart disease. Arrhythmia develops mostly in response to an alteration in adrenergic tone. The individual at risk may have an excessive response to catecholamines, which may provoke a fatal arrhythmia. There are many options for treating the individual at risk, including beta blockers, other cardiac therapy, and other biobehavioral therapy. Future developments will involve further descriptions of the links between the nervous and cardiovascular systems.

ACKNOWLEDGMENTS

The authors thank Colleen Ford for her timely response to repetitive deadlines.

REFERENCES

1. Lown B. Mental stress, arrhythmias and sudden death. Am J Med 1982; 72: 177–180.
2. Kligfield P. John Hunter, angina pectoris and medical education. Am J Cardiol 1980; 45:367–369.
3. Cannon W B. "Voodoo" death. Am Anthropol 1942; 44: 169–181.
4. Moritz A R, Zamcheck N. Sudden and unexpected deaths of young soldiers. Arch Pathol 1946; 42:459–494.
5. Strassman H D, Thaler M B, Schein E H. A prisoner of war syndrome: apathy as a reaction to severe stress. Am J Psychol 1956; 112:998–1003.
6. Engel G L. Sudden and rapid death during psychological stress. Ann Intern Med 1971; 74:771–782.
7. Myers A, Dewar H A. Circumstances attending 100 sudden deaths from coronary artery disease with coroner's necropsies. Br Heart J 1975; 37: 1133–1143.
8. Reich P, DeSilva R A, Lown B, Murawski B J. Acute psychological disturbances preceding life-threatening ventricular arrhythmias. JAMA 1981; 246:233–235.
9. Trichopoulos D, Katwouyanni K, Zavitsanos X, Tzonou A, Dalla-Vorgia P. Psychological stress and fatal heart attack: the Athens (1981) earthquake natural experiment. Lancet 1983; 1:441–444.
10. Spain D M, Bradess V A, Mohr C. Coronary atherosclerosis as a cause of unexpected and unexplained death. JAMA 1960; 174:384–388.
11. Black D W, Warrack G, Winokur G. Excess mortality among psychiatric patients. JAMA 1985; 253:58–61.

12. Rosenman R H, Brand R J, Jenkins D, Friedman M, Straus R, Wurm M. Coronary heart disease in the western collaborative group study. JAMA 1975; 233:872–877.

13. Williams R B Jr, Lane J D, Kuhn C M, Melosh W, White A D, Schanberg S M. Type A behavior and elevated physiological and neuroendocrine responses to cognitive tasks. Science 1982; 218:483–485.

14. Zyanski S J, Jenkins C D, Ryan T J, Flessas A, Everist M. Psychological correlates of coronary angiographic findings. Arch Intern Med 1976; 136: 1234–1237.

15. Kaplan J R, Manuck S B, Clarkson T B, Lusso F M, Taub D M, Miller E W. Social stress and atherosclerosis in normocholesterolemic monkeys. Science 1983; 220:733–735.

16. Cinciripini P M. Cognitive stress and cardiovascular reactivity. I. Relationship to hypertension. Am Heart J 1986; 112:1044–1050.

17. Talbott E, Kuller L H, Detre K, Perper J. Biologic and psychosocial risk factors of sudden death from coronary disease in white women. Am J Cardiol 1977; 39:858–864.

18. Talbott E, Kuller L H, Perper J, Murphy P A. Sudden unexpected death in women: biological and psychosocial origins. Am J Epidemiol 1981; 114: 671–682.

19. Ruberman W, Weinblatt E, Goldberg J D, Chaudhary B S. Psychosocial influences on mortality after myocardial infarction. N Eng J Med 1984; 311:552–559.

20. Rahe R H, Romo M, Bennett L, Stilanen P. Recent life changes, myocardial infarction, and abrupt coronary death. Arch Intern Med 1974; 133:221–228.

21. Jacobs S, Ostfeld A. An epidemiological review of the mortality of bereavement. Psychosom Med 1977; 39:344–357.

22. Bruhn J G, Paredes A, Adsett C A, Wolf S. Psychological predictors of sudden death in myocardial infarction. J Psychosom Res 1973; 18:187–191.

23. Deanfield J E, Shea M, Kensett M, et al. Silent myocardial ischaemia due to mental stress. Lancet 1984; 2:1001–1005.

24. Specchia G, de Servi S, Falcone C, et al. Mental arithmetic stress testing in patients with coronary artery disease. Am Heart J 1984; 108:56–63.

25. Rozanski A, Bairey C N, Krantz D S, et al. Mental stress and the induction of silent myocardial ischemia in patients with coronary artery disease. N Eng J Med 1988; 318:1005–1012.

26. Schiffer F, Hartley L H, Schulman C L, Abelmann W H. Evidence for emotionally-induced coronary arterial spasm in patients with angina pectoris. Br Heart J 1980; 44:62–65.

27. Levine S P, Towell B L, Suarez A M, Knieriem L K, Harris M. M, George J N. Platelet activation and secretion associated with emotional stress. Circulation 1985; 71:1129–1134.

28. Verrier R L, Hagestad E L, Lown B. Delayed myocardial ischemia induced by anger. Circulation 1987; 75:249–253.

29. Rabb W, Chaplin J P, Bajusz E. Myocardial necroses produced in domesticated rats and in wild rats by sensory and emotional stress. Proc Soc Exp Biol Med 1964; 116:665–669.
30. Johansson G, Jonsson L, Lannek N, Blomgren L, Lindberg P, Poupa O. Severe stress-cardiopathy in pigs. Am Heart J 1974; 87:451–457.
31. Rona G. Catecholamine cardiotoxicity. J Mol Cell Cardiol 1985; 17:291–306.
32. Own B, Verrier R L, Rabinowitz S T. Neural and psychologic mechanisms and the problem of sudden cardiac death. Am J Cardiol 1977; 39:890–902.
33. Skinner J E, Lie J T, Entman M L. Modification of ventricular fibrillation latency following coronary artery occlusion in the conscious pig. The effects of psychological stress and beta-adrenergic blockade. Circulation 1975; 51:656–667.
34. Stevenson I P, Duncan C H, Wolf S, Ripley H S, Wolff H G. Life situation, emotions, and extrasystoles. Psychosom Med 1949; 11:257–272.
35. Sigler L. Abnormalities in the electrocardiogram induced by emotional strain. Am J Cardiol 1961; 8:807–814.
36. Sigler L H. Emotion and athersclerotic heart disease. Br J Med Psychol 1967; 40:55–64.
37. Moss A J, Wynar B. Tachycardia in house officers presenting cases at grand rounds. Ann Intern Med 1970; 72:255–256.
38. Taggart P, Gibbons D, Somerville W. Some effects of motor-car driving on the normal and abnormal heart. Br Med J 1969; 4:130–134.
39. Taggart P, Carruthers M, Somerville W. Electrocardiogram, plasma catecholamines and lipids, and their modification by oxprenolol when speaking before an audience. Lancet 1973; 2:341–346.
40. Lown B, DeSilva R A, Lenson R. Roles of psychologic stress and autonomic nervous system changes in provocation of ventricular premature complexes. Am J Cardiol 1978; 41:979–985.
41. Orth-Gomer K, Edwards M E, Erhardt L, Sjogren A, Theorell T. Relation between ventricular arrhythmias and psychological profile. Acta Med Scand 1980; 207:31–36.
42. Katz C, Martin R D, Landa B, Chadda K D. Relationship of psychologic factors to frequent symptomatic ventricular arrhythmia. Am J Med 1985; 78:589–594.
43. Follick M J, Gorkin L, Capone R J, et al. Psychological distress as a predictor of ventricular arrhythmias in a post-myocardial infarction population. Am Heart J 1988; 116:32–36.
44. Harvey W P, Levine S A. Paroxysmal ventricular tachycardia due to emotion. JAMA 1952; 150:479–480.
45. Levine S A. Benign atrial fibrillation of forty years' duration with sudden death from emotion. Am Intern Med 1962; 58:681–684.
46. Lown B, Temte J V, Reich P, Gaughan C, Regestein Q, Hai H. Basis for recurring ventricular fibrillation in the absence of coronary heart disease and its management. N Engl J Med 1976; 294:623–629.

47. Vlay S C. Ventricular tachycardia/fibrillation on the first day of medical school. Am J Cardiol 1986; 57:483.
48. Brodsky M A, Sato D A, Iseri L T, Wolff L J, Allen B A. Ventricular tachyarrhythmia associated with psychological stress. JAMA 1987; 257: 2064–2067.
49. Moss A J, Schwartz P J, Crampton R S, Locati E, Carleen E. The long QT syndrome: a prospective international study. Circulation 1985; 71:17–21.
50. Wellens H J J, Vermeulen A, Durrer D. Ventricular fibrillation occurring on arousal from sleep by auditory stimuli. Circulation 1972; 46:661–665.
51. Baron R C, Thacker S B, Gorelkin L, Vernon A A, Taylor W R, Choi K. Sudden death among Southeast Asian refugees. JAMA 1983; 250:2947– 2951.
52. Otto C M, Tauxe R V, Cobb L A, et al. Ventricular fibrillation causes sudden death in Southeast Asian immigrants. Ann Intern Med 1984; 100: 45–47.
53. Kinzie J D, Fredrickson R H, Ben R, Fleck J, Karls W. Posttraumatic stress disorder among survivors of Cambodian concentration camps. Am J Psychiatry 1984; 141:645–650.
54. Tavazzi L, Zotti A M, Rondanelli R. The role of psychologic stress in the genesis of lethal arrhythmias in patients with coronary artery disease. Euro Heart J 1986; 7(Suppl A):99–106.
55. Richter C P. On the phenomenon of sudden death in animals and man. Psychosom Med 1957; 19:191–198.
56. Wolf S. The bradycardia of the dive reflex—a possible mechanism of sudden death. Condit Reflex 1967; 2:88–95.
57. Dimsdale J E, Moss J. Plasma catecholamines in stress and exercise. JAMA 1980; 243:340–342.
58. Morady F, Kou W H, Kadish A H, et al. Antagonism of quinidine's electro-physiologic effects by epinephrine in patients with ventricular tachycardia. J Am Coll Cardiol 1988; 12:388–394.
59. Topaz O, Castellanos A, Grobman L R, Myerburg R J. The role of arrhythmogenic auditory stimuli in sudden cardiac death. Am Heart J 1988; 116: 222–226.
60. Scott N A, DeSilva R A, Lown B, Wurtman R J. Tyrosine administration decreases vulnerability to ventricular fibrillation in the normal canine heart. Science 1981; 211:727–729.
61. Friedman M, Powell L H, Thoresen C E, et al. Effect of discontinuance of type A behavioral counseling on type A behavior and cardiac recurrence rate of post myocardial infarction. Am Heart J 1987; 114:483–490.
62. Ragland D R, Brand R J. Type A behavior and mortality from coronary heart disease. N Eng J Med 1988; 318:65–111.
63. Benson H, Alexander S, Feldman C L. Decreased premature ventricular contractions through use of the relaxation response in patients with stable ischaemic heart-disease. Lancet 1975; 2:380–382.
64. Wheatley D. Comparative effects of propranolol and chlordiazepoxide in anxiety states. Br J Psychiatry 1969; 115:1411–1412.

65. Mazzuero G, Galdangelo F, Zotti A M, Bertolotti G, Tavazzi L. Effects of propranolol, atenolol, and chlordesmethildiazepam on response to mental stress in patients with recent myocardial infarction. Clin Cardiol 1987; 10:293–302.

66. Goldstein D S, Dionne R, Sweet J, Gracely R, et al. Circulatory, plasma catecholamine, cortisol, lipid, and psychological responses to a real-life stress (third molar extractions): effects of diazepam sedation and of inclusion of epinephrine the local anesthetic. Psychosom Med 1985; 44:259–272.

67. Stratton J R, Halter J B. Effect of a benzodiazepine (alprazolam) on plasma epinephrine and norepinephrine levels during exercise stress. Am J Cardiol 1985; 56:136–139.

68. Lane R D, Schwartz G E. Induction of lateralized sympathetic input to the heart by the CNS during emotional arousal: a possible neurophysiologic trigger of sudden cardiac death. Psychosom Med 1987; 49:274–284.

69. Michelson E L. Canine models for ventricular tachyarrhythmia. Ann Intern Med 1981; 95:648–649.

70. Rowsell H C, Mustard J F, Downie H G. Experimental atherosclerosis in swine. Ann NY Acad Sci 1965; 127:743–762.

71. Factor S M, Sonnenblick E H. The pathogenesis of clinical and experimental congestive cardiomyopathies: recent concepts. Prog Cardiovasc Dis 1985; 31:395–420.

23

MENTAL STRESS AND THE INDUCTION OF MYOCARDIAL ISCHEMIA

Alan Rozanski

Cedars–Sinai Medical Center, University of California School of Medicine, Los Angeles, California

David S. Krantz

Uniformed Services University of the Health Sciences, Bethesda, Maryland

Jacob Klein

Cedars-Sinai Medical Center, University of California School of Medicine Los Angeles, California

John S. Gottdiener

University of Maryland School of Medicine, Baltimore, Maryland

To the lay person, mental stress is conceived of as both a risk factor for the development of coronary atherosclerosis and as a causal agent for acute cardiac events, such as myocardial infarction and sudden death. Much of the lay folklore and observations regarding mental stress and cardiac events have been reviewed by Engel and others (1,2). Despite such observations, scientific efforts attempting to prove causal links between mental stress and coronary artery disease have often been hindered by important methodological considerations. Recently, technical breakthroughs have provided investigators with new opportunities to assess the potential relationship between mental stress and coronary artery disease. These opportunities include the use of cardiac imaging techniques for laboratory investigation, ambulatory monitoring of the electrocardiogram and cardiac function, and methods of assessing dynamic coronary vascular changes during mental stress through the use of coronary angiography. Using such techniques, we and others have studied the relationship between mental stress and myocardial ischemia, which is an important functional marker of coronary artery disease. The rationale for our approach and the results of recent studies are reviewed in this chapter.

PRIOR STUDIES AND LIMITATIONS

Mental Stress as a Stimulus for Coronary Atherosclerosis

The Framingham study and other epidemiological investigations established four major coronary risk factors: family history, hypercholesterolemia, arterial hypertension, and smoking. Epidemiological investigations of biobehavioral mechanisms that may also contribute to coronary risk have examined social indicators (e.g., socioeconomic status), characteristics of the environment (e.g., occupational demands and social support), psychological factors (e.g., type A behavior, hostility), and psychophysiological reactivity to stress. The reader is referred to work by Krantz et al. (3), Matthews and Haynes (4), Ostfeld and Eaker (5), and chapters in this volume by Galosy and by Verrier for reviews of the broader human and animal literature on behavioral stress and coronary artery disease.

The potential role of psychological stress as a "risk factor" for coronary atherosclerosis is difficult to determine by relying solely on epidemiological methodology. This is because of the long time course over which coronary disease develops and difficulties in defining and quantitating stress. Epidemiological investigations in this area are also limited by their correlational nature and the presence of numerous confounding variables, including the fact that one or more of the major Framingham risk factors are often present among individuals being evaluated for psychological stress. Because they provide a high degree of experimental control, animal models designed to assess the direct effects of psychosocial stress on the state of the coronary vasculature may represent the most conclusive means of studying whether psychosocial stress is independently related to coronary atherosclerosis. Animal studies, such as those by Kaplan et al. (6), have demonstrated a strong association between psychosocial stress and the development of atherosclerosis under conditions in which diet is controlled.

It is now generally hypothesized that the initiating event in the atherosclerotic process involves injury to the endothelium of the coronary intima: the "response-to-injury" hypothesis of atherosclerosis (7,8). Defining the factors that result in injury to the endothelium is needed for an understanding of the potential causes of atherosclerosis. Many factors are now implicated in this process, including hyperlipidemia, altered rheological forces (e.g., as accompanies arterial hypertension), hormonal factors, and endothelial effects induced by other factors such as smoking and diabetes (7,8). For the reasons cited earlier, animal studies are needed to determine if and how neuroendocrine correlates of stress promote endothelial injury. Some research suggests that endothelial injury can be potentiated by the cardiovascular and neuroendocrine correlates of sympathetic nervous system or pituitary–adrenal–cortical activity associated with stress (9,10). The pathogenetic role of stress-related sympathetic nervous activity is suggested, indirectly, by a recent animal study, which showed that the beta-adrenergic blocking drug propranolol was able to ablate the atherogenic effects of psychosocial stress (11). The precise mechanism of this protective action (whether central or peripheral) still remains unclear. Work with animal models will continue to remain crucial to the development of a basic science understanding of the mechanisms by which psychosocial stress might injure the coronary endothelium. Furthermore, as the sensitive monitoring techniques described in this chapter are utilized in suitable animal models, it should become possible to further our understanding of the relationship between coronary arterial changes and resultant pathophysiological effects. For a further discussion of the role of stress in the pathogenesis of atherosclerosis, the reader is referred to work by Clarkson et al. (12). The remainder of this chapter will examine the pathophysiological effects of mental stress in humans under conditions of preexisting atherosclerosis.

Mental Stress and the Precipitation of Cardiac Events

Several epidemiological studies have suggested a relationship between mental stress and the occurrence of clinical cardiac events, such as myocardial infarction and cardiac death (13-15). When examined together, the published data in this area are contradictory, and the relative importance of stress as a precipitator of cardiac events remains unclear. Methodological limitations in this area of investigation are similar to those noted earlier: the multifactorial nature of coronary disease and difficulties in the definition and measurement of stress. Another problem with epidemiological research on coronary disease results from limitations associated with the use of conventional epidemiologic end points: "hard" cardiac events such as myocardial infarction and cardiac death. These cardiac events occur relatively infrequently in stable patients, so that a large population must be evaluated over a long period of time to reveal significant associations. Furthermore, patients who are identified at risk of infarction or death now commonly undergo coronary bypass surgery or coronary angioplasty. Such patients are then either excluded from follow-up studies (thus falsely lowering the potential event rate) or are included as having experienced cardiac "events" (thus overestimating the true event rate). This "intervention bias" is a potent factor in diminishing the overall frequency of observed cardiac events.

The decision to perform coronary bypass surgery or coronary angioplasty in patients with stable coronary artery disease is now often based, in large part, on the presence and magnitude of myocardial ischemia (16). Myocardial ischemia occurs transiently, whenever there is inadequate myocardial supply to meet myocardial oxygen demand. Its metabolic consequences include a temporary diminution in cardiac contraction, electrophysiological derangements, and the development of anginal chest pain. Even when coronary disease is advanced, however, myocardial ischemia may not be present under resting conditions. During physical stress, a period of heightened metabolic demand, myocardial ischemia may, however, be induced with high frequency in patients with angiographically significant coronary disease. Many studies have established the prognostic significance of exercise-induced myocardial ischemia (16), and cardiac events increase exponentially with an increase in the magnitude of myocardial ischemia (17). Thus, when myocardial ischemia is extensive, patients are at high risk for cardiac events, and aggressive intervention, such as coronary bypass surgery is warranted. Conversely, when exercise-induced ischemia is absent, patients with coronary artery disease are at low risk for cardiac events (16) and display comparable survival rate whether treated medically or surgically (18).

IMPORTANCE OF MYOCARDIAL ISCHEMIA AS A MEASURE FOR BIOBEHAVIORAL RESEARCH

Because myocardial ischemia is prognostically significant and is often the proximate indicator for surgical intervention, it represents a reasonable end point for assessing the efficacy of therapeutic behavioral interventions. For example, investigators recently used the magnitude of exercise-induced myocardial ischemia to assess the efficacy of a diet-exercise intervention program in patients with coronary disease (19). The practice of using myocardial ischemia as a biobehavioral end-point is likely to increase, for three reasons:

1. Myocardial ischemia is *easily measured*, by any of a variety of imaging and monitoring techniques. The various methods that may be used to assess myocardial ischemia are illustrated in Figure 1.

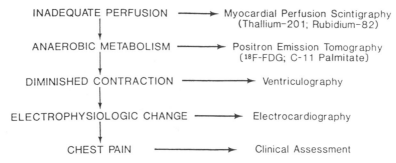

FIGURE 1 The consequences of inadequate perfusion, leading to myocardial ischemia, are listed on the left side. Inadequate perfusion and contractile abnormalities generally precede the onset of surface ECG changes; chest pain is generally a late and inconstant finding during myocardial ischemia. Noninvasive methods for assessing each aspect of the ischemic process now exist. These are listed on the right (from ref. 26, with permission).

2. Myocardial ischemia is *easily provoked*. With the use of sensitive techniques, it is now apparent that in patients with coronary artery disease, a variety of physiological stimuli including exercise, mental stress (20,21), cold stimulation (22), and smoking (23) can induce ischemia. The conventional clinical coronary disease end points (myocardial infarction, cardiac death, angina pectoris) do not share this feature. Unlike myocardial ischemia, angina pectoris is not easily provoked. It represents instead a late and inconstant correlate of ischemia. The absence of angina does not exclude the presence of myocardial ischemia during laboratory provocation, as is discussed in a later section. Thus, myocardial ischemia is the only functional marker of coronary artery disease that is readily studied in a controlled manner.
3. As noted earlier, myocardial ischemia is *highly relevant* to clinical assessment and treatment, based on its prognostic significance.

OBJECTIVE ASSESSMENT OF MYOCARDIAL ISCHEMIA

Until recently, studies of psychological stress and myocardial ischemia had to rely on reports of chest pain. In the absence of objective markers of myocardial ischemia, the development of angina was the only means of determining links between mental stress and ischemia. It has long been recognized that intense emotion can precipitate angina (24), but exercise is a far more frequent trigger of anginal pain. Based on this observation, there had been relatively little interest in exploring the potential relationship between mental stress and myocardial ischemia. Recently, however, a technology has been validated for performing an *objective* assessment of myocardial ischemic activity out of the hospital. Continued refinements in ambulatory electrocardiography have resulted in the ability to detect changes in the ST segment (used to assess myocardial ischemia). Until now, ambulatory (or Holter) electrocardiography has been used solely to assess the R waves (high-frequency component of the electrocardiogram) for analyses of cardiac arrhythmias in coronary patients. By contrast, the ST segment is a low-frequency signal that is not detectable by older Holter equipment. The occurrence of ST segment depression, which is a conventional marker of myocardial ischemia, is a reliable indicator of ischemia when ambulatory electrocardiography (ECG) is used in patients with a high likelihood of or documented coronary artery disease. This was demonstrated by work of Deanfield et al., who compared Holter ECG changes to changes in myocardial perfusion during positron emission tomographic imaging in coronary patients (22). However, caution should be applied to interpreting the results of ambulatory ECG in patients without a high likelihood of coronary disease, since many factors besides ischemia may cause depression of the ST segment (25,26). Using ambulatory electrocardiography for ST segment analysis, investigators have recently made a series of observations (see Table 1) that have provided important insights into myocardial ischemia.

    1. Most episodes of ST segment depression are "silent." Studies indicate that 75-90% of episodes of ST segment depression occur in the *absence* of chest pain in patients with coronary artery disease (26). These data serve to underscore the limitation of earlier field studies that relied on angina as a clinical end point for biobehavioral research.

    2. ST segment changes manifest a typical circadian tendency, with the greatest density of episodes occurring between 6 a.m. and 12 p.m. (27). This rhythm parallels that noted for myocardial infarction (28), heart rate (29,30), blood pressure (29,30), and catecholamine secretion (31,32). Rocco et al. have demonstrated that when the heart threshold for the development of ischemic ST segment depression is assessed for patients undergoing ambulatory ECG, patients are more likely to develop ischemia when their heart rate reaches this threshold in the morning hours than in the evening (27). It is not yet clear whether the circadian tendency of myocardial ischemia is an endogenous process (e.g., related to cortisol or other endogenous secretions), exogenously related to mental and physical activity levels, or both. Intrinsic morning surges in plasma catecholamine levels may result in increased heart rate, blood pressure, and cardiac contractility. Rising catecholamine levels might also increase the sensitivity of epicardial coronary vessels to vasoconstrictor stimuli (33) and promote a hypercoagulable state, by promoting platelet aggregability (34) and decreasing the function of the fibronolytic system (35,36). More work is needed to investigate these potentially important physiological processes in the circadian tendency of transient ischemia.

    4. There is a significant variability within a given patient regarding the heart rate threshold for the onset of ST segment depression. When patients who develop ST segment depression during exercise electrocardiography undergo ambulatory ECG, ST segment depression is noted at heart rates approximately

TABLE 1 Reported Observations of Myocardial Ischemia During Ambulatory ECG

Most ischemic episodes (i.e., episodes of ST depression) are "silent."
Ischemic episodes show a circadian tendency.
There is significant variability in the heart rate threshold for ischemia.
There is significant variability in the frequency of ischemia over time.
Ischemic episodes may occur during mental activity in the absence of strenuous exercise.
Transient ischemia during Holter monitoring signifies an increased risk of cardiac events.

---

25 beats/min lower than the exercise threshold (37–41). The reason for this lower threshold is not well understood.

5. There is also a significant variability over time (e.g., day to day, month to month) in the frequency of ST segment depression on ambulatory ECG (38,42). The reasons for this variability are also not presently well understood.

6. ST segment depression frequently occurs during nonexertional activities, including activities involving mental stress (43,44). For example, Barry et al. investigated the relationship between patients' perceived level of physical and mental activity with the occurrence of ST depression during daily life (43). When ischemic activity was normalized for the percentage of the day spent in a given state, there was an incremental increase in the likelihood of having ischemia when patients were engaged in "stressful" mental activity compared with "usual" mental activity. Freeman et al. further examined the relationship of life stress to transient ischemia in coronary disease patients during periods of uncertainty (i.e., following coronary angiography but prior to finding out the results of this diagnostic test), and subsequently, during a less stressful period when patients had the time to adjust to their diagnosis (44). In addition to ambulatory ECG monitoring and diary ratings of distress, measurements of urinary catecholamines were obtained. In this study, silent ischemia was significantly more frequent during the first stressful period than the second, less stressful period. Correspondingly, there was greater emotional upset and more urinary norepinephrine excretion during the first period. These data provide further evidence of an association between mental stress and myocardial ischemia. Furthermore, these data suggest that emotional states may account for some of the unexplained within-patient variability in the occurrence of transient ischemia over time.

7. The occurrence of ST-segment depression during ambulatory ECG has prognostic significance. This has been demonstrated by a number of recent studies, including studies in patients with stable coronary disease (45–47) and with unstable angina (48).

In revealing new insights concerning the characteristics of myocardial ischemia during daily life, these recent studies have also raised many pertinent questions about the pathophysiology of myocardial ischemia, especially as it relates to the potential role of mental stress in this process. In particular, the causes of ischemia during relatively low heart rate elevations and the surprising variability in the threshold for ischemic onset have raised questions regarding the relative role of "demand" factors (e.g., heart rate elevation) and "supply" factors (e.g., coronary vasospasm) in precipitating myocardial ischemia. Furthermore, the observation that ischemia sometimes occurs during periods of mental stress has furthered speculations of a causal link between mental stress and myocardial ischemia. Laboratory studies have addressed these issues.

LABORATORY INDUCTION OF MYOCARDIAL
ISCHEMIA DURING MENTAL STRESS

Initial studies involving the laboratory provocation of myocardial ischemia
during mental stress relied on ECG as a sole ischemic marker (49–53). The
results of these studies are summarized in Table 2. The observed frequency of
mental stress-induced ST segment depression varied widely, from 0% in two
studies (51,52) to 86% during a public speaking task in a small group of seven
coronary disease patients (49). Both the potency of the different stressors and
differences in the populations studied could have contributed to these differences. For instance, only 30% of the 20 patients studied by DeBusk et al. had
exercise-induced ST segment depression (51), whereas 75% of the 122 patients
studied by Specchia et al. had exercise-induced ST segment depression (53). In
recent years, with the advent of radionuclide imaging, it has become apparent
that ECG is a relatively insensitive index for the identification and quantification
of myocardial ischemia. For instance, during exercise testing, ischemic changes
can be detected in 80–90% of patients with angiographically significant coronary
disease when radionuclide stress testing is used (16). By comparison, the sensitivity of exercise ECG is only 60–65%. For this reason, investigators have
become interested in applying radionuclide imaging techniques to the study of
laboratory-induced mental stress.

Assessment by Radionuclide Ventriculography

Our interest in mental stress testing in patients with coronary artery disease was
twofold. First, in order to assess a causal relationship between mental stress and
ischemia, laboratory provocation of myocardial ischemia during mental stress
was necessary, since ambulatory findings linking mental stress to ST segment
depression represent only a correlational association. Second, we sought to use
the controlled laboratory situations to study the pathophysiology of myocardial
ischemia.

Radionuclide ventriculography is very well suited to the assessment of cardiac
function during mental stress. The equipment and material needed to perform
radionuclide ventriculography are illustrated in Figure 2. The technique involves
the injection of a small amount of radioactive agent (25 mc: technetium 99m)
labeled to red blood cells. Hence, all blood-pool-containing organs or structures
are labeled with technetium 99m and emit radioactivity, in proportion to their
blood volume. A scintillation camera captures the emitted radiation, and converts the emitted photons into photoelectric energy. If one places the scintillation camera over the chest, the blood-pool-containing structures of the heart can
be imaged, including the right and left atrium and both ventricules. Since the
heart is a dynamic organ, static images would provide useless information on
cardiac function. It is necessary instead to assess cardiac function in dynamic

TABLE 2 Electrocardiographic Studies Examining Effects of Laboratory-Induced Mental Stress

Reference	Subjects	Procedure	Major findings
49	7 CAD patients	Public speaking task. Double-blind technique of giving either placebo or 40 mg oxyprenolol on two different occasions	ST depression either appeared or worsened in six subjects during public speaking while on placebo, but not on oxyprenolol
50	24 patients with angina, 19 controls	BP and ECG measurements during rest, exercise, and an IQ quiz. Patients were taken off cardiovascular medications for 72 h	No controls had ST depression ⩾1mm. Seven of 24 patients had ST depression ⩾1.0mm. Ischemia during IQ quiz occurred at lower rate of pressure products than during exercise
51	20 patients 3–7 weeks after acute myocardial infarction	Patients underwent an exercise test and three psychological stressors: open-ended interview, videotape of stressful scenes, and difficult, time-pressured puzzle.	30% of patients displayed ischemic abnormalities during exercise
52	11 CAD patients	Harrassing mental arithmetic test. Aortic BP, thermodilution coronary sinus flow, BP, ECG	No ST segment changes occurred during mental arithmetic stressor, despite a 40% increase in consumption and coronary sinus blood flow
53	122 patients undergoing diagnostic coronary angiography	Mental arithmetic stress test and exercise testing. BP and ECG measurements	Of 90 patients with a positive exercise ECG, 22 (24%) showed mental stress-induced ST abnormalities. Eight had angina during mental stress. Thirty showed negative results on both exercise and mental stress tests

SCINTIGRAPHIC DATA

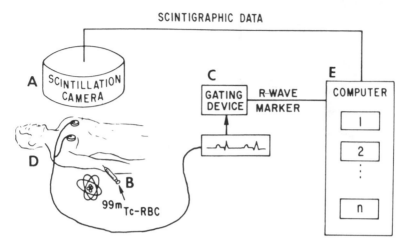

FIGURE 2 The material and equipment needed to perform multiple gated equilibrium blood pool ventriculography are listed schematically. These include a scintillation camera (A), radiopharmaceutical used to tag the red blood cells (B), and a gating device (C), which synchronizes events from the R wave of the ECG, recorded from electrodes (D). A computer (E) records the scintographic data and anlayzes it (reprinted by permission from Berman DS. Clinical nuclear cardiology, Chapter 4, Grune & Stratton, Inc.).

mode. This is made possible by using a "gating device"—a physiological synchronizer—that times the recording of radioactivity to physiological events. The R wave of the ECG, which corresponds to end-diastole, is used to trigger the gating device. The cardiac cycle is then divided into 20 equal frames, so that the amount and location of emitted radiation is recorded for each 1/20th of the cycle. Since there are not sufficient counts in one heart cycle to obtain accurate counting statistics, information over sequential heart beats are summed until sufficient counts per frame are available (approximately 100,000 counts/frame). It requires approximately 2 min to obtain sufficient counts; hence, radionuclide images using the gated equilibrium technique are collected over a minimum of 2 min.

Two principal variables are assessed by radionuclide ventriculography: segmental wall motion and global left ventricular ejections fraction. To assess segmental wall motion, sequential frames are placed into a flicker-free continuous cineloop, with the images viewed on the computer's video display. The ventricle is usually divided into five segments, as shown in Figure 3, with each segment scored using a five-point system, as illustrated. The ejections fraction, which is the percentage of the cardiac blood volume that is ejected with each heart beat, can be calculated readily using radionuclide ventriculography, since the counts emanating from the left ventricle during radionuclide ventriculo-graphy are proportional to the blood volume. By determining the counts ejected with each heart beat (end-diastolic counts minus end-diastolic counts), and expressing this as a percentage of the end-diastolic counts, the ejection fraction can be determined.

Radionuclide ventricolography has been used to assess cardiac function during exercise in patients with coronary artery disease since the late 1970s. Ischemic effects include the development of segmental wall motion abnor-malities during exercise and the development of a fall in the measured ejection fraction. In normal persons, segmental wall motion remains normal or becomes hypercontractile during exercise and the ejection fraction typically rises.

For our research, we selected four qualitatively different mental tasks: mental arithmetic, the Stroop color–word task, a personally relevant speaking task, and a reading task. The first two tasks were selected as cognitive stressors, designed to elicit both mental arousal and an element of frustration. For the speaking stressor, patients were asked to talk about personal faults or undesirable habits in front of two observers for 5 min. This task was designed to be both emotion-ally arousing and personally relevant. Following this, patients were asked to read from a prose passage, to assess whether nonemotional speech per se could pro-duce ischemic effects.

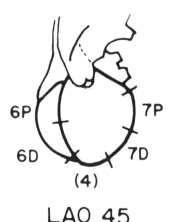

LAO 45

FIGURE 3 Schematic representation of the division of a radionuclide scinti-gram of the left ventricle (LV) in the 45° left anterior oblique view. For scoring purposes, the LV is divided into five segments: upper septum (6P), distal septum (6D) inferoapex (4), distal posterolateral wall (7D), and proximal posterolateral wall (7P). For each segment, the LV is scored on a five-point scale: 3 = normal, 2 = mild hypokinesis, 1 = hypokinesis, 0 = akinesis, and –1 = dyskinesis.

We evaluated 39 patients with a high likelihood of or known coronary artery disease and 12 normal persons during our protocol to compare the effects of mental stress and exercise during radionuclide ventriculography (20). Among the 29 patients with exercise-induced wall motion abnormalities, 21 (72%) experienced the induction of wall motion abnormalities during one or more mental tasks as well (see still frame example in Fig. 4). Wall motion abnormalities also occurred in 2 (20%) of the 10 patients who failed to exercise to 85% of maximal predicted heart rate. Abnormalities in the normal patients were rare. One normal patient had an abnormal response to exercise and one had an abnormal response during mental stress testing.

Most of the wall motion abnormalities induced by mental stress occurred "silently": only 4 (17%) of the 23 patients with mental stress-induced wall motion abnormalities developed concomitant chest pain. Wall motion abnormalities during mental stress occurred at relatively low heart elevations compared to exercise testing. Both of these aspects of mental stress-induced ischemia simulate the characteristics of ischemia noted during ambulatory ECG.

Electrocardiography was a relatively insensitive tool for assessing the effects of myocardial ischemia in our study (Fig. 5), which was not dissimilar from the frequency noted by Specchia et al. in their large study of 122 patients during mental stress testing. These data underscore the need to use a sensitive index to assess myocardial ischemia induced by mental stress. The relative insensitivity of electrocardiography would appear to relate to the transmission of the electrical signal across the chest wall. When surface ECG changes are compared to either

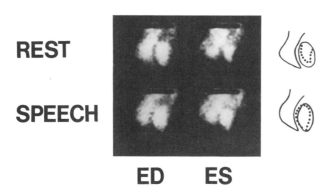

FIGURE 4 Still frame example of mental stress-induced wall motion abnormality. For rest (top) and speech (bottom), the end-diastolic (ED) are on the left, end-systolic (ES) images in the middle, and superimposed edges are on the right. This patient developed frank septal dyskinesis while discussing a topic of personal stress (from ref. 20, with permission).

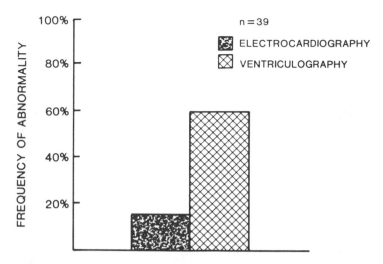

FIGURE 5 Frequency (vertical axis) of abnormality for ECG monitoring and radionuclide ventriculographic imaging in 39 patients undergoing mental stress testing. In contrast to the high frequency of abnormality during radionuclide ventriculography, the frequency of abnormality during ECG monitoring was low.

intracoronary ECG or endocardial electrograms, it is evident from investigations (54,55) that the latter methods detect significantly more ischemic abnormalities, and earlier, than does surface ECG.

Our results also revealed significant differences in ischemic-producing potency among the various mental tasks. The personally relevant speaking task was more potent than the other mental tasks in inducing wall motion abnormalities, and the magnitude of induced abnormality was also greater (Fig. 6). Other ischemic indices, including the induction of chest pain and ECG change, were also more common during the speech task (Fig. 7). These data suggest that personally relevant mental stress may be more potent than nonspecific mental arousal in inducing myocardial ischemia. In individual patients, however, cognitive tasks such as math may also be emotionally stressful. Further work is needed to assess the nature of psychophysiological determinants of ischemia during mental stress.

Assessment by Other Imaging Modalities

A number of other imaging or monitoring modalities besides radionuclide ventriculography are well suited for assessing the pathophysiological effects of mental stress (Table 3). Each of these techniques has already been applied by one or more investigators and is reviewed below.

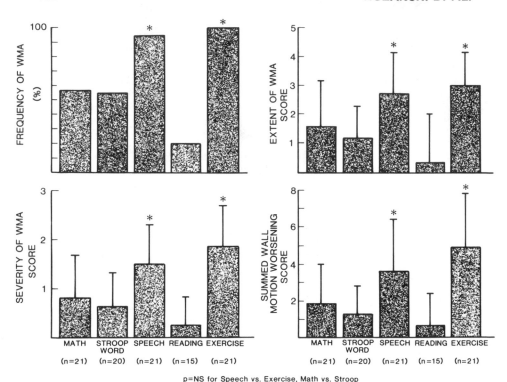

FIGURE 6 Comparative responses to four mental tasks and exercise in 21 CAD patients who demonstrated wall motion worsening (WMA) during one or more mental tasks and during exercise. The top left graph demonstrates the frequency of WMA during each of the four mental tasks and exercise. The top right graph represents the score for the extent of WMA (i.e., the number of segments, out of five potential segments, that showed worsening) under stress. The bottom left graph demonstrates the change in score (on a five-point scale) for the segment demonstrating the greatest degree of wall motion worsening. The bottom right graph represents the summed wall motion worsening score, equal to the difference in the scores for wall motion in the five segments at rest and during stress. Each bar represents the mean +/- S.D. The wall motion scores induced by speech were more frequent, extensive, and severe than those induced by the other mental tasks, and comparable in magnitude to those induced by exercise (from ref. 20, with permission).

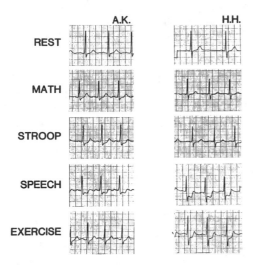

FIGURE 7 Strips from ECG studies recorded during mental tasks and exercise in two patients. Patient A.K. demonstrated 2 mm of downsloping ST segment depression during public speech, but not during other mental tasks. There was no ST segment depression during exercise, despite a slightly higher heart rate than during the speech task. Patient H.H. demonstrated an ischemic electrocardiographic response during public speech (3 mm of downsloping ST segment depression) but no significant change during the other mental tasks.

Positron Emission Tomography

This technique involves the use of short-lived radiotracers that decay by the emission of positrons, which are antielectrons. When combined with an electron, the masses of the electron and positron annihilate to form 511 KeV photons that are emitted simultaneously 180 degrees apart. These photons easily penetrate the bodily tissues and are recorded by external radiation detectors. When a circumferential array of detectors is used, radionuclide data can be recorded simultaneously from different angles around a cross-section of the body. This technique can be used to assess myocardial perfusion, glucose metabolism, free fatty metabolism, and other metabolic processes. Myocardial perfusion is commonly assessed using rubidium 82, which has a short physical half-life of only 78 s. Thus, this radionuclide can be used to assess myocardial perfusion at rest and during sequential interventions. Deanfield et al. used this radiotracer to assess the comparative effects of mental stress and exercise in patients with coronary artery disease, positive exercise tests, and typical angina (21). Of 16 patients all of whom developed perfusion abnormalities and ST segment depression with exercise, 12 (75%) also developed transient perfusion defects during

TABLE 3   Techniques for Assessing Myocardial Ischemia During Mental Stress

Laboratory techniques	Ambulatory technique
Radionuclide ventriculography	Ambulatory ECG
Positron emisson tomography	Ambulatory ventricular function
Echocardiography	monitor (VEST)
Stationary radionuclide probe	
Ambulatory ventricular function	
monitor (VEST)	
ECG	

mental stress, in correspondence to the defect elicited with exercise. By comparison, ECG abnormalities were only half as common.

Echocardiography

This commonly used technique uses ultrasound to delineate cardiac structures and assess cardiac wall motion. While conventionally used at rest, it has also been used during mental stress testing by Gottdiener et al. (56), who assessed cardiac wall motion at rest and during mental stress and exercise in 14 patients with coronary artery disease (CAD) and in 6 normal individuals. The preliminary results from this ECG study are similar to those previously cited using radionuclide ventriculography. Among the 11 patients with exercise-induced wall motion abnormalities, 8 (73%) also developed wall motion abnormalities during mental stress testing. None of the three CAD patients without exercise-induced abnormalities and none of the normal patients developed wall motion abnormalities during mental stress. Again, mental stress-induced abnormalities occurred at relatively low heart elevations compared to exercise, were typically silent, and not accompanied by ECG abnormalities.

Radionuclide Probe

This modification of the equilibrium blood pool imaging technique relies on a specially collimated nonimaging nuclear probe and dedicated microprocessor. It is used only for assessing left ventricular ejection fraction, but does not assess wall motion. The nuclear probe is 2 inches in diameter with a ½ inch thick crystal and converging collimator. The recorded scintillation data and ECG are input simultaneously and sampled at 10 ms intervals by the microprocessor. Averaged data may be sampled for ejection fraction intervals at intervals as short as 8 s. LaVeau et al. recently used this technique to assess the time course of ejection fraction changes during mental stress in patients with coronary disease (57). The study revealed that reductions in ejection fraction occur rapidly during mental stress in patients with coronary disease, tend to be sustained during the mental stress period, and rebound quickly following stress (57). These data emphasize the importance of maintaining a high level of mental stress throughout the imaging period. Reductions in ejection fraction were not observed during mental stress in their normal population. As in prior studies, the observations of LaVeau et al. confirmed the generally silent nature of mental stress-induced ischemia.

Ambulatory Ventricular Function Monitor

An ambulatory version of the radionuclide probe has been developed. This ambulatory ventricular function monitor (VEST, Capintec Inc.) contains a small radionuclide detector, which is positioned over the left ventricle under direct gamma camera supervision. It is immobilized against the chest wall by using a tight-fitting garment. Like the stationary probe, the VEST permits beat-to-beat analysis of left ventricular ejections fraction (Fig. 8). Data 30 s in duration are usually summed continuously and expressed on a trend plot as a function of time, as shown in Figure 9. Changes in heart rate, systolic volume, and diastolic

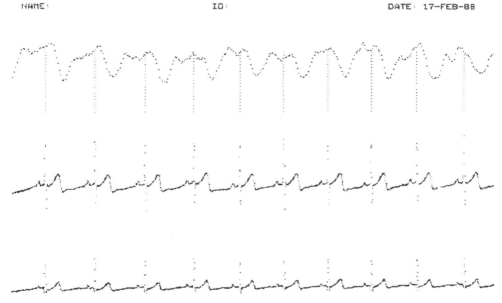

FIGURE 8 The top graph illustrates the best-by-beat time–activity curves obtained using the ambulatory left ventricular function monitor. The vertical dotted line represents end diastole, corresponding to the R wave of the ECG. The bottom two graphs represent the corresponding ECG tracings from a precordial and inferior lead positions.

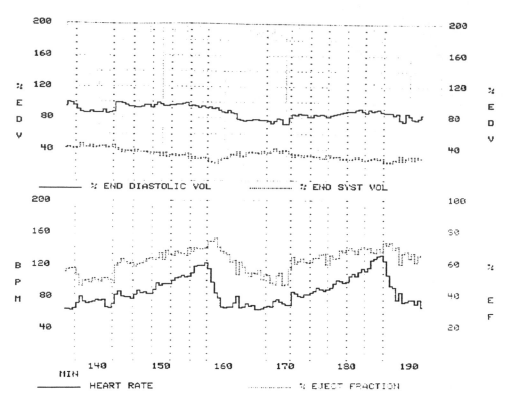

FIGURE 9 Trend plots as a function of time (on bottom horizontal axis from
<140 to 190 min). For the top graph, the solid line represents the trend in
end-diastolic volume and the dotted line represents the end-systolic volume
trend. The volume change (%) is indicated on the vertical axis. For the bottom
graph, heart rate (HR) trend is represented by the solid line and ejection fraction
trend on the dotted line. The vertical axis on the left indicates HR in beats/min
(BPM); the axis on the right represents ejection fraction (0–100%). As the subject began exercising (at approximately 140 and 170 min into the study), the
heart rate increased, to approximately 120 BPM. In both instances, the ejection
fraction rose substantially, which is a typically normal response.

volume are expressed simultaneously. Breisblatt et al. recently assessed changes in ejection fraction during mental stress and exercise in patients with coronary artery disease (58). As in the prior studies, falls in ejection fraction (of 5% or more) occurred commonly in patients with exercise-induced falls in ejection fraction (present in 12 [55%] of 22 patients), but not in those without exercise-induced falls (present in only 1 [8%] of 13 patients).

Cinecoronary Angiography During Mental Stress

Cardiac imaging modalities can evaluate the end result of myocardial ischemia during mental stress. Another question concerns the underlying coronary arterial pathophysiology responsible for permiting the induction of mental stress-induced ischemia. Coronary arteries normally dilate to physiological stimuli such as exercise or mental stress. Research suggests, however, that the coronary vasculature is capable of paradoxical vasoconstriction during physiological stimulation in patients with underlying coronary artery disease (59,60). In a preliminary study, Rebecca et al. performed serial coronary angiography, at rest and during the performance of mental arithmetic, in patients with coronary artery disease (61). This work indicated that the coronary vessels may paradoxically vasoconstrict during mental stress, in association with underlying atheroma. These data lend support to the hypothesis that the occurrence of myocardial ischemia during mental stress involves, in part, a primary reduction in myocardial oxygen supply.

Mental Stress and Cardiac Arrhythmias

As with ischemia, research indicates that laboratory-induced mental stress can increase both the frequency and severity of cardiac arrhythmias (62–65). Animal model studies linking psychological stress to the pathogenesis of cardiac arrhythmias are reviewed by Verrier in this volume. In human studies, psychological stress, but not manipulations of peripheral autonomic reflexes by maneuvers such as hyperventilation or tilting, can provoke increases in ventricular premature beats in predisposed patients with myocardial electrical instabilities (66). Other research suggests that mental stress may trigger life-threatening arrhythmias in patients with coronary artery disease. The occurrence of ventricular ectopy is often not clinically important in patients without underlying heart disease. The combined presence of arrhythmias and ischemia, however, is considered particularly troublesome, since ischemia per se results in a transient lowering of the ventricular fibrillatory threshold. More work is needed to examine the interrelationship between cardiac arrhythmias, myocardial ischemia, and mental stress during daily life activity.

DETERMINATION OF THE PATHOPHYSIOLOGY OF MYOCARDIAL ISCHEMIA: INTEGRATION OF RECENT STUDIES

The reports of ischemia occurring with relatively low heart rate elevations during ambulatory monitoring has fueled speculation regarding the potential importance of coronary vasospasm as opposed to an increase in myocardial oxygen demand as an inciting cause of ischemia. Our laboratory studies, however, indicate a substantial increase in systolic and diastolic blood pressure during laboratory-provoked mental stress. Thus, the increase in myocardial oxygen demand during nonphysical stress may be higher than that indicated by the elevation in heart rate changes alone. In our previously described study (20), diastolic blood pressure elevations were larger during mental than physical stress, and systolic blood pressure elevations were comparable. Furthermore, mental stress causes catecholamine secretion (67), which may have a direct effect on cardiac contractility. Other "demand" factors may include changes in cardiac volume and the rate of onset of mental and physical stress. Several studies suggest that the effects of "sudden" physical stress may be different from that of gradual physical stress (68–70), but the relevance of this potential variable relative to mental and physical stress testing has not yet been evaluated.

A growing body of knowledge may help to explain the phenomenon of coronary vasoconstriction during mental stress in patients with coronary artery disease. Healthy coronary endothelium contains endogenous "endothelium-derived relaxant factors" (EDRF), which cause the coronary vessel to vasodilate during physiological stimulation such as exercise or cold stimulation. Furchgott et al. were the first researchers to identify a paradoxical and abnormal vasoconstriction of the coronary artery after induced coronary endothelial injury (58). It is now recognized that as part of the coronary atheromatous process the endothelium overlying the atheromata becomes dysfunctional and loses the ability to release EDRF. When they cannot interact with EDRF, "endothelial-dependent" vasodilators, such as acetylcholine, can cause paradoxical coronary vascoconstriction. Endothelial dysfunction can now be identified indirectly in humans. If acetylcholine is applied during serial angiography in humans, coronary vasodilation will be elicited in smooth coronary arteries and paradoxic vasoconstriction will be elicited in zones containing atheromata (60). Abnormal coronary vasoconstriction occurs during such physiological stimuli as exercise (71), cold pressor stimulation (72), and mental stress (61) in humans. The response parallels that obtained with acetylcholine in the same patients.

Thus, based on the aforementioned data, it is now possible to postulate how "demand" and "supply" factors might interrelate with neurohumoral stimulation to cause myocardial ischemia during mental stress. At the initiation of mental stress, catecholamine stimulation leads to increased myocardial oxygen demand by causing increases in heart rate, blood pressure, cardiac contractility, and cardiac volume (increased venous return). Simultaneously, neurohumoral stimulation leads to coronary vasoconstriction and a primary reduction in myocardial supply. Much more work is needed to better define the exact role of neurohumoral factors in the pathogenesis of ischemia.

FUTURE DIRECTIONS

The aforementioned technological and methodological advances have enabled investigators to further our understanding of the pathophysiology of mental stress-induced ischemia and to begin to characterize the frequency of this phenomenon. More work is needed to characterize the frequency of transient ischemia during ambulatory ECG monitoring. "Lab–field" correspondence studies are required to determine whether the occurrence of silent ischemia on Holter monitoring predicts the induction of ischemia during laboratory-induced mental stress or vice versa. The circadian variation in myocardial ischemia requires investigation and the factors governing the variability in frequency of ischemic episodes need to be delineated. The prognostic significance of silent ischemia is now becoming evident (45–48), but determination of the clinical importance, if any, of mental stress-induced ischemia requires the follow-up of patients being identified in current investigations. Furthermore, more studies on the pathophysiology of ischemia during mental stress need to be performed. An important issue is the identification of means by which stress-related factors (e.g., catecholamines) interact with the complex cell biology of atherosclerosis (e.g., coronary receptors). Exploration of this latter issue may require interplay between human and animal studies. The ultimate goal of these investigations should be a basic science explanation for the means by which mental stress aggravates the cell biology of atherosclerosis and induces myocardial ischemia in patients with underlying coronary artery disease.

ACKNOWLEDGMENT

This work was supported in part by a research grant from the John D. and Catherine T. MacArthur Foundation, the KROC Foundation, NIH SCOR grant 17561, and USUHS grant R07233.

REFERENCES

1. Engel GL. Sudden and rapid death during psychological stress. Folklore or folk wisdom? Ann Intern Med 1971;74:771–782.
2. Dimsdale JE. Emotional causes of sudden death. Am J Psychiatry 1977; 134:1361–1366.

3. Krantz DS, Contrada RJ, Hill DR, Friedler E. Environmental stress and bio-behavioral antecedents of coronary heart disease. J Consult Clin Psychol 1988; 56:333-341.
4. Matthews KA, Haynes SG. Type A behavior pattern and coronary disease risk: update and control evaluation. Am J Epidemiol 1986; 123:923-960.
5. Ostfeld A, Eaker E. (eds). Measuring psychosocial variable in epidemiologic studies of cardiovascular disease. NIH Pub. No. 85-2270, Bethesda, MD: NIH.
6. Kaplan JR, Manuck SB, Clarkson TB, Lusso FM, Taub DM, Miller EW. Social stress and atherosclerosis in normocholesterolemic monkeys. Science 1983; 220:733-735.
7. Ross R, Glomset J. Atherosclerosis and the arterial smooth muscle cell. Science 1973; 180-1332.
8. Ross R, Glomset JA. The pathogenesis of atherosclerosis. N Engl J Med 1976; 295:369-377.
9. Manuck SB, Henry JP, Anderson DE, et al. Task force 4: biobehavioral mechanisms in coronary artery disease. Circulation 1987; 76 (Suppl. I): I158-I163.
10. Abboud FM. Effects of sodium, angiotension, and steroids on vascular reactivity in man. Fed Proc 1974; 33:143-149.
11. Kaplan JR, Manuck SB, Adams MR, Weingand KW, Clarkson TB. Propranolol inhibits coronary atherosclerosis in behaviorally predisposed monkeys fed on atherogenic diet. Circulation 1987; 76: 1364-1372.
12. Clarkson T, Clarkson B, Weingand KW, Kaplan JR, Adams MR. Mechanisms of atherogenesis. Circulation 1987; 76: Suppl II 120-128.
13. Greene WA, Goldstein SS, Moss AJ. Psychological aspects of sudden death: a preliminary report. Arch Intern Med 1972; 129:725-731.
14. Rahe RH, Romo M, Bennett L, Stilanen P. Recent life changes, myocardial infarction, and abrupt coronary death: sudden studies in Helsinki. Arch Intern Med 1974; 132:221-228.
15. Myers A, Dewar HA. Circumstances attending 100 sudden deaths from coronary artery disease with coroners' necropsies. Br Heart J 1975; 37: 133-143.
16. Rozanski A, Berman DS. The efficacy of cardiovascular nuclear medcine exercise studies. Semin Nucl Med 1987; 17:104-120.
17. Ladenheim ML, Pollack BH, Rozanski A, et al. Extent and severity of myo-cardial hypoperfusion as orthogonal indices of prognosis in patients with suspected coronary artery disease. J Am Coll Cardiol 1986; 7:464-471.
18. Jones RH, Floyd RD, Austin EH, Sabiston DC. The role of radionuclide angiocardiography in the preoperative prediction of pain relief and pro-longed survival following coronary artery bypass grafting. Ann Surg 1983; 197:743-754.
19. Schuler G, Schlierf G, Wirth A, et al. Low-fat diet and regular supervised physical exercise in patients with symptomatic coronary artery disease: reduction of stress-induced myocardial ischemia. Circulation 1988; 77: 172-181.

20. Rozanski A, Bairey CN, Krantz DS, et al. Mental stress and the induction of silent myocardial ischemia in patients with coronary artery disease. N Engl J Med 1988; 318:1005–1012.

21. Deanfield JE, Kensett M, Wilson RA, et al. Silent myocardial ischemia due to mental stress. Lancet 1984; 2:1001–1004.

22. Deanfield JE, Shea M, Ribiero P, et al. Transient ST-segment depression as a marker of myocardial ischemia during daily life. Am J Cardiol 1984; 54: 1195–1200.

23. Deanfield JE, Shea MJ, Wilson RA, Horlock P, de Landsheere CM, Selwyn AP. Direct effects of smoking on the heart: silent ischemic disturbances of coronary flow. Am J Cardiol 1986; 57:1005–1009.

24. Williams J, Edwards G. John Hunter's last pupil. Ann R Coll Surg Engl 1968; 42:69–70.

25. Berman DS, Rozanski A, Knoebel SB. The detection of silent ischemia: cautions and precautions. Circulation 1987; 75:101–105.

26. Rozanski A, Berman DS. Silent myocardial ischemia. I. Pathophysiology, frequency of occurrence, and approaches toward detection. Am Heart J 1987; 114:615–626.

27. Rocco MB, Barry J, Campbell S, et al. Circadian variation of transient myocardial ischemia in patients with coronary artery disease. Circulation 1987; 75:395–400.

28. Muller JE, Stone PH, Turi ZG, et al. Circadian variation in the frequency of onset of acute myocardial infarction. N Engl J Med 1985; 313:1315–1322.

29. Millar-Craig MW, Bishop CN, Raftery EB. Circadian variation of blood pressure. Lancet 1978; 1:795–797.

30. Floras JS, Jones JV, Johnston JA, Brooks DE, Hassan MO, Sleight P. Arousal and the circadian rhythm of blood pressure. Clin Sci Mol Med 1978; 55:395s–397s.

31. Weitzman E, Fukushima D, Nogeire C, Roffwarg H, Gallagher TF, Hellman L. Twenty-four hour pattern of the episodic secretion of cortisol in normal subjects. J Clin Endocrinol Metab 1971;33:14–22.

32. Turon MB, Deegan T. Circadian variations of plasma catecholamine, cortisol and immunoreactive insulin concentration in supine subjects. Clin Chim Acta 1974;55:389–397.

33. Rocco MB, Nabel EG, Selwyn AP. Circadian rhythms and coronary artery disease. Am J Cardiol 1987; 59:13C–17C.

34. Tofler GH, Czeisler CA, Rutherford J, Williams GH, Muller JE. Increased platelet aggregability after arising from sleep (abstr). J Am Coll Cardiol 1986;7(suppl A):116A.

35. Rosing DR, Brakman P, Redwood DR, et al. Blood fibrinolytic activity in man. Diurnal variation and the response to varying intensities of exercise. Circ Res 1970; 27:171–184.

36. Petralito A, Maniafico RA, Gibino S, Cuffari MA, Miano MF, Fiore CE. Daily modifications of plasma fibrinogen platelets aggregation. Howell's time, PTT, TT and antithrombin III in normal subjects and in patients with vascular disease. Chronobiologia 1982;9:195–201.

37. Schang SJ Jr, Pepine CJ. Transient asymptomatic ST segment depression during activity. Am J Cardiol 1977;39:396–402.
38. Deanfield JE, Selwyn AP, Chierchia S, et al. Myocardial ischemia during daily life in patients with stable angina: its relation to symptoms and heart rate changes. Lancet 1983;2:753–758.
39. Cecchi AC, Dovellini EV, Marchi F, Pucci P, Santoro GM, Fazzini PF. Silent myocardial ischemia during ambulatory electrocardiographic monitoring in patients with effort angina. J Am Coll Cardiol 1983:1934–1993.
40. Quyyumi AA, Mockus L, Wright C, Fox KM. Morphology of ambulatory ST-segment changes in patients with varying severity of coronary artery disease investigation of the frequency of nocturnal ischemia and coronary spasm. Br Heart J 1985:53;186–191.
41. Carboni GP, Celli P, D'Ermo M, Santoboni A, Zanchi F. Combined cardiac cinefluoroscopy, exercise testing and ambulatory ST-segment monitoring in the diagnosis of coronary artery disease: a report of 104 symptomatic patients. Int J Cardiol 1985;9:91–101.
42. Nabel EG, Barry J, Rocco MB, et al. Variability of transient myocardial ischemia in ambulatory patients with coronary artery disease. Circulation 1988;78:60–67.
43. Barry J, Selwyn AP, Nabel EG, et al. Frequency of ST-segment depression produced by mental stress in stable angina pectoris from coronary disease. Am J Cardiol 1988;61:979–983.
44. Freeman LJ, Nixon PG, Sallabank P, Reaveley D. Psychological stress and silent myocardial ischemia. Am Heart J 1987; 114:447–482.
45. Tzivoni D, Gavish A, Zin D, et al. Prognosis significance of ischemic episodes in patients with previous myocardial infarction. Am J Cardiol 1988; 62:661–664.
46. Tzivoni D, Weisz G, Ganish A, Zin D, Keren A, Stern S. Comparison of mortality and myocardial infarction rates in stable angina pectoris with and without ischemic episodes during daily activities. Am J Cardiol 1989; 63: 273–276.
47. Rocco MB, Nabel EG, Campbell S, et al. Prognostic importance of myocardial ischemia detected by ambulatory monitoring in patients with stable coronary artery disease. Circulation 1988; 78:877–884.
48. Gottlieb SO, Weisfeldt ML, Duyang P, Mellits ED, Gerstenblith G. Silent ischemia as a marker for early unfavorable outcomes in patients with unstable angina. N Engl J Med 1986;314:1214–1219.
49. Taggart P, Caruthers M, Somerville W. Electrocardiogram plasma catecholamines and lipids and their modification by oxyprenolol when speaking before an audience. Lancet 1973;2:341–346.
50. Schiffer F, Hartley LH, Schulman CL, Abelmann WH. The quiz electrocardiogram: a new diagnostic and research technique for evaluating the relation between emotional stress and ischemic heart disease. Am J Cardiol 1976;37:41–47.
51. DeBusk RF, Taylor CB, Agras WS. Comparison of treadmill exercise testing and psychologic stress testing soon after myocardial infarction. Am J Cardiol 1979;43:907–912.

52. Bassan MB, Marcus HS, Ganz W. The effect of mild-to-moderate mental stress on coronary hemodynamics in patients with coronary artery disease. Circulation 1980; 62:933-935.
53. Specchia G, dc Servi S. Falcone C, et al. Mental arithmetic stress testing in patients with coronary artery disease. Am Heart J 1984;108:56-63.
54. Friedman PL, Shook T, Kirschenbaum JM, Selwyn AP, Ganz P. Value of the intracoronary electrocardiogram to monitor ischemia during percutaneous coronary angioplasty. Circulation 1986;74:330-339.
55. Nabel EG, Shook TL, Meyerovitz M, Ganz P, Selwyn AP, Friedman PL. Detection of pacing-induced myocardial ischemia by endocardial electrograms recorded during cardiac catheterization. J Am Coll Cardiol 1988;11: 938-992.
56. Gottdiener JS, Krantz DS, McGee A, et al. Echocardiographic assessment of mental stress induced wall motion abnormalities (abstr). J Am Coll Cardiol 1989;
57. LaVeau P, Rozanski A, Krantz DS, et al. Ischemic left ventricular performance during provocative mental stress testing. Am Heart J, in press
58. Breisblatt LUM, Weiland FL, McLain JR, Tomlinson GC, Burns MJ, Spaccavento LJ. Usefulness of ambulatory radionuclide monitoring of left ventricular function early after acute myocardial infarction after predicting residual myocardial ischemia. Am J Cardiol 1988;62:1005-1010.
59. Furchgott RF, Zawadzki JV. The obligatory role of endothelial cells in the relaxation of arterial smooth muscle by acetylcholine. Nature 1980;288: 373-376.
60. Ludmer PL, Selwyn AP, Shook TL, et al. Paradoxical vasoconstriction induced by acetylcholine in atherosclerotic coronary arteries. N Engl J Med 1986;315:1046-1051.
61. Rebecca G, Wagner R, Zebede T, et al. Pathogenetic mechanisms causing transient myocardial ischemia with mental arousal in patients with coronary artery disease (abstr). Clin Res 1986; 34:338A.
62. Stevenson JP, Duncan CII, Wolf S, Ripley HS, Wolff HG. Life situations, emotions and extrasystoles. Psychosom Med 1949; 11:257-272.
63. Lown B, Verier R, Corbalan R. Psychologic stress and threshold for repetitive ventricular response. Science 1973; 182:834-836.
64. Reich P, DeSilva RA, Lown B, Murawski BJ. Acute psychological disturbances preceding life-threatening ventricular arrhythmias. JAMA 1981; 246:233-235.
65. Tavazzi L, Zotti AM, Rondanelli R. The role of psychologic stress in the genesis of lethal arrhythmias in patients with coronary artery disease. Eur Heart J 1986; 7:Suppl A:99-106.
66. Lown B. Sudden cardiac death: biobehavioral perspective. Circulation 1987;76 (Suppl II) I186-I196.
67. Dimsdale JE, Moss J. Plasma catecholamines in stress and exercise. JAMA 1980;243:340-342.
68. Barnard RJ, Gardner GW, Diaco NV, MacAlpin RN, Kattus AA. Cardiovascular responses to sudden strenous exercise - heart rate, blood pressure, and ECG. J Appl Physiol 34;833-837, 1973.

69. Foster C, Anholm JD, Hellman CK, Carpenter T, Pollock ML, Schmidt DH. Left ventricular function during sudden strenuous exercise. Circulation 1981; 63:592–596.

70. Duncan HW, Barnard RJ, Grimditch GK, Vinten-Johansen J, Buckberg GD. Cardiovascular response to sudden strenuous exercise. Basic Res Cardiol 1987; 82:226–232.

71. Gordon JB, Zebede J, Wayne RR, Mudge GH, Ganz P, Selwyn AP. Coronary constriction with exercise: possible role for endothelial dysfunction and alpha tone (abstr). Circulation 1986; 74:Suppl 2:II-481.

72. Nabel EG, Ganz P, Gordon JB, Alexander RW, Selwyn AP. Dilation of normal and constriction of atherosclerotic arteries caused by the cold pressor test. Circulation 1988; 77:43–52.

24

STRESS-INDUCED HYPERGLYCEMIA AND ITS RELATION TO DIABETES MELLITUS

Gerald J. Taborsky, Jr. and Daniel Porte, Jr.
Veterans Administration Medical Center and University of Washington, Seattle, Washington

This chapter explains how hyperglycemia occurs during stress in normal individuals and how stress contributes to hyperglycemia in diabetics. Toward that end, we will review the actions of stress-induced neural and endocrine factors on the organs of glucose production and utilization; the different mechanisms by which hyperglycemia occurs during different types of stress; and the contribution of stress to the causes and exacerbation of diabetic hyperglycemia.

ACTION OF NEUROENDOCRINE FACTORS ON GLUCOSE HOMEOSTASIS

The hormones and neurotransmitters released during stress influence carbohydrate metabolism, either by their actions on the primary organ of glucose production—the liver—or by their actions on insulin-sensitive organs of glucose utilization: muscle and adipose tissue. Certain of the actions are indirect, mediated by effects on the endocrine pancreas, whose hormones insulin and glucagon are major controllers of both glucose production and utilization.

It is useful to separate the control of glucose production and utilization into factors that act acutely, producing a minute-to-minute regulation, and other factors that have slower, more permissive effects responsible for longer term regulation. The acute or minute-to-minute regulation acts by cellular mechanisms that are usually already expressed in liver, muscle, and adipose tissue, whereas the permissive, long-term regulators usually induce or enhance cellular expressions of enzymes in the pathways of carbohydrate metabolism.

Increased Hepatic Glucose Production

Minute-to-Minute Regulators

SYMPATHETIC NERVOUS SYSTEM

Epinephrine   The adrenal hormone epinephrine (EPI) has an acute glycogenolytic effect at the liver, which increases hepatic glucose production and therefore the plasma glucose level. The action of EPI is rapid, producing a transient increase of hepatic glucose production that then returns to a near basal rate despite continued EPI administration. The adrenergic receptors mediating this response have been characterized as alpha-1 in some studies and beta-2 in others (1), depending on the species or conditions of the study. Alpha-1 adrenergic activation increases intramembrane turnover of phosphatidylinositol and generates intracellular inositol triphosphate and diacylglycerol, which, in turn, release calcium from intracellular stores. The increased calcium quickly leads to activation of phosphorylase and glycogen breakdown. Beta-2-adrenergic activation stimulates adenylate cyclase, raising intracellular levels of cAMP. The increased cAMP leads to a series of phosphorylations via cAMP-dependent protein kinase, ultimately activating phosphorylase and inactivating glycogen synthetase.

Although EPI has the direct effects on the liver described above, its major effects to stimulate hepatic glucose production are indirect, mediated through inhibition of insulin and stimulation of glucagon secretion (see below for the actions of insulin and glucagon on hepatic glucose production). Epinephrine's inhibitory action on insulin secretion is mediated by activation of alpha 2-adrenergic receptors. Epinephrine's stimulatory actions on glucagon secretion can be mediated by either alpha- or beta-adrenergic receptors depending on the conditions of the experiment. Activation of the adrenergic receptors on the pancreatic A and B cell impairs the normal ability of glucose both to stimulate insulin secretion and inhibit glucagon release. This decrease in the sensitivity of the pancreatic islet to plasma glucose is a critical factor in the generation and maintenance of hyperglycemia during stress, since pancreatic islets with normal sensitivity respond to hyperglycemia by secreting sufficient insulin and reducing glucagon sufficiently to restore euglycemia quickly. In contrast, during stress-induced EPI secretion, this same hyperglycemic level produces less stimulation of insulin and less inhibition of glucagon secretion so that the glucose level returns not to normal but to an elevated level. Thus, the actions of catecholamines on the islet actually reset the level of glucose around which carbohydrate metabolism is regulated, resulting in sustained hyperglycemia.

Norepinephrine Norepinephrine (NE), like EPI, is a dual agonist with both alpha- and beta-adrenergic actions. Exogenous NE can produce the same qualitative glycogenolytic response as EPI, but NE may be a less effective alpha 2-adrenergic agonist. Studies in vivo suggest that the *circulating* levels of NE necessary to achieve such effects are not usually produced except during very severe stress (2). Instead, NE is usually considered a local sympathetic neurotransmitter, and several studies have demonstrated that electrical stimulation of the sympathetic nerves to the liver can increase hepatic glucose production (3–5). There have been no major studies directly measuring the activation of hepatic noradrenergic nerve during stress, perhaps because such determinations are complex, requiring measurement of both local and circulating NE, hepatic NE extraction, and hepatic blood flow in order to calculate hepatic NE spillover (6). Several indirect studies suggest that the liver nerves are activated during stress. For example, hepatic NE content is decreased after exercise (7), suggesting local release of NE, and hepatic denervation results in less hyperglycemia in adrenalectomized animals (8). However, other, apparently similar, studies suggest little effect of hepatic denervation on the glycogenolytic response to stress (9).

Just as EPI exerts its major glycogenolytic action indirectly via the endocrine pancreas, so also may NE. Activation of the sympathetic nerves to the pancreas results in impaired insulin and stimulated glucagon secretion, leading to the same elevation of the glucose set point described above for EPI. Although NE can activate the same alpha 2-inhibitory adrenergic receptor on the B cell and the alpha- and beta-adrenergic stimulatory receptors on the pancreatic A cell, other nonadrenergic neurotransmitters may also be involved in these neurally mediated changes of insulin and glucagon secretion (see below).

Sympathetic Neuropeptides The discovery of the neuropeptides neuropeptide Y (NPY) and, more recently, galanin, in certain sympathetic nerves raises the possibility that they might mediate neurally induced changes in carbohydrate metabolism. NPY appears to be released primarily during high-frequency neural activation (10), when apparently it helps to prolong the vasoconstriction initiated by coreleased NE (10). NPY is released during stress (11), but its release from the nerves innervating the liver has yet to be investigated.

Another neuropeptide, galanin, has been proposed as a sympathetic neurotransmitter in the pancreas (12). In the dog, galanin-like immunoreactivity is present in fibers innervating the islet cells and galanin is released during activation of pancreatic nerves (13). Splanchnic nerve stimulation releases galanin into both the pancreatic venous blood and the systemic circulation (14). Preliminary data suggest that circulating levels of galanin-like immunoreactivity increase during the stress of exercise (15). Its localization and release from the nerves innervating the liver has yet to be investigated.

POSTERIOR PITUITARY HORMONES: Vasopressin Vasopressin is not usually considered a major controller of hepatic glucose production, but it is released during certain types of stress and in vitro studies have suggested that it is a potent glycogenolytic agent (16). Vasopressin acts at a V_1 receptor to accelerate phosphatidyl inositol turnover in the liver (17), which in turn increases cytosolic calcium levels. The increased intracellular calcium activates specific phosphorolyses and kinases that lead ultimately to activation of glycogen phosphorylase and inactivation of glycogen synthetase (1). Despite the potency of vasopressin compared to other glycogenolytic agents, it is not clear that the levels of vasopressin in the systemic circulation during stress reach the concentrations necessary to affect hepatic glycogenolysis significantly.

PANCREATIC HORMONES

Insulin Insulin secretion is usually impaired during stress by catecholamines, cortisol, and/or neuropeptides, leading to a fall in the portal venous levels to which the liver is exposed. Since insulin is a tonic and potent inhibitor of hepatic glucose production, insulin deficiency produces a rapid increase in hepatic glucose production (18). Even if the hypoinsulinemia is sustained during stress, the increase of hepatic glucose production is transient because marked hyperglycemia directly suppresses further glucose production by the liver. Thus, the *magnitude* of hyperglycemia can be self-limiting. The *duration* of the hyperglycemia can be long, however, if insulin secretion remains inhibited, since the insulin response to glucose is a major factor in accelerating the clearance of glucose from blood (see below).

Withdrawal of the tonic inhibitory effect of insulin not only directly stimulates hepatic glucose production but also enhances the responsiveness of the liver to the glycogenolytic agents glucagon (see below) and EPI (see above). Insulin deficiency enhances stimulated glycogenolysis by preventing activation of phosphodiesterase, which would increase the cAMP breakdown and thus lower the intracellular cAMP response to these agents. In addition, insulin deficiency eliminates the stimulation of glycogen synthetase and therefore eliminates the diversion and futile cycling of the newly formed glucose back into the synthesis of new glycogen (4).

In addition to its effect on hepatic glycogenolysis, insulin deficiency contributes to hyperglycemia by enhancing hepatic gluconeogenesis both directly at the liver and indirectly via effects on the organs supplying gluconeogenic substrates. For example, insulin deficiency increases lipolysis in adipose tissue, which supplies glycerol and augments proteolysis in muscle that increases plasma amino acids.

Glucagon Many stresses stimulate glucagon secretion from the A cell of the pancreatic islets, resulting in marked increases in the portal venous glucagon concentrations to which the liver is exposed. Such increases of glucagon can produce rapid and large increases in hepatic glucose production (18). This increment is initially due to glycogenolysis. However, the resultant hyperglycemia directly suppresses hepatic glucose production and helps return hepatic glucose production to basal levels within a few hours despite sustained hyperglucagonemia. Glucagon produces this increase in hepatic glucose production via activation of adenylate cyclase, which increases intracellular cyclic cAMP. Through a series of phosphorylations, increased intracellular cAMP levels lead to activation of phosphorylase, the rate-limiting enzyme for glycogen breakdown, and inactivation of glycogen synthetase, the rate-controlling enzyme for glycogen synthesis (1). The glucagon-induced increase of cAMP also leads, indirectly, to an increase in gluconeogenesis by decreasing the activity of the key glycolytic enzymes: pyruvate kinase and 6-phosphofructo 1-kinase (1).

Long-Term Regulators

ANTERIOR PITUITARY HORMONES

Growth Hormone and Insulin-Like Growth Factor 1   While most studies have concentrated on the chronic effects of growth hormone to produce *peripheral* insulin resistance, growth hormone also antagonizes insulin action at the liver (19). The increased hepatic glucose production, however, is partially offset by increased basal insulin levels secondary to the insulin resistance produced by growth hormone (20). Although insulin-like growth factor 1 (IGF-1) has been implicated in mediating the growth effects of growth hormone administration, it is unlikely that IGF-1 mediates the insulin resistance effects of growth hormone since infusions of recombinant IGF-1 have an insulin-like, not an insulin-antagonistic, action.

ACTH and Glucocorticoids   ACTH levels increase during a variety of stresses and increase the secretion of adrenal glucocorticoids. Glucocorticoids in turn increase hepatic glucose production (21) by a number of effects. Glucocorticoids accelerate proteolysis at the muscle, which releases amino acids for use as gluconeogenic precursors. They also increase the activation, and later the synthesis, of key enzymes in the gluconeogenic pathway. Although glucocorticoids acutely stimulate glycogen synthetase and glycogen repletion in formerly glucocorticoid-deficient animals, in normal animals glucocorticoids seem to stimulate glycogenolysis (22). In addition, glucocorticoids enhance the effect of both EPI and glucagon to stimulate hepatic glucose production (23) and convert their normally transient effect into a sustained stimulation (24) that results in marked and sustained elevation of plasma glucose levels.

Thyroid-Stimulating Hormone and Thyroid Hormones   Levels of thyroid-stimulating hormone (TSH) are increased during stress, leading to increased plasma levels of T_3 and T_4. Given the slow onset and long-lasting effects of thyroid hormones on metabolism, they would not be expected to participate in the *acute* regulation of hepatic glucose production. They can, however, change an organ's responsiveness to acute regulators such as catecholamines. For example, thyroid hormone deficiency enhances the beta 2-adrenergic responsiveness (1) and diminishes alpha 1-adrenergic responsiveness of the liver. Since these actions antagonize each other, the net effect on glycogenolysis per se is unclear.

Decreased Glucose Utilization

Minute-to-Minute Regulators

PANCREATIC HORMONES: INSULIN In the presence of many stresses, insulin secretion is impaired. Since insulin is a major physiological stimulator of the uptake of glucose from plasma into muscle and adipose tissue, such impairment contributes to the hyperglycemia of stress by preventing the rapid clearance of glucose from plasma. The stress-induced increase of plasma catecholamines is most often invoked as the mediator of impaired insulin secretion during stress. Such impairment is mediated by activation of alpha 2-adrenergic receptors on the pancreatic B cell. Other factors contribute to the impairment of insulin secretion during stress and therefore the absolute or relative decrease in glucose utilization. These include cortisol, which is released during stress and has direct inhibitory effects on pancreatic B-cell function and stimulatory effects on pancreatic A-cell function (25). Other putative factors include neuropeptides such as galanin whose pancreatic release has been postulated during stress (12) and whose insulin-inhibitory action has been demonstrated (13).

Several stress hormones, in addition to decreasing glucose utilization by impairing insulin *secretion*, can also impair the *action* of the insulin that is secreted and thereby further decrease glucose utilization. These factors and their effects are described below.

SYMPATHETIC NERVOUS SYSTEM: EPINEPHRINE AND NOREPINEPRHINE Early in vitro studies demonstrated that beta-adrenergic effects of epinephrine antagonized the action of insulin to transport glucose into skeletal muscle (26). When insulin levels are low (e.g., fasting), this effect of epinephrine is minor, since most of peripheral glucose uptake goes to insulin-independent tissues such as the brain. When insulin levels are high (e.g., during or immediately after meals), this effect may be sizable, explaining in large part the effect of stress in impairing glucose tolerance.

Long-Term Regulators: Anterior Pituitary Hormones

GROWTH HORMONE. Growth hormone has both an acute insulin-like effect and a chronic insulin-antagonist effect. The insulin-like effect is more prominent in growth-hormone-deficient animals and lasts only a few hours. The insulin-antagonistic action is apparent 6–12 h after growth hormone treatment and may persist even though growth hormone levels have returned to baseline. This effect of growth hormone to antagonize insulin-stimulated glucose uptake results in an impairment of glucose tolerance (20) and exaggerates the hyperglycemia of stress. Recent studies have focused on its potential to explain increased insulin requirements or hyperglycemia in diabetics (27).

ADRENOCORICOTROPIC HORMONE AND CORTISOL. Many stresses release adrenocorticotropic hormone (ACTH), which in turn stimulates the adrenal cortex to secrete cortisol. Glucocorticoid excess has long been known to produce resistance to insulin's actions and a compensatory increase in insulin secretion. Indeed, just 1 day of cortisol treatment is sufficient to impair insulin-stimulated glucose utilization. Although the mechanism of this effect is not clear, insulin binding is increased, not decreased, so a postreceptor effect is likely. Whatever the mechanism, the net result is a decrease in glucose transporters and an impairment of insulin's ability to stimulate the uptake of glucose from plasma into muscle and adipose tissue.

MECHANISMS OF HYPERGLYCEMIA DURING DIFFERENT TYPES OF STRESS

Surgery

Major surgery is a common clinical stress, but it is usually complicated by the presence of other independent stresses. For example, surgical procedures that produce substantial blood loss are complicated by the stress of hemorrhage hypotension (see below). Major thoracic or abdominal surgery can produce heat loss and since many anesthetics impair autonomic thermoregulation, mild hypothermia can occur (see below). Indeed, in pediatric cardiac surgery, hypothermia is intentional and beneficial. Postsurgical infections can significantly complicate the type of stress response following surgery (see below).

Even without these complications, the stress response to surgery is complex because it is determined by two opposing factors. The first is anesthesia, which, depending on the type and depth, can limit the magnitude of the sympathetic and counterregulatory hormone response. The other major factor is nociceptive activation, which can stimulate the sympathetic and counterregulatory hormone response in relation to the extent and severity of the painful stimulus. Two generalizations are worthy of note in this regard. First, anesthetics capable of producing full surgical anesthesia vary in their suppressive effects on the sympathetic activation and hyperglycemia produced by stress. For example, pentobarbital anesthesia in dogs abolishes both the moderate plasma catecholamine response and moderate hyperglycemia produced by central glucopenia present in the conscious animal (28). In contrast, low-dose halothane anesthesia, which can produce a full surgical anesthesia, allows both a plasma catecholamine and plasma glucose response to moderate glucopenia similar to that of the conscious animal (29).

The second generalization relates to the actual stimulus for the sympathetic activation during surgery. Although the common perception is that general anesthetics prevent the recognition of pain, it is clear that major surgery activates pain fibers and that nociceptive stimulation is a major factor in the sympathetic activation that occurs during surgical stress. For example, experiments in dogs have shown that during pentobarbital anesthesia, laparatomy clearly increases plasma catecholamine levels (30), despite the known suppressive effect of this agent on sympathetic activation (28). The analgesic morphine lowers this surgery-induced rise in plasma catecholamine levels, but not the rise induced by central glucopenia (30). In addition, the effect of morphine itself is reversed by the mu-receptor antagonist, naloxone. Other studies suggest the same conclusion. For example, the plasma catecholamine response to surgery on the lower extremities is blocked by low spinal anesthesia, which eliminates neural afferent signals from the site of surgery. Thus surgery activates the sympathetic nervous system and other stress responses by activating nociceptive input to the brain.

Predicting the extent of activation of the sympathetic nervous system and other stress responses during surgery is difficult because it will depend on the type and extent of surgery; the general sympathetic suppression by anesthesia, which is critically dependent on the type and level of anesthetic used; and the more selective suppressive effects of analgesics on the nociceptive stimulation.

After the surgery is over and the anesthesia has been discontinued, the stress response can, in fact, increase because much of the nociceptive stimulation is still present whereas the suppressive effect of the anesthesia is not. Therefore, there can be an increase in plasma catecholamine, cortisol, and growth hormone levels during the immediate recovery phase. The immediate increase in plasma catecholamine levels and the delayed effect of cortisol and growth hormone can sometimes lead to hyperglycemia but more often to glucose intolerance, all of which may resolve when the nociceptive stimulation of the counterregulatory hormones wanes. Therefore, analgesics in the postoperative period would be expected to normalize plasma catecholamine, growth hormone, and cortisol levels, and accelerate the restoration of normal glucose tolerance.

Hypotension

Defense of blood pressure is essential to avoid the acute brain lesions, respiratory failure, and heart failure that occur when blood pressure falls below 25 mmHg for extended periods of time (31). Since the brain is dependent on glucose as its primary metabolic fuel, and since the heart becomes dependent on glucose during periods of anoxia or hypoperfusion, the hyperglycemia that occurs in response to hypotension may represent a mechanism to compensate for the decreased rate of glucose delivery to the brain and heart. If the hypotension is severe and prolonged, even this compensatory mechanism fails. The hypoperfusion and decreased rate of oxygen delivery, reflected in a fall of venous oxygen levels (32), results in anaerobic glycolysis, accumulation of lactic acid (32,33) and local and systemic acidosis (31,32,34). The local acidosis is exacerbated by inadequate removal of locally generated carbon dioxide (32).

Hyperglycemia has been found in a number of clinical (33,34) and experimental (32,35) situations in which hypotension is present. For example, hyperglycemia is present in injured combat soldiers in shock (36) as well as in patients with acute myocardial infarction with associated hypotension or shock (34). Although the interpretation of these clinical studies is complicated by the presence of stresses in addition to hypotension, controlled studies in experimental animals make it clear that hypotension per se can cause hyperglycemia (32, 35). Thus hypotension induced by controlled hemorrhage increases blood glucose levels in dogs (32,37,38) cats, (35,39), and monkeys (31,38). Hemorrhagic hypotension is also complicated by the metabolic acidosis it usually produces (31,32). It is likely, however, that hyptotension, rather than acidosis, produces the hyperglycemic response, since the simulated hypotension of unloading the carotid baroreceptor, in the presence of a normal systemic blood pressure, and absence of acidosis can also elicit substantial hyperglycemia (35).

The general mechanism by which hypotension leads to hyperglycemia can be deduced from the available literature. First, moderate hypotension (arterial pressure of 50 mmHg) does not seem to produce hyperglycemia by a direct effect of hypotension or hypoperfusion on the organs of glucose production (the liver), glucose utilization (the brain), or glucose regulation (the pancreas) (35). Second, central and peripheral sympathetic pathways are involved. Elegant neuroanatomical studies have shown that only certain brain areas are activated during hemorrhagic hypotension in the rat (40). Indeed glucose utilization, which is a presumed index of neuronal activity, increases in most of these areas proportional to the degree of hypotension (40). These discrete areas of the central nervous system presumably control the peripheral autonomic response to hypotension, which includes activation of the sympathetic nervous system and elevation of plasma catecholamines, EPI, and NE (6). In addition to this well-recognized role in controlling blood pressure, catecholamines also contribute to the hyperglycemia of hypotension since combined adrenergic blockade substantially lessens the hyperglycemic response (32).

The endocrine pancreas probably has a substantial role in the hyperglycemia as well, since the pancreatic hormones change in a direction that produces glycogenolysis and hyperglycemia in normal animals (18). Insulin release is inhibited during hypotension, especially the insulin response to secretagogues (34,38). Since glucose is the major insulin secretagogue, such inhibition allows hyperglycemia to develop as well as to persist. The alpha 2-adrenergic effects of catecholamines are presumed to mediate this inhibition of insulin release. If so, circulating epinephrine is the likely mediator since the local noradrenergic nerves to the pancreas are not activated by moderate hypotension (6). Others (34) have suggested that hypoperfusion of the pancreas itself explains the impaired insulin secretion. It is likely, however, that both mechanisms contribute. During moderate hypotension (blood pressure of 50 mmHg), it is likely that catechol-amines mediate the inhibition, since the hypoperfusion of the pancreas is not severe and since cutting splanchnic nerves to eliminate the peripheral sympa-thetic activation reverses the inhibition of insulin release (41). During marked hypotension, it seems possible that the severe hypoperfusion may produce the local organ dysfunction and tissue damage in the pancreas that has been docu-mented for the brain and heart (31). Glucagon secretion is also increased during marked hemorrhagic hypotension (37,41), partly by a beta-adrenergic mecha-nism (37), and undoubtedly contributes to the hyperglycemic response. Sym-pathetic mechanisms are involved since cutting the splanchnic nerves lessens the glucagon response (41). It is also important to recognize that high levels of circulating catecholamine levels present during hemorrhagic hypotension can stimulate glycogenolysis by the liver and thereby increase the plasma glucose level directly. Locally released catecholamines may also contribute under certain conditions, since hepatic denervation can reduce the hyperglycemic response to hypotension (42). Other factors may also contribute. For example, there is some evidence that vasopressin can increase glucagon secretion (43) as well as directly stimulate hepatic glucose production (16). Vasopressin secretion is stimulated during hemorrhagic hypotension (44) and its contribution to the increased glucagon secretion has been suggested (45).

Hypoxia

Acute hypoxia can produce a classic activation of stress hormone release. The resultant hyperglycemia depends on the severity of the hypoxemia and the age of the subject (46,47). In anesthetized dogs, the threshold for the hyperglycemic effects of hypoxia appears to be blood oxygen levels of 40 mmHg, with unequivocal responses produced at 30 mmHg (46). The hyperglycemic effects of hypoxia are more pronounced in younger animals. The sympathetic response to acute hypoxia is pronounced, with peripheral catecholamine levels in the range of 1,000 pg/ml. Despite the magnitude of the general sympathetic activa-tion, the noradrenergic nerves to the pancreas may not be activated by hypoxia (6). The insulin and glucagon responses to hypoxia are consistent with the marked sympathetic activation, that is, relative inhibition of insulin is more than expected for the circulating levels of epinephrine. For example, epinephrine infusion in normal subjects produces an impairment of the acute insulin response to glucose, but not such a severe impairment of the acute insulin response to arginine as seen during hypoxia. The marked inhibition of insulin secretion during hypoxia is reminiscent of selective activation of alpha-adrenergic recep-tors that are inhibitory for insulin release, and lack of any beta-adrenergic receptor activation that is stimulatory to insulin release. Indeed, the acute insu-lin response to the selective beta-adrenergic agonist isoproterenol is abolished by hypoxia (50), are the beta-adrenergic effects at other organs (i.e., lipolysis at adipose tissue [51] and chronotropism at the heart [48]). The stimulation of glucagon secretion produced by hypoxia is not mediated by a beta-adrenergic mechanism, which seems to contribute to other stress-induced glucagon responses in the dog, but rather by an alpha-adrenergic mechanism (49). These findings indicate that there is a dysfunction of the beta-adrenergic receptor during hypoxia such that the marked release of the mixed alpha- and beta-adrenergic receptor agonists EPI and NE leads to selective activation of alpha-adrenergic pathways. This in turn produces larger than expected inhibition of insulin release, alpha-adrenergically dependent glucagon release, and marked hyperglycemia. Although other stress hormones such as growth hormone, ACTH (52) glucocorticoids (52,53), and vasopressin (52) are released during hypoxia, their role in the acute phase of hyperglycemia appears to be minimal.

Hypothermia

Hypothermia is used clinically to suppress metabolism in children undergoing open heart surgery. A variety of measurements have been made in this clinical situation that suggest an impairment of insulin secretion, insulin action, and glucose metabolism leading to glucose intolerance and hyperglycemia (54–57). However, it is not clear from these studies whether the changes of carbohydrate metabolism are due to anesthesia, surgical stress, or the hypothermia per se. Studies in animals have clarified the mechanisms for these effects. In general, hypothermia impairs insulin secretion (58). Whether or not this is a direct effect of hypothermia per se to induce a hypofunction of pancreatic B cells or an effect mediated by circulating levels of catecholamines may depend on the level of hypothermia achieved. For example, severe hypothermia can impair insulin secretion in the isolated perfused pancreas (36). More moderate hypothermia, on the other hand, clearly increases plasma catecholamine levels (59) that mediate a significant part of the impairment of insulin secretion in intact animals, since this is partially reversed by alpha-adrenergic blockade (56,58).

A resistance to insulin action in hypothermic animals and humans probably has two causes: a direct suppressive effect of hypothermia on insulin-sensitive tissues and a beta-adrenergically mediated inhibition of insulin-stimulated glucose uptake. The impaired insulin secretion and impaired insulin action combine to produce severe glucose intolerance in hypothermic subjects. Indeed, patients undergoing hypothermia for surgery become markedly hyperglycemic when given relatively modest glucose infusions. Even without exogenous glucose, most hypothermic animals and patients are at least mildly hyperglycemic despite a suppressive effect of hypothermia on hepatic glucose production (57). Although all the factors listed above can contribute to this hyperglycemia, in moderate hypothermia it is likely that increased glucagon secretion (56) and increased plasma levels of catecholamines (59) make the major contributions. Levels of other stress hormones such as glucocorticoids (60) and growth hormone are also elevated and may contribute to the long-term metabolic changes following an episode of acute hypothermia.

Sepsis

Metabolic responses to sepsis can be qualitatively different depending on the magnitude of the septic insult and the amount of time elapsed after the initial exposure. Sepsis initially produces a transient hyperglycemia that resolves in 4-8 h (61). If the sepsis is mild and prolonged, plasma glucose levels can be normal (62). However, despite these unchanged glucose levels, glucose turnover is increased as reflected in increased glucose utilization and increased hepatic glucose production. During mild sepsis the increased glucose turnover is not accompanied by any signficiant change in insulin, glucagon, or glucocorticoids. Since plasma catecholamine levels are not even doubled at this time, it is not surprising that adrenergic blockade does not affect this elevated glucose turnover (62). Other factors secreted from the macrophage in response to infections, such as tumor necrosis factor (TNF) and interleukin-1 might be responsible for the increased glucose turnover seen during mild, acute infection.

During more chronic infection, glucose production and utilization can be depressed despite normal glucose levels. Such depression occurs despite a doubling or tripling of glucagon, cortisol, and plasma catecholamine levels (63). A suprising finding is that insulin levels are also increased. Studies with adrenergic blockade indicate that the increased level of plasma catecholamines supports even this low level of glucose turnover (63).

When the infection is severe, the plasma level of glucose can be lower than normal. The significant elevation in glucagon and plasma catecholamine levels that occurs is important to maintain even this low level of plasma glucose in order to counteract the higher plasma insulin level and possibly the direct suppresive effects of endotoxin on hepatic glucose production (64). The low levels of glucose seen late during severe sepsis can have a critical role in the outcome. For example, it has been noted that people or animals who die in septic or endotoxin shock invariably have extreme hypoglycemia at the time of death. More recently it has been noted that glucose infusions in anesthetized animals can prevent some of the mortality associated with extreme sepsis. (65,66). Furthermore, if one classifies groups of animals into those that are able to mount a sufficient counterregulatory response and prevent hypoglycemia and those that are not, the latter are the ones who die. Thus, the ability to mount a counterregulatory response to increase hepatic glucose production is critical for offsetting the effects of endotoxins and related factors to cause hypoglycemia. Such studies dramatically illustrate the importance of glucose counterregulatory mechanisms in normal animals and humans.

Thus, although the exact pattern is far from certain, it appears that initially sepsis produces a hyperglycemia that may be dependent on the macrophage factors released in response to the infection. As sepsis worsens, the classic stress factors are activated in an attempt to counterregulate the suppressive effects of elevated insulin and endotoxin levels on hepatic glucose production so that the precarious balance of euglycemia is struck. If sepsis worsens and marked endotoxemia occurs, the activity of the sympathetic nervous system, and the release of glucagon and cortisol, are increased but are overwhelmed, and hypoglycemia and death may ensue.

Burns

Burns produce an obvious and sustained metabolic stress that is reflected in a prolonged increase of the resting metabolic rate. This hypermetabolic state is not due to thyroid hormones, which, in fact, are suppressed in burn patients (67). The resting metabolic rate is elevated in proportion to the area of the burn (67) and gradually normalizes over 1-2 months following the injury (67). The rate of glucose production is usually increased in burn states (69,108) and accounts for the 1-2 weeks of mild hyperglycemia seen after severe burns (50% of the body surface area) (67). The rate of glucose disappearance is also usually elevated after burns (69,70) sometimes accounting for the euglycemia seen in the face of increased glucose production following less severe burns. The turnover of gluconeogenic amino acids (e.g., alanine) is increased in burn states (70) and reflects accelerated net protein catabolism in peripheral tissues. This negative nitrogen balance and the potential loss of vital muscle is a significant problem in burn patients.

Levels of stress hormones are usually elevated after severe burns. Thus plasma catecholamine levels are increased (69,71), reflecting activation of the sympathetic nervous system, including the adrenal medulla. The adrenal cortex is also stimulated by ACTH since glucocorticoids are increased markedly in burn stress (69,70). Elevated glucocorticoid levels may account for the increased proteolysis and contribute to the increased hepatic glucose production by accelerating gluconeogenesis. Growth hormone levels are not usually elevated (70) but levels of another pituitary hormone, vasopressin, are (72). Baseline glucagon levels are consistently elevated (70,69,71) as are glucagon responses to the amino acid arginine (73).

It is likely that all of the stress hormones contribute to the hypermetabolism and increased glucose production characteristic of burn stress. For example, reduction of catecholamine action by combined adrenergic blockade tends to normalize the elevated resting metabolic rate (68). Likewise, administration of an antagonist to platelet-activating factor reduces the plasma catecholamine response to burn stress and partially prevents the mild hyperglycemic response, despite preservation of the elevated glucagon levels (71). Conversely, selective suppression of glucagon secretion, by infusing somatostatin with insulin replacement, not only reverses the elevated rate of glucose production but also necessitates the infusion of glucose to prevent hypoglycemia (70). Finally, the high plasma levels of glucocorticoids probably contribute to the increased glucose production by prolonging the glycogenolytic and gluconeogenetic actions of glucagon.

Despite the elevated levels of catecholamines, plasma insulin levels are normal or even elevated in burn stress (69,70,71,73). These elevated levels of plasma insulin contribute significantly to the increased rate of glucose uptake in burn stress, since suppression of insulin secretion with somatostatin leads to a significant fall in the metabolic clearance rate for glucose (70). Despite the clear effect of elevated insulin on glucose uptake, the other major anabolic effects of insulin (i.e., inhibition of lipolysis and proteolysis) do not appear to be fully expressed, as indicated by increased plasma levels of free fatty acids and increased turnover of plasma alanine. Perhaps sympathetic stimulation of adipose tissue and glucocorticoid stimulation of muscle partially overcomes these inhibitory effects of insulin.

Although burn stress can be characterized by the features listed above, it is important to recognize that these responses can be partially due to the presence of other stresses. For example, severe burns can produce an acute shock-like hypotension (71), which, by itself (see above) can activate the sympathetic nervous system. Indeed, volume and electrolyte replacement are recognized as essential for the management of burn patients (74). Platelet-activating factor has been implicated in the hypotension and activation of the sympathetic nervous system accompanying burn stress (71). In addition, the loss of large amounts of burned skin removes an extremely important barrier to infection. Thus, infection and sepsis are common later complications of burn stress. As reviewed above, sepsis evokes a set of stress responses that include many of those described for burn stress. It is natural, therefore, to wonder to what extent sepsis has complicated the interpretation of clinical studies of burn stress.

STRESS AND DIABETES MELLITUS

Type I, Insulin-Dependent Diabetes Mellitus

Insulin-dependent diabetes is characterized by an islet lesion leading to markedly impaired insulin secretion, with eventual death and loss of almost all of the B cells. It often presents as diabetic coma with ketoacidosis. This was originally thought to indicate the rapid onset of almost total permanent destruction of the islet B cells at the time of diagnosis. In this section we review evidence for a longer premorbid course and the participation of stress-related factors in the causes, pathophysiology, and plasma glucose control in this type of diabetes.

Causes

Islet injury and destruction are now known to precede the onset of clinical hyperglycemia and take place over a much longer period of time than is clinically apparent. This immune injury is indicated by the presence of islet cell antibodies and insulin autoantibodies, which appear several years before the diagnosis of type I diabetes mellitus (75,76). In addition, reduced insulin responses to intravenous glucose also appear months to years prior to severe hyperglycemia (77).

The reasons for the activation of this destructive process are unknown but are believed to represent the activation of an autoimmune state followed by an imbalance between T-helper and T-suppressor cells and the susceptibility or resistance of islet B cells to injury (78). Since some stress hormones (particularly cortisol) are known to modulate the immune system and others to alter islet B-cell activity (epinephrine, glucagon, cortisol) there has been speculation regarding the potential role of such modulation on the development and progress of islet injury. Thus, neurohormonal changes associated with stress have been proposed as one of the environmental factors that interacts with hereditary factors associated with the human leukocyte antigen (HLA)-D region of chromosome 6 important to immune response mechanisms known to be associated with risk of the development of type I diabetes. A recent hypothesis has suggested that lymphokines produced by activated macrophages and helper T cells are toxic to insulin secreting islet B cells and therefore that regulation of antigen presenting cells and/or regulation of helper T-cell production of interleukin (IL-1), interferon-gamma (IFN-γ) and tumor necrosis factor (TNF) can increase destruction of B cells (78). Hormonal regulation of suppressor cells that normally minimize or prevent immune injury is another potential mechanism by which stress hormones (particularly cortisol) and the sympathetic nerves may contribute to the likelihood of autoimmune B-cell destruction of type I diabetes. For example, it has been shown that suppressor T cells are more sensitive to glucocorticoids than T-helper cells (79). Thus, at moderate cortisol dosages, immune injury could be increased by steroids. An example of this phenomenon may be the increased rate of development of an autoimmune form of diabetes induced in mice by low-dosage streptozocin when they are housed 10/cage compared with mice housed 1/cage, since crowded housing is associated with higher circulating adrenal steroid levels (80). A similar phenomenon may explain the observation that cyclophosphamide-treated NOD mice (a model of type I diabetes) have an increased prevalence of diabetes (81). Cyclophosphamide, which is known to be an immune suppressant, markedly increases the eventual development of diabetes in this mouse model of autoimmunity and diabetes. Evidence presented so far suggests that this increased incidence of diabetes is related to cyclophosphamide's immune modulatory effects and seemed to be best explained by postulating a toxic effect of the drug on suppressor T-cell function (82,83).

As an alternative, immune related damage of islet B cells has been shown to be related to the islet B cells' insulin secretory activity at the time of exposure to IL-1 (78). Thus, increased secretion of insulin seems to be followed by an enhanced ability of IL-1 to impair B-cell function. Since increased B-cell secretion of insulin has been found during physical stress and infection, it has been postulated that the B cells would be more sensitive to injury at that time. This increase in insulin level is usually associated with insulin resistance. Glucocorticoids, growth hormone, and the catecholamines all cause insulin resistance and it has been hypothesized that they are the cause of insulin resistance during stress. Because catecholamines also impair insulin secretion, the activity level of the B cell of a stressed individual can be highly varied. However, the temporal pattern of the stress response can often be characterized by an early excess of catecholamines and a late excess of glucocorticoids and growth hormone (74). Therefore the early response to stress may be characterized by reduced insulin secretion, while the later recovery phase is often characterized by insulin resistance, and a compensatory increase in B-cell activity with increased insulin secretion. In fact, studies in vitro and in vivo have suggested that the sensitivity to both immune (84) and nonimmune (85) injury may be increased when insulin secretion is increased. Thus, an alternative explanation for the increased sensitivity of crowded mice to low-dosage streptozocin discussed above could be related to an increased sensitivity of activated islet B cells to injury rather than a decrease in suppressor T-cell function. Such changes in islet B-cell secretory activity could explain why type I diabetes occurs with greater frequency in the fall and winter than during spring and summer. This was originally thought to be due to the increased likelihood of a specific infection causing islet destruction, but the association is without relation to any specific infection. Thus, it may be that the neurohumoral stress response to infection per se causes insulin resistance and increased islet B-cell insulin activity, which in turn sensitizes the B cell to autoimmune injury. The increased activity of the B cell during puberty (86) may provide a similar explanation for the increased incidence of type I diabetes in susceptible subjects at that time of life. Reducing islet number by pancreatectomy (another way of activating residual B cells) has been found to increase the likelihood of permanent diabetes in stressed rats (87) Thus, there are a variety of mechanisms by which stress could contribute to the onset of type I diabetes.

A role for psychological stress in the causes and/or onset of human type I diabetes has also been postulated. Major life events have been found to be more frequent in diabetic children prior to diagnosis than controls (88), but no prospective study has been carried out.

Pathophysiology

In contrast to the speculation reviewed above, the data supporting participation of stress hormones in the hyperglycemia and ketoacidosis of the acutely ill person presenting with recent onset of type I diabetes are unequivocal. Elevated levels of catecholamines, cortisol, growth hormone, and glucagon are characteristic of diabetic ketoacidosis (89). Treatment with intravenous fluids alone, without insulin, will reduce these hormone levels and the hyperglycemia, fatty acid mobilization, and ketogenesis (90). These findings suggest that elevation of these counterregulatory hormones is responsible for much of the metabolic disturbance. We have suggested that they are the major factors in converting insulin deficiency without ketoacidosis to decompensated hyperglycemia with ketoacidosis. Confirming this concept, it has been shown that beta-adrenergic blocking agents are effective in reducing elevated fatty acid mobilization in ketoacidosis (89). Since many insulin-dependent diabetics present to the physician without ketoacidosis, we have suggested that insulin deficiency of the magnitude usually observed is a necessary but not a sufficient explanation for the ketoacidosis syndrome (91). We believe that volume depletion and activation of baroreceptor-mediated stimulation of the autonomic nervous system and the hypothalamopituitary axis are necessary additional factor(s) in initiating ketoacidosis. We have suggested that B-cell injury leads to impaired insulin secretion that is partially compensated by the hyperglycemia that follows.

When the hyperglycemia becomes a sufficient magnitude to lead to glycosuria and electrolyte loss, the subsequent volume depletion associated with the excretion of glucose and electrolytes activates the counterregulatory hormones EPI, glucagon, growth hormone, and cortisol, which, in the presence of insulin deficiency, produce the full-blown diabetic ketoacidosis syndrome. This concept may explain why it has been possible to use lower dosages of insulin in recent years for the treatment of ketoacidosis. It may be largely because therapy is now focused on vigorous replacement of fluid and electrolyte losses. This volume replacement treatment minimizes volume depletion and restores elevated counterregulatory hormone levels towards normal (90). Such fluid replacement reduces the insulin resistance induced by these hormones and possibly allows for improved insulin secretion from residual B cells. Thus, ketoacidosis in insulin-dependent diabetes would be characterized as a sequence of events in which B-cell damage causes insulin deficiency, which leads to hyperglycemia, which leads to glycosuria, volume depletion, activation of the autonomic and pituitary hypothalamic axes, mobilization of fatty acids, increased hepatic glucose and ketone production, and eventually ketoacidosis. In this context, severe hyperglycemia in itself is a form of stress, and there is a vicious circle in which the underlying pancreatic abnormality in type I diabetes leads to hyperglycemia, which leads to a neuroendocrine stress response, which leads to more hyperglycemia and eventual ketoacidosis. This cycle is more likely to occur in patients with insulin-dependent diabetes because of the efficient excretion of glucose in younger persons, coupled with the greater severity of insulin deficiency compared to the older noninsulin-dependent group. In some circumstances, it would appear that ketoacidosis can occur even in the presence of "normal" levels of basal insulin being overwhelmed by increased levels of catecholamines, growth hormone, cortisol, and glucagon. We have documented such an instance in a patient who had basal insulin levels that were apparently normal but in fact were low, given the associated hyperglycemia. This patient went from hyperglycemia and glycosuria without ketosis to full-blown ketoacidosis without any further decline in plasma insulin levels (91). This would seem to indicate that the transition from simple hyperglycemia to ketoacidosis may occur as a result of increased stress hormone stimulation of lipolysis and gluconeogenesis rather than further insulin deficiency.

Some experimental efforts have been directed to the study of whether psychological stress can influence the development of ketoacidosis in susceptible patients. Based on the observation that poorly controlled juvenile-onset-type diabetics develop elevated ketone body levels during stress interviews (92,93), two difficult-to-manage patients with recurrent acidosis thought to be related to psychological factors in their environment were treated with oral propranolol (beta-adrenergic blocker) (94). The rationale was that catecholamine-induced lipolysis would be prevented, so that episodes of poor diabetes control would not be associated with ketoacidosis. In these two patients, this treatment was associated with marked reduction in the frequency of hospitalization for ketoacidosis, in contrast to other forms of therapy directed at reducing the environmental stress factors in these patients' lives. This form of therapy has obvious problems because of its potential to enhance unawareness of hypoglycemia in insulin-treated patients and is not recommended as routine therapy for such individuals. However, it does indicate, as do observations made during stress interviews, that insulin-dependent diabetics are particularly sensitive to activation of the autonomic and hypothalamopituitary systems. Attempts to quantitate this phenomenon in insulin-dependent diabetics have been made and are consistent with such a hypothesis. It has been shown, for example, that hyperglycemia induced by cortisol, EPI, or glucagon is exaggerated in insulin-dependent diabetics (95), and this is particularly true during periods of relatively poor diabetes control. For this reason, a variety of stress states are associated with an increased need for insulin in insulin-dependent diabetic patients. It is also a commonly observed phenomenon that deterioration of diabetes control is likely during episodes of sepsis, burn, hypoxia, hypotension, or vascular accidents in insulin-treated diabetic patients. The assumption is that the islet will tend to adapt in normal subjects to maintain insulin secretion due to the ability of beta-adrenergic stimulation and glucose to stimulate insulin secretion. In insulin-dependent diabetes, the ability of beta-adrenergic stimulation to increase hepatic glucose production and impair peripheral insulin-mediated glucose uptake will be present but there will be no compensatory islet response and therefore more severe hyperglycemia would be predicted.

Chronic Glucose Control

In addition to precipitating ketoacidosis, stress has been hypothesized to play a role in day-to-day blood glucose regulation in insulin-treated type I diabetics. When insulin levels are fixed by the injection pattern of the patient, factors that influence endogenous insulin secretion become unimportant to glucose levels, but factors that change insulin sensitivity become exaggerated because there is no compensatory islet response to modulate them. Thus, one can expect major changes in insulin need whenever catecholamines, steroids, or growth hormone levels are increased in type I diabetes. In normal subjects this modulation amounts to a two- to fivefold increase in insulin level during administration of stress hormones that produce insulin resistance. Since this change in insulin secretion cannot take place in a person with type I diabetes, severe hyperglycemia or even ketoacidosis can occur during stress despite continued treatment with the usual dose of insulin. While an increased sensitivity of type I diabetes to cortisol, EPI, and glucagon hormones has been demonstrated (95) controlled clinical studies to define which hormones are contributing to stress hyperglycemia in type I diabetic patients under ordinary clinical treatment have not been performed. However, in poorly controlled patients an inverse relation between circulating norepinephrine levels and plasma CO_2 has been shown, and higher basal levels of norepinephrine were correlated with greater norepinephrine responses to exercise (96). Thus, once activated (probably by hypovolemia in this case), the same external stimulus (exercise) caused a greater concentration of the counterregulatory (stress) hormone, which would be expected in turn to produce more hyperglycemia and/or fatty acid mobilization and ketosis.

In addition to physical stress, psychological factors that increase stress hormones in type I diabetes have been postulated to play a role in glucose control. For example, stress interviews in type I diabetics have been shown to lead to exaggerated increases in free fatty acids (FFA) and ketones (92,93). However, despite a general clinical belief and an association between anxiety scores and diabetes control (97), or correlations between psychological testing and glycosuria in children at camp (98), experimental documentation that psychological factors can have major effects on blood glucose levels is not available, and there are many studies with negative results (99). Thus, variation in neuroendocrine effectors associated with stress is suspected to contribute to the wide fluctuations in plasma glucose that occur in treated type I diabetic patients unrelated to variations in food intake and insulin dosages, but unambiguous identification and documentation of this concept remain an important unresolved problem.

Type II, Noninsulin-Dependent Diabetes Mellitus

Noninsulin-dependent diabetes mellitus (NIDDM) is characterized by a generalized impairment of the islet A- and B-cell response to glucose. Insulin release is reduced and glucagon suppression by glucose is less effective. Most patients also have insulin resistance and obesity (100).

Causes

We have suggested that glucose recognition by a number of neuroendocrine cells is abnormal in patients with type II diabetes and that it may explain some of the abnormal neuroendocrine and islet findings in patients with this syndrome (101). The poor suppression of glucagon by glucose, the elevation of catecholamine levels unrelated to any ketoacidosis, and the supersensitivity to exercise-induced increases of growth hormone or a paradoxical increase in growth hormone by oral glucose in individuals with mild hyperglycemia may be part of the underlying disease. Although these abnormalities may be due to intrinsic structural or metabolic defects, they may be secondary to the metabolic disorder, or it is possible that neuroendocrine factors known to influence the islet sensitivity to glucose are primarily involved. Evidence for a role of neuroendocrine factors in type II diabetes is provided by studies that show increased insulin release in NIDDM during infusion of the alpha-adrenergic receptor blocking agent phentolamine, implying increased alpha-adrenergic receptor activity or sensitivity in such subjects (102). In fact, an alpha-adrenergic blocking agent has been developed that appears to be clinically successful in lowering plasma glucose levels in humans (103). It is of great interest therefore, that a well-described mouse model of diabetes and obesity (ob/ob) has also been found to be supersensitive to catecholamines and to stress-induced hyperglycemia. In fact, these animals may only have significant elevations of plasma glucose when stressed (104). Since mice are traditionally bled from the retro-orbital sinus, this bleeding stress may be an important contributor to the presence of hyperglycemia in this model. Classic conditioning can also be used to produce hyperglycemia in these animals, and the investigators have hypothesized that autonomic nervous system dysfunction plays a significant role in the pathogenesis of hyperglycemia in this model of type II diabetes (105).

There are other possibilities for neuroendocrine factors involved in type II diabetes. Studies have shown that the serotonin-blocking agent methysergide and the prostaglandin synthesis inhibitor sodium salicylate increase insulin secretion in NIDDM (106). The effects of centrally injected morphine or related analogues to cause hyperglycemia has even raised the possibility that endogenous morphine-related peptides may underlie hyperglycemia in some patients with NIDDM (107). In addition, we have shown that infusion of a synthetic B-cell selective somatostatin analogue in dogs produces hyperglycemia due to impairment of glucose-induced insulin release, which is analogous to that found in

NIDDM (108). A similar phenomenon has been observed during infusion of the neuropeptide galanin, which is also a selective inhibitor of insulin secretion and present in pancreatic nerves (12). Its release has been stimulated by activation of the sympathetic pancreatic neural innervation (13). Thus, several inhibitory B-cell neuroendocrine factors can produce a syndrome that resembles NIDDM and may contribute to some clinical cases.

Pathophysiology

Although none of the above findings are conclusive regarding a primary role for abnormalities of nervous system function in causing type II diabetes, it is apparent that activation of neuroendocrine systems can impair glucose sensitivity of the islet B cell and produce a syndrome functionally similar to NIDDM. There is accumulating evidence that such activation may be an important part of the hyperglycemia observed in NIDDM. Thus, regardless of considerations of cause, it is clear that activation of these systems during stress in such patients is almost certain to produce more severe hyperglycemia than in normal subjects.

During this discussion of stress hyperglycemia, we have emphasized the key role that islet B cells must play in any hyperglycemic state. Due simply to the feedback nature of islet regulation, it appears that increased hepatic glucose production and/or decreased peripheral glucose utilization alone or together cannot lead to sustained hyperglycemia unless the islet fails to adapt (100). Therefore, on theoretical grounds one would expect that hyperglycemia in NIDDM must be associated with an abnormality of islet function. Nevertheless, the presence of such an islet abnormality has been somewhat controversial because during standard oral glucose tolerance testing, insulin levels may appear to be normal or even elevated in some noninsulin-dependent diabetics. The presence of apparently normal amounts of insulin is partly related to the fact that control groups of equivalent body weight have not always been used to evaluate the appropriateness of the insulin response; but, which is more important, the insulin levels have not been compared at matched glucose levels (see below). To confuse the issue further, insulin secretory responses to a variety of nonglucose stimulants are apparently normal in many NIDDM patients. Thus, if fasting plasma glucose is less than 200 mg/dl, most of these patients have apparently normal basal insulin levels for body weight and normal insulin responses to intravenous arginine, secretin, isoproterenol, and tolbutamide (109). Only an abnormal response to intravenous glucose can be consistently demonstrated. However, it is now recognized that the basal insulin levels and responses to nonglucose stimulants are only "normal" because of the associated hyperglycemia. Thus at *matched* glucose levels there is a severe reduction of basal insulin secretion and the insulin responses to all nonglucose secretagogues. The hyperglycemia compensates for a reduced basal glucose sensitivity of the islet B cell and impaired response to the nonglucose inputs and provides the apparently "normal" insulin level observed (100). Because of this defect in glucose sensing, any metabolic change that tends to impair insulin action or accelerate hepatic glucose production will be more effective in elevating glucose in NIDDM patients because it would require a greater degree of hyperglycemia to compensate for the increase in insulin demand. In addition, it has now become apparent that islet B cells are probably more sensitive to the inhibitory actions of epinephrine in NIDDM because the ability of epinephrine to impair islet function is also sensitive to glucose (110). Thus, in normal individuals, the initial suppression of basal insulin by EPI is reversed by the hyperglycemia produced by EPI. This restores basal insulin secretory rates to pretreatment levels and modulates the hyperglycemia induced by epinephrine. In patients with NIDDM, much greater degrees of hyperglycemia are required to overcome the inhibitory effects of EPI. Thus, the same amount of stress hormone during baroreceptor, chemoreceptor, pain receptor, or psychological stimulation would be expected to produce greater increments of glycemia in patients with NIDDM. These impairments of the islet responses to glucose, with their attendant effects on the sensitivity of islet B cells to nonglucose stimulants, probably explains why some patients with NIDDM develop ketoacidosis during stress due to burn, trauma, surgery, or vascular occlusive events and require insulin treatment transiently (91). Not only is there increased mobilization of fatty acids by stress hormones but there is also a simultaneous exaggerated impairment of insulin secretion. After the stress activation of the autonomic nervous system is over and counterregulatory hormone levels decline, these same patients may then be able to maintain reasonable blood sugar levels with the usual diet or oral drug therapy.

Chronic Glucose Control

In patients with NIDDM, plasma glucose levels are reregulated to a stable level greater than in the normal population. The usual regulatory mechanisms for maintaining a constant plasma glucose level are present, although impaired. That is, the B cell still secretes insulin and it responds to glucose, but the capacity of the B cell to respond to glucose is reduced. Therefore any nutrient challenge or challenge from an increased output of counterregulatory hormones will result in greater degrees of hyperglycemia for longer periods of time. But, just as in the normal individual, these mechanisms will tend to stabilize plasma glucose levels even during stress. Thus, with mild forms of stress, the reregulated plasma glucose level will tend to remain constant.

The degree to which hyperglycemia will be increased by a particular stress in a patient with NIDDM is difficult to predict. It will depend on the sensitivity of that individual to all of the stress-related hormones, the basic nature of his or her islet impairment, and the responsiveness of the counterregulatory hormones to the stressful event. Very little is known about changes in sensitivity or responsiveness of this neuroendocrine regulatory system in patients with NIDDM. Nevertheless, since glucose sensitivity of the islet is clearly impaired and many of these subjects are insulin-resistant to begin with, it seems clear that greater degrees of glycemic increments are going to occur if the stress produces similar elevations in stress hormones. This sensitivity will presumably depend on the degree of hyperglycemia prior to the stressful event. Therefore, individuals under relatively poor control will be expected to become much worse and perhaps be unable to reregulate if volume depletion occurs due to the increased glycosuria. This may then lead to a vicious circle in which stress leads to glycosuria, which increases stress and leads to more hyperglycemia. This positive feedback presumably explains the development of ketoacidosis during sepsis, trauma, and/or surgical interventions, in patients with relatively poorly controlled NIDDM. On the other hand, the use of oral hypoglycemic agents to lower plasma glucose levels and improve islet function and peripheral sensitivity to insulin results in a patient who has reregulated his or her plasma glucose level to a more normal value. In this case, it has been the general experience that maintaining the individual on oral agents allows for reasonable responses to the modest stress associated with elective surgical procedures without the need to switch to insulin. However, in any patient a severe episode of bacterial sepsis or myocardial infarction, burn, major trauma or other stress may lead to a stress response that overwhelms the islet and produces a stimulus beyond the ability of the impaired islet to counteract. Thus, severe degrees of hyperglycemia and ketoacidosis are not uncommon in NIDDM during stress. It has been a general clinical impression that psychological factors also play a role in day-to-day blood sugar levels. However, documentation of this belief and identification of the specific hormone mechanisms which might be involved remain for the future.

REFERENCES

1. Exton JH. Mechanisms of hormonal regulation of hepatic glucose metabolism. Diabetes Metab. Rev 1987; 3(1):163–183.
2. Silverberg AB, Shah SD, Haymond MW, Cryer PE. Norepinephrine:hormone and neurotransmitter in man. Am J Physiol 1978; 234 (Endocrinol Metab Gastrointest Physiol 3):E252–256.
3. Hartmann H, Beckh K, Jungermann D. Direct control of glycogen metabolism in the perfused rat liver by the sympathetic innervation. Eur J Biochem 1982; 123:521–526.
4. Edwards AV. The hyperglycemic response to stimulation of the hepatic sympathetic innervation in adrenalectomized cats and dogs. J Physiol London 1972; 220:697–710.
5. Seydoux J, Brunsmann MJA, Jeanrenaud B, Girardier L. a-Sympathetic control of glucose output of mouse liver perfused in situ. Am J Physiol 1979; 236 (Endocrinol Metab Gastrointest Physiol 5):E323–E327.

6. Havel PJ, Veith RC, Dunning BE, Taborsky GJ Jr. Pancreatic noradrenergic nerves are activated by neuroglucopenia but not by hypotension or hypoxia in the dog: evidence for stress-specific and regionally-selective activation of the sympathetic nevous system. J Clin Invest 1988; 82:1538–1545.
7. Winder WW, Beattie MA, Picquette C, Holman RT. Decrease in liver norepinephrine in response to exercise and hypoglycemia. Am J Physiol 1983; 244:R845–R849.
8. Lautt WW, Divan PD, Singh RR. Control of the hyperglycemic response to hemorrhage in cats. Can J Physiol Pharmacol 1982; 60:1618–1623.
9. Sonne B, Mikines KJ, Richter EA, Christensen NJ, Galbo H. Role of liver nerves and adrenal medulla in glucose turnover of running rats. J Appl Physiol 1985; 59(5):1640–1646.
10. Lundberg JM, Pernow J, Lacroix JS. Neuropeptide Y: sympathetic cotransmitter and modulator? NIPS 1989; 4:13–17.
11. Pernow J. Co-release and functional interactions of neuropeptide Y and noradrenaline in peripheral sympathetic vascular control. Acta Physiol Scand 1988; 133, Suppl. 568:1–56.
12. Dunning BE, Taborsky GJ Jr. Galanin: sympathetic neurotransmitter in endocrine pancreas? Diabetes 1988; 37(9):1157–1162.
13. Dunning BE, Taborsky GJ Jr. Galanin release during pancreatic nerve stimulation is sufficient to influence islet function. Am J Physiol 1989; 256:E191–198.
14. Dunning BE, Havel PJ, Veith RC, Taborsky GJ Jr. Pancreatic and extrapancreatic galanin release during sympathetic neural activation. Am J. Physiol 1990; 258:E436–444.
15. Dunning BE, Karlsson S, Ahren B. Galanin contributes to stress-induced inhibition of insulin secretion in swimming mice. Diabetes 1989; 38(2): 48A.
16. Hems DA, Whitton PD. Stimulation by vasopressin of glycogen breakdown and gluconeogenesis in the perfused rat liver. Biochem J 1973; 136:705–709.
17. Litosch I, Lin SH, Fain JN. Rapid changes in hepatocyte phosphoinositides induced by vasopressin. J Biol Chem 1983; 258:13727–13732.
18. Cherrington AD, Stevenson RW, Steiner KE, et al. Insulin, glucagon, and glucose as regulators of hepatic glucose uptake and production in vivo. Diabetes Metab Rev 1987; 3(1):307–332.
19. Rizza RA, Mandarino LJ, Gerich JE. Effects of growth hormone on insulin action in man. Mechanisms of insulin resistance, impaired suppression of glucose production, and impaired stimulation of glucose utilization. Diabetes 1982; 31:663–669.
20. Press M. Growth hormone and metabolism. Diabetes Metab Rev 1988; 4: 391–414.
21. Rizza R, Mandarino L, Gerich J. Cortisol-induced insulin resistance in man: impaired suppression of glucose production and stimulation of glucose utilization due to a post-receptor defect of insulin action. J Clin Endocrinol Metab 1982; 54:131–138.

22. McMahon M, Gerich J, Rizza R. Effects of glucocorticoids on carbohydrate metabolism. Diabetes Metab Rev 1988; 4:17-30.
23. Shamoon H, Hendler R, Sherwin R. Synergistic interaction among anti-insulin hormones in the pathogenesis of stress hyperglycemia in humans. J Clin Endocrinol Metab 1981; 52:1235-1241.
24. Eigler N, Sacca L, Sherwin RS. Synergistic interactions of physiologic increments of glucagon, epinephrine, and cortisol in the dog: a model for stress-induced hyperglycemia. J Clin Invest 1979; 63:114-123.
25. Barseghian C, Levine R. Effect of corticosterone on insulin and glucagon secretion by the isolated perfused rat pancreas. Endocrinology 1980; 106: 547-552.
26. Abramson EA, Arky RA. Role of beta-adrenergic receptors in counterregulation to insulin-induced hypoglycemia. Diabetes 1968; 17:141-146.
27. Gerich JE. Glucose counterregulation and its impact on diabetes mellitus. Diabetes 1988; 37:1608-1617.
28. Taborsky GJ Jr, Halter JB, Baum D, Best JD, Porte D Jr. Pentobarbital anesthesia suppresses basal and 2-deoxy-D-glucose-stimulated plasma catecholamines. Am J Physiol 1984; 247:R905-R910.
29. Havel PJ, Flatness DE, Halter JB, Best JD, Veith RC, Taborsky GJ Jr. Halothane anesthesia does not suppress sympathetic activation produced by neuroglucopenia. Am J Physiol 1987; 252:E667-E672.
30. Taborsky GJ Jr, Halter JB, Porte D Jr. Morphine suppresses plasma catecholamine responses to laparotomy but not to 2-deoxyglucose. Am J Physiol 1982; 242:E317-E322.
31. Selkoe DJ, Myers RE. Neurologic and cardiovascular effects of hypotension in the monkey. Stroke 1979; 10(2):147-157.
32. Zierott G, Pappova E, Lundsgaard-Hansen P. Combined adrenergic blockade in experimental hemorrhagic hypotension. Pflugers Arch 1969; 24:310 (1):1-15.
33. Carey LC, Cloutier CT, Lowery BD. Growth hormone and adrenal cortical response to shock and trauma in the human. Ann Surg 1971; 174(3):451-460.
34. Taylor SH, Saxton C, Majid PA, Dykes JR, Ghosh P, Stoker JB. Insulin secretion following myocardial infarction with particular respect to the pathogenesis of cardiogenic shock. Lancet 1969; 27:2(635):1373-1378.
35. Järhult J, Holmberg J, Lundvall J. Reflex plasma hyperglycemia and hyperosmolality evoked by unloading of the carotid baroreceptors. Acta Physiol Scand 1977; 101(1):105-111.
36. Carey LC, Cloutier CT, Lowery BD. Blood sugar and insulin response of humans in shock. Ann Surg 1970; 172:342.
37. Lindsey CA, Faloona GR, Unver RH. Plasma glucagon levels during rapid exsanguination with and without adrenergic blockade. Diabetes 1975; 24 (4):313-316.
38. Hiebert JM, Kieler C, Soeldner JS, Egdahl RH. Species differences in insulin secretory responses during hemorrhagic shock. Surgery 1976; 79(4):451-455.

39. Järhult J, Holmberg J, Lundvall J, Mellander S. Hyperglycemic and hyperosmolar responses to graded hemorrhage. Acta Physiol Scand 1976; 97(4): 470–475.
40. Savaki HE, Macpherson H, McCulloch J. Alterations in local cerebral glucose utilization during hemorrhagic hypotension in the rat. Circ Res 1982; 50(5):633–644.
41. Järhult J, Falck Bengt F, Ingemansson S, Anders N. The functional importance of sympathetic nerves to the liver and endocrine pancreas. Ann Surg 1978; 2:96–100.
42. Lautt WW. Afferent and efferent neural roles in liver function. Prog Neurobiol 1983; 21:323–348.
43. Dunning BE, Moltz JH, Fawcett CP. Actions of neurohypophysial hormones on pancreatic hormone release. Am J Physiol 1984; 246:E108–E114.
44. Zerbe RL, Feurstein G, Kopin IJ. Effect of captopril on cardiovascular, sympathetic and vasopressin responses to hemorrhage. Eur J Pharmacol 1981; 72:391–395.
45. Dunning BE, Verbalis JG, Fawcett CP. Evidence for participation of the neurohypophysial hormones in the hyperglucagonemic response to hemorrhage in the rat. Neuroendocrinology 1985; 41:385–389.
46. Baum D, Porte D Jr. Stress hyperglycemia and the adrenergic regulation of pancreatic hormones in hypoxia. Metabolism 1980; 29(11 Suppl 1):1176–1185.
47. Bouissou P, Peronnet F, Brisson G, Helie R, Ledoux M. Metabolic and endocrine responses to graded exercise under acute hypoxia. Eur J Appl Physiol 1986; 55:(3):290–294.
48. Baum D, Griepp R, Porte D Jr. Glucose-induced insulin release during acute and chronic hypoxia. Am J Physiol 1979; 237(1):E45–E50.
49. Baum D, Porte D Jr, Ensinck J. Hyperglucahonemia and a-adrenergic receptor in acute hypoxia. Am J Physiol 1979; 237:E404–408.
50. Baum D, Porte D Jr. Beta adrenergic receptor dysfunction in hypoxic inhibition of insulin release. Endocrinology 1976; 98:359–366.
51. Baum D. The inhibition of norepinephrine-stimulated lipolysis by acute hypoxia. J Pharmacol Exp Ther 1969; 169:87–94.
52. Jones CT, Roebuck MM, Walker DW, Johnston BM. The role of the adrenal medulla and peripheral sympathetic nerves in the physiological responses of the fetal sheep to hypoxia. J Dev Physiol 1988; 10:17–36.
53. Mlekusch W, Paletta B, Truppe W, Paschke E, Grimus R. Plasma concentrations of glucose, corticosterone, glucagon and insulin and liver content of metabolic substrates and enzymes during starvation and additional hypoxia in the rat. Horm Metab Res 1981; 13:612–614.
54. Baum D, Dillard DH, Porte D Jr. Inhibition of insulin release in infants undergoing deep hypothermic cardiovascular surgery. N Engl J Med 1968; 12:279(24):1309–1314.
55. Shida H, Morimoto M, Inokawa K, Tsugane J. Studies on lipid and carbohydrate metabolism during surface-induced deep hypothermia with circulatory arrest for open-heart surgery. Jpn J Surg 1977; 12:7(4):211–216.

56. Helman A, Gilbert M, Pfister-Lemaire N, Reach G, Assan R. Glucagon and insulin secretion and their biological activities in hypothermic rats. Endocrinology 1984; 115(5):1722-1728.
57. Kuntschen FR, Galletti PM, Hahn C. Glucose-insulin interactions during cardiopulmonary bypass. Hypothermia versus normothermia. J Thorac Cardiovasc Surg 1986; 91(3):451-459.
58. Baum D, Porte D Jr. Alpha-adrenergic inhibition of immunoreactive insulin release during deep hypothermia. Am J Physiol 1971; 221(1):303-311.
59. Therminarias A, Pellerei E. Plasma catecholamine and metabolic changes during cooling and rewarming in dogs. Exp Biol 1987; 47 (2):117-123.
60. Wang LC, Peter RP. Changes in plasma glucose, FFA, corticosterone, and thyroxine in He-02-induced hypothermia. J Appl Physiol 1977; 42(5):694-698.
61. Wolfe RR, Burke JF. Glucose and lactate metabolism in experimental septic shock. Am J Physiol 1978; 235(5):R219-R227.
62. Hargrove DM, Bagby GJ, Lang CH, Spitzer JJ. Adrenergic blockade does not abolish elevated glucose turnover during bacterial infection. Am J Physiol 1988; 254:E16-E22.
63. Durkot MJ, Wolfe RR. Effects of adrenergic blockade on glucose kinetics on septic and burned guinea pigs. Am J Physiol 1981; 241:R222-227.
64. Wolfe RR, Shaw JHF. Glucose and FFA kinetics in sepsis: role of glucagon and sympathetic nervous system activity. Am J Physiol 1985; 248:E236-E243.
65. Hinshaw LB. The role of glucose in endotoxin shock. Circ Shock 1976; 3:1-10.
66. Hinshaw LB, Peyton MD, Archer LT, Black MR, Coalson JJ, Greenfield LJ. Prevention of death in endotoxin shock by glucose administration. Surg Gynecol Obstet 1974; 139:851-859.
67. Vaughan GM, Becker RA, Unger RH, et al. Nonthyroidal control of metabolism after burn injury: possible role of glucagon. Metabolism 1985; 34:637-641.
68. Wolfe RR, Durkot MJ. Evaluation of the role of the sympathetic nervous system in the response of substrate kinetics and oxidation to burn injury. Circ Shock 1982; 9:395-406.
69. Durkot MJ, Wolfe RR. Effects of adrenergic blockade on glucose kinetics in septic and burned guinea pigs. Am J Physiol 1981; 241:R222-R227.
70. Jahoor F, Herndon DN, Wolfe RR. Role of insulin and glucagon in the response of glucose and alanine kinetics in burn-injured patients. J Clin Invest 1986; 78:807-814.
71. Lang C, Dobrescu C. Attenuation of burn-induced changes in hemodynamics and glucose metabolism by the PAF antagonist SRI 63-675. J Pharmacol 1988; 156:207-214.
72. Morgan R, Martyn JAJ, Philbin D, Coggins, C, Burke J. Water metabolism and antidiuretic hormone (ADH) response following thermal injury. J Trauma 1980; 20:468-472.

73. Shuck JG, Eaton RP, Shuck LW, Wachtel TL, Schade DS. Dynamics of insulin and glucagon secretions in severely burned patients. Trauma 1977; 17:706–713.
74. Wolfe RR. Acute versus chronic response to burn injury. Circ Shock 1981; 8:105.
75. Palmer J, Lernmark A. Pathophysiology of type I (insulin-dependent) diabetes. In: Rifkin H, Porte D Jr, eds. Diabetes mellitus theory and practice, 4th ed. 1990 pp 414–435.
76. Tarn AC, Smith CP, Spencer KM, Bottazzo GF, Gale EAM. Type I (insulidependent) diabetes: a disease of slow clinical onset? Br Med J 1987; 294:342–345.
77. Srikanta S, Ganda OP, Gleason RE, et al. Pre-type I diabetes: linear loss of beta cell response to intravenous glucose. Diabetes 1984; 33:717–720.
78. Nerup J, Mandrup-Poulson T, Mølvig J, Helqvist S, Wogensen L, Egeberg J. Mechanisms of pancreatic β-cell destruction in type I diabetes. Diabetes Care 1988; 11 (Suppl 1):16–23.
79. Bradley LM, Mishell RI. Differential effects of glucocorticosteroids on the functions of helper and suppressor T lymphocytes. Proc Natl Acad Sci 1981; 78(5):3155–3159.
80. Mazelis AG, Albert D, Crisa C, et al. Relationship of stressful housing conditions to the onset of diabetes mellitus induced by multiple, sub-diabetogenic doses of streptozotocin in mice. Diabetes Res 1987; 6:195–200.
81. Harada M, Makino S. Promotion of spontaneous diabetes in nonobese diabetes-prone mice by cyclophosphamide. Diabetologia 1982; 27:604–606.
82. Juenaga K, Yoon JW. Association of β-cell-specific expression of endogenous retrovirus with development of insulitis and diabetes in NOD mouse. Diabetes 1988; 37:1722–1726.
83. Charlton B, Bacelj A, Slattery RM, Mandel TE. Evidence for suppression in spontaneous autoimmune diabetes mellitus. Diabetes 1989; 38:441–447.
84. Spinas GA, Palmer JP, Mandrup-Poulsen T, Andersen HI, Nielson JH, Nerup J. The bimodal effect of interleukin-1 on rat pancreatic beta-cells—stimulation followed by inhibition—depends upon dose, duration of exposure and ambient glucose concentration. Diabetologia 1988; 31:168–174.
85. West DB, Seino Y, Woods SC, Porte D Jr. Ventromedial hypothalamic lesions increase pancreatic sensitivity to streptozotocin in rats. Diabetes 1980; 29:948–951.
86. Block CA, Paed FC, Clemons SAP, Sperling MA. Puberty decreases insulin sensitivity. J Pediatr 1987; 110:481–487.
87. Capponi R, Kawada ME, Varela C, Vargas L. Diabetes mellitus by repeated stress in rats bearing chemical diabetes. Horm Metab Res 1980; 12:411–412.
88. Robinson N, Fuller JH. Role of life events and difficulties in the onset of diabetes mellitus. J Psycho Res 1985; 29(6):583–591.
89. Porte D Jr, Robertson RP. Control of insulin secretion by catecholamines, stress, and the sympathetic nervous system. Fed Proc 1973; 32:1792–1798.

90. Waldhausl W, Kleinberger G, Korn A, et al. Severe hyperglycemia effects of rehydration on endocrine derangements and blood glucose concentrations. Diabetes 1979; 28:577–584.

91. Porte D Jr. Sympathetic regulation of insulin secretion and its relation to diabetes mellitus. Arch Intern Med 1969; 123:252.

92. Hinkle LE, Wolf S. A summary of experimental evidence relating life stress to diabetes mellitus. J Mt Sinai Hosp 1953; 19(4):537–570.

93. Hinkle LE, Conger GB, Wolf S. Studies on diabetes mellitus: the relation of stressful life situations to the concentration of ketone bodies in the blood of diabetic and nondiabetic humans. J Clin Invest 1950; 29:754–769.

94. Baker L, Barcai A, Kaye R, et al. Beta adrenergic blockade and juvenile diabetes: acute studies and long-term therapeutic trial. Evidence for the role of catecholamines in mediating diabetic decompensation following emotional arousal. J Pediatr 1969; 75:19–29.

95. Shamoon H, Hendler R, Sherwin RS. Altered responsiveness to cortisol, epinephrine, and glucagon in insulin-infused juvenile-onset diabetes. Diabetes 1980; 29:284–291.

96. Christensen NJ. Catecholamines and diabetes mellitus. Diabetologia 1979; 16:211–224.

97. Mazze RS, Lucido D, Shamoon H. Psychological and social correlates of glycemic control. Diabetes Care 1979; 7:360–366.

98. Hanson SL, Pichert JW. Perceived stress and diabetes control in adolescents. Health Psychol 1986; 5:439–452.

99. Drash AL, Becker DJ. Behavioral issues in patients with diabetes mellitus with special emphasis on the child and adolescent. In: Rifkin H, Porte D Jr, eds. Diabetes Mellitus Theory and Practice, 4th ed, 1990, pp. 922–934.

100. Kahn SE, Porte D Jr. The pathophysiology of type II (non-insulin dependent) diabetes mellitus: implications for treatment. In: Rifkin H, Porte D Jr, eds. Diabetes Mellitus Theory and Practice, 4th ed, 1990; pp. 436–456.

101. Porte D Jr, Robertson RP, Halter JB, et al. Neuroendocrine recognition of glucose: the glucoreceptor hypothesis and the diabetic syndrome. In: Katsuki Sato M, Takagi SF, Oomura Y, eds. International symposium on food intake and chemical senses. Tokyo: University of Tokyo Press, 1977: 331–342.

102. Robertson RP, Halter JB, Porte D Jr. A role for alpha adrenergic receptors in abnormal insulin secretion in diabetes mellitus. J Clin Invest 1976; 57:791–795.

103. Kawazu S, Suzuki K, Negishi T, Ishii J. Studies of midaglizole (DG-5128). Diabetes 1987; 36:216–220.

104. Surwit RS, Feinglos MN, Livingston EG, Kuhn CM, McCubbin JA. Behavioral manipulation of the diabetic phenotype in ob/ob mice. Diabetes 1984; 33:616–618.

105. Surwit RS, Feinglos MN. Stress and autonomic nervous system in type II diabetes. Diabetes Care 1988; 11:1 83–85.

106. Robertson RP, Chen M. A role for prostaglandin E2 in defective insulin secretion and carbohydrate intolerance in diabetes mellitus. J Clin Invest 1977;60:747–753.

107. Pyke DA. Diabetes: the genetic connections. Diabetologia 1979;17:333–343.

108. Taborsky GJ, Porte D Jr. Endogenous hyperglycemia restores insulin release impaired by somatostatin analogue. Am J Physiol 1981; 240: E407–E413.

109. Pfeifer MA, Halter JB, Porte D Jr. Insulin secretion in diabetes mellitus. Am J Med 1980; 70:579–588.

110. Halter JB, Beard JC, Porte D Jr. Islet function and stress hyperglycemia: plasma glucose and epineprhine interaction. Am J Physiol 1984; 247: E47–E52.

25

EFFECT OF STRESS ON GASTRIC ULCER FORMATION

YVETTE TACHÉ

*Veterans' Administration Medical Center and University of
California School of Medicine, Los Angeles, California*

Selye's publication (1) describing "a syndrome produced by diverse nocuous agents" brought the first experimental evidence in 1936 that exposure to various "noxious stimuli" elicits acute gastric mucosal lesions. Furthermore, Selye established that gastric injury along with adrenal hypertrophy and thymolymphatic involution were characteristic bodily responses to what he defined as the "stress syndrome" (2). These pioneer observations stimulated numerous investigations on the pathogenesis and treatments of stress ulcers (2–4).

This chapter will focus on the various experimental models used to cause stress-related gastric lesions and how they relate to human pathological conditions. The pathophysiological mechanisms involved in stress ulcer formation will be outlined, with special emphasis on the role of the central nervous system (CNS).

EXPERIMENTAL MODELS OF STRESS ULCERS

Gastric Ulcers Induced by Exposure to Physical Stressors

Since Selye's original observations, a plethora of experimental models have been developed mainly in the rat to produce acutely stress-related gastric ulcers. Gastric mucosal lesions have been initially induced by a wide variety of stressful physical procedures such as restraint combined with cold exposure or immersion in water at $23°C$ (5,6), prolonged motor activity by swimming or running through an exercise wheel (7), inescapable and unpredictable or predictable tail or foot shocks (8), trauma such as spinal cord transection (9). Hemorrhagic shock (10), or 40% burn (2). Prior to the application of all these stressors, a necessary prerequisite to inducing gastric pathological conditions is a period of starvation ensuring emptiness of the stomach (6,11). Among these different experimental models, the most widely used to study the pathogenesis and the antiulcer effects of drugs are the water immersion or cold restraint stress (4) and hemorrhagic shocks (10).

Gastric Ulcers Induced by Exposure to Psychological Stressors

The ulcerogenic effect of psychological stressors has been clearly established in experimental animals using nonphysical, emotional stimuli such as conflict situations (12). Ichimura et al. (13,14) described a model based on visual, olfactory, and auditory distress communications sent to untreated mice through a communication box by mice exposed to foot shock. Such a paradigm causes gastric lesions in both groups. Mine et al. (15) reported the formation of gastric hemorrhagic erosions in a nontreated, nonfasted rat following 1 h exposure to a rat made aggressive by intracerebroventricular injection of 6-hydroxydopamine followed by 1 month of isolated housing and continuous tail pinching during the pair-housing with the nontreated, nonfasted rats.

CHARACTERISTICS OF STRESS ULCERS
Morphological Features

Gastric hemorrhagic lesions developed within 1-6 h of exposure to the stressors described above, except in the shock paradigm model, which required a minimum of 2 h rest period in the home cage at the end of stress application (16). Histological examination of the gastric mucosa revealed that all these procedures cause essentially similar gastric damage consisting of acute, superficial, punctuated or elongated, hemorrhagic mucosal erosions, localized mainly in the glandular portion of the stomach (5). Because these gastric lesions rarely penetrate the muscularis mucosa layer, as such, they are not true gastric ulcers. Scanning electromicroscopic studies revealed, within 30 min of stress, exposure, extensive damage to the apical membranes of the surface epithelial cells occurring prior to the initiation of macroscopically visible hemorrhagic lesions (5). The epithelial cells exfoliate to expose the lamina propria (5). Takeuchi et al. (17) reported that pyloric ligation combined with water immersion restraint modify the features of gastric ulcers. The formation of the lesions extends to the antrum as well as the corpus and can penetrate the muscularis mucosa (17).

Incidence

The occurrence of gastric ulcerations produced by stress is influenced by several factors recently reviewed by Pare (4), including genetic factors (18,19) and age. Rats 130 days old develop more gastric ulcers in response to cold restraint or water restraint than 45-day-old rats (20). Other factors include circadian variations shown by a peak incidence of gastric lesions during the dark period (21). Dietary influence has been demonstrated in studies showing that dietary deprivation of linoleic acid (polyunsaturated fatty acid involved in the biosynthesis of prostaglandin) increases the occurrence of stress-induced gastric lesions. Conversely, rats fed a diet enriched with linoleic acid have reduced cold restraint stress ulcers (22). These effects are mediated through modulation of prostaglandin levels (22). Intragastric hyperosmolar glucose prevents stress ulceration by a mechanism unrelated to prostaglandin pathways (23). The outcome of gastric ulcerations is also related to the stressors used (4,20) as well as developmental or environmental variables. For instance, early weaning (15 instead of 21 days) increases susceptibility to ulcer formation in response to restraint or activity stress (7,24,25) and early handling influences the ulcerogenic response to restraint (26). Repeated exposures to mild stressors in adult rats provide a partial immunity to subsequent similar ulcerogenic procedure, although some cross-protection with other stressors has also been observed (27).

Clinical Correlation

The closest correlation between experimental acute gastric damage elicited by exposure to physical or psychological stressors and a clinical disease is the human stress ulcer rather than peptic ulcer disease. However, recent studies indicate that peptic ulcer disease tends to be correlated with stressful life events and psychosocial factors (28). Stress ulcers in humans closely simulate morphologically acute stress-related experimental gastropathy and consist of multiple erosive lesions with various depths of penetration in the mucosa localized in the acid–peptic secreting portion of the stomach. They occur in patients who experienced episode of shocks related to hemorrhage or sepsis or other stressful conditions including trauma, surgery, extensive thermal or neurological injury, or serious illnesses (29–31). Progression or coalescence of these lesions, in the absence of treatment, can result in acute hemorrhagic gastritis and massive bleeding of life-threatening severity.

ROLE OF THE CENTRAL NERVOUS SYSTEM IN THE PATHOGENESIS OF EXPERIMENTAL STRESS ULCERS

Surgical and Electrophysiological Evidence

The central nervous system has long been suspected of being implicated in the development of gastric ulceration. Schiff in 1867 (32) and Brown-Sequard in

1876 (33) showed that cerebral lesions were associated with gastric ulcerations in experimental animals. Initial clinical observations by Cushing in 1932 (34) indicated a high incidence of gastritis in patients with head injury, cerebral stroke, or tumor. Since then, numerous investigations using electrical stimulation or lesions of discrete brain area targeted by stereotactic approach pointed out the telencephalic limbic system, inclusive of the hypothalamus, as neuroanatomical substrates in the formation of gastric ulcers (35-37). In nonrestrained or restrained rats, gastric ulcers have been induced or aggravated by acute electrical lesions of the posterior cingulate and enthorhinal cortex (38), hippocampus (38), median raphe nucleus (40), lateral hypothalamus (39,41) or ventral tegmental area (42) and by electrical stimulation of the medial and centromedial amygdala (43) or paraventricular nucleus (44). Electrical lesions of the centromedial amygdala or ventroamygdalofugal pathways or electrical stimulation of the medial forebrain bundle-posterior hypothalamus attenuate the incidence of gastric ulcers elicited by stress or lateral hypothalamic lesions (41,45). These and other findings have allowed us to establish a correlation between amygdalar activity and susceptibility to stress ulceration (43).

Pharmacological Evidence

Psychoactive Drugs

A CNS component in stress-induced gastric ulceration was further demonstrated using pharmacological approach. Centrally active drugs including antidepressants, sedatives, hypnotics, and antipsychotics were first shown to exert a protective effect against stress-related experimental ulcers (46). Now it is well established that pentobarbital, imipramine, chlorpromazine, chlorbenzoxamine, meprobamate, diazepam, and other central benzodiazepan receptor agonists, clcnazepam, lorazepam, oxazolam, and chlordiazepoxide protect against restraint-induced ulcers (4,14,47,48).

Brain Peptides

The recognition that specific brain nuclei identified by electrical stimulation or lesioning and psychoactive drugs influence the formation of stress ulceration has triggered investigations to elucidate biochemical substrates in the brain mediating or influencing stress-related gastric lesions. Recent studies have shown that specific peptides act in the brain to induce, promote, or prevent gastric ulcer formation in the rat (49,50). In particular, convergent information indicates that brain thyrotropin-releasing factor (TRH) may be involved in mediating gastric ulcers induced by cold restraint stress.

ROLE OF BRAIN TRH IN MEDIATING COLD RESTRAINT STRESS-INDUCED GASTRIC EROSIONS Gastric hemorrhagic erosions can be rapidly induced by injection into the cerebrospinal fluid of TRH or various stable TRH analogs such as RX 77368 or DN-1417 in 24 h fasted rats (51-53). The stable analogs are more potent than TRH to induce gastric pathological lesions (51, 52). Lesions are visible within 2 h and maximal at 4-6 h after injection (51-53) and are similar macroscopically and histologically to those elicited by stress (51, 53). The effect of TRH is CNS mediated since the intravenous route of administration is ineffective (51-53) and peptide specific, as shown by the inactivity of a number of other neuropeptides tested under the same conditions, including growth hormone releasing factor, corticotropin-releasing factor (CRF), bombesin, neurotensin, somatostatin, substance P, calcitonin, calcitonin gene-related peptide (CGRP), and opioid peptides (49). Specific brain sites on which TRH acts to trigger ulcer formation have been localized in the central amygdala and dorsal motor nucleus (43,54).

The neural mechanisms through which central TRH induces gastric ulcerations appear to be related to increased parasympathetic activity (55). This contention is supported by the fact that injection of TRH into the cerebrospinal fluid or the dorsal vagal complex enhanced the parasympathetic outflow from the cervical and gastric branches of the vagus (56,57). Electrical stimulation of the vagus nerve induced similar gastric lesions (58). Moreover, peripheral blockade of cholinergic muscarinic receptors, unlike blockade of dopaminergic or adrenergic receptors, prevented the ulcerogenic effects of central injection of TRH or TRH analogues (51-53). CNS injection of TRH induces a vagally mediated and atropine-sensitive stimulation of gastric acid, pepsin, and serotonin secretion and contractility, and histamine release (55,59-62). Which of these alterations of gastric function by itself or in combination contributes to the development of gastric lesions remains to be established.

Neuroanatomical and functional findings have strengthened the concept that these neuropharmacological observations may have physiological relevance, particularly in relation to gastric ulcers elicited by cold restraint. High concentrations of TRH immunoreactivity and specific receptors have been localized in the dorsal vagal complex, nucleus ambiguus, and amygdala (63-66). TRH immunoreactivity in the dorsal vagal complex is mostly contained in nerve fibers arising from the raphe nucleus (64) and is correlated with preganglionic neurons contributing projections to the stomach (67,68). Further evidence for the role of brain TRH in this gastric lesion model is the finding that cold exposure is known to release brain TRH (69), and passive immunization with TRH antiserum injected intracerebroventricularly prevented gastric lesions elicited by cold restraint stress (70). Taken together, these studies suggest that the initiating neural pathways involved in cold restraint stress model may be related to the activation of the parasympathetic outflow to the stomach by medullary TRH (Fig. 1). To what extent medullary TRH may be involved as a final common pathway mediating the ulcerogenic response to other stressors needs to be investigated. Furthermore, these findings validate the use of TRH or stable TRH analog injections

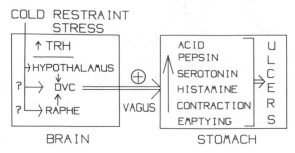

FIGURE 1 Possible role of brain TRH in cold-restraint stress-induced gastric lesions in rats. DVC, dorsal vagal complex; ?, pathways to be investigated.

into the CSF as a simple chemical method leading to acute gastric lesions. Such an experimental model represents a new relevant tool to explore both the central and peripheral mechanisms involved in the pathogenesis of cold restraint stress ulcers.

PEPTIDES ACTING IN THE BRAIN TO INHIBIT STRESS-INDUCED GASTRIC EROSIONS The influence of brain peptides over stress ulcer formation was first established in 1979 by the demonstration that bombesin injected into the CSF prevents cold restraint stress ulceration (71). Since then, a number of peptides, namely, calcitonin, CGRP, CRF, bombesin, opioid peptides, and neurotensin, have been shown to act in the brain to inhibit gastric lesions induced by cold restraint stress or central TRH when injected into the CSF (49, 72-74).

Previous neuropharmacological, physiological, and neuroanatomical studies have substantiated the fact that central CRF mediates in part the endocrine, behavioral, and autonomic responses to stress (75-79) and the alterations of gastrointestinal transit and gastric acid secretion induced by restraint or surgical stress in the rat (80-83). By contrast, existing evidence supports a protective rather than causative role of brain CRF in the ulcerogenic response to stress. Injection of CRF into the cerebrospinal fluid or the ventromedial hypothalamus did not induce gastric erosions in 24 h fasted rats (51,53,84). Furthermore, instead of acting synergistically with cold restraint to promote ulcer formation, central injection of CRF prevented the development of gastric erosions in cold-restraint-stressed rats (84,85).

Brain sites of action have been localized for some peptides and correlated with the distribution of peptide-immunoreactivity and receptors (49). For instance, microinjections of calcitonin or CRF into the ventromedial hypothalamic nucleus (84,86), calcitonin into the paraventricular nucleus or lateral hypothalamus (86), and neurotensin, β-endorphin and enkephalin analogs into the central amygdala (87,88) prevented or attenuated restraint or cold restraint stress ulcerations.

For most of these peptides, the central mechanism of their action is still poorly understood. The prevention of cold restraint gastric ulcers elicited by neurotensin microinjected in the central amygdala required integrity of the dopaminergic system (87). This and other studies using pharmacological approaches have suggested that neurotensin action involves an interaction with central dopamine (87,89) and norepinephrine (90) pathways. Bombesin-induced inhibition of cold restraint stress may involve central interaction with TRH. Bombesin injected into the CSF blocks TRH release induced by cold (91) and simultaneous microinjection of bombesin with TRH in the dorsal motor nucleus prevented the stimulatory effect of TRH on gastric acid secretion (92,93).

The peripheral mechanisms by which these peptides prevent stress-related gastric lesions elicited by cold restraint may be related to the integrated changes in gastric secretory and motor function leading to the inhibition of aggressive factors together with stimulation of defensive factors. For instance, central injection of bombesin, CRF, calcitonin, or CGRP at dosages that prevent stress ulcer, inhibits gastric acid and pepsin secretion and high-amplitude gastric contractions, and stimulates gastric bicarbonate and mucus secretion (94,95).

The precise nature of the relationship between peptide activity in specific brain regions and gastric ulcer prevention remains to be further established through the use of specific antagonists. Henke et al. demonstrated that microinjection of the opiate antagonist naloxone into the central amygdala aggravates cold restraint stress ulcers, whereas injection of beta-endorphin or enkephalin analogue exerts a naloxone-reversible preventive effect (88). These results suggest a possible role of opioid peptides in the maintenance of gastric mucosal integrity. Brain CRF is released during stress (96) and triggers alterations in gastric secretory and motor function (82,95) for effective "coping" with the ulcerogenic effect of stress, and may play a modulatory role in the formation of stress lesions.

Brain Biogenic Amines

The possible role of central biogenic amines in stress ulceration has recently been reviewed by Hernandez et al. (97). Among the classic neurotransmitters, circumstantial evidence indicates that the dopaminergic system, mostly in the mesocorticolimbic system, exerts an inhibitory influence leading to the attenuation of stress ulcerogenesis (42). This is substantiated by several facts. Stress activates the brain dopamine system (97). Injection of dopamine into the amygdala protects against cold-restraint gastric ulcers in rats (87), whereas dopamine depletion by neurotoxin or dopamine receptor blockade has the opposite effect (42,87). Lesions of the ventral tegmental area, which contains dopamine cell bodies projecting to the mesocorticolimbic system, induced or aggravated ulcer formation (42). Moreover, dopaminergic mechanisms have been implicated in the antiulcerogenic effect of central neurotensin (87,98).

Some evidence also supports the likelihood that brain norepinephrine pathways are implicated in stress ulceration. Acute stress restraint decreases norepinephrine levels and increases its turnover mostly in the hypothalamus (99). Selective depletion of brain noradrenergic pathways exacerbated stress ulcer formation (100), although opposite results have also been reported (101).

PERIPHERAL MECHANISMS INVOLVED IN STRESS ULCERATION

More than 50 years after Selye's recognition of stress ulcer formation, and despite being the focus of extensive investigations, the exact peripheral mechanisms and sequence of events leading to the formation of gastric ulceration remain poorly understood. Stress ulcer development is, however, now known to be related to interactions between various circulating or local pathogenic factors. Their relative importance and the interplay in causing these lesions are still to be further defined and may vary depending on the experimental model under study. All or part of such alterations as peripheral sympathetic and parasympathetic activation, stimulation of the pituitary–adrenal axis leading to the discharge of catecholamine and corticosterone, increased gastric acid, histamine and serotonin secretion, and high-amplitude gastric contractions, decreased gastric mucus or bicarbonate secretion and blood flow, disturbance of gastric mucosal microcirculation, inhibition of prostaglandins biosynthesis, formation of oxygen-derived free radicals, and deficit in mucosal energy metabolism, may contribute to ulcer formation.

The importance of acid in the pathogenesis of mucosal injury elicited by stress is clear in most models. While acid may be considered the sine qua non for stress ulcer genesis, several studies have clearly demonstrated that the presence of acid alone does not solely determine gastric ulceration. First, the increase in gastric acid secretion elicited by pentagastrin, histamine, or behanechol does not lead to ulcer formation (107,108). Second, most of the stressors except cold restraint induce a decrease rather than an increase in gastric acid secretion (109). The reduction of defensive factors such as prostaglandins, bicarbonate, and mucus secretion; inadequate microcirculation; and inhibition of cell renewal may play as major a role as aggressive factors (105). In particular, levels of four prostaglandins were found to be decreased by 70% in the immersion cold re-restraint stress model (104). Moreover, a reciprocal correlation exists between ulcer index and the activity of the enzyme phospholipase, which is involved in the biosynthesis of prostaglandin (104).

In hemorrhagic shock-induced gastric ulcers, oxygen-derived free radicals generated by reperfusion following ischemia appear to play an important role (10,88). They cause lipid peroxidation and damage to the cellular membranes and release of intracellular components such as lysosomal enzymes, leading to further damage by disruption of the interstitial matrix (88).

SUMMARY

The underlying central and peripheral mechanisms involved in stress gastric ulcer development and healing are still not fully understood despite intensive investigations using various experimental models of stress-related gastric ulcers. The cause is multifactorial, although the relative importance and sequential contribution of the various factors are not clearly established. The demonstration that specific peptides act centrally to induce or prevent stress ulceration has resulted in a recent surge of interest in studies of the CNS components involved in stress ulceration. Through the use of TRH, CRF, calcitonin, CGRP, neurotensin, and opioid peptides and their antagonists, when available, new insight has and will continue to be gained regarding brain sites, neural pathways, and peripheral mechanisms involved in stress ulcer formation. The characterization of such brain mechanisms may lead to new approaches to the treatment of stress ulcers.

ACKNOWLEDGMENTS

The author thanks David Claus for helping with the preparation of the manuscript. The author's work is supported by the National Institute of Mental Health Grant MH-00663 and the National Institute of Arthritis, Metabolism and Digestive Disease, Grants DK-33061 and 30110.

REFERENCES

1. Selye H. Syndrome produced by diverse nocuous agents. Nature 1936; 138:32.
2. Selye H. Theories. In Stress in health and disease. Boston, London: Butterworths, 1976: 928–1148.
3. Silen W. Experimental models of gastric ulceration and injury. Am J Physiol 1988;255:G395–G402.
4. Paré W P, Glavin G B. Restraint stress in biomedical research: a review. Neurosci Biobehav Rev 1986; 10;339–370.
5. Ohno T, Hirose N, Uramoto H, Ishihara T, Okabe S. Surface epithelial cell damage induced by restraint and water-immersion stress in rats effects of 16,16-dimethyl prostaglandin E2 on stress-induced gastric lesions. Jpn J Pharmacol 1986;45:405–415.
6. Senay E C, Levine R J. Synergism between cold and restraint for rapid production of stress ulcers in rats. Proc Soc Exp Biol Med 1967; 124:1221–1223.
7. Glavin G B, Paré W P. Early weaning predisposes rats to exacerbated activity-stress ulcer formation. Physiol Behav 1985; 34:907–909.
8. Garrick T, Minor T R, Buack S, Weiner H, Guth P. Predictable and unpredictable shock stimulates gastric contractility and causes mucosal injury in rats. Behav Neurosci 1989; 103:

9. MacLellan D G, Shulkes A, Hardy K J. Profile of gastric stress ulceration following acute cervical cord injury: an animal model. Aust NZ J Surg 1986; 56:499–504.

10. Wadhwa S S, Perry M A. Gastric injury induced by hemorrhage, local ischemia, and oxygen radial generation. Am J Physiol 1987; 253:G129–G133.

11. Mikhail A, Hirschberg J. Ulceration in the rat's forestomach: its reduction by non-nutritive bulky substances. Physiol Behav 1972; 8:769–770.

12. Sawrey W L, Weisz J D. An experimental method of producing gastric ulcers. J Comp Physiol Psychol 1956; 49:269–270.

13. Ichimaru Y, Gomita Y. A new screening method for anti-ulcer agents: psychological stress produced by intraspecies emotional communication. Pharmacology 1987; 34:176–180.

14. Ichimaru Y, Moriyama M, Gomita Y. Gastric lesions produced by conditioned emotional stimuli in the form of affective communication and effects of benzodiazepines. Life Sci 1984; 34:187–192.

15. Mine K, Nakagawa T, Fujiwara M, Ito Y, Kataoka Y, Watanabe S, Ueki S. A new experimental model of stress ulcers employing aggressive behavior in 6-OHDA-treated rats. Physiol Behav 1981; 27:715–721.

16. Desiderato O, MacKinnon J R, Hissom H. Development of gastric ulcers in rats following stress termination. J Comp Physiol Psychol 1974; 87:208–214.

17. Takeuchi K, Okabe S, Takagi K. A new model of stress ulcer in the rat with pylorus ligation and its pathogenesis. Am J Dig Dis 1976; 21:782–788.

18. Paré W P, Schimmel G T. Stress ulcer in normotensive and spontaneously hypertensive rats. Physiol Behav 1986; 36:699–705.

19. Glavin G B, Mikhail A A. Stress duration, gastric emptying, and ulcer development in three strains of rats. Biochem Med 1977; 18:58–63.

20. Paré W P. A comparison of two ulcerogenic techniques. Physiol Behav 1988; 44:417–420.

21. Waldrop R D, Rubin N H, MacLellan D G, Rayford P L, Thompson J C. Daily variations in the formation of gastric ulcers caused by cervical cord transection in the rat. Gastroenterology 1988; 94:1080–1082.

22. Schepp W, Steffen B, Ruoff H J, Schusdziarra V, Classen M. Modulation of rat gastric mucosal prostaglandin E2 release by dietary linoleic acid: effects on gastric acid secretion and stress-induced mucosal damage. Gastroenterology 1988; 95:18–25.

23. Ephgrave K, Horton J W, Burns D K. Hyperosmolar glucose prevents stress ulceration in the rat restraint model despite inhibition of endogenous prostaglandins. Surg Gynecol Obstet 1987; 164:9–16.

24. Ackerman S H. Premature weaning, thermoregulation, and the occurrence of gastric pathology. In: Weiner H, Hofer MA, Stunkard AJ, eds. Brain, behavior, and bodily disease. New York: Raven Press, 1981: 67–86.

25. Ackerman S H. Early life events and peptic ulcer susceptibility: an experimental model. Brain Res Bull 1980; 5 (Suppl.1):43–49.

26. Winokur G, Stern J, Taylor R. Early handling and group housing effect on development and response to stress in the rat. J Psychosom Res 1959; 4: 1-4.
27. Paré W P. Prior stress and susceptibility to stress ulcer. Physiol Behav 1986; 36:1155-1159.
28. Feldman M, Walker P, Green J L, Weingarden K. Life events stress and psychosocial factors in men with peptic ulcer disease. A multidimensional case-controlled study. Gastroenterology 1986; 91:1370-1379.
29. Skillman J J, Bushnell L S, Goldman H, Silen W. Respiratory failure, hypotension, sepsis, and jaundice. A clinical syndrome associated with lethal hemorrhage from acute stress ulceration of the stomach. Am J Surg 1969; 117:523-530.
30. Lucas C E, Sugawa C, Riddle J, Rector F, Rosenberg B, Walt A J. Natural history and surgical dilemma of "stress" gastric bleeding. Arch Surg 1971; 102:266-273.
31. Butterfield W C. Experimental stress ulcers: a review. Surg Annu 1975; 7: 261-278.
32. Schiff M. In: Loescher FH, ed. Leçons sur la physiologie de la digestion. 1867: 416-452.
33. Brown-Sequard C E. Des altérations qui surviennent dans la muqueuse de l'estomac, consécutivement aux lesions cérébrales. Prog Med 1876; 4:136-137.
34. Yoshihara T, Kitaoka T, Tomihara K, Kiya K, Nomura M. Gastrointestinal bleeding in patients with severe head injury, hypertensive intracerebral hemorrhage, and ruptured cerebral aneurysm. Hiroshima J Med Sci 1983; 32:35-40.
35. Grijalva C V, Londholm E, Novin D. Physiological and morphological changes in the gastrointestinal tract induced by hypothalamic intervention: an overview. Brain Res Bull 1980; 5:19-31.
36. Salim A S. The hypothalamus and gastric mucosal injuries: origin of stress-induced injury. J Psychiatr Res 1988; 22:35-42.
37. Henke P G. The telencephalic limbic system and experimental gastric pathology: a review. Neurosci Biobehav Rev 1982; 6:381-390.
38. Henke P G, Savoie R J, Callahan B M. Hippocampal deafferentation and deefferentation and gastric pathology in rats. Brain Res Bull 1981; 7:395-398.
39. Grijalva C V, Deregnaucourt J, Code C F, Novin D. Gastric mucosal damage in rats induced by lateral hypothalamic lesions: Protection by propantheline, cimetidine and vagotomy. Proc Soc Exp Biol Med 1980; 163:528-533.
40. Hoshino K, Sugizaki M. Ulcerogenic effect of the lesion of the median raphe nucleus in fasted rats. Braz J Med Biol Res 1986; 19:123-130.
41. Grijalva C V, Taché Y, Gunion M W, Walsh J H, Geiselman P J. Amygdaloid lesions attenuate neurogenic gastric mucosal erosions but do not alter gastric secretory changes induced by intracisternal bombesin. Brain Res Bull 1986; 16:55-61.

42. Ray A, Henke P G, Sullivan R M. Central dopamine systems and gastric stress pathology in rats. Physiol Behav 1988; 42:359–364.
43. Henke P G. Recent studies of the central nucleus of the amygdala and stress ulcers. Neurosci Biobehav Rev 1988; 12:143–150.
44. Ferguson A V, Marcus P, Spencer J, Wallace J L. Paraventricular nucleus stimulation causes gastroduodenal mucosal necrosis in the rat. Am J Physiol 1988; 255:R861–R865.
45. McCutcheon N B, Guile M N, McCormick R. Electrical stimulation of the medial forebrain bundle-posterior lateral hypothalamus attenuates gastric lesions. Physiol Behav 1986; 37:435–440.
46. Bonfils S, Dubrasquet M. Psychotropic drugs in experimental peptic ulcer induced by psychological stress. In: Pletscher A, Marino A, eds. Psychotropic drugs in internal medicine. Amsterdam: Excerpta Medica Foundation, 1969: 80–94.
47. Kunchandy J, Kulkarni S K. Involvement of central type benzodiazepine and GABAA receptor in the protective effect of benzodiazepines in stress-induced gastric ulcers in rats. Arch Int Pharmacodyn Ther 1987; 285:129–136.
48. File S E, Pearce J B. Benzodiazepines reduce gastric ulcers induced in rats by stress. Br J Pharmacol 1981; 74:593–599.
49. Taché Y, Ishikawa T. Role of brain peptides in the ulcerogenic response to stress. In: Taché Y, Morley JE, Brown MR, eds. Symposia Hans Selye: neuropeptides and stress. New York: Springer-Verlag, 1989: 146–157.
50. Taché Y. The peptidergic brain–gut axis: influence on gastric ulcer formation. Chronobiol 1987; 4:11–17.
51. Goto Y, Taché Y. Gastric erosions induced by intracisternal thyrotropin-releasing hormone (TRH) in rats. Peptides 1985; 6:153–156.
52. Maeda-Hagiwara M, Watanabe H. Intracerebroventricular injection of a TRH analogue, y-butyrolactone-y-carbonyl-L-histidyl-prolinamide, induces gastric lesions and gastric acid stimulation in rats. Naunyn Schmiedebeergs Arch Pharmacol 1985; 330:142–146.
53. Nakane T, Kanie N, Audhya T, Hollander C S. The effects of centrally administered neuropeptides on the development of gastric lesions in the rat. Life Sci 1985; 36:1197–1203.
54. Hernandez D E, Emerick S G. Thyrotropin-releasing hormone: medullary site of action to induce gastric ulcers and stimulation acid secretion. Brain Res 1988; 459:148–152.
55. Taché Y, Maeda-Hagiwara M, Goto Y, Garrick T. Central nervous system action of TRH to stimulate gastric function and ulceration. Peptides 1988; 9 (Suppl.1):9–13.
56. Taché Y, Goto Y, Hamel D, Pekary A, Novin D. Mechanisms underlying intracisternal TRH-induced stimulation of gastric acid secretion in rats. Regul Peptides 1985; 13:21–30.
57. Somiya H, Tonoue T. Neuropeptides as central integrators of autonomic nerve activity: effects of TRH, SRIF, VIP and bombesin on gastric and adrenal nerves. Regul Peptides 1984; 9:47–52.

58. Cho C H, Hung K M, Ogle C W. The aetiology of gastric ulceration induced by electrical vagal stimulation in rats. Eur J Pharmacol 1985; 110:211–217.

59. Stephens R L, Ishikawa T, Weiner H, Novin D, Taché Y. TRH analog, RX 77368, injected into the dorsal vagal complex stimulates gastric secretion in rats. Am J Physiol 1988; 254:G639–G643.

60. Okuma Y, Osumi Y, Ishigawa T, Mitsuma T. Enhancement of gastric acid output and mucosal blood flow by tripeptide thyrotropin releasing hormone microinjected into the dorsal motor nucleus of the vagus in rats. Jpn J Pharmacol 1987; 43:173–178.

61. Rogers R C, Hermann G E. Dorsal medullary oxytocin, vasopressin, oxytocin antagonist, and TRH effects on gastric acid secretion and heart rate. Peptides 1985; 6:1143–1148.

62. Stephens R L, Taché Y. Intracisternal injection of TRH analogue, RX 77368, stimulates serotonin release into the gastric lumen in the rat. Am J Physiol 1989; 256:G377–G383.

63. Kubek M J, Rea M A, Hodes Z I, Aprison M H. Quantitation and characterization of thyrotropin-releasing hormone in vagal nuclei and other regions of the medulla oblongata of the rat. J Neurochem 1983; 40:1307–1313.

64. Palkovits M, Mezey E, Eskay R L, Brownstein M J. Innervation of the nucleus of the solitary tract and the dorsal vagal nucleus by thyrotropin-releasing hormone-containing raphe neurons. Brain Res 1986; 373:246–251.

65. Manaker S, Winokur A, Rostene W H, Rainbow T C. Autoradiographic localization of thyrotropin-releasing hormone receptors in the rat central nervous system. J Neurosci 1985; 5:167–174.

66. Mantyh P W, Hunt S P. Thyrotropin-releasing hormone (TRH) receptors Localization by light microscopic autoradiography in rat brain using [3H]-[3-Me-His2]TRH as the radioligand. J Neurosci 1985; 5:551–561.

67. Takayama K, Ishikawa N, Miura M. Sites of origin and termination of gastric vagus preganglionic neurons: an HRP study in the rat. J Auton Nerv Syst 1982; 6:211–223.

68. Shapiro R E, Miselis R R. The central organization of the vagus nerve innervating the stomach of the rat. J Comp Neurol 1985; 238:473–488.

69. Arancibia S, Assenmacher I. Sécrétion de TRH dans le troisième ventricle cérébral lors de l'exposition aigue au froid chez le rat non anesthésie. Effect des drogues a-adrénergiques. C R Soc Biol (Paris) 1987; 181:323–331.

70. Basso N, Bagarini M, Pekary E, Genco A, Materia A. Role of thyrotropin-releasing hormone in stress ulcer formation in the rat. Dig Dis Sci 1988; 33:819–823.

71. Taché Y, Simard P, Collu R. Prevention by bombesin of cold-restraint stress induced hemorrhagic lesions in rats. Life Sci 1979; 24:1719–1725.

72. Morley J E, Levine A S, Silvis S E. Intraventricular calcitonin inhibits gastric acid secretion. Science 1981; 214:671–673.

73. Taché Y, Kolve E, Maeda-Hagiwara M, Kauffman G. CNS action of calcitonin to alter experimental gastric ulcers in rats. Gastroenterology 1987; 41:651–655.

74. Kolve E, Taché Y. Intracisternal CGRP prevents gastric ulcer formation in the rat (abstr). Gastroenterology 1989; 96:A266.
75. Rivier J, Rivier C, Vale W. Synthetic competitive antagonists of corticotropin-releasing factor: effect on ACTH secretion in the rat. Science 1984; 224:889–891.
76. Berridge C W, Dunn A J. A corticotropin-releasing factor antagonist reverses the stress-induced changes of exploratory behavior in mice. Horm Behav 1987; 21:393–401.
77. Rivier C, Rivier J, Vale W. Stress-induced inhibition of reproductive functions: role of endogenous corticotropin-releasing factor. Science 1986; 231: 607–609.
78. Brown M R, Gray T S, Fisher L A. Corticotropin-releasing factor receptor antagonist: effects on the autonomic nervous system and cardiovascular function. Regul Peptides 1986; 16:321–329.
79. Brown M R, Fisher L A, Webb V, Vale W W, Rivier J E. Corticotropin-releasing factor: a physiologic regulator of adrenal epinephrine secretion. Brain Res 1985; 328:355–357.
80. Lenz H J, Raedler A, Greten H, Vale W W, Rivier J E. Stress-induced gastrointestinal secretory and motor responses in rats are mediated by endogenous corticotropin-releasing factor. Gastroenterology 1988; 95: 1510–1517.
81. Williams C L, Peterson J M, Villar R G, Burks T F. Corticotropin-releasing factor directly mediates colonic responses to stress. Am J Physiol 1987; 253:G582–G586.
82. Stephens R L, Yang H, Rivier J, Taché Y. Intracisternal injection of CRF antagonist blocks surgical stress-induced inhibition of gastric secretion in the rat. Peptides 1988; 9:1067–1070.
83. Taché Y, Kolve E, Stephens R L, Rivier J E. Role of corticotropin-releasing factor in mediating gastric ileus. Gastroenterology 1989; 96:A499.
84. Gunion M W, Kauffman G L, Taché Y. Intrahypothalamic corticotropin-releasing factor elevates gastric bicarbonate and inhibits stress ulcers in rats. Am J Physiol 1990; 258:G152–157.
85. Krahn D D, Wright B, Billington C J, Levine A S. Exogenous corticotropin-releasing factor inhibits stress-induced gastric ulceration (abstr). Soc Neurosci 1986; 12:1063.
86. Ishikawa T, Taché Y. Intrahypothalamic microinjection of calcitonin prevents stress-induced gastric lesions in rats. Brain Res Bull 1988; 20:415–419.
87. Ray A, Henke P G, Sullivan R M. The central amygdala and immobilization stress-induced gastric pathology in rats: neurotensin and dopamine. Brain Res 1987; 409:398–402.
88. Ray A, Henke P G, Sullivan R M. Opiate mechanisms in the central amygdala and gastric stress pathology in rats. Brain Res 1988; 442:195–198.
89. Hernandez D E, Stanley D A, Melvin J A. Prange A J Jr. Involvement of brain dopamine systems on neurotensin-induced protection against stress gastric lesions. Brain Res 1986; 381:159–163.

90. Zhang J, Washington J, Seaton J, Kauffman G. Central nervous system norepinephrine is involved in cold water restraint-induced gastric mucosal injury and central neurotensin-induced protection (abstr). Gastroenterology 1988; 94:A516.

91. Brown M, Vale W. Peptides and thermoregulation. In Cox B, Lomax P, Milton AS, Schonbaum E, eds. Thermoregulatory mechanisms and their therapeutic implications. S Karger, 1980: 186–194.

92. Taché Y, Marki W, Rivier J, Vale W, Brown M. Central nervous system inhibition of gastric secretion in the rat by gastrin-releasing peptide, a mammalian bombesin. Gastroenterology 1981; 81:298–302.

93. Ishikawa T, Taché Y. Bombesin microinjected into the dorsal vagal complex inhibits vagally stimulated gastric acid secretion in the rat. Regul Peptides 1989; 24:187–194

94. Taché Y, Ishikawa T, Gunion M, Raybould H. Central nervous system action of bombesin to influence gastric secretion and ulceration. Ann NY Acad Sci 1988; 547:183–193.

95. Taché Y, Gunion M M, Stephens R. CRF: central nervous system action to influence gastrointestinal function and role in the gastrointestinal response to stress. In: De Souza EB, Nemeroff CB, eds. Corticotropin-releasing factor: basic and clinical studies of a neuropeptide. Boca Raton: CRC Press, 1989; 299–307

96. Plotsky P M, Vale W. Hemorrhage-induced secretion of corticotropin-releasing factor-like immunoreactivity into the rat hypophysial portal circulation and its inhibition by glucocorticoids. Endocrinology 1984; 114:164–169.

97. Hernandez D E. Neuroendocrine mechanisms of stress ulceration: focus on thyrotropin-releasing hormone (TRH). Life Sci 1986; 39:279–296.

98. Hernandez D E, Stanley D A, Melvin J A, Prange A J Jr. Role of brain neurotransmitters on neurotensin-induced gastric cytoprotection. Pharmacol Biochem Behav 1985; 22:509–513.

99. Tsuda A, Tanaka M, Kohno Y, et al. Marked enhancement of noradrenaline turnover in extensive brain regions after activity-stress in rats. Physiol Behav 1982; 29:337–341.

100. Glavin G B. Selective noradrenaline depletion markedly alters stress responses in rats. Life Sci 1985; 37:461–465.

101. Bakke H K, Murison R, Walther B. Effect of central noradrenaline depletion on corticosterone levels and gastric ulcerations in rats. Brain Res 1986; 368:256–261.

102. Murakami M, Lam S K, Inada M, Miyake T. Pathophysiology and pathogenesis of acute gastric mucosal lesions after hypothermic restraint stress in rats. Gastroenterology 1985; 88:660–665.

103. Kivilaakso E. Pathogenetic mechanisms in experimental gastric stresss ulceration. Scand J Gastroenterol Suppl 1985; 110:57–62.

104. Takano K I, Sugiyama S, Nakazawa S, Ozawa T. The role of phospholipase in the genesis of gastric ulcers in rats. Scand J Gastroenterol 1987; 22: 577–584.

105. Yabana T, Yachi A. Stress-induced vascular damage and ulcer. Dig Dis Sci 1988; 33:751–761.
106. Galibrea J L, Canela M, Salva J A, Puig M, Schwartz S, Rull M. Gastric mucosal energy metabolism in stress ulcer. Eur Surg Res 1982; 14:377–385.
107. Takeuchi K, Ohtsuki H, Okabe S. Pathogenesis of compound 48/80-induced gastric lesions in rats. Dig Dis Sci 1986; 31:392–400.
108. Maeda-Hagiwara M, Watanabe H, Watanabe K. Enhancement by intra-cerebroventricular thyrotropin-releasing hormone of indomethacin-induced gastric lesions in the rat. Br J Pharmacol 1983; 80:735–739.
109. Taché Y, Stephens R L, Ishikawa T. Stress-induced alterations of gastro-intestinal function: involvement of brain CRF and TRH. In: Weiner H, Florin I, Hellhammer D, Murison M, eds. IV. New frontiers of stress research. Huber, Berns 1989: 1–11.

26

ROLE OF STRESS IN THE DEVELOPMENT OF DISORDERS OF GASTROINTESTINAL MOTILITY

Thomas F. Burks

University of Arizona College of Medicine, Tucson, Arizona

Unavoidable stress can cause profound functional changes in the gastrointestinal tract. The relationship between stress and gastrointestinal motility has long been recognized intuitively by laypersons, but scientific and clinical studies of the gastrointestinal effects of stress are somewhat more recent. A relationship between stress and intestinal motility was first demonstrated by Walter Cannon (1), who observed changes in the flow of intestinal contents in cats exposed to a growling dog. Fright in a human volunteer was noted over 30 years ago to produce increased colonic motility (2). However, experimental investigations of stress's effects on gastrointestinal motility were delayed by failure to appreciate adequately the control of the brain over gastrointestinal motility and unwarranted assumptions about the role of gastrointestinal hormones in producing specific patterns of motility. It is now increasingly appreciated that the central nervous system (CNS), the brain and the spinal cord, modulate neural activity of the enteric nervous system of the gastrointestinal tract, which directly regulates gastrointestinal motility.

For a stimulus to be perceived as stressful, it is believed that the stressful stimulus must be received, appreciated, and processed in the brain (3). That is, a decerebrate human or animal would not be able to perceive a stimulus (or at least a nonphysical stimulus) as a stressor. Indeed, insofar as stress involves the threat or disturbance of well-being or homeostasis of the whole organism, the role of the CNS is a requirement. A stimulus can only be a true source of stress, or a stressor, through mediation by the CNS (3). However, contemporary studies of the regulation of gastrointestinal motility have emphasized the autonomy of the enteric nervous system (ENS) in the regulation of gastrointestinal motility and propulsion (4). The enteric nervous system is a complex network of intrinsic neurons that regulate, by means of local reflex arcs, the motor activity of the esophagus, stomach, small intestine, and colon, as well as intestinal and colonic mucosal transport processes. The ENS is arranged in two major plexuses: the myenteric plexus, between the longitudinal and circular muscle layers, and the submucous plexus, between the circular muscle and mucosa. Motor impulses that regulate contractions of longitudinal and circular smooth muscle are believed to originate primarily in the myenteric plexus, whereas the submucous plexus receives input from fibers serving sensory receptors and regulates functions of mucosal epithelial cells. Neurons of the ENS utilize a variety of neurotransmitter chemicals: acetylcholine, 5-hydroxytryptamine, cholecystokinin, enkephalin, neurotensin, somatostatin, gamma-aminobutyric acid, and others. The ENS is thought to contain over 5×10^6 neurons. It also contains the neural machinery necessary for integrating sensory and extrinsic information and for programming particular patterns of gastrointestinal motility. The CNS, even in response to stress, does not directly regulate contractions of gastrointestinal smooth muscle. As shown in Figure 1, the main role of the CNS in regulating motility is probably the ability to select ENS programs that provide particular desired patterns of motility.

In response to disturbing or threatening sights, sounds, and other sensory stimuli, including somatosensory signals, that initiate the stress reaction, the brain can direct patterns of motility that provide a response to the perceived stressor. The information is conveyed from the brain to the ENS primarily by means of the parasympathetic and sympathetic divisions of the autonomic

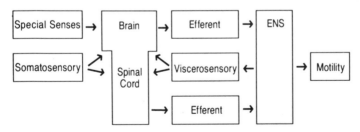

FIGURE 1 Schematic representation of relationship of the central nervous system (brain and spinal cord) and ENS to gastrointestinal motility. The central nervous system receives sensory input from the special senses, the somatosensory system, and from the viscerosensory system, includng the gastrointestinal tract. Efferent (motor) signals from the brain and spinal cord modulate neural activity of the ENS, which is responsible for integrating intrinsic neural influences and programming specific patterns of motility.

nervous system. It is now recognized that the brain and spinal cord contain chemosensitive sites at which neuropeptides and other chemicals involved in stress can act to influence gastrointestinal motility (5,6).

The gastrointestinal tract also has viscerosensory connections to the CNS. Vagal afferent nerves serving mechanoreceptors and chemoreceptors in the wall of the stomach, for example, project centrally to the tractus and nucleus solitarius of the brainstem and initiate sensory signals that travel rostrally to higher structures in the brain (7,8). Primary afferents from the intestine that terminate in the dorsal horn of the spinal cord may send collaterals to the ENS and to prevertebral sympathetic ganglia as well (9). Both the CNS and ENS can respond to sensory information arising from the organs of digestion.

Stimuli perceived by the brain as stressors can result in CNS-directed neural and hormonal signals to the gastrointestinal tract (Fig. 2). These signals reach the ENS to influence the selection of programs that regulate patterns of motility. The particular patterns of motility determine the rate of flow or propulsion of luminal contents through the different portions of the digestive tube. Pharmacological studies indicate that propulsion, measured as gastric emptying, small intestinal transit, or colonic transit, can be regulated differently in the stomach, small intestine, and colon (10), thereby providing regional specificity in CNS influences on motility.

Studies of the effects of stress on gastrointestinal motility have been complicated by technical limitations in the ability to measure with precision motility in all parts of the gastrointestinal tract, different contractile states associated with fed or fasting conditions of subjects, differences in responses to different stressors, and inadequate understanding of functional diseases that can alter motility. Until very recently, most attempts to study the effects of stress on gastrointestinal motility were carried out in humans rather than animals, thereby introducing complexities of variations in conditions between studies and restricted ability to collect quantitative data. For these reasons, there has been conflict in the results of some studies. Overall, however, several important and relatively consistent changes in gastrointestinal motility in response to stress have been observed in normal human subjects, patients with stress-related functional bowel disease, and in animal models.

HUMAN STUDIES

Stress-Induced Changes in Gastrointestinal Motility

Experimental stress has been shown in many studies to alter specific aspects of gastrointestinal motility in human subjects. Wolf has provided an interesting historical account of observations carried out in individual subjects with gastric fistulas (11). More recent observations are summarized in Table 1. Several types

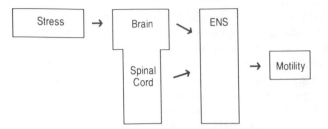

FIGURE 2   Schematic representation of the effects of stress on gastrointestinal motility. Psychic and physical stressors evoke responses in the brain, and efferent signals are conveyed by nerves and hormones to the ENS to influence integration and programming of motility.

of experimental stressors have been used in studies of gastrointestinal motility. For example, labyrinthine stimulation and vertigo produced by instilling cold water into the external auditory canal of one ear was found to decrease gastric emptying in healthy volunteers and to decrease contractions of the antrum of the stomach (12). The same authors also used painful immersion of one hand in ice water as a stressor to document delayed gastric emptying brought about by stress (13). Labyrinthine stimulation with cold water and painful immersion of one hand in cold water were also found in other studies to decrease antral contractions (14). Dichotomous listening to recordings, a nonnoxious stressor, was found to inhibit the development of the migrating motility complexes of the jejunum that is characteristic of the fasting motility pattern in humans (15). Electronic video games, driving in traffic, and other psychological stressors were also found to decrease the incidence of fasting migrating motor complexes in normal subjects (16). However, another study with fed subjects found that labyrinthine stimulation tended to convert random duodenal postprandial contractions to migrating motor complexes characteristic of fasting (12). An earlier study had suggested that stressful interviews produced increased jejunal contractions in 7 of 27 subjects examined (17). It should be noted that this study was carried out before the migrating motor complexes of the small intestine had been recognized and it is possible that the presence of unrecognized motor complexes complicated interpretation of the motility recordings. Experimental stress can produce changes in gastrointestinal propulsion as well as changes in patterns of motility. Two preliminary studies have indicated that painful immersion of one hand in cold water reduces orocecal transit of intestinal contents in humans (18,19). Experimental stress has usually been found to increase the incidence and amplitudes of contractions of the colon in humans. Immersion of one hand in ice water increased colonic contractions (20,21). Induction of headache by a device that compressed the head also increased contractions of the colon (20). Card-sorting and ball-sorting psychological stress was also found to increase the number of colonic contractions (21). In another study, exposure of normal subjects to a stressful interview was not found to induce consistent changes in colonic motility (22). Overall, most studies in human subjects indicate that experimental psychological and painful stressors decrease gastric emptying, affect small intestinal patterns of motility, and usually increase the incidence or amplitude of colonic contractions.

Functional Bowel Disease

The pathological motility disorder most associated with stress is irritable bowel syndrome, also known as irritable colon or spastic colon. Irritable bowel syndrome consists of abdominal pain or discomfort usually related to defecation, episodic constipation or diarrhea, passage of mucus, and a feeling of incomplete evacuation. A large proportion of patients give a strong history of stress-related or stress-evoked symptoms (23).

Among the abnormalities of gastrointestinal motility noted in patients with irritable bowel syndrome, summarized in Table 2, increased colonic responses to stress are a prominent feature (21). In comparison with normal controls, patients with irritable bowel syndrome usually display normal rates of gastric emptying (24). However, motor abnormalities of the small intestine and colon have been observed in a number of studies. For example, prolonged recordings of motility of the small intestine documented suppression of migrating motor complexes in some 30% of patients with irritable bowel syndrome, abnormal

TABLE 1 Effects of Experimental Stressors on Gastrointestinal Motility in Humans

Stressors	Effects	References
Labyrinthine stimulation	↓ Gastric emptying	12
Cold water pain	↓ Gastric emptying	13
Labyrinthine stimulation	↓ Antral contractions	12,14
Cold water pain	↓ Antral contractions	14
Dichotomous listening	↓ Migrating complexes	15
Psychological	↓ Migrating complexes	16
Stressful interview	↑ Jejunal contractions	17
Cold water pain	↓ Orocecal transit	18,19
Cold water pain	↑ Colonic contractions	20
Head compression pain	↑ Colonic contractions	20
Psychological	↑ Colonic contractions	21
Cold water pain	↑ Colonic contractions	21

↓, Decreased; ↑, increased.

TABLE 2   Abnormalities of Gastrointestinal Motility in
Patients with Irritable Bowel Syndrome

Small intestine	Colon
↓ Migrating complexes (15,23)	↑ Contractions (22)
↑ Irregular contractions (23)	↑ Stress response (21)

spontaneous contractions in 40–50% of patients, and abnormal contractile activity in response to stress in nearly 50% of patients (23). In a study carried out over 36 h, 19 of 22 patients with irritable bowel syndrome showed motility abnormalities in the small intestine (23). An important feature of the study carried out with prolonged recordings is that motility abnormalities in patients were found to be intermittent and paroxysmal. Intermittent motility abnormalities are consistent with the episodic symptoms associated with this disorder. Patients with irritable bowel syndrome characterized by episodes of diarrhea were found to have shorter small intestinal transit times than controls, whereas patients with constipation were found to have prolonged small intestinal transit times (24). In 74% of 34 patients who experienced pain after a test meal, the onset of pain was associated with arrival of the meal residue in the cecum (24). In a study with similar methodology carried out in eight normal subjects, dichotomous listening stress was found to increase the rate of small intestinal transit (25). In other studies, pain stress induced by immersion of a hand in cold water was found to decrease small intestinal transit (18,19). It can be concluded that different stressors in normal human subjects or patients produce different changes in small intestinal motility.

Patients with irritable bowel syndrome displayed higher rates of colonic contractions than normal patients (22), and exaggerated contractile responses to stress (21). In normal subjects or patients with irritable bowel syndrome, the most consistent motility alteration associated with stress is an increase in colonic contractions.

ANIMAL STUDIES

It is evident from human and animal studies that the type of stressor used is a key variable in experimental stress. We have compared a number of stress models in rats and the effects of the stressors on gastrointestinal transit, which is a measure of propulsive motor activity. Also, because analgesia frequently accompanies stress responses in rats (26), antinociceptive responses in standard hot plate or tail-flick tests were also evaluated. The results of these studies are summarized in Table 3. As expected, different stressors produced different effects. Partial restraint of unanesthetized rats produced by wrapping the foreshoulders and thorax with paper tape ("wrap restraint") was found consistently to induce analgesia and to decrease small intestinal transit (27). Electroconvulsive shock (28) and electrical foot shock (29) induced analgesia, but had no effect on small intestinal transit. In a cold water swimming test, rats were required to swim intermittently for 10 s periods in water maintained at 4°C (27). Other animals were required to swim similarly in water maintained at 20°C. The cold water swimming test resulted in both analgesia and decreased small intestinal transit, whereas the warm water swimming test did not induce analgesia or alter small intestinal transit. The effects of cold were assessed by maintaining animals for 1 h at an ambient temperature of 4°C. Other rats were restrained in wire mesh restraints for 1 h at an ambient temperature of 4°C. Cold exposure alone neither induced analgesia nor altered small intestinal transit. Cold restraint did not induce analgesia, but produced significant inhibition of small intestinal transit. A purely psychological stressor, exposure to a cat, produced a behavioral response but not analgesia or changes in small intestinal transit. Rats exposed to vapors of diethyl ether for 5 min developed analgesia and decreased small intestinal transit. The analgesia induced by wrap restraint, electroconvulsive shock, and foot shock was blocked or reversed by naloxone (3 or 10 mg/kg). The initial analgesia associated with exposure to ether was not sensitive to naloxone, but late analgesia (20–40 min after ether exposure) was sensitive to naloxone. The analgesia associated with cold water swimming was not blocked by naloxone. Thus, different stressors produced different combinations of analgesia and inhibition of small intestinal transit. Also analgesia associated with different stressors showed differences in sensitivity to naloxone. It is known that

TABLE 3 Ability of Stressors to Induce Analgesia and to Alter Small Intestinal Transit (SIT) in Unanesthetized Rats

Stressor	Analgesia	SIT
Wrap restraint	Yes	↓
Electroconvulsive shock	Yes	0
Footshock	Yes	0
Cold water swim	Yes	↓
Warm water swim	No	0
Cold exposure	No	0
Cold restraint	No	↓
Exposure to cat	No	0
Diethyl ether vapors	Yes	↓

0, No effect.

stress-induced analgesia in animals can be produced by both opioid and non-opioid mechanisms (26).

Strain and Gender Differences

In humans, stress-related disorders of gastrointestinal motility are thought to affect female more often than male subjects (30). Acute wrap restraint and chronic wrap restraint (72 h) were evaluated for effects on small intestinal transit in Sprague-Dawley rats (27). Acute wrap restraint was found to inhibit small intestinal transit equally in male and female rats. However, chronic wrap restraint (72 h) inhibited small intestinal transit only in female rats. It was interesting that prior (10 days) gonadectomy abolished the antitransit effects of chronic wrap restraint in female rats, but caused male rats to become more susceptible to the antitransit effects of wrap restraint.

Another variable involved in determining the response of an animal to stress is its strain. The effects of acute wrap restraint were evaluated in female Sprague-Dawley and Fischer 344 rats at two different times of day, 1:00 p.m. and 5:00 p.m. In the 1:00 p.m. test, acute wrap restraint decreased small intestinal transit only in Fischer 344 rats, not in Sprague-Dawley rats. However, in the 5:00 p.m. test, both strains of rat displayed decreased small intestinal transit in response to acute wrap restraint.

These studies indicate that animals, like humans, are sensitive to multiple factors that influence responses to stress. It is noteworthy that gonadal extirpation reversed the gender difference in responsiveness to chronic wrap restraint, which suggests that sex hormones may have an influence on stress-induced gastrointestinal changes. Estrogen has been shown to inhibit small intestinal transit (31).

Release of Adrenocortiocotropic Hormone and Beta-Endorphin

To ascertain that the changes in transit induced by wrap restraint were associated with accepted markers of stress, plasma levels of adrenocorticotropic hormone (ACTH) and beta-endorphin were measured by radioimmunoassay (32). Figure 3 shows the peak changes in ACTH and beta-endorphin levels in wrap-restrained and control animals. Wrap restraint resulted in a rapid, eightfold increase in plasma ACTH levels within 20 min, levels remained elevated for 30 min, and returned to control values by 60 min. The pattern of release of beta-endorphin was similar. Wrap restraint stress resulted in a rapid increase in plasma beta-endorphin concentrations that peaked 20 min after application of stress, and remained elevated for 60 min. These results indicated that wrap restraint is a true stress stimulus. Both endocrine changes and analgesia are hallmark responses to stress.

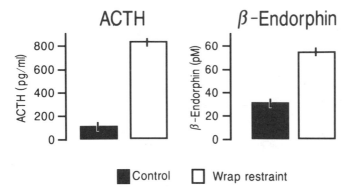

FIGURE 3   Effects of wrap restraint on plasma levels of ACTH and β-endorphin in rats. Blood samples were taken 20 min after wrapping or sham wrapping (control) (n = 4 per group).

Effect of Time of Day

The effect of stress on small intestinal transit was strongly dependent on the time of day when the experiment was performed (Table 4). Effects of wrap restraint stress on inhibition of small intestinal transit and plasma levels of ACTH were assessed at nine different times of day in female Sprague-Dawley rats on a 12 h (7 a.m.–7 p.m.) light schedule. The animals were relatively refractory to stress-induced changes in small intestinal transit during the morning and midday tests. The greatest changes in intestinal transit and plasma ACTH concentrations occurred in the late afternoon hours. Animals tested at 5:00 p.m., immediately before the beginning of the dark phase, showed the greatest response in both stress-induced inhibition of intestinal transit and release of ACTH. The similarity of the two responses to wrap restraint stress was striking and there was a pronounced correlation (r = 0.95) between the inhibition of small intestinal transit and stimulation of ACTH release over the entire 24 h period.

The degree of intestinal dysfunction produced by stress was dependent on the time of day that the animals were stressed, which suggested a circadian influence on stress-induced changes in intestinal propulsion. Others have reported a similar circadian influence on stress-induced analgesia in mice (33). Moreover, the gastrointestinal tract itself exhibits different circadian patterns in secretory and motor functions that persist in fasted animals, which suggests that the patterns are not due to feeding cycles (34). Also, circadian variability has been reported in the susceptibility of the gastric mucosa to aspirin-induced lesions (35). It is of interest to note that a close correlation occurred between

TABLE 4   Influence of Time of Day on Wrap-Restraint-Induced Inhibition of Small Intestinal Transit and Plasma Levels of ACTH

Time	Inhibition of transit (%)	Plasma ACTH pg/ml)[a]
1:00 a.m.	10 ± 6	312 ± 144
4:00	17 ± 4	395 ± 95
7:00[b]	33 ± 17	453 ± 13
10:00	22 ± 9	390 ± 32
1:00 p.m.	15 ± 7	344 ± 26
4:00	25 ± 5*	500 ± 35
5:00	46 ± 10**	822 ± 38
7:00[c]	10 ± 6	253 ± 64
10:00	13 ± 7	279 ± 103

[a]Control (nonstressed) level = 95 ± pg/ml.
[b]Lights on.
[c]Lights off.
Significant, * p < 0.05; ** p < 0.01.

stress induced inhibition of small intestinal transit and stress-induced release of ACTH. Rats were most sensitive to the effects of stress in the late afternoon, at a time when circadian variations in plasma levels of ACTH are maximum, and when stress-induced release of endocrine factors is most prominent. It has been reported that symptoms are most severe for patients with irritable bowel syndrome in the early morning, the equivalent of late afternoon in rats and other nocturnal species, which may suggest a circadian influence on the sensitivity of the human bowel to stress (36,37).

Effects of Wrap Restraint Stress on Gastric Emptying, Small Intestinal Transit, and Colonic Transit

In humans, experimental stress affects gastric emptying, small intestinal motility, and colonic motility. Patients with irritable bowel syndrome often exhibit abnormalities in both small intestinal motility and motility of the colon. Studies were carried out in female Sprague-Dawley rats to determine effects of wrap restraint stress on gastric emptying, small intestinal transit, and colonic transit (32). Small intestinal and colonic transit were measured by the geometric center method (38). Wrap restraint stress did not affect the rate of gastric emptying in rats (Table 5). As observed in other studies, wrap restraint stress inhibited small intestinal transit, reducing the geometric center of transit from 5.4 to 4.1 (a geometric center of 1 indicates no transit, a geometric center of 10 indicates complete transit through the small intestine). Wrap restraint stress greatly increased colonic transit and also resulted in an increase in fecal excretion.

The changes in intestinal transit induced by wrap restraint stress in the rat are similar to changes in intestinal motility induced by stress in humans. Physical stress in humans, such as immersion of a hand in cold water, delays orocecal transit (18). Stress increases colonic motility in both normal subjects and patients with irritable bowel syndrome (21). Diarrhea is a common symptom of stress, and the increased fecal excretion associated with wrap restraint in rats apparently results from increased colonic transit. When wrap restraint stress is the type of stimulus used, the resultant changes in gastrointestinal motor function in rats (decreased small intestinal transit, increased large intestinal transit, and increased fecal output) are very similar to symptoms reported in humans in response to stress, or symptoms associated with functional bowel disease thought to be induced or exacerbated by stress.

Effects of Stress on Motility

Wrap restraint stress in rats was found to produce changes in transit in the small intestine and colon that mimic, in some respects, stress-induced changes in transit in humans. Stress in humans has been observed to be associated also with changes in motility. For example, stressful interviews caused increased contractions in the small intestine (17), and noxious stimuli or psychological stress caused increased contractions of the colon (20,21). Patients with irritable bowel syndrome may exhibit fewer organized migrating complexes and more irregular contractions in the small intestine than healthy controls (23) and more contractile activity in the colon (22).

To determine the effects of stress on intestinal motility in an animal model, we have measured intraluminal pressure in the small intestine and colon of rats before and after wrap restraint (Fig 4). Wrap restraint stress consistently caused increased incidence and amplitude of contractions in the small intestine and

TABLE 5 Effects of Wrap Restraint Stress on Gastric Emptying, Small Intestinal Transit, and Colonic Transit in Unanesthetized Rats

Function measured	Control	Wrap restraint
Gastric emptying (%)	54 ± 5	53 ± 9
Small intestinal transit (GC)	5.4 ± 0.4	4.1 ± 0.2*
Colonic transit (GC)	2.9 ± 0.2	5.0 ± 0.6**

*Significant, $p < 0.05$; ** $p < 0.01$.
GC, Geometric center.

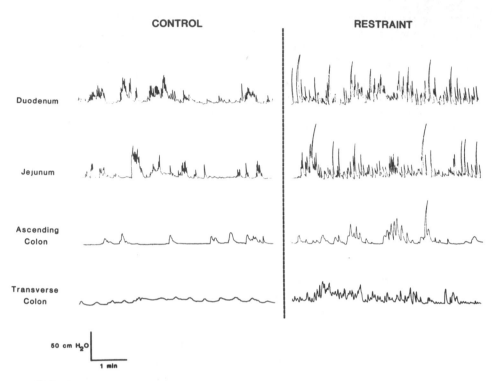

FIGURE 4   Stress-induced changes in motility in the small intestine and colon in the rat wrap restraint model. Intraluminal pressure was recorded from indwelling catheters by means of a low-compliance perfusion system. Records illustrate motility before and after wrap restraint.

colon (JM Peterson, TF Burks, unpublished observations, 1990). Wrap restraint stress was associated with reduction or abolition of migrating motor complexes in the small intestine and increased regular or irregular contractions. Wrap restraint stress caused an increase in the frequency of contractions in the colon and often in the amplitude of contractions. It is not certain at present why the increased contractions in the small intestine are associated with decreased propulsive activity and the increased contractions in the colon may be associated with increased propulsive activity. However, it is of interest that the changes in motility in the animal model seem to mimic those reported to be associated with experimental stress and stress-related disease in humans.

MEDIATORS OF STRESS RESPONSES

The observation that stress-induced changes in ACTH levels and intestinal transit in rats occur in parallel suggests that endocrine messengers may play a role in mediating the effects of stress on the gastrointestinal tract. The hypothalamic-pituitary–adrenal axis is the endocrine system most central to the stress response (39). ACTH and beta-endorphin are released concomitantly from the pituitary in response to stress (40). Beta-endorphin and other opioid peptides with actions at mu opioid receptors can act in the brain and spinal cord to inhibit gastrointestinal motility (41,42). However, endogenous opioid peptides administered peripherally generally do not alter gastrointestinal motility in vivo (42). ACTH can stimulate the adrenal glands to secrete glucorticoid hormones, principally corticosterone in the rat (39). Corticotropin-releasing factor (CRF) also acts at extrapituitary sites to alter plasma concentrations of norepinephrine and epinephrine (43). Thus, CRF-mediated stress effects could result either from pituitary–adrenal or extrapituitary actions of CRF. Experiments have been carried out to determine what endogenous substances might mediate gastrointestinal motility changes brought about by stress.

Surgical ablation of the adrenal glands and pituitary did not alter wrap restraint stress-induced inhibition of small intestinal transit in rats (32). Moreover, intravenously administered ACTH or beta-endorphin did not affect small intestinal transit, even when the dosages administered were much greater than those required to reach plasma concentrations of the hormones under stress conditions. Therefore, stress-induced changes in gastrointestinal transit in rats seem not to be mediated by pituitary or adrenally derived factors. While stress-induced endocrine function and intestinal dysfunction are highly correlated, they appear not to be causally related.

Alterations in stress-induced gastrointestinal transit in humans were reduced by administration of a beta adrenergic antagonist, thus suggesting a possible mediator role of catecholamines (18,19). However, suppression of gastric motor complexes induced in dogs by acoustic stress was not sensitive to blockade by the adrenergic antagonists phentolamine and propranolol (44,45).

Evidence for a direct mediator role of CRF in stress-induced changes in gastrointestinal motility in rats has recently been presented (46). CRF, administered intravenously (iv) or intracerebroventricularly (icv) produced significant changes in the propulsive activity of the gastrointestinal tract. Gastric emptying was inhibited in a dose-dependent manner, at dosages of 1.0–10.0 μg iv or icv. In addition, CRF, in dosages of 0.3–10.0 μg, inhibited small intestinal transit and increased colonic transit, resulting in increased fecal output. At higher dosages, CRF induced diarrhea. Thus, there was a striking parallelism between gastrointestinal effects of stress and exogenously administered CRF, especially when

CRF was administered at an icv dosage of 0.3 μg (Table 6). Low dosages of CRF, like stress, decreased small intestinal transit, increased colonic transit, and increased fecal excretion, without affecting gastric emptying. To determine whether endogenously released CRF might mediate gastrointestinal motility responses to stress in vivo, a CRF antagonist, alpha-helical CRF-(9-41) (47), was used. The CRF antagonist given iv or icv at a dosage of 50 μg had no effect alone on small intestinal transit or colonic transit. However, it effectively antagonized the effects of exogenous CRF on small intestinal and colonic transit when CRF and the antagonist were administered via the same route. Administration of the CRF antagonist icv or iv immediately before wrap restraint stress completely blocked the stress-induced increase in colonic transit and significantly diminished the stress-induced increase in fecal excretion. However, the CRF antagonist did not antagonize stress-induced inhibition of small intestinal transit. The results of these studies obviously suggest that endogenous CRF may mediate the effects of stress on intestinal motility and transit, particularly in the colon. Blockade of endogenous CRF can prevent the response of the colon to stress, which suggests that CRF may be directly responsible for mediating the effects of stress on colonic function. CRF can stimulate the pituitary to release ACTH and beta-endorphin. However, exogenously administered ACTH and beta-endorphin did not alter small intestinal or colonic transit. It therefore appears that neither pituitary nor adrenally derived factors are involved in mediating the effects of stress on the intestine. CRF released by stress may act in the brain to alter autonomic nervous system outflow or may act directly within the enteric nervous system of the gastrointestinal tract to alter propulsive activity (Fig. 5).

A CRF link in stress-induced changes in gastrointestinal motility has been supported in subsequent reports. Application of partial restraint in rats, like CRF administered icv (48), was found to decrease gastric emptying, inhibit small intestinal transit, and increase colonic transit (49). Effects of both exogenously administered CRF and stress, including effects on the small intestine, were antagonized by alpha-helical CRF-(9-41) administered icv (49). In dogs, CRF given icv suppressed cyclic motor complexes in the gastric antrum but not in the

TABLE 6 Similarities of Effects of Wrap Restraint Stress and CRF on Gastrointestinal Functions

Function	Wrap restraint stress	CRF (0.3 μg icv)
Gastric emptying	0	0
Small intestinal transit	↓	↓
Colonic transit	↑	↑
Fecal excretion	↑	↑

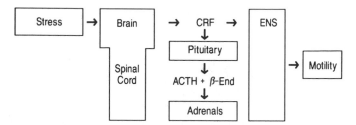

FIGURE 5 Schematic representation of the possible central role of CRF in mediating certain effects of stress on gastrointestinal motility. A potential extra-pituitary action of CRF on ENS-regulated motility is postulated. The pituitary actions of CRF result in secretion of ACTH and β-endorphin (β-End). ACTH acts on the adrenal glands to stimulate secretion of glucocorticoid hormones.

jejunum (50). Acoustic stress produced identical effects (45). In mice fed a milk powder meal containing fat, acoustic stress (rock music played through loud-speakers) and cold stress (ambient temperature of 10°C) were found to increase gastric emptying (51). In this case, the stressors evidently reversed fat-induced decreases in gastric emptying. Administration of CRF antiserum intraperitone-(ip) blocked the effects of acoustic and cold stress on gastric emptying. An interesting finding was that administration of CRF antiserum by ip injection also blocked the effects of icv CRF on gastric emptying. These important experiments suggest that the stress-induced alterations of gastric emptying were abolished by immunoneutralization of circulating CRF. Since CRF-like immuno-reactivity also occurs in the stomach, adrenals, lung, liver, and pancreas (52,53), it is not certain whether the CRF released by stress that affects gastrointestinal motility arises from the brain or from a peripheral site. Experiments both with a CRF antagonist and CRF antiserum suggest the possibility of peripheral actions of CRF that affect motility (32,51).

CONCLUSIONS

Stress is a complex reaction characterized by centrally directed activation of both endocrine and autonomic systems. Since gastrointestinal motility is controlled directly by the enteric nervous system, stress-induced effects on motility apparently result from brain and spinal cord selection of specific motility programs directed by the enteric nervous system. Stressors may influence the central nervous system to select stereotype motility programs.

Experimental stress in humans can affect gastric emptying, small intestinal motility, and colonic motility. The most consistent documented alteration in gastrointestinal motility associated with experimental stress in humans is increased contractile activity of the colon. Altered colonic and small intestinal contractions have also been associated with motility changes in functional bowel disease, such as irritable bowel syndrome.

Many stress models have been tested in rats to determine the effects of stress on gastrointestinal motility. In several respects, acute wrap restraint stress mimics the effects of experimental and pathological stress in humans: there is inhibition of small intestinal transit, stimulation of colonic transit, stimulation of small intestinal and colonic motility, and increase in fecal excretion, but no change in gastric emptying. Acute wrap restraint stress fulfills the criteria of a true stress response in that plasma levels of ACTH and beta-endorphin are increased and the procedure is accompanied by naloxone-sensitive analgesia. Other restraint models and acoustic stress in animals also affect gastrointestinal motility. It is important that test models represent true stress responses and mimic, to the extent possible, stress responses in humans if the models are to be useful for studies of stress mechanisms.

Evidence has been put forward that some components of the gastrointestinal response to stress may be mediated by extrapituitary actions of CRF. The CRF link may be in the central nervous system or in the periphery. Additional experimentation will be required to determine the precise site of CRF action. Identification of CRF as a critical link in the effect of stress on gastrointestinal motility and transit provides new opportunities to understand one of the most typical responses of the body to stress.

ACKNOWLEDGMENTS

The author is particularly indebted to Cynthia L. Williams and Julie M. Peterson for their valuable contributions to many of the studies cited in this chapter. I am grateful to Ms. Rita Sainz for preparation of the manuscript. Work from the author's laboratory was supported by USPHS grants DA02163 and DK36289.

REFERENCES

1. Cannon WB. The movement of the intestines studied by means of the roentgen rays. Am J Physiol 1902; 6:251–277.

2. Almy TP. Experimental studies on irritable colon. Am J Med 1951; 10: 60–67.

3. Wingate DL, Kumar D. Stress and gastrointestinal motility. In: Kumar D, Gustavsson S, eds. An illustrated guide to gastrointestinal motility. Chichester: John Wiley, 1988: 255–264.

4. Johnson LR. (ed). Physiology of the digestive system, 2nd ed. New York: Raven Press, 1987.

5. Burks TF. Central sites of action of gastrointestinal drugs. Gastroenterology 1978; 74: 322–324.

6. Porreca F, Burks TF. The spinal cord as a site of opioid effects on gastrointestinal transit in the mouse. J Pharmacol Exp Ther 1983; 227: 22-27.

7. Barber WD, Burks TF. Brain stem response to phasic gastric distention. Am J Physiol 1983; 245: G242-G248.

8. Ewart WR. Sensation in the gastrointestinal tract. J Comp Physiol Biochem 1985; 82A: 489-493.

9. Kruger L, Rodin BE. Peripheral mechanisms involved in pain. In: Kitchell RL, Erickson HH, eds. Animal pain—perception and alleviation. Bethesda, MD: American Physiological Society, 1983: 1-26.

10. Porreca F, Burks TF. Centrally administered bombesin affects gastric emptying and small and large bowel transit in the rat. Gastroenterology 1983; 85: 313-317.

11. Wolf S. The psyche and the stomach—a historical vignette. Gastroenterology 1981; 80: 605-614.

12. Thompson DG, Richelson E, Malagelada J-R. Perturbation of gastric emptying and duodenal motility through the central nervous system. Gastroenterology 1982; 83: 1200-1206.

13. Thompson DG, Richelson E, Malagelada J-R. Perturbation of upper gastrointestinal function by cold stress. Gut 1983; 24: 277-283.

14. Stanghellini V, Malagelada J-R, Zinsmeister AR, Go VLW, Kao PC. Stress-induced gastroduodenal motor disturbances in humans: possible humoral mechanisms. Gastroenterology 1983; 85: 83-91.

15. McRae S, Younger K, Thompson DG, Wingate DL. Sustained mental stress alters human jejunal motor activity. Gut 1982; 23: 404-409.

16. Valori RM, Kumar D, Wingate DL. Effects of different types of stress and of "prokinetic" drugs on the control of the fasting motor complex in humans. Gastroenterology 1986; 90: 1890-1900.

17. Roth HP, Ferreri RN, Petti MA, Evans MW. Motility of the small intestine during emotional reactions. Ann Intern Med 1953; 38: 38-53.

18. O'Brien JD, Thompson DG, Holly J, Burnham WR, Walker E. Stress disturbs human gastrointestinal transit via a beta-1 adrenoreceptor mediated pathway. Gastroenterology 1985; 88: 1520.

19. O'Brien J, Thompson DG, Holly J, Burnham W, Walker E. Beta-blockers can protect human upper gastrointestinal function from disturbances by stress. Gut 1985; 26: A559.

20. Almy TP, Tulin M. Alterations in colonic function in man under stress: experimental production of changes simulating the "irritable colon." Gastroenterology 1947; 8: 616-626.

21. Narducci F, Snape WJ, Battle WM, London RL, Cohen S. Increased colonic motility during exposure to a stressful situation. Dig Dis Sci 1985; 30: 40-44.

22. Latimer P, Sarna S, Campbell D, Latimer M, Waterfall W, Daniel EE. Colonic motor and myoelectrical activity: a comparative study of normal subjects, psychoneurotic patients, and patients with irritable bowel syndrome. Gastroenterology 1981; 80: 893-901.

23. Kumar D, Wingate DL. Irritable bowel syndrome. In: Kumar D, Gustavsson S, eds. An illustrated guide to gastrointestinal motility. Chichester: John Wiley, 1988: 401–410.

24. Cann PA, Read NW, Brown C, Hobson N, Holdsworth CD. Irritable bowel syndrome: relationship of disorders in the transit of a single solid meal to symptom patterns. Gut 1983; 24: 405–411.

25. Cann PA, Read NW, Cammack J, et al. Psychological stress and the passage of a standard meal through the stomach and small intestine in man. Gut 1983; 24: 236–240.

26. Mayer DJ. Stress, analgesia and neuropeptides. In: Taché Y, Morley JE, Brown MR, eds. Neuropeptides and stress. New York: Springer-Verlag, 1989: 175–187.

27. Williams CL, Burks TF. Stress, opioids, and gastrointestinal transit. In: Morley JE, Brown MR, eds. Neuropeptides and stress. New York: Springer-Verlag, 1989: 175–187.

28. Galligan JJ, Porreca F, Burks TF. Dissociation of analgesic and gastrointestinal effects of electroconvulsive shock-released opioids. Brain Res 1983; 271: 354–357.

29. Galligan JJ, Porreca F, Burks TF. Footshock produces analgesia but no gastrointestinal motility effects in the rat. Life Sci 1983; 33 (Suppl. 1): 473–475.

30. Whitehead WE, Engel BT, Schuster MM. Irritable bowel syndrome. Physiological and psychological differences between diarrhea predominant and constipation predominant patients. Dig Dis Sci 1980; 25: 404–413.

31. Ryan JP, Bhojwani A. Colonic transit in rats: effect of ovariectomy, sex steroid hormones, and pregnancy. Am J Physiol 1986; 251: G46–G50.

32. Williams CL, Villar RG, Peterson JM, Burks TF. Stress-induced changes in intestinal transit in the rat: a model for irritable bowel syndrome. Gastroenterology 1988; 94: 611–621.

33. Puglisis-Allegra S, Castellano C, Oliverio A. Circadian variation in stress-induced analgesia. Brain Res 1982; 252: 373–376.

34. Stevenson NR, Sitren HS, Furuya S. Circadian rhythmicity in several small intestinal functions is independent of use of the intestine. Am J Physiol 1980; 238: G203–G207.

35. Olson CE, Soll AH, Guth PH. Circadian variation of susceptibility to gastric mucosal injury by acidified aspirin or absolute ethanol in the rat. Gastroenterology 1986; 91: 1192–1197.

36. Kumar D, Wingate DL. IBS: a paroxysmal disorder. Lancet 1985; 2: 973–977.

37. Kumar D, Wingate DL, Ruckebusch Y. Circadian variation in the propagation velocity of the migrating motor complex. Gastroenterology 1998; 91: 926–930.

38. Miller MS, Galligan JJ, Burks TF. Accurate measurement of intestinal transit. J Pharmacol Methods 1981; 6: 211–217.

39. Rivier CL, Plotsky PM. Mediation by corticotropin releasing factor (CRF) of adrenohypophysial hormone secretion. Annu Rev Physiol 1986; 48: 475–494.

40. Guillemin R, Vargo T, Rossier J, et al. β-endorphin and adrenocorticotropin are secreted concomitantly by the pituitary gland. Science 1977; 197: 1367–1369.
41. Galligan JJ, Burks TF. Opioid peptides inhibit intestinal transit in the rat by a central mechanism. Eur J Pharmacol 1982; 85: 61–68.
42. Burks TF, Galligan JJ, Hirning LD, Porreca F. Brain, spinal cord and peripheral sites of action of enkephalins and other endogenous opioids on gastrointestinal motility. Gastroenterol Clin Biol 1987; 11: 44B–51B.
43. Brown MR, Fisher LA. Corticotropin-releasing factor: effects on the autonomic nervous system and visceral systems. Fed Proc 1985; 44: 243–248.
44. Gué M, Bueno L. Diazepam and muscimol blockade of the gastrointestinal motor disturbances induced by acoustic stress in dogs. Eur J Pharmacol 1986; 131: 123–127.
45. Gué M, Fioramonti J, Frexinos J, Alvinerie M, Bueno L. Influence of acoustic stress by noise on gastrointestinal motility in dogs. Dig Dis Sci 1987; 32: 1411–1417.
46. Williams CL, Peterson JM, Villar RG, Burks TF. Corticotropin-releasing factor directly mediates colonic responses to stress. Am J Physiol 1987; 253: G582–G586.
47. Rivier J, Rivier C, Vale W. Synthetic competitive antagonists of corticotropin-releasing factor induced ACTH secretion in the rat. Science 1985; 224: 889–891.
48. Lenz HJ, Burlage M, Raedler A, Greten H. Central nervous system effects of corticotropin-releasing factor on gastrointestinal transit in the rat. Gastroenterology 1988; 94: 598–602.
49. Lenz HJ, Raedler A, Greten H, Vale WW, Rivier JE. Stress-induced gastrointestinal secretory and motor responses in rats are mediated by endogenous corticotropin-releasing factor. Gastroenterology 1988; 95: 1510–1517.
50. Bueno L, Fargeas MJ, Gué M, Peeters TL, Bormans V, Fioramonti J. Effects of corticotropin-releasing factor on plasma motilin and somatostatin levels and gastrointestinal motility in dogs. Gastroenterology 91: 1986; 884–889.
51. Bueno L, Gué M. Evidence for the involvement of corticotropin-releasing factor in the gastrointestinal disturbances induced by acoustic and cold stress in mice. Brain Res 1988; 441: 1–4.
52. Nieuwenhuyzen-Kruseman AC, Linton EA, Lowry PJ, Rees LH, Besser GM. CRF-like immunoreactivity in the human gastrointestinal tract. Lancet 1982; 2: 1245–1246.
53. Petrusz P, Merchenthaler I, Maderdrut JL, Heitz PU. Central and peripheral distribution of corticotropin-releasing factor. Fed Proc 1985; 44: 229–235.

27

STRESS-INDUCED IMMUNE DYSFUNCTION IN HUMANS

Michael Irwin

*Veterans Administration Medical Center and University of California
School of Medicine, San Diego, California*

The role of stress or threatening life events in inducing immunological disturbances in humans has been the subject of keen interest over the last several years. This chapter will review the studies that describe an association between adverse life events, psychological responses, and altered immunity. To facilitate the organization and understanding of the evidence supporting a relationship between stress and immune dysfunction, a hypothetical model is proposed and discussed briefly.

MODEL OF STRESS-INDUCED IMMUNE DYSFUNCTION

One model with which to frame and understand the clinical research that describes the association between stress and immune dysfunction in humans is illustrated in Figure 1. This basic model is a simplified ideal that suggests how several social, psychological, and biological domains might be related to immune dysfunction following adverse life events, while recognizing that the relationship among these psychosocial and psychological domains is certain to be more complex than what is shown. Furthermore, the available data, based mainly on cross-sectional studies, are not yet able to characterize fully the causal pathways between these domains that result in immune changes or potential development of disease in persons subject to stress. Longitudinal studies are needed to test these proposed paths. Nevertheless, this model emphasizes some of the specific

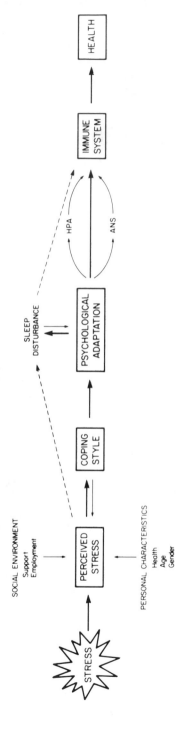

FIGURE 1 Hypothetical model to explain association between stress and immune alterations in humans.

hypothesized relationships that have been examined in a series of studies over the last decade.

This model predicts that certain combinations of stressors and buffers in the social environment will act through individual adaptation to produce biological changes in the endocrine and immune systems that can result in illness. For example, personal characteristics such as age and health, and psychosocial and environmental factors such as social support and employment status, converge with the individual's personality to predict the person's level of coping and psychological adaptation to stress. Alterations in that psychological adaptation, as measured by symptoms of insomnia, anxiety, and/or depression, are then postulated to mediate changes in neuroendocrine and autonomic efferent pathways from the brain to alter immune function. Such decrements in immunological competence are hypothesized to produce an increased susceptibility to disease and changes in health outcome. Of course, health changes in and of themselves may be psychologically stressful, can actually change the social environment (e.g., levels of social support), and may have independent effects on such biological variables as neuroendocrine and immune function.

The following sections will review the clinical findings that link stressful events, disruption of social supports, and poor psychological adaptation to altered immune function. The hypothesized relationships between altered immunity and stress with regard to each of these broad domains will be outlined and organized according to the proposed model, given the limitations of conclusions based on retrospective data. Furthermore, no single study has yet described the rich complexity of all these interrelationships. First, however, a brief overview of the immune system and its relevance to health status will be provided. This overview is an attempt to place the data linking psychological processes and immune function in the broader context of the psychobiology of health and disease.

LIFE STRESS AND HEALTH OUTCOME

Morbidity and Mortality in Bereavement

Experimental and epidemiological evidence link adverse life events, psychological distress, and depressive symptoms to the development and course of many human diseases. One of the most stressful life experiences, the death of a spouse, has been researched since the 19th century. In the past 20 years, studies of conjugal bereavement have demonstrated an elevated mortality rate among bereaved spouses that varied with age, sex, and time elapsed after the loss (1–11). Despite the heterogeneity of the results, there appears to be an excess mortality during the early periods after the loss, particularly among widowers up to the age of 75. However, one well-conducted study failed to show this effect

(3), and another recent study found no association between bereavement and mortality due to cancer (13).

One possible explanation that has been suggested for the premature death of a bereaved spouse involves the "broken heart effect." While more inquiry is needed, this hypothesis has been supported by several studies that have demonstrated that object loss and depression are the setting in which disease can occur. For example, Schmale and Iker interviewed 42 patients admitted to a general medical service and documented that 31 of 42 patients experienced the onset of an illness within 1 week of a significant loss (14). Other studies have shown an association between depressive profiles and development of cancer. In 40 women hospitalized for cone biopsies having class III Pap smears, feelings of hopelessness identified at interview correctly classified 8 of the 14 women with cancer and 23 of the 26 women without cancer (15). Grossarth-Maticek et al. similarly noted that feelings of hopelessness and depression at baseline were associated with an increased incidence of cancer among 1353 persons examined in a Yugoslav village and evaluated for a total of 10 years (16). The Western Electric Health Study has demonstrated, with 20 years of follow-up, an association between depression as measured by the Minnesota Multiphasic Personality Inventory and an increased mortality due to cancer (17). Even after adjustment for age, number of cigarettes smoked, alcohol intake, occupational status, and family history of cancer, the relationship between depressive personality and cancer persisted. Together these results are consistent with the hypothesis that psychological depression or response to loss may provoke the development of disease, in particular, spread of malignant neoplasms (18).

Depression and Cancer

To establish further this link between psychological states and malignant disease, several follow-up studies have demonstrated that affective disorders and clinical depression are related to increased cancer morbidity and mortality. In a 4 year follow-up of patients with primary diagnoses of affective disorders, men over age 40 had a higher mortality rate, particularly from carcinoma, than similar-aged men in the general population (19). Varsamis has confirmed these observations in a 6 year follow-up of psychiatric patients (20). In addition, older patients (mean age, 76.5 years) with affective disorders had a higher incidence of malignant disease than other geriatric patients (21). However, Anisman and Vacharko have provided a review of studies of stress and cancer in human subjects and concluded that studies "at best provided a mixed bag of results and the factors contributing to diverse outcome across studies have yet to be identified" (22). Thus, future approaches need to adopt an experimental sophistication that involves well-controlled, prospective, and prognostic evaluations in which the analyses are based on types of tumors and include social, cultural and demographic variables.

Caregiving Stress: Health Impact

Aside from studies of the effects of bereavement and loss, there has been little systematic work on the health impact of other major life stresses. However, recent studies have begun to describe the physical and mental health risks associated with the distress of caring for ill spouses. For example, Satariano et al. (23) found that elderly people who reported their spouses as being ill in the last 6 months were more likely to report their own health as poor compared to those whose spouses were not previously ill (23). Fengler and Goodrich reported that elderly wives caring for disabled husbands suffered many health problems and should be considered "hidden patients" (24). Although George and Gwyther failed to find deterioration in physical health for caregivers of memory-impaired adults, they did find them especially vulnerable to psychological distress (25). Living with the patient was associated with decreased mental health, social participation, and financial resources (25).

Influences of Coping and Social Support

Style of coping and quality of social support are thought to be determinants of whether such severe adversities as bereavement or caregiving become translated into psychological and physical morbidity. As the Greek philosopher Epictetus noted, "We are disturbed not by events but by our opinions of events." An event is a stressor only if some mediator meaning converts it into a noxious stimulus. Thus, if coping strategies and social supports influence the response to adverse events, these factors should buffer the health-related effect of stressful events. Green et al. showed in 50 males with periodontal disease that as the number of what many observers would consider to be stressors in their lives increased, severity and spread of disease increased in most of the subjects, but not in all (26). Some of the patients, who did not feel threatened by their experiences, did not show progression of disease. Temoshok has also found that one factor influencing survival among patients with acquired immune deficiency syndrome (AIDS) was the degree of control they experienced over their lives; those who felt they could exert little control died more quickly (27).

In summary, severe stressful life events, particularly loss, are associated with decrements in health. Evidence suggests that when a person is in psychological distress or coping poorly with life stress, he or she is at risk for changes in health.

RELEVANCE OF IMMUNE SYSTEM TO HEALTH

One hypothesis to explain why the morbidity and mortality of stressed or depressed persons are increased proposes that changes in the immune system may occur that account for an increase in infectious, neoplastic, or autoimmune disease. However, some of the disorders reported to follow stress are not obviously immune related; the increased mortality rate in bereaved spouses is due at least in part to an increased incidence of cardiac disease such as arrhythmias (28). Nevertheless, a number of stress-related disorders are associated with either a decrement in immunological competence or an alteration in the regulation of the immune system (29). The increased incidence of mononucleosis (30), influenza, pneumonia, tuberculosis (31,32), streptococcal (33), and herpes (34) infections in stressed persons is thought to be associated with immunological hypoactivity, whereas the stress-related increase in the rates of arthritis (35,36) and other autoimmune disorders along with allergies (37) may reflect immune hyper-activity.

Limitations of Current Studies

The relationship between adverse life events, depressive symptoms, immune alterations, and health status is complex and largely unexplored. No study has yet delineated a causal chain showing that a particular psychological state produces an immunological response that then results in an altered clinical outcome. Elliott and Eisdorfer argue that to understand the relationship be-tween stress and disease all the processes involved in an "X" to "Y" to "Z" model must be studied (38). Most studies have demonstrated that psychological processes can result in immune changes. Others have shown that psychological processes can influence the development of disease. What is missing are studies that have examined all these links simultaneously (39).

Furthermore, it may be an oversimplification to suggest that stress-related decreases in any one, or even several, in vitro immune measures may accurately reflect immunological competence and predict an increased susceptibility to illness (40,41). For example, a decrease in one immune parameter, T-helper cell function, may result in an increased risk for acute viral infections but a de-creased risk for autoimmune processes. Thus, an association between suscepti-bility to illness and immune changes depends not only on the magnitude of immune change but also on the specific immune parameter involved and its relationship to and function within the immune system. To highlight the com-plexity of the immune system, a review of the major components of the immune system and their relation to a variety of illnesses are presented briefly in the following section. Elements of the immune system that have been studied in persons undergoing stress will be emphasized.

The Immune System

The immune system is a surveillance mechanism that discriminates self from nonself (42). Immunological defenses against foreign antigens protect the individual from disease-causing microorganisms such as bacteria and viruses, parasites, and cancer cells (40). This resistance is subserved by a dual system: the cellular and humoral immune responses (40).

Humoral Immunity

The humoral immune response leads to the production of specific antibodies directed against foreign antigens. The pathway of this response involves a complex interaction between immune cells including T lymphocytes, B lymphocytes, and accessory cells such as macrophages. One kind of T lymphocyte, the T-helper cell, responds to the presence of nonself antigen, binds to it, and presents it to B cells, causing them to differentiate and secrete a specific antibody. Deficiencies of any component in this pathway will lead to a diminished humoral response to antigen and thus a decreased resistance to infection (40,43). For example, destruction of T-helper cells by the human immunodeficiency virus (HIV) occurs in individuals with acquired immunodeficiency syndrome, leading to their infection with viruses, bacteria, fungi, and parasites (44).

The B cells that differentiate into plasma cells produce five classes of antibodies or immunoglobulins (IgG, IgM, IgA, IgE, and IgD) (45). IgG, the major circulating antibody, enters most tissue spaces and functions by coating microorganisms, making it possible for polymorphonuclear neutrophils and macrophages to recognize, engulf, and destroy foreign antigens such as bacteria (45). IgM is confined to the vascular compartment and is capable of directly annihilating bacteria (45). IgA concentrates in body fluids such as tears, saliva, and secretions of the respiratory and gastrointestinal tracts, functioning to protect these mucosal entrances to the body (46). IgE attaches itself to foreign antigens and then to the surface of the specialized tissue cells such as basophils and mast cells (47). Little is known of IgD, which is present in B-cell surfaces and thought to facilitate the process of lymphocyte activation by an unknown mechanism.

Cellular Immunity

The cellular immune response is characterized by the ability of various killer cells to seek out and destroy either cells infected with viruses or tumor cells that have acquired foreign nonself antigenic characteristics. One type of killer effector cell, the cytotoxic T cell, interacts with T-helper cells to proliferate and then kill cells specific for given antigens such as virally infected cells. Another type of killer cell, the natural killer (NK) cell, demonstrates killer cell activity that is immunologically nonspecific (40,48). These cells are presumably of T-cell lineage and do not require sensitization to specific antigens to lyse a wide variety of cell types. Loss of NK cell function impairs host resistance against viral illness and tumor cell growth (49–53). In animals, studies of levels of NK cytotoxicity are correlated with resistance against tumor growth and metastatic spread. Inhibition of an effective NK response results in a growth of primary metastatic carcinomas (54), selective depletion of NK cells renders mice unable to regulate the growth of an NK susceptible lymphoma (55), and mice congenitally deficient in NK cells have a marked increase in metastases following tumor transplantation (56). In human malignant disease, NK cells also play a role. Patients with a genetic deficiency of NK cells have an increased incidence of a fatal lymphoma-like disorder (57) and persons at risk for cancer have lower NK activity than that found in individuals of control families (58). Augmentation of killer cells using interleukin-2 (IL-2) has been shown to have therapeutic potential in cancer victims even in patients with metastatic disease (59). A reduction in NK activity precedes viral reactivation and development of symptoms (60). Finally, aged subjects (61) and patients with AIDS who are known to be at risk for virus infection (44) have lower NK activity than that found in control subjects.

Immune Regulation

Another aspect of immunological integrity involves its regulation. Failure in immune regulation or a tendency of the system to respond inappropriately to autoantigens (self-antigens) can result in immune responses directed against one's own organs (40). These autoimmune responses can involve both the humoral and cellular immune systems, including autoantibodies produced by B lymphocytes and destruction by T-killer cells and macrophages. Autoimmune reactions that reflect the interaction of lymphocytes are hypothesized to occur because helper T cells are induced or suppressor T cells are inhibited (62). Self-directed immune responses are characterized in a variety of disorders including thyroiditis, rheumatoid arthritis, myasthenia gravis, and systemic lupus erythematosus (40, 63). Thus, the proper regulation of immune responsiveness is crucial for physical health.

Lymphokines

Regulation of the humoral and cell-mediated immune responses also involves the secretion of humoral mediators or lymphocytes by T cells or macrophages (64). For example, the lymphokine interleukin-1 (IL-1) is produced by antigen-activated macrophages (65). Its release leads to the activation of T lymphocytes and their production of interleukin-2 (IL-2) (66). IL-2, which is secreted from these antigen-stimulated lymphocytes, in turn functions to switch T cells from G1 (resting) into the S (DNA replication) phase of the cell cycle, thus serving as a mediator of T-cell clonal expansion (67). Furthermore, previous studies have indicated that IL-2 receptor density may be one of the critical variables that determine the extent of T-cell proliferation. IL-2 receptors are only expressed on activated T cells (e.g., after exposure to either mitogens such as concanavalin A or IL-1) (68). Interferon, which is also produced by antigenically stimulated peripheral blood lymphocytes, activates NK cells and NK lysis (53). Interferon has been postulated to play a protective role against viral infections and tumor cell growth (69). In summary, it is likely that factors that influence the expression of IL-1, IL-2, or gamma interferon would have an impact on the responsiveness of lymphocytes to antigens and, thus, the regulation of the immune system.

Inadequate production of lymphokines has been observed in several disease states, including deficits in nutritional status, the development or progression of

AIDS, autoimmune diseases, diabetes mellitus, and certain types of cancer (64). However, it is not clear whether the failure to produce a particular lymphokine in vitro reflects what occurs in vivo.

We have reviewed the various components of the immune system. We now turn to studies that describe alterations in immunological functioning among persons undergoing stress.

STRESS AND IMMUNE DYSFUNCTION

Clinical Studies of Bereavement

The loss of a spouse is a tragic experience: it is accorded premiere status of all stressful life experiences, rank-ordered in terms of their impact (70). Clinical studies of immune function in bereavement have demonstrated altered immunity, including suppression of lymphocyte responses to mitogenic stimulation, reduced natural killer cell activity, and alterations of T-cell subpopulations.

In 1977, Bartrop and colleagues first reported a relationship between bereavement and immunological function (71). Measures of lymphocyte responses to mitogen stimulation were compared in 26 men and women whose spouses had died and in 26 age- and sex-matched control subjects. T cell responses to low dosages of phytohemagglutinin (PHA) and concanavalin A (con A) were reduced both at 3 weeks and at 6 weeks after the death of the spouses, during which time active bereavement occurred. T- and B-cell numbers did not differ between groups. In addition, lymphocyte function in vivo was evaluated using several specific antigens (streptokinase, mumps antigen, and purified protein derivative of tuberculin) known to produce characteristic delayed hypersensitivity reactions on routine skin testing. No differences between the bereaved subjects and controls were obtained using these skin testing procedures. However, anergy on skin testing implied a more profound compromise of the immunological apparatus than abnormal responses to mitogen stimulation.

In the second study, Schleifer et al. prospectively measured white blood cell count, T- and B-lymphocyte populations, and responses to PHA, con A, and pokeweed mitogen stimulation in 15 men before and after the death of their wives from metastatic breast cancer (72). Schleifer and colleagues confirmed Bartrop et al.'s finding of suppressed mitogen stimulation responses in bereavement, demonstrating a significant suppression of lymphocyte responses during the first 2 months following the death of a spouse. An intermediate level of mitogen responsivity was found during the 4–14 month period after bereavement. Neither total white blood cell count nor T- and B-cell subpopulations differed from before to after bereavement.

These two studies documented an association between bereavement and suppressed lymphocyte responses to mitogens and raised new questions. Does bereavement affect not only lymphocyte responses to mitogenic stimulation but also other parameters of humoral and cell-mediated immunity? For example, assessment of plasma immunoglobulin levels, NK cell activity, or T-cell subpopulations would extend these observations and further characterize the association between bereavement and changes in other components of immunity. Second, are immunological changes in bereavement confined to subjects who respond to the loss with demonstrable depressive symptoms? Thus, the psychological response to the loss, not merely the event, may mediate alterations in immune function.

Linn et al. examined immunocompetence during bereavement using various measures of humoral and cell-mediated immunity (73). Severity of depressive symptoms was assessed using the depression subscale of the Hopkins symptom checklist. Reduced lymphocyte responses to the mitogen PHA were found in bereaved subjects who had high depression scores but not in those who had few signs of depression. Lymphocyte responses to con A and pokeweed mitogen did not differ between those with and without depressive symptoms. Moreover, analyses of serum levels of IgG, IgA, and IgM, in vivo responses to skin tests, and neutrophilic chemotaxis in the bereaved subjects were comparable to those found in the controls. Based on these observations, the authors concluded that abnormal lymphocyte responses in bereaved persons were more likely in those with depressive symptoms.

To extend these earlier observations and clarify further the effect of psychological processes on immune function, Irwin et al. conducted a series of clinical studies that addressed the role of bereavement and depressive symptoms in altering T-cell subpopulations and NK activity (74–78). In the first study, measures of total lymphocyte counts, T-helper, and T-suppressor cell numbers, and NK cytotoxicity were compared among three groups of women: those whose husbands were dying of lung cancer, those whose husbands had recently died, and women whose husbands were in good health (77). The 37 women who formed this study population were free of chronic medical disorders associated with altered immune function and did not abuse drugs or alcohol. Current changes in marital relationships and other life experiences were assessed using the Social Readjustment Rating Scale (SRS) and the severity of depressive symptoms was rated using the Hamilton Depression Rating Scale (HDRS). Subjects and controls were studied at least 3 times over a 1–3 month period and results of the immune assays were expressed as means for the individual subjects, to minimize the influence of interassay variability in comparisons of these groups.

On the basis of their overall mean SRS scores, subjects were assigned to one of three groups: those with low SRS scores, moderate SRS scores, or high SRS scores. Women whose husbands were healthy were more likely to be classified in the low SRS group, whereas women who either were anticipating or had experienced the death of their husband were likely to be in the middle or high SRS groups, respectively. Neither mean age of the subjects nor ethnic composition was significantly different between these groups. On the average, depressive symptoms as measured by HDRS were significantly more severe in the moderate and high SRS groups than in the low SRS group. NK activity expressed in lytic units was significantly different between the three groups; the groups with moderate and high SRS scores were found to have reduced NK activity compared to low SRS control subjects (Fig. 2). Neither the absolute number of lymphocytes nor the T-cell subpopulations, including number of T-helper, T-suppressor/cytotoxic cells, and the ratio of T-helper to T-suppressor cytotoxic cells, was different between the groups.

To explore the contribution of psychological responses to immune changes in persons experiencing bereavement, the relationship between intensity of

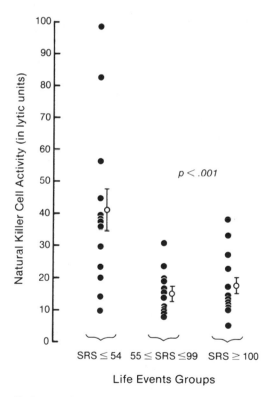

FIGURE 2   Natural killer cell activity in women with low, moderate, and high social readjustment rating scale (SRS) scores. Each point represents the individual mean of multiple measures.

depressive symptoms and alterations of immune variables was evaluated in this cross-sectional study (77). Reduced NK activity was significantly correlated with the HDRS total score and also with the HDRS subscales for depressed mood and insomnia. In addition, the severity of depressive symptoms as measured by total HDRS score was related to a loss of T-suppressor/cytotoxic cells and an increase in the ratio of T-helper to T-suppressor cytotoxic cells.

When taken together, these studies of immunity in bereavement have demonstrated that measures of cell-mediated immunity, including lymphocyte responses to mitogenic stimulation, natural killer cell activity, and T-cell subpopulations, are altered in men and women undergoing major life changes such as bereavement. Furthermore, severity of depressive symptoms in response to the loss appears to be an important determinant of the magnitude of change in these cellular immune measures. Bereavement is a process in which spouses differ in their psychological responses. Some women are more distressed while others are relieved compared with the distress of acute anticipation. Thus, as our model illustrates, these changes in depressive symptoms, not merely the death of the spouse, might predict and potentially determine the reduction in cell-mediated immunity. The important role of psychological processes in mediating altered immunity will be discussed further in a following section.

These studies were conducted to evaluate the relationship between acute severe life changes, such as bereavement, and alterations in immune function. Thus, no data were generated regarding the association between these stress-related immune changes and health outcome. For example, the alterations in the number of T-suppressor cells and in the ratio of T-helper to T-suppressor cells were within the normal range and do not necessarily have clinical significance. However, it is known that lower T-suppressor cell levels are associated with the emergence of autoantibodies (62) and it has been reported that auto-antibodies occur more often in depressed patients than in control subjects (79–82).

In summary, studies of immune function in bereavement have shown that severe acute psychological stress has a significant impact on cellular immunity. Relatively minor aversive events are also associated with altered immunity.

Effect of Examination Stress

Academic examinations are associated with a suppression of lymphocyte responses to mitogen stimulation, reduced NK cell activity, increased plasma titers of Epstein-Barr and herpes viral antigens, alterations in T-cell subpopulations, and increased plasma levels of circulating immunoglobulins.

Dorian et al. first reported alterations in lymphocyte subpopulations and mitogen responses during academic examinations (83). In 8 psychiatry trainees taking their oral examinations and 16 psychiatrists not taking exams, psychological distress was assessed and measures of T-cell subpopulations, B-cell numbers, mitogen reactivity, NK activity, and plaque-forming cell responsiveness were obtained. The "high stress" examinees (based on their ratings on a 10 cm visual analogue scale) exhibited higher white blood cell counts, an increased absolute lymphocyte count, a reduction in PHA reactivity, and a reduction in plaque-forming cell response (an index of B-cell function) than the control subjects and the low-stress examinees.

In a series of other studies conducted by Glaser and Kiecolt-Glaser and colleagues, the initial observations of exam-related alterations in cellular immunity have been confirmed and extended. Medical students demonstrated significantly lower levels of NK activity (84) and blastogenesis (using both con A and PHA) during final examinations as compared to baseline samples taken 1 month earlier (85). Stress-related decreases in the percentages of total T lymphocytes, helper T lymphocytes, and suppressor T cells have been found (85), and examination stress is also associated with significant increases in plasma levels of IgG, IgM, and IgA (86). Although these immunological changes were within the normal range, a similar pattern—hypergammaglobulinemia and decreased cellular immune response (but with changes that are not normal)—has been found in patients with immunosuppressive diseases such as AIDS.

Based on findings that link examination stress and altered immunity and that describe the role of immunity in controlling the recurrence of latent herpes virus infections, further studies of medical students were conducted to determine whether the expression of herpes viral antigens is influenced by examination stress. Antibody titers to Epstein-Barr virus (EBV), cytomegalovirus (CMV), and herpes simplex virus (HSV) were significantly increased during the first day of examination compared to either the month before examination or upon students' return from summer vacation (87). These increased antibody titers against latent herpes viruses were presumed to reflect poorer immune system control of the virus, thus providing empirical support for clinical speculation linking stress and herpes virus infections.

In summary, even a relatively common stressor such as academic stress can downregulate cellular immunity. These changes in immune responses are associated with a reactivation of one or more latent herpes viruses.

Chronic Stress and Immune Dysfunction

Most human behavioral immunology research has focused on the effects of acute stressors and demonstrated that both severe and relatively minor aversive events can alter cellular immunity. It also appears that chronic stressors (lasting over 1 or more years) can result in alterations in immune function.

Kiecolt-Glaser and Glaser et al. have addressed the immunological sequelae of longer-term or chronic stress in the study of caregivers of a patient with

Alzheimer's disease (88). The stresses of caring for a patient with Alzheimer's disease often leave family members at risk for depression (89) and are associated with decreased life satisfaction (25) and increased levels of psychiatric symptoms (25). To understand the health-related effects of caregiving, psychological and immunological analyses were carried out in 34 caregivers and 34 matched controls. The caregivers were found to be more distressed as measured by self-report of depressive symptoms and to have poorer immune function than controls (88). The caregivers showed significantly higher antibody titers to EBV and reduced percentages of total T lymphocytes and helper T cells. Numbers of neither T-suppressor cells nor natural killer cells differed between the two groups.

The stress of job loss and long-term unemployment has also been found to be associated with psychological distress and reduced cellular immune responses (90). Unemployment for more than 9 months was accompanied by a decrease in lymphocyte reactivity to PHA and PPD in vitro compared to the response in control women. Despite an active psychosocial intervention program aimed at those who were unemployed, immunological function was found to remain decreased during the study interval.

These data suggest that chronically stressed individuals, as well as those who are acutely stressed, show poor psychological adaptation and altered immunity compared to well-matched, similarly aged peers. With regard to the immunological changes associated with either acute or chronic stress, it appears that functional assays such as mitogen responses, NK activity, or antibody titers to herpes viruses are more likely to be consistently associated with adverse life events than are changes in quantitative assessments. While the critical connections between stress-related immunologic alterations and actual health changes were not established in any of these investigations, the data have increasingly suggested that these immune decrements may have their most important consequences in persons with other, preexisting immunological impairments, such as aged persons.

Role of Social Support

Social support has been hypothesized to be a key factor in buffering stress, acting to ameliorate the depressive symptoms during stress. In subjects experiencing the stress associated with caring for a patient with Alzheimer's disease, Scott et al. found the support system to be an effective resource in improving caregivers' ability to cope with chronic stress, as measured by severity of psychological symptoms (91). Morycz similarly found the availability of support to be the best predictor of level of caregiver stress, compared to the demographic characteristics of the caregiver and severity of dementia in the patient (92). These studies further emphasize that social support is not simply defined as the count of resource persons, but should also include the types of supports provided, as well as the consistency and emotional satisfaction related to those supports.

Although disruption of social attachments, especially marital relationships, is likely to be associated with more psychological symptoms (93), reduced immunological functioning (71–77), and greater health risks (94), few studies have examined health-related correlates of marital *quality* within the married population. Kiecolt-Glaser et al. hypothesized that marital discord or dissatisfaction related to the spouse may represent a chronic stressor and have important psychological and physiological consequences, including effects on immune function (95). Increased emotional distress is reliably associated with poorer marriage, and unmarried people are happier than those in troubled marriages (96). Furthermore, unhappily married individuals report poorer health than do married or divorced people (97), showing as well greater physiological arousal (98). Kiecolt-Glaser et al. extended these observations and first reported on the association between poor marital quality and reduced immunological functioning among married women (95) and men (99).

In the first study of women (95), 38 separated or divorced women were compared with 38 married women using three functional assays including mitogen responses to con A and PHA and antibody titers to the latent herpes virus, EBV. Quantitative evaluations of T-lymphocyte subsets including numbers of NK cells were also obtained. Consistent with previous findings regarding the immunological effects of marital disruption due to death (71,72,77), separated or divorced women had significantly lower percentages of NK and helper cells, poor mitogen responsiveness, and higher antibodies to EBV than the married women (95). Poor marital quality in the married subjects was also associated with greater depression and a poorer response on the three qualitative or functional immunological assays, lymphocyte responses, and antibody titers to EBV. In summary, these data emphasize that the quality of the marital relationship is associated with immune function; the simple presence of a partner appears not to be equivalent to a supportive relationship.

In a second study, self-report data and blood samples were obtained from 32 separated or divorced men and 32 matched married men (99). Similar to the findings in women, separated or divorced men were more distressed and lonelier and had significantly poorer values on two functional indices of immunity (antibodies to two herpes viruses). T-cell subpopulations did not differ between the groups. Poor marital quality was again associated with greater distress and a poorer response on one functional immunological measure (EBV antibody titers).

In summary, evidence suggests that psychological resources such as supportive relationships moderate distress and may buffer against stress-related immunological changes. Dissatisfaction with relationships, including poor marital quality, is associated with psychological distress and altered immunological functioning, similar to the findings described with other psychological stressors.

Coping and Immune Function

Style of coping is hypothesized to be a determinant of whether severe adversity becomes translated into psychological and physical morbidity. Research on coping and health has been influenced by the work of Lazarus and associates, who defined coping responses into two general categories; problem-focused coping and emotion-focused coping (100). Problem-focused coping includes activities such as information seeking, planning alternative strategies, and actually doing something to change existing poblems. Emotion-focused coping is directed more toward easing inner distress and includes emotional reactions, withdrawal, and drug use.

The potential usefulness of these classifications is illustrated by several reports that found outcomes differing based on the dominant coping strategy used. In a study of older adults coping with chronic illnesses, problem-focused strategies such as information search had a positive effect on adjustment whereas emotion-focused strategies such as wish fulfilling, fantasy, avoidance, and blame are related to poor adjustment and negative affect (101,102). Self-blame combined with perceived loss of control have been found by Pagel to predict worsened depression in caregivers of spouses of Alzheimer's patients in a significant way (103). Levine and associates found that caregivers who used problem solving and positive self-talk were more highly skilled copers with demented relatives than those who did not use such strategies (104).

Despite the clearly demonstrated link between coping and psychological adjustment during stress, few if any studies have evaluated the role of coping responses as defined by Lazarus et al. (100) in mediating stress-induced alterations in immune function. Most have evaluated coping responses indirectly, postulating that a diminished capacity to adapt, as indicated by psychiatric symptoms, is a measure of coping. For example, Locke et al. rated the severity of life events in 114 students and, on the basis of these reports and measures of psychiatric symptoms, organized the sample into four groups: low stress/low symptoms, high stress/high symptoms, high stress/low symptoms, and low stress/ high symptoms (105). Those subjects with few psychological symptoms in the face of large amounts of stress ("good copers") had significantly higher NK activity than those experiencing high levels of both symptoms and stress. Consistent with these data, Irwin et al. found in a small longitudinal study of women experiencing bereavement that the severity of depressive symptoms, not merely the death of the spouse, was correlated with a reduction of NK activity (76). Relaxation techniques have been suggested as a coping intervention to reduce stress (106). In 35 medical students undergoing examination stress, the frequency of relaxation practice was a significant predictor associated with the percentage of T-helper indices. This finding might indicate, according to Kiecolt-Glaser et al., that relaxation techniques are capable of enhancing immunological changes or at least buffering against them during stress (107).

PSYCHOLOGICAL DEPRESSION AND IMMUNE DYSFUNCTION

Alterations in immune function are associated with distressing life events and it appears that the psychological response to these events is an important correlate of immune dysfunction. Since bereaved subjects and distressed persons often manifest depressed mood and symptom patterns consistent with major depressive disorder (108), it has been hypothesized that psychological depression or anxiety may itself be associated with immunological change.

Alterations in T-cell subpopulations have also been characterized in depressed patients compared to control subjects. Consistent with the findings of Irwin et al., who found a relationship between the severity of depressive symptoms and an increase in the ratio of T-helper to suppressor/cytotoxic cells in bereaved women (77), Syvalahti et al. found that depressed patients have a lower percentage of T-suppressor/cytotoxic cells and a higher ratio of T-helper to T-suppressor cytotoxic cells than in control subjects (113). However, other studies have found no depression-related differences in quantitative measures of lymphocytes including number of T cells, B cells, T-helper, T-suppressor, and NK cells (114, 115).

To clarify the role of depression in reducing cell-mediated immunity, several studies have compared immune responses in depressed patients and control subjects. Cappel et al. (109) reported that PHA responses were lower in psychotically depressed patients during the first days of illness than following clinical remission. Kronfol and colleagues replicated these observations in 26 drug-free depressed patients and found blunted lymphocyte responses to mitogenic stimulation with con A, PHA, and pokeweed during depression (110). Schleifer et al. also found suppressed lymphocyte reactivity in severely depressed patients and further described abnormalities of lymphocyte subpopulations in patients with depression. Absolute and T- and B-lymphocyte cell counts were reduced, although relative percentages were unchanged (111). Since no differences in immune measures were found in mildly depressed outpatients (112), Schleifer and colleagues have concluded that the severity of depressive symptoms is an important factor associated with altered lymphocyte responses in depression.

Irwin et al. have extended these observations of altered immunity in depression by measuring the cytolytic activity of peripheral lymphocytes and quantitating the total differential and absolute white blood cell counts in two groups of subjects: medication-free, hospitalized acutely depressed patients and age- and sex-matched control subjects studied on the same day as the patients. In the study of 19 hospitalized male patients who met research diagnostic criteria (RDC) for major depressive disorder, the patients who were acutely depressed showed significantly more depressive symptoms than those in the RDC-never mentally ill control group (116). Neither group included men who were currently abusing alcohol. Figure 3 shows that NK cell activity was significantly

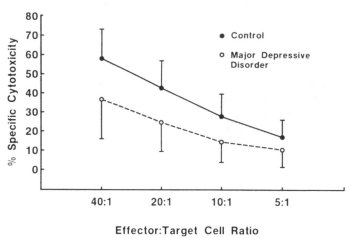

FIGURE 3 Natural killer cytotoxicity in depressed subjects and controls. Each point represents the mean of the percentage specific cytotoxicity for each group (n = 19) across the four effector to target cell ratios.

lower in the depressed patients than in the control subjects, a finding that has been replicated by Urich et al. (117) and Mohl and colleagues (118). In addition, severity of depressive symptoms was correlated with a reduction in NK activity.

The total white blood cell (WBC) count and absolute counts of each cell type were also compared between the two groups. The depressed patients showed both a significantly higher WBC count and a higher number of neutrophils than control subjects, but concentrations of lymphocytes, monocytes, and eosinophils were not significantly different between the two groups. Thus, the present study using a cross-sectional matched-pair design confirms the retrospective report of Kronfol et al., which describes an increased number of neutrophils in depressed patients compared to controls (119).

Altered immunity involving reduced NK activity, neutrophilia, changes in T-cell subpopulations, and suppressed lymphocyte responses to mitogenic stimulation appears to be a biological concomitant of affective disorders. While these data support the role of psychological processes and depressive symptoms in mediating alterations in immune function, the mechanisms by which these immunological abnormalities occur in stressed and depressed patients remain largely unexplored.

MECHANISMS OF IMMUNE DYSFUNCTION: CLINICAL STUDIES

The following sections will briefly review evidence that stress might be associated with alterations in the release of lymphokines important in the regulation of cellular immune responses; changes in a number of behavioral factors, such as sleep patterns and activity or exercise levels, that can affect immune function; and perturbations of the endocrine system. Clinical studies will be highlighted that describe the potential role of these various factors in mediating immune changes during stressful psychological events.

Stress and Changes in Lymphokine Regulation

As has been discussed, psychological stress can have a negative impact on cell-mediated immune responses and it is possible that stress induces alterations in either the release of lymphokines or the response of T and B cells to these humoral immune regulators. Based on considerable evidence that NK lysis is reduced during stress, studies have begun to focus on the impact of stress on immunological modulators of NK cell activation and lysis. To this end, Glaser et al. have found that total interferon production by con-A-stimulated lymphocytes is decreased during stress (120). Gamma interferon, which is important in controlling viral infections, augments NK lysis (64). Future studies might examine stress-related difference in the production of IL-1 and IL-2 or the expression of IL-2 receptors by lymphocytes.

Influence of Behavioral Factors

Both sleep disturbances and reduced activity levels occur in depressed patients and stressed persons and changes in each of these behavioral factors could potentially produce alterations in immune function. In investigating the role of sleep disturbance, Palmblad et al. found in 12 male students that sleep deprivation for 48 h produced a significant decrease in lymphocyte responses to PHA stimulation (121). These responses increased to baseline levels after the vigil. Based on the findings of Moldofsky et al., which describe an association between slow-wave sleep onset and dramatic increases in IL-1 activity and changes in both lymphocyte reactivity to PHA and NK activity (122), future studies might evaluate the relationship between depression-associated changes in sleep architecture and immune abnormalities.

Moderate exercise has been found to produce increases in the population of circulating cells that can lyse NK targets (123). Data from 10 volunteers demonstrated an increase in the number of *activated* killer cells, suggesting a recruitment of circulating inactive cells to become active killer cells. While the mechanism of this effect is not known, exercise facilitates the release of interferon and B-endorphin and both hormones can augment NK cytotoxicity.

Endocrine Responses and Immune Function

Endocrine changes concomitant with stress and depression may mediate alterations in immunity. First, hypercortisolism has been postulated to play a governing role in the immunological deficits during stress and depression. Munck and colleagues (124) have hypothesized that glucocorticoids act to suppress the primary defense reactions, including immune reactivity, following stress. However, the in vivo immunoregulatory effects of corticosteroids in humans have not been clearly defined. For example, in vitro studies are frequently performed with suprapharmacological dosages of corticosteroids that are not attainable in humans following in vivo administration (125). Moreover, the results of studies done in rats, a steroid-sensitive species, may not be relevant to the immunological actions of corticosteroids in a steroid-resistant species such as humans. Thus, with these caveats in mind, several recent studies in humans have examined the role of stress-induced increases in adrenal cortical activity to modulate immune function.

Irwin et al. investigated the relationship between NK activity and plasma cortisol in three groups of subjects: women who were anticipating the death of their husbands, women whose husbands had recently died, and controls. Bereaved women showed reduced NK activity and increased plasma cortisol levels compared to controls (126). However, anticipatory bereaved women who also showed significant reductions in NK activity had levels of cortisol comparable to those of controls (Fig. 4). Increases in plasma cortisol levels were not correlated with a reduction of NK activity during bereavement. A similar lack of association between adrenal activity and immune function has been found in depressed patients. Suppressed lymphocyte responses to mitogen has been associated with neither dexamethasone nonsuppression (127) nor increased secretion rates of urinary free cortisol (128). Furthermore, in animals, shock has been found to reduce lymphocyte responses to mitogens in both adrenalectomized and control groups (129). In summary, it appears that increased secretion of glucocorticoids is not required for stress-related suppression. Instead, alterations in other neurohormones, neurotransmitters, and neuropeptides may reduce cell-mediated immune responses.

The autonomic nervous system is another pathway by which the brain or psychological states may alter immunological functioning. Nervous fibers are distributed throughout lymphoid tissues including both primary (thymus, bone marrow) and secondary (spleen, lymph nodes) organs and are localized in the vasculature and parenchyma of these tissues (130). Thus, regions of lymphoid tissues in which lymphocytes reside receive direct nervous innervation by fibers containing predominantly norepinephrine (131). Lymphocytes are capable of receiving signals from the sympathetic nervous system, and Hellstrand et al. have shown that direct in vitro application of norepinephrine inhibits NK activity, an effect that is antagonized by preincubation with the beta antagonist propranolol (132). The functional relationship between sympathetic nerves, monoamine neurotransmitters, and immune responses has only begun to be studied. No clinical studies have yet examined the relationship between stress-induced increases in catecholamines and altered immune function. However, in rats either surgical denervation of the spleen or chemical sympathectomy using 6-hydroxydopamine produces augmented antibody responses and altered T- and B-cell responsiveness to mitogen stimulation (131).

The release of neuropeptides or neurotransmitters within the brain may

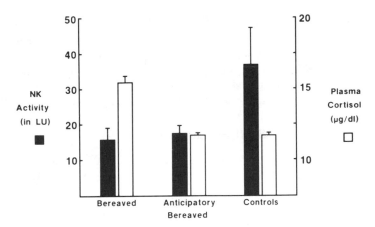

FIGURE 4 Natural killer cell activity and plasma cortisol levels in three groups of women: those mourning the loss of their husbands (n = 9), those anticipating his death (n = 11), and control subjects (n = 8). Range shown is mean ± SEM of multiple measures of NK activity and plasma cortisol.

coordinate activation of the pituitary adrenal axis and the autonomic nervous system to reduce immune function during stress. Corticotropin-releasing factor (CRF) has been hypothesized to act as a central nervous system regulator of biological responses to stress. Irwin et al. have recently posed an animal model to test whether central CRF is involved in stress-related immune suppression (133). Central administration of CRF produces a dose-dependent suppression of NK activity that appears to be specific and independent of direct systemic mechanisms. The autonomic nervous system is likely to be one pathway by which central CRF reduces natural killer cytotoxicity. Pharmacological manipulations that prevent CRF-induced increases in plasma norepinephrine levels also significantly antagonize the reduction of NK activity by CRF (134). In addition, CRF-induced increases in plasma norepinephrine are correlated with the reduction of NK activity (134). Based on the finding that increased concentrations of CRF have been found in the cerebrospinal fluid of depressed patients (135), it is tempting to consider the possibility that alterations of CRF in depression or stress might be operating to reduce immune function.

SUMMARY

We have reviewed evidence for diminished cell-mediated immune function during threatening life events and clinical depression. A model has been formulated to organize the clinical research relevant to the association between stress and immune dysfunction. To characterize the mechanisms by which the brain influences immune cells, an interdisciplinary approach involving the efforts of researchers with expertise in the neuroendocrine and autonomic physiology of the stress response is needed. An additional challenge for medicine is to use longitudinal data to test the pathways by which psychological responses alter immune function. Furthermore, no conclusions can yet be reached concerning the clinical relevance of these perturbations of the immunological apparatus in producing health risks and increased vulnerability to disease in patients experiencing stress.

ACKNOWLEDGMENT

This work was partly supported by NIMH grants #MH44275-01, #MH30914, the San Diego VA Clinical Research Center on Alcoholism, and a VA Merit Review.

REFERENCES

1. Rees W D, Lutkins S G. Mortality of bereavement. Br Med J 1967; 4:13–16.
2. Kraus A S, Lilienfeld A M. Some epidemiologic aspects of the high mortality rate in the young widowed group. J Chron Dis 1959; 10:207–217.
3. Helsing K J, Szklo M. Mortality after bereavement. Am J Epidemiol 1981; 114:41–52.
4. Young M, Benjamin B, Wallis C. The mortality of widowers. Lancet 1963; 2:454–456.
5. Cox P R, Ford J R. The mortality of widows shortly after widowhood. Lancet 1964; 1:163–164.
6. Parkes C M, Benjamin B, Fitzgerald R G. Broken heart: a statistical study of increased mortality among widows. Br Med J 1969; 1:740–743.
7. Ward A W M. Mortality of bereavement. Br Med J 1976; 1:700–702.
8. Bowling A, Benjamin B. Mortality after bereavement: a follow-up study of a sample of elderly widowed people. Biol Soc 1985; 2:197–203.
9. Ekblom B. Significance of socio-psychological factors with regard to risk of death among elderly persons. Acta Psychiatr Scand 1963; 39:627–633.
10. Mellstrom D, Nilsson A, Oden A, Rundgren A, Svanborg A. Mortality among the widowed in Sweden. Scand J Soc Med 1982; 10:33–41.
11. Karpio J, Koskenvuo M, Rita H. Mortality after bereavement: a prospective study of 95,647 widowed persons. Am J Public Health 1987; 77:283–287.
12. Clayton PJ. Mortality and morbidity in the first year of widowhood. Arch Gen Psychiatry 1974; 30:747–750.
13. Jones DR, Goldblatt PO, Leon DA. Bereavement and cancer: some data on deaths of spouses from the longitudinal study of Office of Population Censuses and Surveys. Br Med J 1984; 289:461–464.
14. Schmale AH, Iker H. Hopelessness as a predictor of cervical cancer. Soc Sci Med 1966; 5:95–100.
15. Schmale AH, Iker HP. The effect of hopelessness and the development of cancer. I. Identification of uterine cervical cancer in women with atypical cytology. Psychosom Med 1966; 28:714–721.
16. Grossarth-Maticek R, Kanazir DT, Vetter H, Schmidt P. Psychosomatic factors involved in the process of cancerogenesis. Psychother Psychosom 1983; 40:191–210.

17. Persky VW, Kempthorne-Rawson J, Shekelle RB. Personaltiy and risk of cancer; 20-year follow-up of the Western Electric study. Psychosom Med 1987; 49:435–449.
18. Engel GL. A life setting conducive to illness: the giving-up given-up complex. Arch Intern Med 1968; 69:293–300.
19. Whitlock FA, Siskind M. Depression and cancer: a follow-up study. Psychol Med 1979; 9:747–752.
20. Varsamis J, Zuchowski T, Main KK. Survival rate and causes of death of geriatric psychiatric patients. Can Psychiatr Assoc J 1972; 17:17–21.
21. Kerr TA, Schapiro K, Roth M. Relationship between premature death and affective disorders. Br J Psychiatry 1969; 115:1277–1282.
22. Anisman H, Zacharko RM. Stress and neoplasia: speculations and caveats. Behav Med Update 1983; 5:27–35.
23. Satariano W, Minkler MA, Langhauser C. The significance of an ill spouse for assessing health differences in an elderly population. J Am Geriatr Soc 1984; 32:187–190.
24. Fengler AP, Goodrich N. Wives of elderly disabled men: the hidden patients. Gerontologist 1979; 19:175.
25. George LK, Gwyther LP. Caregiver well-being: a multidimensional examination of family caregivers of demented adults. Gerontologist 1986; 26: 253–259.
26. Green LW, Tryon WW, Marks B, Huryn J. Periodontal disease as a function of life events stress. J Hum Stress 1986; 12:32–36.
27. Temoshok L, Fox BH (eds). International issue. Advances 1986; 3(4):1–179.
28. Jacobs S, Ostfeld A. An epidemiological review of the mortality of bereavement. Psychosom Med 1977; 39:Z344–357.
29. Melnechuk T. Emotions, brain immunity, and health: a review. In: Clynes M, Panksepp J, eds. Emotions and Psychopathology. New York: Plenum Press, 1988: 181–247.
30. Kasl SV, Evans AS, Niederman JC. Psychosocial risk factors in the development of infectious mononucleosis. Psychosom Med 1979; 41:445–446.
31. Plaut SM, Friedman SB. Psychosocial factors, stress, and disease processes. In: Ader R, ed. Psychoneuroimmunology. New York: Academic Press, 1981:3–30.
32. Plaut SM, Friedman SB. Biological mechanisms in the relationship of stress to illness. Pediatr Annu 1985; 14:563–567.
33. Meyer RJ, Haggerty R. Streptococcal infections in families: factors altering individual susceptibility. Pediatrics 1962; 29:539–549.
34. Cohen F. Stress and bodily illness. Psychiatr Clin North Am 1981; 4:267–286.
35. Baker GBH, Brewerton DA. Rheumatoid arthritis: a psychiatric assessment. Br Med J 1981; 282:2014.
36. Solomon GF. Emotional and personality factors in the onset and course of autoimmune disease, particularly rheumatoid arthritis. In: Ader R, ed. Psychoneuroimmunology. New York: Academic Press, 1981: 159–182.
37. Barnes DM. Nervous and immune system disorders linked in a variety of diseases. Science 1986; 232:160–161.

38. Elliott GR, Eisdorfer C. Stress and human health. New York: Springer, 1982.
39. Braveman N. Immunity and aging: immunological and behavioral perspectives. In: MW Riley, Matarazzo JM, Baum A, eds. The aging dimension. Hillsdale, NJ: Lawrence Erlbaum, 1987: 93–124.
40. Hood LE, Weisman IL, Wood WB, Wilson JH. Immunology. Menlo Park, CA: Benjamin Cummings.
41. Calabrese JR, Kling MA, Gold PW. Alterations in immunocompetence during stress, bereavement, and depression: focus on neuroendocrine regulation. Am J Psychiatry 1987; 144:1123–1134.
42. Cohn M. What are the elements of immune responsiveness? In: Guillemin R, Cohn M, Melnechuk T, eds. Neural modulation of immunity. New York: Raven Press, 1985: 3–25.
43. Blumberg RS, Schooley RT. Lymphocyte markers and infectious disease. Semin Hematol 1985; 22:31–114.
44. Creemers PC, Sterk DF, Boyko WJ. Evaluation of natural killer cell activity in patients with persistent generalized lymphadenopathy and acquired immunodeficiency syndrome. Clin Immunol Immunopathol 1985; 36:414–450.
45. Spiegelberg HL. Biological activities of immunoglobulins of different classes and subclasses. Adv Immunol 1974; 19:259–270.
46. Hanson LA, Ahlstedt S, Anderson B, et al. The biological properties of secretory IgA. J Reticuloendothel Soc 1980; 28(suppl):1S–9S.
47. Lichtenstein LM, Norman PS. Human allergic reactions. Am J Psychiatry 1969; 46:163–171.
48. Marx JL. How killer cells kill their targets. Science 1986; 231:1367–70.
49. Burnet FM. The concept of immunological surveillance. Prog Exp Tumor Res 1970; 13:1–2.
50. Henney CS, Gillis S. Cell-mediated cytotoxicity. In: Paul WE, ed. Fundamental immunology. New York: Raven Press, 1984.
51. Herberman RB. Natural cell mediated immunity against tumors. New York: Academic Press, 1980.
52. Herberman RB, Otaldo JR. Natural killer cells: their role in defense against disease. Science 1981; 214:24.
53. Herberman RB. Natural killer cells. Hosp Pract 1982; 4:93–103.
54. Reid LM, Minato N, Gresser I, et al. Influence of antimouse interferon serum on the growth and metastasis of tumor cells persistently injected with virus and human prostatic tumor athymic mice. Proc Natl Acad Sci USA 1981; 78:1171.
55. Kawase I, Urdol DL, Brooks CG. Selective depletion of NK cell activity in vivo and its effect on the growth of NK sensitive and NK resistant tumor cell variants. Int J Cancer 1982; 29:507.
56. Talmadge JE, Myers KM, Prien DJ, et al. Role of NK cells in tumor growth and metastases in beige mice. Nature 1980; 224:622.
57. Roder JC, Haliotis T, Klein M, et al. A new immunodeficiency disorder in humans involving NK cells. Nature (Lond) 1980; 284:553.
58. Strayer DR, Carter WA, Mayberry SD, Pequignot E, Brodsky I. Low natural

cytotoxicity of peripheral blood mononuclear cells in individuals with high familial incidences of cancer. Cancer Res 1984; 44:370–374.

59. Rosenberg SA, Lotze MT, Muul LM, et al. A progress report on the treatment of 157 patients with advanced cancer using lymphokine-activated killer cells and interleukin-2 or high-dose interleukin-2 alone. N Engl J Med 1987; 316:899–906.

60. Pleszcynski MR, Lieu H. Natural cytotoxic cell activity linked to time of recurrence of herpes labialis. Clin Exp Immunol 1984; 55:224–228.

61. Facchini A, Marian E. Increased number of circulating Leu 11+(CD16) large granular lymphocytes and decreased NK activity during human aging. Clin Exp Immunol 1987; 68:340–347.

62. Makinodan R, Kay MMB. Age influence on the immune system. Adv Immunol 1980; 29:307.

63. Smith HR, Steinberg AD. Autoimmunity: a perspective. Ann Rev Immunol 1983; 1:197–205.

64. Dinarello CA, Mier JW. Medical intelligence current concepts: lymphokines. N Engl J Med 1987; 317:940–945.

65. Oppenheim JJ, Stadler BM, Siranganian RP, et al. Lymphokines: their role in lymphocyte responses—properties of interleukin-1. Fed Proc 1982; 41: 257–262.

66. Gillus S. Interleukin-2: biology and biochemistry. J Clin Immunol 1983; 3: 1–13.

67. Ruscetti FW. Biology of interleukin-2. Surv Immunol Res 1984; 3:122–126.

68. Cantrell DA, Smith KA. Transient expression of interleukin-2 receptors. J Exp Med 1983; 158:1895–1911.

69. Young HA, Ortaldo JR. One signal requirement for interferon-gamma production in large granular lymphocytes. J Immunol 1987; 139:724–727.

70. Holmes T, Rahe R. The social readjustment rating scale. J Psychosom Res 1967; 11:213–218.

71. Bartrop RW, Lazarus L, Luckherst E, Kiloh LG. Depressed lymphocyte function after bereavement. Lancet 1977; 1:834–386.

72. Schleifer SJ, Keller SE, Camerino M, Thorton JC, Stein MM. Suppression of lymphocyte stimulation following bereavement. JAMA 1983; 250:374–377.

73. Linn MW, Linn BS, Jensen J. Stressful events, dysphoric mood, and immune responsiveness. Psychol Rep 1984; 54:219–222.

74. Irwin M, Daniels M, Bloom E, Weiner H. Life events, depression, and natural killer cell function. Psychopharmacol Bull 1986; 22:1093–1096.

75. Irwin M, Daniels M, Bloom E, Weiner H. Depression and changes in T-cell subpopulations. Psychosom Med 1986; 48:303–304.

76. Irwin M, Daniel M, Smith TL, Bloom E, Weiner H. Impaired natural killer cell activity during bereavement. Brain Behav Immunity 1987; 1:98–104.

77. Irwin M, Daniels M, Bloom E, Smith TL, Weiner H. Life events, depressive symptoms and immune function. Am J Psychiatry 1987; 144:437–441.

78. Irwin M, Daniels M, Weiner H. Immune and neuroendocrine changes during bereavement. Psychiatr Clin North Am 1987; 10:449–465.

79. Shopsin B, Sathananthan GL, Chan TL, Kravitz H, Gershon S. Antinuclear factor in psychiatric patients. Biol Psychiatry 1973; 7:81–87.

80. Deberbt R, Hooren JV, Biesbrouck M, Amery W. Antinuclear factor-positive mental depression: a single disease entity? Biol Psychiatry 1976; 11: 69–74.

81. Johnstone EC, Whaley K. Antinuclear antibodies in psychiatric illness: their relationship to diagnosis and drug treatment. Br Med J 1975; 28:724–725.

82. Nemeroff CB, Simon JS, Haggerty JJ, Evans DL. Antithyroid antibodies in depressed patients. Am J Psychiatry 1985; 142:840–843.

83. Dorian B, Garfinkel P, Brown G, Gladman D, Keystone E. Aberrations in lymphocyte subpopulations and function during psychological stress. Clin Exp Immunol 1982; 50:132–138.

84. Kiecolt-Glaser R. Psychosocial modifiers of immunocompetence in medical students. Psychosom Med 1984; 46:7–23.

85. Glaser R, Kiecolt-Glaser JK, Stout JC, Tarr KL, Speicher CE, Holliday JE. Stress-related impairments in cellular immunity. Psychiatry Res 1985; 3:249–260.

86. Glaser R, Mehl VS, Penn G, Speicher CE, Kiecolt-Glaser JK. Stress-associated changes in plasma immunoglobulin levels. Int J Psychosom 1986; 33: 41–42.

87. Glaser R, Kiecolt-Glaser JK, Speicher CE, Holliday JE. Stress, loneliness, and changes in herpes virus latency. J Behav Med 1985; 3:249–260.

88. Kiecolt-Glaser JK, Glaser R, Dyer C, Shuttleworth E, Ogrocki P, Speicher CE. Chronic stress and immunity in family caregivers of Alzheimer's disease victims. Psychosom Med 1987; 49:1–277.

89. Eisdorfer C, Kennedy G, Wisnieskiew A, Cohen D. Depression and attributional style in families coping with the stress of caring for a relative with Alzheimer's disease. Gerontologist 1983; 23:115–116.

90. Arnetz BB, Wasserman J, Petrini B, et al. Immune function in unemployed women. Psychosom Med 1987; 19:3–12.

91. Scott JP, Roberto KA, Hutton JT. Families of Alzheimer's victims: family support to the caregivers. J Am Geriatr Soc 1986; 34:348–354.

92. Morcyz RK. Caregiving strain and the desire to institutionalize family members with Alzheimer's disease. Res Aging 1985; 7:329–361.

93. Bloom BL, Asher AJ, White SW. Marital disruption as a stressor: a review and analysis. Psychol Bull 1978; 85:867–894.

94. Vanbragge LM. Marital status and health. J Marriage Fam 1979; 41: 267–285.

95. Kiecolt-Glaser JK, Fisher LD, Ogrock P, Stout JC, Speicher CE, Glaser R. Marital quality, marital disruption, and immune function. Psychosom Med 1987; 49:13–34.

96. Glenn ND, Weaver CN. The contribution of marital happiness to global happiness. J Marriage Fam 1981; 43:161–168.

97. Renne KS. Health and marital experience in an urban population. J Marriage Fam 1971; 23:338–350.

98. Levenson RW, Gottmann VM. Physiological and affective predictors of change in relationship satisfaction. J Pers Soc Psychol 1985; 49:85–94.

99. Kiecolt-Glaser JK, Kennedy S, Malkoff S, Fisher L, Speicher CE, Glaser R.

Marital disorder and immunity in males. Psychosom Med 1988; 50:213–219.

100. Lazarus RS, Folkman S. Stress, appraisal and coping. New York: Springer, 1984.

101. Felton BJ, Revenson RA. Coping with chronic illness: a study of illness controllability and the influence of coping strategies on psychological adjustment. J Consult Clin Psychol 1984; 53:343–353.

102. Felton BJ, Revenson RA, Hintrichsen GA. Stress and coping in the explanation of psychological adjustment among chronically ill adults. Soc Sci Med 1984; 18:889–898.

103. Pagel MD, Bicher J, Coppel DB. Loss of control, self-blame, and depression: an investigation of spouse caregivers of Alzheimer's disease patients. J Abnorm Psychol 1985; 94:169–182.

104. Levine N, Dastover DP, Gendron C. Coping with dementia: a pilot study. J Am Geriatr Soc 1983; 30:12–18.

105. Locke SE, Kraus L, Leserman L, Hurst MW, Heisel SJ, Williams RM. Life change, stress, psychiatric symptoms, and NK activity. Psychosom Med 1984; 46:441–453.

106. Edmonton WE. Hypnosis and relaxation. New York: John Wiley, 1981.

107. Kiecolt-Glaser JK, Glaser R, Strain EC, et al. Modulation of cellular immunity in medical students. J Behav Med 1986; 9:5–21.

108. Clayton PJ, Halikes JA, Maurice WL. The depression of widowhood. Br J Psychiatry 1972; 120:71–78.

109. Cappell R, Gregoire F, Thiry L, Sprecher S. Antibody and cell mediated immunity to herpes simplex virus in psychotic depression. J Clin Psychiatry 1978; 39:266–268.

110. Kronfol Z, Silva J, Greden J, Dembinski S, Gardner R, Carroll B. Impaired lymphocyte function in depressive illness. Life Sci 1983; 33:241–247.

111. Schleifer S, Keller SE, Meyerson AT, Raskin MD, Davis KL, Atein M. Lymphocyte function in major depressive disorder. Arch Gen Psychiatry 1984; 41:484–486.

112. Schleifer SJ, Keller SE, Siris SG, Davis KL, Stein M. Lymphocyte function in ambulatory depressed patients, hospitalized schizophrenic patients, and patients hospitalized for herniorrhaphy. Arch Gen Psychiatry 1985; 42:129–134.

113. Syvalahti E, Eskola J, Ruuskanen O, Laine T. Nonsuppression of cortisol in depression and immune function. Prog Neuropsychopharmacol Biol Psychiatry 1985; 9(4):413–422.

114. Darko DF, Gillin JC, Rock SC, et al. Immune cells and the hypothalamic-pituitary axis in major depression. Psychol Res 1988; 25:173–179.

115. Wahlin A, vonKnorring L, Roos G. Altered distribution of T lymphocyte subsets in lithium-treated patients. Neuropsychobiology 1984; 11:243.

116. Irwin M, Smith TL, Gillin C. Reduced natural killer cytotoxicity in depressed patients. Life Sci 1987; 41:2127–2133.

117. Urich A, Muller C, Aschauer H, Resch F, Zilinski CC. Lytic effector cell function in schizophrenia and depression. J Neuroimmunol 1988; 18:291–301.

118. Mohl PC, Huang L, Bowden C, Fischbach M, Vogtsberger K, Talal N.

Natural killer cell activity in major depression (letter). Am J Psychiatry 1987; 144:1619.

119. Kronfol Z, Turner R, Nasrallah H, Winokur G. Leukocyte regulation in depression and schizophrenia. Psychiatry Res 1984; 13:13–18.

120. Glaser R, Rice J, Speicher CE, Stout JC, Kiecolt-Glaser JK. Stress depresses interferon production by leukocytes concomitant with a decrease in natural killer cell activity. Behav Neurosci 1986; 100:675–678.

121. Palmblad J, Petrini B, Wasserman J, Akerstedt T. Lymphocyte and granulocyte reactions sleep deprivation. Psychosom Med 1979; 41: 273–278.

122. Moldofsky H, Lue FA, Eisen J, Keystone E, Gorczynski RM. The relationship of interleukin-1 and immune functions to sleep in humans. Psychosom Med 1986; 48:309–318.

123. Targan S, Bitran L, Doug F. Activation of human NKCC by moderate exercise: increased frequency of NK cells with enhanced capability of effector-target lytic interactions. Clin Exp Immunol 1981; 45:352–360.

124. Munck A, Guyre PM, Holbrook NJ. Physiological functions of glucocorticoids: their relation to pharmacological actions. Endocr Rev 1984; 5:25–44.

125. Cupps TR, Fauci AS. Corticosteroid-mediated immunoregulation in man. Immunol Rev 1982; 65:133–155.

126. Irwin M, Daniels M, Risch SC, Bloom E, Weiner H. Plasma cortisol and natural killer cell activity during bereavement. Biol Psychiatry 1988; 24: 173–178.

127. Kronfol Z, House JD. Depression, hypothalamic–pituitary–adrenocortical activity, and lymphocyte function. Psychopharmacol Bull 1985; 21:476–478.

128. Kronfol Z, Hover JD, Silva J, et al. Depression, urinary free cortisol excretion, and lymphocyte function. Br J Psychiatry 1986; 148:70–73.

129. Keller SE, Weiss JM, Schleifer SJ, et al. Stress-induced suppression of immunity in adrenalectomized rats. Science 1983; 221:1301–1304.

130. Livnat S, Felten SY, Carlson SL, Bellinger DL, Felten DL. Involvement of peripheral and central catecholamine systems in neural-immune interactions. J Neuroimmunol 1985; 10:5–30.

131. Felten DL, Felten SY, Carlson SL, Oilschowka JA, Livnat S. Noradrenergic and peptidergic innervation of lymphoid tissue. J Immunol 1985; 135: 755s–765s.

132. Hellstrand K, Hermodsson S, Strannegard O. Evidence for a B-adrenoceptor-mediated regulation of human natural killer cells. J Immunol 1985; 134:4095–4099.

133. Irwin MR, Vale W, Britton KT. Central corticotropin-releasing factor suppresses natural killer cytotoxicity. Brain Behav Immunity 1987; 1: 81–87.

134. Irwin MR, Hauger RL, Brown MR, Britton KT. Corticotropin-releasing factor activates the autonomic nervous system and reduces natural cytotoxicity. Am J Physiol 1988; 255:R744–R747.

135. Nemeroff CB, Widerlov E, Bissette G, et al. Elevated concentrations of CSF corticotropin-releasing factor-like immunoreactivity in depressed patients. Science 1984; 226:1342–1344.

Stress Management

28

DEVELOPING STRATEGIES FOR STRESS MANAGEMENT

Ronald H. Cox
Miami University, Oxford, Ohio

Diseases of the heart and cerebrovascular system account for over 1 million deaths a year in the United States (1). The contributions of lifestyle, behavior, and stress to this deadly fact have been documented by investigations in both epidemiology and the experimental sciences. Attempts to modify lifestyle variables or manage stress offer the potential for high returns in both human life and its quality. The classic, nonpharmacological approaches to this concern, and the management of stress in particular, involve relaxation and biofeedback training. Both have been in use for a number of years and have proven effective for many individuals (2). Exercise training is now garnering considerable interest as a potential stress management tool (30).

The utility of exercise training for stress management is suggested by a large body of evidence, albeit indirect. The lower rates of cardiovascular morbidity and mortality found in physically active populations compared to more sedentary groups is the most compelling (4,5). Although it lends itself to a number of interpretations, the one of most ubiquity and relevance is that physical fitness reduces the insult of pathogenic environmental insults, one of which is stress (6–9). Efforts to document this effect and establish exercise training as a viable stress management strategy have followed two routes.

The sine qua non of success in stress management is the interdiction of the pathological condition (e.g., hypertension) resulting from repeated (chronic) exposure to stress. However, the relatively long time periods involved before chronic stress can result in deleterious health effects, ethical considerations, and the multitude of extraneous variables (i.e., genetics, diet) operating in the lives of human beings have limited the data generated from this group, which bears on this criterion. Animal models that directly address the issue of stress-induced disease and thus lend themselves to studies of exercise interdiction have been limited, until recently (9–13). James E. Lawler and colleagues at the University of Tennessee have demonstrated the utility of the borderline hypertensive rat (BHR) as a model for studies of this type. The BHR is the first filial (F_1) generation of the spontaneously hypertensive rat (SHR) and its normotensive genetic control the Wistar Kyoto (WKY). The sensitivity of this animal to environmental influences on blood pressure is most clearly expressed in its response to daily shock–shock conflict. This chronic stress elevates the blood pressure of the BHR to hypertensive levels (6,10). Moreover, exercise training will block the majority of this pathogenic effect (6; see Fig. 1). The potential of the BHR to explore the mechanisms of stress-induced hypertension and exercise-mediated protection is now being exploited experimentally in a number of laboratories (12,14,15).

This chapter will focus on the second and most common experimental approach used to establish the efficacy of physical training as a stress management strategy. This has involved assessing the effects of training on the physiological responses elicited by acute stress (reactivity). In this regard, cardiovascular and endocrine variables have received the greatest attention and these will be the emphasis here. This chapter is not a review of the literature as much as an examination of the rationale, assumptions, and evidence that underlie this approach and the issues and questions that have arisen as a result of it.

Foremost is the recognition that drawing conclusions about the vulnerability to chronic stress based on assessments of the acute response to stress may not be simple. The nature and degree of relationship between the *acute* effects of stress and the *chronic* sequelae remain ill-defined. For example, does a large pressor response to initial stress exposure portend a greater vulnerability to stress-induced hypertension? It is interesting that the interdisciplinary studies of training–stress response interactions discussed here are providing data and insights that bear on this traditional question of the psychosomatic area.

The multidisciplinary approach resulting from the collaborations of exercise physiologists, psychologists, and psychophysiologists has impinged on other theoretical and methodological issues and questions posed by the "mother disciplines." The most prominent involves defining the nature of the physiological mechanisms involved in exercise-training adaptations. The insights to be gained from studies of the physiological response to nonexercise stress in trained individuals has only recently been appreciated. Other issues include progress in identifying and refining the search for the pathogenic stimulus or factor(s) triggered by stress and justifying the physiological variables chosen to define stress reactivity and determining the extent to which high reactivity is

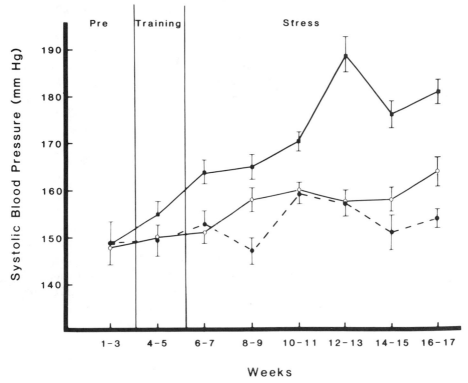

FIGURE 1   Mean (±SEM) tail cuff systolic blood pressure for each 2 week period before the chronic stress was imposed (PRE), during the 2 weeks when the stress was being progressively lengthened to the 2 h daily maximum (TRAINING), and during the 12 weeks of daily swim and/or tail shock (STRESS). Exercise-shock animals are represented by open circles, shock-only animals by closed boxes, and control animals with closed circles (from ref. 6).

deleterious. Concomitant with the interdisciplinary observations bearing on these questions comes the formulation of new perspectives about stress, exercise, and the physiological mechanisms that lend themselves to successful stress management strategies.

The treatment of these possibilities requires an excursion into the speculative realm, into which I have plunged quite freely and, perhaps in some cases, with too much enthusiasm. My intentions were never to be provocative for the sake of provocation, but to show the value of assuming a mechanistic physiological perspective toward exercise and its effects. This will allow consideration of previously ignored and even contraindicated strategies for managing and modulating the effects of stress on cardiovascular health and function.

EXERCISE TRAINING AS A MODULATOR OF STRESS

Despite the labor of many investigators, we still cannot identify with certainty a particular stress response (e.g., a large pressor response or high heart rate) responsible for the development of stress-induced cardiovascular pathological changes. If it exists, this particular response or responses would become the ultimate target of our management techniques. In the interim, the goal has been to attenuate the cardiovascular and sympathoadrenal responses and, if possible, all the physiological responses elicited by stress. The prevailing wisdom has assumed that the larger the physiological response to stress, the greater the pathogenic potential (16-19). The larger responses seen in those at genetic risk of hypertension support such a view (20-22). (Evidence is presented below that may qualify and limit the scope of this assumption.)

Techniques to manage stress, such as relaxation and biofeedback training, attempt to interdict the deleterious effects of stress by attenuating its physiological responses. Dynamic exercise has also lent itself to such a strategy. Dynamic exercise, also referred to as rhythmic, endurance, or aerobic activity, involves repeated rhythmic movement of large muscle groups with minimal resistance. The classic examples include distance running, swimming, and cycling. The basis for a belief in the utility of this form of exercise for modifying the acute physiological response to stress is not difficult to understand. The adaptations that occur in cardiovascular, endocrine, and sympathetic nervous system function as a result of repeated exercise stress (i.e., physical training) are well documented (23-27). Foremost in the minds of most exercise physiologists is an increase in maximal oxygen uptake (VO_2 max), which is usually considered the best index of physical fitness (3,23). This change reflects an increase in the O_2 transport capacity of the cardiovascular system, primarily via a larger maximal cardiac output. This greater cardiac reserve or capacity is often *assumed* to be the mediator of the vitality and lower coronary heart disease (CHD) risk associated with active people, and the basis for many of the other adaptations observed subsequent to training (28-30).

Two of the most striking adaptations are the relative bradycardia and diminished plasma catecholamine responses observed during a given exercise effort. The experiments by Winder and colleagues illustrate this point very well (Fig. 2). The progressively lower heart rate and plasma norepinephrine and epinephrine levels seen during an exercise session after repeated exposure are readily apparent even though the exercise workload remained constant. We can therefore conclude that the "stress" produced by this exercise elicited a smaller cardiovascular and sympathetic nervous system response as a result of physical training.

This phenomenon has not gone unnoticed and there have been many attempts to see if the effect "generalizes" to other stress situations (i.e., is a smaller response seen to other, non-exercise challenges?). In this quest, physically

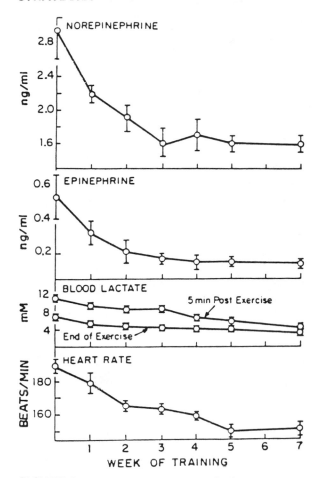

FIGURE 2 As training progresses the heart rate response and plasma catechola-mine levels elicited by a 5 min exercise bout (1483 kpm/min) are seen to de-crease. The smaller cardiovascular and autonomic responses elicited by the same workload have suggested to many that the response to other stressors will be attenuated (from ref. 27).

trained individuals and their sedentary counterparts have been shown movies, shocked, gassed, quizzed, immersed, tilted, squeezed, vacuumed, and drugged in an effort to demonstrate a difference in their physiological and autonomic nervous system responses (8,20,31-41). The results, in general, have been equivocal, if not absolutely surprising to those expecting a smaller physiological response in trained individuals.

From the vantage point of more recent work in this area (12,14,42,43) and the assumption of a more critical appraisal of training-induced adaptations, the only surprising thing is expecting to see a smaller response. I believe the mistake has three parts. The first is assuming that a large max VO_2 lends itself to a reduced responsiveness; the second and related mistake is an overinterpretation of the basis for the relative bradycardia and attenuated catecholamine responses observed during exercise after training; and the third has consisted of not recognizing the nature of the adaptations that do occur in neural and endocrine systems with repeated use, particularly that elicited by exercise. The present discussion will focus on the latter two reasons. VO_2 max and its relationship to stress management will be considered along with alternative strategies.

The reductions in heart rate and circulating catecholamines observed during exercise obviously reflect a change in the activity of either or both the parasympathetic and sympathetic branches of the autonomic nervous system. If the change in activity indicates some fundamental alteration in the structure of the autonomic or central nervous system itself, a generalization to other situations that provoke the same structures should have been observed. This clearly is not the case. A possible explanation lies in recognizing that the effector response (autonomic activity) is a function not only of the integrity and inherent capacities of the system itself but also of the afferent branch of the response system. As a consequence, a change in the internal environment of a trained muscle or a different recruitment pattern could alter the type and intensity of afferent information conveyed to a central controller of autonomic activity (44-46). This possibility is strikingly demonstrated by individuals training one leg on a bicycle ergometer. With this experimental design, the peripheral, metabolic adjustments induced by training are all confined to the leg exercised each day, yet central cardiovascular and neural adaptations may still occur because the heart and autonomic nervous system are activated with each and every exercise session. Changes in cardiovascular and plasma catecholamine responses can be monitored across the course of training one leg in a manner similar to that documented by Winder et al. shown in Figure 2.

The results of this type of experiment are shown in Figures 3 and 4. Heart rate and plasma catecholamine responses to the exercise with one leg show large reductions from the first to the 13th day of training. The most striking observation, however, is the response when the untrained leg is subjected to the exercise. Cardiovascular and catecholamine responses are at the original level. Thus

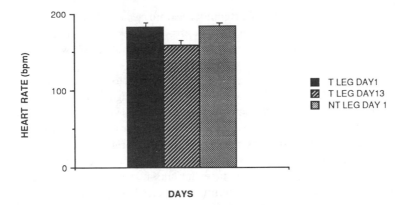

FIGURE 3 When one leg is exercised daily on a bicycle ergometer the heart rate response to the exercise is seen to decrease from the first day (solid) to the thirteenth day of training (cross-hatch). However, when the nontrained leg is subjected to the exercise (after the trained leg has adapted) the heart rate is at the original level seen on day 1 (last bar) (courtesy R.P. Claytor).

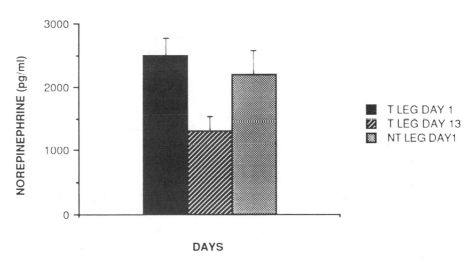

FIGURE 4 When one leg is exercised daily on a bicycle ergometer the plasma catecholamine levels produced by the exercise bout are significantly smaller on day 13 (cross-hatch) than on the first day (solid). However, if the contralateral leg is then exercised (last bar), the catecholamine levels show no significant reduction (courtesy R.P. Claytor).

no "carry over" or generalization of attenuated cardiovascular and autonomic activity is seen from one leg to another. This is surprising because the heart and sympathetic nervous system were activated at training threshold levels when the trained leg was undergoing its exercise.

The interpretation of these experiments is still the center of vigorous debate in the exercise science field, but there is agreement that a significant contribution to the cardiovascular and autonomic response to exercise must arise from local adaptations in the trained muscles. In other words, many of the cardiovascular changes associated with training are "peripheral" in origin as opposed to strictly "central" (the heart or nervous system itself). One can therefore ask if endurance exercise is the only way to induce the muscular adaptations conducive to changes in cardiovascular and autonomic function (47).

Observations of the highly specific nature of exercise training adaptations show clearly the problems of expecting a simple carryover of reduced responsiveness to stress through exercise training. In fact, one could argue that unless the new stress engages or depends upon exercise-trained muscles, no change in physiological response is possible. This is not an unreasonable position and the contribution of peripheral factors, particularly the musculature, to both the physiological and emotional responses of an individual has had a revered place in psychological theories of emotion since the James–Lange theory was proposed in the 19th century. Even if this was the only mechanism by which training could exert a "braking" influence on autonomic function, most stresses, even emotional ones, are attendant with some behavioral (i.e., muscular) activity and a recommendation for exercise would be warranted. However, before we assume that this is the only potential mechanism for exercise to alter the expression of stress or effect its management, we must consider several points.

First "central" adaptations have been documented for exercise training. Therefore, changes in stress response to new provocations are theoretically possible. The central adaptations include ventricular hypertrophy and increases in myocardial performance (26,48,49). Changes in central nervous system (CNS) function, although lacking compelling documentation, are certainly possible and are suggested by reports of enhanced endogenous opiate activity in endurance athletes and increased cholinergic tone and alterations of hypothalamic–pituitary function in female athletes (26,50). Second, some changes resulting from exercise training, while not "central" in the respect of signifying alterations of the heart or CNS, are pervasive in their possible effects on physiological adjustments to stress. These include the well-documented changes in insulin sensitivity that accompany exercise and training, adrenal hypertrophy, and enhanced secretory adrenal capacity, expanded plasma volume, and changes in tissue sensitivity to adrenergic stimulation (14,43,51-53).

Third, we must recognize that the acute cardiovascular (CV) and sympathetic nervous system responses to stress can be attenuated in trained animals (6) and perhaps humans (41) under *some* conditions. These conditions are not clearly defined but appear to be ones in which repeated exposure or practice has taken place. This is consistent with the idea that when the novelty and surprise of the stress are minimal, the cardiovascular and autonomic activity will largely reflect the metabolic/behavioral demands of the situation. In the context of the previous discussion, the peripheral factors (i.e., the trained musculature and the altered afferent information arising from it) might now exert an observable effect on autonomic activity. Whereas exercise training will also greatly reduce the hypertension resulting from chronic stress in the BHR model, the temptation to draw a causal connection between these two observations is strong. However, the attenuated responsiveness after repeated exposure is not expressed in all cardiovascular measurements (e.g., heart rate is blunted, but not blood pressure). In addition, the time at which the reduction in reactivity occurs or its mechanisms (e.g., behavioral vs. physiological) are not established. As a consequence, conclusions about reduced reactivity mediating the exercise-induced prophylaxis, or that the central adaptations lead to an attenuated reactivity, must be guarded.

TRAINING AND NOVEL STRESS: A PARADOXICAL EFFECT?

The "central" training adaptations noted above may be incompatible with a decrement in initial stress response. In fact, some adaptations may provide the potential for enhanced physiological responses to stress (e.g., adrenal hypertrophy, increases in tissue sensitivity to adrenergic stimulation). This possibility was anticipated by Kvetnansky almost 20 years ago, although not in relationship to exercise training (54). On the basis of immobilization stress studies in rats (54,55), Kvetnansky hypothesized that sympathoadrenal adaptation to stress involved two basic processes. One involved CNS habituation and the other biochemical alterations. Upon repeated exposure to a stressor, CNS habituation would serve to reduce the activation of the sympathetic nervous system (i.e., the organism becomes accustomed to and is no longer "alarmed" or "surprised" by the situation). From a behavioral perspective, this may correspond to the organism adopting an appropriate coping response. However, because sympathoadrenal activity is still above basal levels while the animals are exposed to the stressor, biochemical adaptations are induced. These adaptations include increased transmitter content of neurons, adrenal hypertrophy, and enhanced catecholamine-synthesizing activity. These changes provide an increased potential for responding and Kvetnansky predicted that exposure to a novel stressor would unmask this increased potential because the "braking" influence of CNS habituation would be absent. There has been little testing of this provocative idea, but many of the biochemical and tissue adaptations Kvetnansky observed for restraint stress have also been documented for exercise training (56,57). They would undoubtedly contribute to an enhanced capacity to endure intense and prolonged exercise efforts, but they also suggest that physically trained organisms will have a larger response to novel stressors than their respective, sedentary controls. Are there any data to support such a view?

A reexamination of data bearing on the response of trained and untrained individuals to stress presents some support for this notion. The study by Sinyor et al. (40) is particularly illustrative. The cardiovascular and biochemical responses of subjects during mental arithmetic, Stroop Color Word task, and a challenging quiz were compared between groups estimated to be high and low in aerobic fitness. This work has been cited extensively in regard to a faster heart rate recovery in the trained group, although the support was limited. Another feature of their observations that is not normally emphasized is shown by the catecholamine responses measured across the stress period in Figure 5 and the cortisol

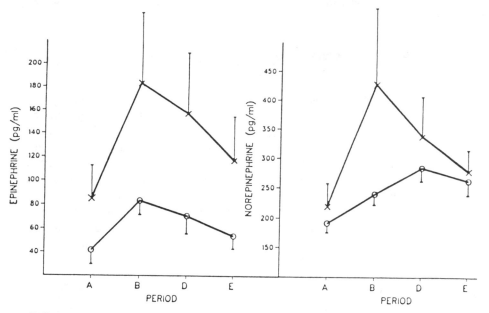

FIGURE 5 Mean (±SEM) catecholamine responses of trained (x) and untrained (o) males to psychologically challenging laboratory tasks. Results of ANOVA showed no overall significant difference between groups; however, the trained group showed a higher norepinephrine level at 1 min. The responses are in the direction predicted by a physiological analysis of exercise training adaptations (from ref. 40).

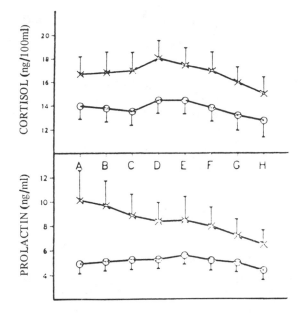

FIGURE 6 Mean (±SEM) cortisol and prolactin values for trained (x) and untrained (o) males during laboratory provocations. As in Figure 5, the trained group shows the tendency for higher values, $p < 0.09$ for cortisol and $p < 0.05$ for prolactin at points A and D (from ref. 40).

and prolactin responses shown in Figure 6. Although the differences observed are often only trends at some sampling points, the trained group does show a significantly greater increase in norepinephrine levels in the first minute and higher prolactin levels. These observations are striking in their contrast with traditional expectations and the responses observed between trained and untrained subjects during exercise. Moreover, the consistency with Kvetnansky's hypothesis is striking. A reanalysis of our own data reveals a similar result (32). The mean norepinephrine responses of a group of highly trained endurance athletes were higher than sedentary volunteers in every challenge used (standing, reaction times, isometric, and cold pressor). When compared with analysis of covariance, the responses to an aversive reaction time shock-avoidance task and handgrip isometrics were significantly higher in the trained group.

Firm support is difficult to garner for the notion of enhanced responsiveness in trained humans because of the relatively mild provocation offered by psychological laboratory situations. This problem can be obviated by recourse to animal models or the use of intense physiological challenges. Experiments involving exposure to 7% carbon dioxide (hypercapnia), hypoxia, or bolus injection of glucagon are in this category. Kjaer & Galbo (43) used these stimuli on men differing in maximum oxygen uptake capacity (VO_2 max) by 43%. The epinephrine responses to these challenges were always higher in the trained group (see Fig. 7). Of additional interest is the cardiovascular response to hypercapnia. Figure 8 is also adapted from the data of Kjaer and Galbo and shows a significantly greater heart rate and blood pressure response in the trained group. This is interesting because in many of the comparisons of trained and untrained individuals in the psychosocial stress experiments the cardiovascular differences are often equivocal or in the direction of lower responses for the trained. The demonstration of greater responses to the physiological provocations could reflect two factors. One, which is unique to the physiological challenges, is the total absence of a behavioral response. This would circumvent any inhibitory influence from activated, trained muscles and allow an enhanced capacity of trained individuals to be expressed. The second appears to be related to the statistical manipulations (e.g., covariance techniques) designed to remove differences between the trained and untrained subjects in baseline values. These are often used or recommended in the psychosocial literature (8,35–38). Although legitimate in principle, the differences in baseline heart rates between trained and untrained individuals reflect a well-documented physiological adaptation of training. The validity of trying to eliminate it must be questioned.

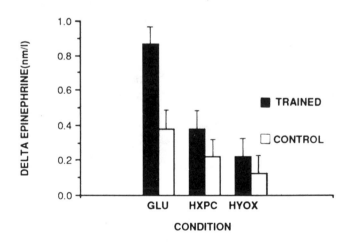

FIGURE 7   The mean epinephrine responses of endurance trained (solid bars) and untrained (open bars) males to hypercapnia (HXPC), hypoxia (HYOX), and bolus injection of glucagon (GLU). The trained group consistently showed significantly higher responses to the physiological challenges (adapted from ref. 43).

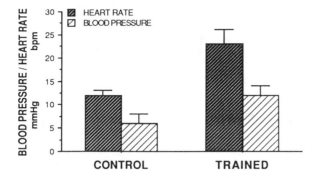

FIGURE 8 (Mean ± SEM) heart rate (solid) and blood pressure (hatched) responses to hypercapnia (7% carbon dioxide) elicited in trained and control subjects. The responses of the trained men were significantly higher than the controls (adapted from ref. 43).

Animal Work: The BHR and Novel Stress

A direct test of the Kvetnansky hypothesis as it bears on exercise training requires the use of animal models. This allows control of several key factors. The first is genetic influences. Several of the laboratory comparisons of fit and sedentary human subjects have used elite endurance athletes: those with VO_2 max values of 70 ml O_2/kg/min or greater. Oxygen uptake capacities of this magnitude are the result of very intense training and a favorable genetic potential for endurance activities. Any differences in cardiovascular and autonomic function observed between these two groups during stress cannot be confidently attributed to the training alone. The control of genetic factors and the random distribution of subjects to exercise and sedentary conditions that is possible with animal experiments minimize the variance contributed by this factor. In a related manner, the influence of differences in training modalities (e.g., cycling vs. swimming vs. running) and intensities that exist among the human studies can be controlled with animal models. The use of animal models allows the application of stress paradigms that have the intensity to elicit significant physiological mobilizations. This factor may be critical for exposing differences in autonomic nervous system activity associated with training. The changes elicited in plasma catecholamine values after laboratory maneuvers in humans usually are less than a doubling of resting levels (32,33), and often are considerably less (41). In contrast, the 10-fold changes elicited in rats (6) by experimental stress paradigms provide a greater range and possibility of detecting functional differences. In addition, the higher values may be closer to the intensity of some real life situations encountered by humans (58,59).

The design of the studies used to address the Kvetnansky hypothesis involved vigorously training female borderline hypertensive rats (BHRs) for 10 weeks before they were exposed to an unsignaled foot-shock stress. The trained animals swam for 2 h each day as previously described (6). This type of protocol results in classic training adaptations, which include a resting bradycardia, hypertrophied left ventricle, enlarged adrenals that contain significantly higher catecholamine levels, and evidence of changes in basal autonomic tone as reflected by altered responses to ganglionic blockade (14). The assessment of cardiovascular activity during the stress sessions involves monitoring the blood pressure and heart rate via an indwelling arterial catheter during a 15 min preshock period, during 15 min of intermittent foot-shock (1 s shock, every 40 s), and during a 15 min recovery period.

Results of this experiment are shown in Figures 9 and 10 and document the dilemma one faces in trying to form conclusions about the effect of exercise training on stress reactivity. Heart rate responses of the two groups show the closest approximation to traditional expectations of training's effects on stress. That is, by the 5th min of the stress the trained group shows a lower heart rate than the controls. However, even this observation is subject to qualification. Because the trained group has a significantly lower resting heart rate than the controls (a difference that disappears by the second min of stress), a greater *reactivity* of heart rate in trained animals could be argued if the responses in the later minutes were not seen.

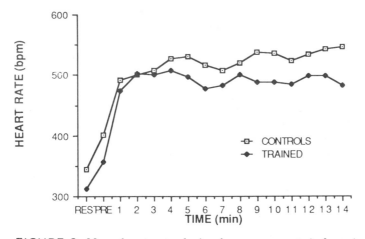

FIGURE 9 Mean heart rate during home cage rest, before shock onset in the grid box (PRE), and during each minute of intermittent foot shock in trained (solid) and untrained (open) female BHRs. The trained group showed significantly lower heart levels after the 4th minute (from ref. 14).

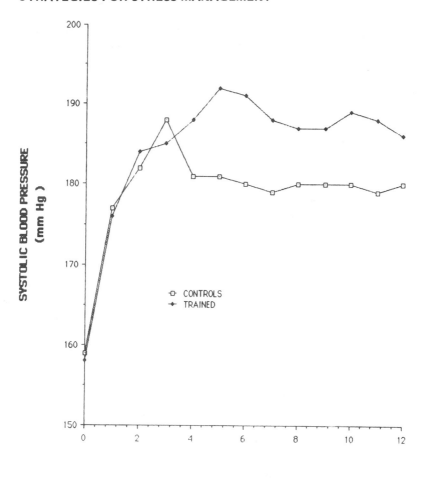

MINUTES

FIGURE 10 Mean systolic blood pressure during home cage rest, before shock onset in the grid box (PRE), and during each minute of intermittent foot shock in trained (solid) and untrained (open) female BHRs. The trained group showed significantly higher blood pressure after the 5th minute of stress (from ref. 14).

The blood pressure differences between the two groups do not require much qualification. The greater response and significantly higher levels achieved by the trained group is clear and has been replicated in recent work (42). The hemodynamic mechanisms (e.g., enhanced cardiac output vs. changes in total peripheral resistance) that serve this response pattern are not currently known but are the object of our investigations. The delineation of these factors will help us to understand the potential value or, conversely, the "drawbacks" of this response. Moreover, it may aid in clarifying the contribution made by acute pressor responses during stress to the elevations in basal blood pressure observed after chronic exposure. If trained animals are more resistant to the long-term effects of stress on blood pressure yet show higher acute responses, a "fusion" of acute stress responses into a tonically high blood pressure level appears untenable. Yet this has been the tacit assumption of many views of the psychosomatic process involved in stress-induced hypertension (16,19,60).

From the perspective of Kvetnansky's hypothesis, the results are not surprising. Nonetheless they present some challenging questions and implications. First, from a methodological standpoint the dependent variable used as an index of stress reactivity, and by extrapolation an index of successful stress management, must be considered with caution. The responses evaluated in the stress reactivity literature include heart rate, blood pressure, biochemical measures, and skin temperature. A single index may give misleading conclusions about the success of exercise training in the management of stress. Second, the evaluation of the effects of exercise training on the long-term pathogenic consequences of stress are clear. Exercise-trained animals tolerate stress better and remain healthier than control animals. The mechanisms that confer this protection are not known, and a simple stress-reduction model does not appear adequate to guide our theoretical and experimental development. The observations of trained and untrained groups during novel, unpracticed stress illustrate the inadequacy of a simple stress-reduction model, but this may be resolved by adaptation studies. In other words, after repeated exposure, when coping strategies have been adopted by the organism and novelty is no longer a salient feature of the situation, a simple stress-reduction model may describe the response of physically trained organisms. However, even this approach may not resolve the apparent paradox. Observations of trained BHRs and SHRs that have been repeatedly exposed to various stress paradigms still show blood pressure levels during the stress that are comparable to their sedentary counterparts (6,12). An analysis of the blood flow distribution and hemodynamic patterns during the stress may differentiate the two groups despite the similarity in blood pressure.

One can legitimately ask if the enhanced reactivity of trained animals observed on the first exposure to stress is a potentially deleterious characteristic. The rebuttal might be that this attribute can be tolerated because the eventual, long-term consequences of training are beneficial if the various organ blood flows are different. However, the potential adaptive value of this characteristic (i.e., high reactivity) must also be considered. An evaluation of this possibility requires an examination of the physiological consequences of the high pressor response and excursion into a different domain, one sometimes ignored by physiologists: behavior.

REACTIVITY: ADAPTIVE VALUE?

Physiological

From a strictly physiological perspective, an acute rise in blood pressure cannot be classified as deleterious. Simply put, blood flow is directly related to the difference in pressure between two points. Therefore, an animal with a higher blood pressure might achieve better organ perfusion. In the case of the kidneys, a higher blood pressure resulting from some hemodynamic patterns might mean maintaining glomerular filtration rate (GFR) during stress. This is fanciful speculation and admittedly a remote possibility, considering the myriad mechanisms, intrinsic and extrinsic to the kidney, that regulate its function in the face of large pressure changes (61). However, all factors being equal, the possibility of better-maintained renal function exists. If we consider the central role of the kidneys in the regulation of blood pressure, it would be ironic if a *higher* acute blood pressure response, by maintaining naturiesis, was associated with a *lower* basal blood pressure in the long term.

A less speculative possibility regarding the benefits of a higher pressure level during stress involves muscle blood flow. Again, all factors being equal, muscle perfusion and work capacity should be better with higher pressure. Some support for this possibility and its adaptive value are found in the exercise literature addressing the "crossover" issue. The particular study addressed this question with methodology similar in principle to the one-leg training studies but differed in actual execution. The subjects in these experiments trained both legs simultaneously on a bicycle ergometer and at fairly high work rates (24). After training, their oxygen uptake capacity was measured during leg work and during work using the arms. As expected, an improvement in VO_2 max was observed when the leg test was administered. More surprising was the reported 10% increase in peak VO_2 attained during work on the arm ergometer. Because the arms could not have undergone any local metabolic improvements during the leg training, the interpretation was that an improvement in myocardial capacity allowed a higher VO_2 to be reached during the arm test. This argument was strengthened by the observation that a higher blood pressure level was reached during the arm test after the leg training. In other words, improved myocardial performance allowed the generation of a greater pressure. This, in turn, forced a greater perfusion and delivery of oxygen to muscle tissue that had not undergone any local adaptations.

In the context of our comparisons of trained and untrained animals in a novel stress situation, a higher blood pressure might be viewed in a similar fashion. The trained animal may be better prepared physiologically to cope with the stressor even if the coping behavior requires musculature that has not undergone any physical training. Thus, the higher pressure during stress, if producing a greater muscle blood flow, would allow a greater workload to be accomplished before fatigue occurred, even if the work involved untrained muscles.

Until the pathogenic significance of differences in the hemodynamic patterns that mediate pressure changes (cardiac output or total peripheral resistance) are established, blood pressure changes during stress can only be considered a crude approximation of vulnerability to disease.

Behavioral

A second potential advantage of enhanced pressor and sympathoadrenal activity during stress is also related to behavior, but via its contribution to learning and attentional capacities. This hypothesis follows from the work of Martinez and colleagues on the mechanisms of amphetamine-induced learning enhancements (62). While the enhancing effects of amphetamines on learning acquisition, particularly one-trial passive avoidance, have been documented, Martinez et al. have shown that much of the effect of amphetamines is lost after adrenal demedullation. Thus peripheral sympathoadrenal activation is necessary for the full manifestation of amphetamines' effects on learning. The contribution of the adrenal medulla to avoidance learning has also been shown by others (63,64).

Since adrenal epinephrine is not thought to cross the blood–brain barrier (65), much of the contribution of adrenal activation to the central nervous system must be indirect (i.e., afferent input via baroreceptors or visceral activity). A logical, although speculative, extrapolation would be that animals or humans with enhanced sympathoadrenal or pressor activity would show better acquisition of avoidance responses. This hypothesis has been applied to rat strains differing in reactivity to stress by Campbell and DiCara (66), with positive findings. They found that SHRs learned a conditioned avoidance response (CAR) faster than normotensive WKYs (66). A comparison of physically trained and sedentary animals for learning acquisition has not been performed, yet the greater pressor response and hypertrophied adrenal glands of trained animals may favor their learning performance.

In a parallel fashion, a higher pressor reactivity may be adaptive to an organism by reducing behavioral reactivity to noxious stimulation. Within a learning context this might allow attention to be focused on salient features of the situation, which, in turn, might help in deciding on an appropriate escape or avoidance response. The latter point is speculative, but a relationship between behavioral responsiveness to noxious stimulation and blood pressure has been demonstrated (67). Dworkin et al. (67) showed that elevations in blood pressure produced by phenylephrine infusions were associated with reduced running to avoid an aversive electrical stimulation of the trigeminal nucleus. Denervating the baroreceptors eliminated the effect. Thus the reduced aversiveness associated with the phenylephrine infusions were not a result of direct actions of the drug on the brain but of afferent information generated by the baroreceptors.

The possible facilitation of cognitive function by physiological reactivity has not been seriously considered, yet it may confer an adaptive advantage to fit organisms. A recent study (68) extends this notion by providing provocative evidence that the structural integrity of the brain is strongly affected by adrenal hormones. The demonstration by Sloviter et al. (68) that adrenalectomy resulted in severe neuronal destruction in the hippocampus strengthens the cogency of the functional effects described above. Although it is a matter of speculative extrapolation, the effect of "hyperfunction" of the adrenals on the maintenance of brain function and neural integrity, particularly in aging animals, is a possibility worthy of investigation.

NEW STRATEGIES

If the protection from stress-induced pathological change afforded by exercise training is not solely related to the classic adaptations of endurance training (i.e., increases in max VO_2), but to other as yet undefined mechanisms (e.g., altered afferent information from trained muscles), perhaps other forms of exercise, not usually associated with attenuated responsiveness to stress, should be considered as management techniques.

Further justification to explore alternative exercise strategies is provided by the limitations inherent in endurance exercise training programs. Kaplan (69) has reviewed these, as they bear on the role of exercise as a nonpharmacological treatment and/or adjunct to traditional medical approaches to high blood pressure. The same shortcomings will mitigate against the use of exercise as a stress management tool. The major reason is that patient acceptance is probably no better than for drug therapies, and long-term compliance with aerobic exercise regimens is not as good. In fact, the low rates of adherence to sustained dynamic exercise protocols are abysmal, usually on the order of 50–80% dropout rates (61), and warrant the exploration of other exercise modalities, which will accommodate an individual's preferences, schedules, and facilities, yet still be efficacious.

Resistance Training

One exercise modality that has largely been ignored by those seeking nonpharmacological methods for interdicting the effects of stress on cardiovascular

health is weight training. Weight training or heavy resistance training is characterized by movements against resistance performed for sets of, usually, 8–12 repe-
titions. The primary goals of this form of training are to increase strength and
muscular mass (i.e., hypertrophy), the extremes of which are illustrated by
competitive weightlifters and bodybuilders, respectively.

Many studies have been performed to evaluate the effect of weight training
on VO_2 max. With few exceptions the results show that weight training produces no change in oxygen uptake capacity (28,70). This is true despite the fact
that cardiovascular activity (heart rate and blood pressure) during training
sessions are extremely high. Heart rates on the order of 150–200 beats/min
(bpm) have been reported (30,71). Thus, the ineffectiveness of weight training
for increasing the capacity of the cardiorespiratory system (max VO_2) is not due
to an insufficient training stimulus, but reflects instead the nature of the training
itself. However, before weight training is disregarded as a potential stress
management tool or adjunct for attempts to reduce the risk of coronary heart
disease, recall that the factors induced by endurance exercise that afford a protection from stress-induced pathological changes or coronary artery disease are
as yet unidentified. Moreover, the contribution of high VO_2 max capacities per
se to the vitality associated with active individuals is even less clear (85). The
characteristics most consistently associated with a reduced risk of CHD found in
active people are caloric expenditure and body leanness (64). Weight training
may lend itself to those characteristics.

Another feature of resistance training that has only recently become clear is
its effect on the functional activity of the sympathoadrenal and cardiovascular
system during the exercise itself. If one considers the many studies that have
examined the cardiovascular and sympathoadrenal responses to submaximal
exercises after endurance training, it is surprising that almost no work exists that
describes the responses to submaximal resistance exercise after resistance training. In an effort to explore this question, a collaborative effort (72) with Dr.
Randal Claytor was undertaken to document the responses of young adult males
to resistance exercise on commercial weight-training machines (Nautilus). The
men trained on the machines 3 days per week for 8 weeks. Each session consisted of 14 exercises and required 28–32 min to complete. A graduate research
assistant supervised each subject to ensure uniformity in the time required to
complete the session and to encourage the men to increase resistance whenever
possible. Every other week the men performed the original workload (first day)
and their heart rate was recorded and blood samples obtained immediately after
the last exercise. This protocol is analogous to the designs used with endurance
exercise discussed previously.

The measurement of aerobic capacity (VO_2 max) before and after 8 weeks of
resistance training showed no change, as expected. However, evidence of reduced
sympathetic nervous system activity was documented by the diminishing catecholamine response to the test workload (Fig. 11).

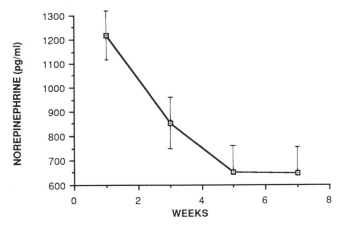

FIGURE 11   Mean (± SEM) plasma norepinephrine levels elicited by a constant resistance exercise regimen over the course of 8 weeks of resistance training (adapted from ref. 72).

We believe that this study has very important implications for stress management. First, most stresses encountered in daily life have a physical component; second, the physical component is seldom a purely rhythmic, endurance-type activity. Examples abound, but shoveling snow, moving furniture, and running after a bus for 30 s while carrying a heavy briefcase are standard scenarios. Even the cheering and emotional investment of a spectator at an athletic event involves jumping up, fits of clapping, squeezing a program or the seat (isometrics), and even Valsalva maneuvers (e.g., holding your breath during that "critical" foul shot or field goal attempt). Therefore, a reduction in the heart rate and sympathetic nervous system response to daily stresses may follow after resistance training.

Although a number of possibilities exist to explain our observations of a reduced catecholamine response (e.g., changes in removal rate), they are consistent with the notion that changes in muscle afferent activity are involved in the cardiovascular and sympathetic nervous system adaptations associated with repeated exercise. Perhaps the methods by which the muscles are conditioned (resistance vs. endurance training) are not absolutely critical (67). For example, Lehmann and Keul have shown that the catecholamine responses of resistance-trained men during submaximal cycle ergometry (endurance exercise) were reduced compared with untrained men (71). If confirmed, this illustrates a striking example of "crossover" of training effects and strong support for the efficacy of weight training to diminish the physiological "tumult" encountered in daily life. Whether or not "crossover" can be demonstrated, the fact remains that many daily stresses involve a physical component that engages the musculature in a way that parallels the activity of resistance exercise. In conjunction with the growing evidence (73) that resistance training can reduce resting blood pressure and blood lipid profiles (two recognized risk factors for CHD), the notion that a resistance training prescription is beneficial is not rash.

Isometric Exercise

Isometric exercise, in contrast to dynamic exercise, is characterized by sustained muscle tension and resistance with minimal alteration in muscle length. Handgrip is a classic example of static exercise and weight lifting can involve a substantial isometric component, but typically has components of both isometric and isotonic exercise. Static or isometric exercise protocols have either been ignored as potential therapeutic or prophylactic actions and/or considered to be contraindicated. The suggestion that isometric exercise might confer a beneficial effect on cardiovascular function (e.g., lower resting blood pressure), and hence an ability to manage stress, while not rash, obviously requires justification and explanation. This can be achieved by an examination of its hemodynamic concomitants, long-term effects on blood pressure, and the putative mechanisms that lend themselves to stress management.

Static exercise, like dynamic exercise, produces an acute rise in systemic blood pressure, which appears to be related to the intensity and duration of the activity (54,74). The belief that isometric exercise is potentially dangerous appears to stem from the view, recently expressed by Kaplan (69), that dramatic systolic pressure increases occurring during isometric exercise raise the potential for acute cardiovascular damage, so that the "prudent course perhaps would be to caution against isometric exercise" (p. 366).

While it is true that *maximal* isometric efforts carried to the *point of fatigue* generate large pressor responses, brief, nonfatiguing static contractions produce only modest elevations in blood pressure. For example, 30% of maximal voluntary contractions (MVC) performed for 2 min elicit changes in systolic and diastolic blood pressure of only 17 and 16 mmHg, respectively. A close examination of the hemodynamic responses elicited by isometric efforts may further dispel some of the reluctance to consider static exercise as a safe and potentially useful exercise modality.

Studies of weight lifters, hammer throwers, and shot putters have provided insights into the hemodynamic changes associated with static exercise (74–77), although none of these are strictly static efforts. With the onset of static exercise the muscular effort is transmitted to the cardiovascular controlling centers of the brain, resulting in decreased vagal activity, a rise in heart rate, and an increased sympathetic noradrenergic outflow. The result is an increase in cardiac contractility and constriction of venous capacitance vessels and splanchnic arterioles. Cardiac output rises due to the concomitant increases in venous return, cardiac contractility, and heart rate (78,79). Although splanchnic arterioles constrict, peripheral resistance appears to remain unchanged, while systemic pressure rises as a result of the increased cardiac output (76).

The blood pressure response to static exercise is considerably greater than that associated with dynamic exercise of equal oxygen consumption for a given muscle mass. This fact has probably contributed to the notion that isometric exercise is potentially deleterious. However, it can be argued that equating static and dynamic exercise by oxygen consumption is inappropriate. For example, it would be impossible to obtain a maximum oxygen uptake (VO_2 max) with an isometric effort. Isometric and isotonic efforts do not cover the same range of muscular activity when expressed in terms of oxygen consumption. Isometric efforts are therefore usually quantified as the percentage of the MVC (% MVC) obtained with a given muscle group. In this way, isometric efforts can be produced that elicit only modest pressor responses.

Although it is easy to demonstrate that properly adjusted isometric efforts produce only mild acute pressor responses, the effect repeated efforts (i.e., training) have on cardiovascular function at rest, specifically blood pressure, is not well documented. Reports addressing the training effects of repeated bouts of static exercise, such as those of Longhurst et al. (77) and Shepherd et al. (80), focus on the responses *during* the static contractions with repetitive efforts and do not report the effects on resting blood pressure. However, several reports suggest that a beneficial hypotensive effect of isometric exercise training can be obtained (73,81,82). Hagberg et al. (81) showed that weight training, which has a large isometric component, was effective in maintaining reduced systolic and diastolic pressures in hypertensive adolescents whose pressure had been lowered with endurance (dynamic) exercises. They also showed a hypotensive effect with one subject who practiced weight training without prior endurance training. These findings have been extended by more recent work (73).

A more direct attempt to assess the effect of strictly isometric exercise on resting blood pressure was reported by Kiveloff and Huber (82). They reported considerable decreases in systolic and diastolic blood pressures in hypertensive patients who practiced isometric contractions 3 times daily for 5-8 weeks. Although their study suffers severe shortcomings in methodology and reporting style, it presents some provocative observations. To extend these observations under well-controlled conditions, two studies were performed by Dr. Ronald Wiley of Miami University that clearly show the effectiveness of isometric handgrip exercises in lowering resting blood pressure in humans. The subjects in these studies showed a range of normal blood pressure levels. Isometric handgrip exercise was practiced 3-5 days per week either in the laboratory or at the home or work place. The isometric training consisted of four bouts of 30% MVC contractions held for 2 min interspersed with 3 min rest periods. The training was maintained for 8 weeks and in one of the studies the blood pressure was evaluated after 8 weeks of detraining. The results are summarized in Figure 12.

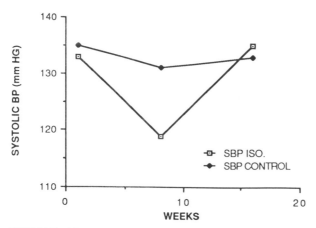

FIGURE 12 Mean resting systolic blood pressure in a nonexercising control group (closed) and a group practicing isometric handgrip 3–5 days per week (open). Blood pressures were taken before, after 8 weeks of training, and after 8 weeks of detraining. The training resulted in a significant reduction in both systolic and diastolic (not shown) blood pressure, which reverted to original levels after training ceased (adapted from ref. 90).

A hypotensive action of the isometric training is clearly demonstrated, which dissipates when training is discontinued. The magnitude of these changes is considerable for a nonpharmacological intervention and equal or exceed those reported for dynamic exercise or dietary modifications (1,83,84).

The animal research literature on isometric exercise and cardiovascular adaptation is unfortunately so sparse as to offer no direct confirmation of these intriguing observations. However, if we take the view that isometric exercise training is not only safe but perhaps even also therapeutic, the few animal studies available relinquish some of their doubt and lend limited support to this strategy.

A recent and direct attempt to show that isometric training is detrimental and produces hypertension in rats was reported by Tipton and colleagues (85). They used a shock avoidance paradigm involving a hanging response to simulate a static exercise condition (rats grabbed a bar and hung there to avoid an electrified grid). Contrary to expectations, repeated exposures *did not* produce an *increase* in resting blood pressure despite the large increases in mean blood pressure elicited by the hanging sessions. The aversive shock avoidance component may have precluded any demonstration of a lowering of blood pressure.

A quite different protocol popularized by Richard Kvetnansky and Irwin Kopin at the NIH, which lends itself to an isometric interpretation, is immobilization stress. This model restrains the rat's head and all limbs to stress the animal for physiological studies. Such whole-body muscular contractions by the rat seem to have many parallels to the whole-body straining (L-1 maneuver) sometimes used by pilots undergoing high "g" forces for the purpose of acutely raising systemic blood pressure (86,87). No documentation of the amount of tension developed by the animals in the immobilization stress has been given, but it must include large isometric components since the animals struggle against the restraint. In one report (55), a significant reduction in resting mean blood pressure was seen after five sessions of daily immobilizations. This is a striking observation considering that the sessions were 2.5 h in duration, involved considerable stress, and used the spontaneously hypertensive rat, a model with a well-documented sensitivity to stress.

The mechanism of action for isometric training's effect on resting blood pressure is not established, but a number of possibilities exist. They are briefly mentioned here to support the validity of these observations and to show a parallel with endurance and resistance training effects. For example, in vitro studies have shown that both isometric and isotonic contractions produce similar increases in glucose uptake, which is an insulin-like effect. An increase in insulin sensitivity is being increasingly linked to lower blood pressure (88). If isometric training increases insulin sensitivity it might lower blood pressure via enhanced sodium and water excretion (88).

The increase in cardiac output and venoconstriction produced during an isometric effort would alter central venous pressure and thus cardiac preload. Repeated increases in preload could produce a hypotensive response through the actions of atrial natriuretic factor (ANF). ANF produces a natriuresis and diuresis through its actions on renal function. In addition, its relaxing effect on vascular smooth muscle would further promote a hypotensive response (89).

Alterations in the afferent inputs to central neural control of cardiovascular function could also contribute to a hypotensive effect. These alterations could arise from changes in the muscular environment, analogous to those posited for endurance and resistance training discussed previously (47,70). A related possibility involves altered baroreceptor sensitivity. Long suspected as an altered factor in rhythmic exercise training, it might also be affected by isometric training.

In summary, there seems to be sufficient rationale and evidence for an effect of isometric exercise on lowering blood pressure to warrant development of models that will allow exploration of this potentially useful approach. An approach which would lend itself to the nonpharmacological management of blood pressure and the management of a prime influence on blood pressure: stress.

SUMMARY AND CONCLUSIONS

The observations and speculations offered here regarding the use of various exercise training modalities as a basis for developing strategies for stress management can be summarized by a few key points. First, the basis for the effects of endurance exercise on cardiovascular mortality and morbidity in general and resistance to stress in particular has not been unequivocally established. Moreover the emphasis on large changes in VO_2 max as the only "true" criteria of a health-promoting and successful exercise program and stress management strategy has been questioned. Because regular endurance exercise produces a variety of other beneficial adaptations (e.g., increases in insulin sensitivity, lower resting blood pressure, lower cholesterol levels, and alterations in muscle afferent information), all of which are shared by resistance training and perhaps by isometric exercise training programs, consideration of these other modalities is warranted.

Second, the observation of exaggerated responses in exercise-trained animals and humans to novel stress points out the need to refine hypotheses concerning the mechanisms of stress-induced pathological changes. The notion that large pressor responses are always associated with greater vulnerability to stress is not consistent with the documented resistance of exercise-trained animals, nor does it recognize the potential of this peripheral activity to influence cognitive function.

The fundamental differences between the first exposure to a stress and the adaptation stage in the magnitude of the responses elicited and mechanisms engaged require careful consideration of the methods and procedures used to explore training-stress interactions. Nonetheless, experimental probes of this fascinating area will reap ample insights into the nature and extent of our adaptative mechanisms.

ACKNOWLEDGMENTS

My appreciation is extended to my colleagues, R.L. Wiley and R.P. Claytor for generously sharing their thoughts and data. This work was supported by National Heart, Lung and Blood Institute Grant HL-34878.

REFERENCES

1. Marx J, Kolta G. Combating the #1 killer: The SCIENCE report on heart research. Washington, DC: American Association for the Advancement of Science, 1978:3-4.
2. Benson H. The relaxation response. New York: William Morrow, 1975.
3. Howley ET, Franks BD. Health/fitness instructors handbook. Champaign, IL: Human Kinetics Publishers, 1986.
4. Montoye HJ. Physical activity and health: an epidemiologic study of an entire community. Progress Report Research Grant HE14712 National Institutes of Health, University of Tennessee, Knoxville, TN; 1972.

5. Slatery M, Jacobs DR, Nichaman MZ. Leisure time activity and CHD death: The US Railroad study. Circulation, 1989; 79:304-311.
6. Cox RH, Hubbard JW, Lawler JE, Sanders BJ, Mitchell VP. Exercise training attenuates stress-induced hypertension in the rat. Hypertension 1985; 7:747-751.
7. Folkins CH, Amsterdam EA. Control and modification of stress emotions through chronic exercise. In: Amsterdam EA, Wilmore JH, DeMaria AN, eds. Exercise in cardiovascular health and disease. New York: Yorke Medical Books, 1977:280-294.
8. Light KC, Obrist PA, James SA, Strogatz DS. Cardiovascular responses to stress: II. Relationships to aerobic exercise patterns. Psychophysiology 1987; 24:79-86.
9. Mills DE, Ward RP. Attenuation of stress-induced hypertension by exercise independent of training effects: an animal model. J Behav Med 1986; 9: 599-605.
10. Lawler JE, Barker GF, Hubbard JW, Schaub RG. Effects of stress on blood pressure and cardiac pathology in rats with borderline hypertension. Hypertension 1981; 3:496-505.
11. Lawler JE, Cox RH, Hubbard JW. An animal model of environmentally produced hypertension. In: Katkin E, Manuck S, eds. Advances in behavioral medicine, Vol 2. J.A.I. Press, 1986:51-96.
12. Lawler JE, Cox RH, Naylor SK, O'Connor EF, Feld JL, Stairs DR. Enhanced blood pressure reactivity to acute tail-shock stress in exercise trained spontaneously hypertensive rats. FASEB J 1988; 2:A1719 (abst).
13. Lawler JE, Cox RH, Sanders BJ, Mitchell VP. The borderline hypertensive rat: a model for studying the mechanisms of environmentally induced hypertension. Health Psychol 1988; 7:137-147.
14. Cox RH, O'Connor EF, Lawler JE. Cardiovascular response to novel stress in swim trained BHR rats. FASEB J 1988; 2:A1719 (abst).
15. Squire JM, Myers MM, Fried R. Cardiovascular responses to exercise and stress in the borderline hypertensive rat. Med Sci Sport Exerc 1987; 19: 11-16.
16. Brod J. Essential hypertension: hemodynamic observationd with a bearing on its pathogenesis. Lancet 1960; 2:273.
17. Davies M. Is high blood pressure a psychosomatic disorder? A critical review of the evidence. J Chron Dis 1971; 24:239.
18. Fleming I, Baum A, Davidson LM, Rectanus E, McArdle S. Chronic stress as a factor in physiological reactivity to challenge. Health Psychology 1987; 6:221-237.
19. Folkow B, Neil E. Circulation. New York: Oxford University Press, 1971.
20. Hull EM, Young SH, Ziegler MG. Aerobic fitness affects cardiovascular and catecholamine responses to stressors. Psychophysiology 1984; 21:353-360.
21. Manuck SB, Giordani G, McQuaid KJ, Garrity SJ. Behaviorally induced cardiovascular reactivity among sons of reported hypertensive and normotensive parents. J Psychosom Res 1981; 25: 261-269.

22. Manuck SB, Proietti JM. Parental hypertension and cardiovascular response to cognitive and isometric challenge. Psychophysiology 1982; 19:481–489.
23. Astrand P, Rodahl K. Textbook of work physiology. New York: McGraw-Hill, 1977.
24. Clausen JP. Effect of physical training on cardiovascular adjustments to exercise in man. Physiol Rev 1977; 57:779–815.
25. Peronnet F, Cleroux J, Perrault H, Cousineau, D, deChamplain J, Nadeau R. Plasma norepinephrine response to exercise before and after training in humans. J Appl Physiol 1981; 51:812–815.
26. Scheur J, Tipton C. Cardiovascular adapations to physical training. Annu Rev Physiol 1977; 39:221–251.
27. Winder WW, Hickson RC, Hagbert JM, Ehsani AA, McLane JA. Training-induced changes in hormonal and metabolic responses to submaximal exercise. J Appl Physiol 1979; 46:766–771.
28. Gettman LR, Pollock ML. Circuit weight training: a critical review of its physiological benefits. Physician Sports Med 1981; 9:44–60.
29. Hurley BF, Seals DR, Ehsani AA, et al. Effects of high-intensity strength training on cardiovascular function. Med Sci Sport Exercise 1984; 16:483–488.
30. Keul J, Haralambi G, Bruder M, Gottstein HJ. The effect of weight lifting exercise on heart rate and metabolism in experienced weight lifters. Med Sci Sports 1978; 10:13–15.
31. Cantor JR, Zillmann D, Day KD. Relationship between cardiorespiratory fitness and physiological responses to films. Percept Motor Skills 1978; 46: 1123–1130.
32. Claytor RP, Cox RH, Howley ET, Lawler KA, Lawler JE. Aerobic power and cardiovascular response to stress. J Appl Physiol 1988; 65:1416–1423.
33. Cleroux J, Peronnet F, deChamplain J. Sympathetic indices during psychological and physical stimuli before and after training. Physiol Behav 1985; 35:271–275.
34. Cox JP, Evans JF, Jamieson JL. Aerobic power and tonic heart rate responses to psychosocial stressors. Pers Soc Psychol Bull 1979; 5:160–163.
35. Holmes DS, Roth DL. Association of aerobic fitness with pulse rate and subjective responses to psychosocial stress. Psychophysiology 1985; 22: 525–529.
36. Jamieson JL, Lavoie NF. Type A behavior, aerobic power, and cardiovascular recovery from a psychosocial stressor. Health Psychol 1987; 4(6):361–371.
37. Lake BW, Suarez EC, Schneiderman N, Tacci N. Type A behavior pattern, physical fitness, and psychophysiological reactivity. Health Psychol 1985; 4:169–187.
38. Perkins KA, Dubbert PM, Martin JE, Faulstich ME, Harris JK. Cardiovascular reactivity to psychological stress in aerobically trained versus untrained mild hypertensives and normotensives. Health Psychol 1986; 5:407–421.
39. Schulhan D, Scher H, Furedy JJ. Phasic cardiac reactivity to psychological stress as a function of aerobic fitness level. Psychophysiology 1986; 23: 562–566.

40. Sinyor D, Schwartz SG, Peronnet F, Brisson G, Seraganian P. Aerobic fitness level and reactivity to psychosocial stress: physiological, biochemical, and subjective measures. Psychosom Med 1983; 45:205-217.
41. Sothmann MS, Horn TS, Hart BA, Gustafson AB. Comparison of discrete cardiovascular fitness groups on plasma catecholamine and selected behavioral responses to psychological stress. Psychophysiology 1987; 24: 47-54.
42. Cox RH, Steele JS, McCoy DE, Wiley RL. Cardiovascular response to stress in swim trained borderline hypertensive rats (BHRs): effects of repeated exposure. FASEB J 1989; 3:A259.
43. Kjaer M, Galbo H. Effect of physical training on the capacity to secrete epinephrine. J Appl Physiol 1988; 64:11-16.
44. Gregory JE, Kennins P, Proske U. Can lactate-evoked cardiovascular responses be used to identify muscle ergoreceptors? Brain Res 1987; 404:375-378.
45. McCloskey DI, Mitchell JH. Reflex cardiovascular and respiratory responses originating in exercising muscle. J Physiol Lond 1972; 224:173-186.
46. Rotto DM, Kaufman MP. Effect of metabolic products of muscular contraction on discharge of group III & IV afferents. J Appl Physiol 1988; 64: 2306-2313.
47. Schantz P. Capillary supply in hypertrophied human skeletal muscle. Acta Physiol Scand 1982; 114:635-637.
48. Dowell R, Cutilleta A, Rudnik M, Sodt P. Heart functional responses to pressure overload in exercised and sedentary rats. Am J Physiol 1976; 230: 199.
49. Schaible TF, Scheuer J. Cardiac function in hypertrophied hearts from chronically exercised female rats. J Appl Physiol 1981; 50:1140-1145.
50. Bonen A, Belcastro AN, Ling WY, Simpson AI. Profiles of selected hormones during menstrual cycles of teenage athletes. J Appl Physiol 1981; 50:545-551.
51. Harri M, Narvola I. Physical training under the influence of beta blockade in rats: Effects on adrenergic responses. Eur J Appl Physiol 1979; 41:199-210.
52. Wyatt HL, Chuck L, Rabinowitz B, Tyberg JV, Parmley WW. Enhanced cardiac responses to catecholamines in physically trained cats. Am J Physiol 1978; 234:H608-613.
53. Yki-Harveinen H, Koivisto VA. Effects of body composition on insulin sensitivity. Diabetes 1983; 32:965-969.
54. Kvetnansky R. Recent progress in catecholamines under stress. In: Usdin ER, Kvetnansky R, Kopin JJ (eds). Catecholamines and stress: recent advances. New York: Elsevier, 1970.
55. Kvetnansky R, McCarty R, Thoa NB, Lake CR, Kopin IJ. Sympatho-adrenal responses of spontaneously hypertensive rats to immobilization stress. Am J Physiol 1979; 236(3):H457-H462.
56. Ostman I, Nyback H. Adaptive changes in central and peripheral noradrenergic neurons in rats following chronic exercise. Neuroscience 1976; 1:41-47.

57. Ostman I, Sjostrand NO. Effects of prolonged physical training on the catecholamine levels of the heart and the adrenals of the rat. Acta Physiol Scand 1971; 82:202–208.

58. Taggart P, Carruthers M, Somerville W. Electrocardiogram, plasma catecholamines and lipids and their modification by orprenolol when speaking before an audience. Lancet 1973; 2:341–346.

59. Wiedeking C, Lake R, Ziegler M, Kowarski A, Money J. Plasma noradrenaline and dopamine-beta-hydroxylase during sexual activity. Psychosom Med 1977; 39:143–147.

60. Hallback M, Weiss L. Mechanisms of spontaneous hypertension in rats. Med Clin North Am 1977; 61:593–609.

61. Vander AJ. Renal physiology, 2nd ed. New York: McGraw-Hill, 1980.

62. Martinez JL, Vasquez BJ, Rigter H, et al. Attenuation of amphetamine-induced enhancement of learning by adrenal demedullation. Brain Res 1980; 195:433–443.

63. Latane B, Schachter S. Adrenalin and avoidance learning. J Comp Physiol Psychol 1962; 55:369–372.

64. Levine S, Soliday S. An effect of adrenal demedullation on the acquisition of a conditioned avoidance response. J Comp Physiol Psychol 1962; 55:214–216.

65. Gilman AG, Goodman LS, Gilman A (eds.) The pharmacological basis of therapeutics, 6th ed. New York: MacMillan, 1980.

66. Campbell RJ, DiCara LV. Running-wheel avoidance behavior in the Wistar/Kyoto spontaneously hypertensive rat. Physiol Behav 1977; 19:473–480.

67. Dworkin BR, Filewich RJ, Miller NE, Craigmyle N, Pickering TG. Baroreceptor activation reduces reactivity to noxious stimulation: implications for hypertension. Science 1979; 205:1299–1301.

68. Sloviter RS, Valequette G, Abrams GM, et al. Selective loss of hypocampal granule cells in the mature rat brain after adrenalectomy. Science, 1989; 243:535–538.

69. Kaplan NM. Non-drug treatment of hypertension. Ann Intern Med 1985; 102:359–373.

70. Stone MH, Wilson GD. Resistive training and selected effects. Med Clin North Am 1985; 109–122.

71. Lehmann M, Keul J. Free plasma catecholamines, heart rates, lactate levels, and oxygen uptake in competition weightlifters, cyclists, and untrained control subjects. Int J Sports Med 1986; 7:18–21.

72. Cox RN, Claytor RP, Howley ET. Cardiovascular and catecholamine adaptations to heavy resistance training. Paper presented at the American College of Sports Medicine. Baltimore, MD, May, 1989.

73. Hurley BF, Hagberg JM, Goldberg AP, et al. Resistive training can reduce coronary risk factors without altering VO_2 max or percent body fat. Med Sci Sports Exercise 1988; 20(2):150–154.

74. Asmussen E. Similarities and dissimilarities between static and dynamic exercise. Circ Res 1981; 48:13–110.

75. Keuhl J, Dickherth HH, Simon G, Lehmann M. Effect of static and dynamic exercise in heart volume, contractility, and left ventricular dimensions. Circ Res 1981; 48:I162–I170.
76. Lind AR, Taylor SH, Humphreys PW, Kennelly BM, Donald KW. The circulatory effects of sustained voluntary muscle contraction. Clin Sci 1964; 27: 229–244.
77. Longhurst JC, Kelly AR, Gonyea WJ, Mitchell JH. Chronic training with static and dynamic exercise: cardiovascular adaptation and response to exercise. Circ Res 1981; 48:I171–I178.
78. Perez-Gonzales JF. Factors determining the blood pressure responses to isometric exercise. Circ Res 1981; 48:I76–I86.
79. Seaman RG, Wiley RL, Zechman FW, Goldey JA. Venous reactivity during static exercise (handgrip) in man. J Appl Physiol 1973; 35:858–860.
80. Shepherd JT, Blomquist CG, Lind AR, Mitchell JH, Saltin B. Static (isometric) exercise. Circ Res 1981; 48:I179–I188.
81. Hagberg JM, Goldring D, Ehsani AA, Hernandez A, Siñacore DR, Holloszy JO. Effect of exercise training on blood pressure and hemodynamics in hypertensive adolescents. J Pediatr 1984; 104:147–151.
82. Kiveloff B, Huber O. Brief maximal isometric exercise in hypertension. J Am Geriatr Soc 1971; 19:1006–1012.
83. Choquette G, Ferguson RJ. Blood pressure reduction in "borderline" hypertensive following physical training. Can Med Assoc J 1973; 108: 699–703.
84. The Joint National Committee on Detection, Evaluation, and Treatment of High Blood Pressure. Arch Intern Med 1984; 144:1045–1057.
85. Tipton CM, McMahon S, Youmans EM, et al. Response of hypertensive rats to acute and chronic conditions of static exercise. Am J Physiol 1988; 254:H592–H598.
86. Cote R, Tripp L, Jennings T, Karl A, Goodyear C, Wiley R. Effect of inspiratory volume on intrathoracic pressure generated by an L-1 maneuver. Aviat Space Environ Med 1986; 57:1035–1038.
87. Williams CA, Lind AR, Wiley RL, Douglas JE, Miller G. Effect of different body postures on the pressures generated during an L-1 maneuver. Aviat Space Environ Med 1988; 59;920–927.
88. DeFronzo RA. The effect of insulin on renal sodium metabolism: a review with clinical implications. Diabetologia 1981; 21:165–171.
89. Atlas SA, Laragh JH. Physiological actions of atrial natriuretic factor. In: Mulrow PJ, Schrier R, eds. Atria hormones and other natriuretic factors. Bethesda, MD: American Physiological Society, 1987: 53–76.
90. Wiley RL, Hueppchen NA. Effect of repeated isometric exercise on resting blood pressure. Fed Proc 1983; 42:742.

29

STRESS TECHNOLOGY MEDICINE

A New Paradigm for Stress and Considerations for

Self-Regulation

David Shannahoff-Khalsa

The Khalsa Foundation for Medical Science, Del Mar, California

Selye defined stress as "the nonspecific response of the body to any demand" (1). Burchfield revised it to include the role of psychological stimuli: "stress is anything which causes an alteration of psychological homeostatic processes" (2). Burchfield's definition is more germane from the perspective of stress management since it is the psychological aspect of people's well-being that is affected first prior to the bodily effects that Selye describes as the "general adaptation syndrome" (GAS) (3). The affective manifestations of stress have drawn attention to stress management, not the classic triad of chronic stress: adrenal enlargement, thymicolymphatic involution, and gastrointestinal ulcers (3). Stress management is a popular concern today due to life's hurried pace and pressures. It seems that the "fight or flight" response, attributed by Cannon to direct physical threats, today arises inappropriately due to psychological stress. The prolonged affective discomforts are now recognized as early warning signs of Selye's "stage of exhaustion" (3).

As people experience these signs and become aware that stress management can help, the tendency is to seek a healthy substitute for psychotropic agents as a solution for anxiety, depression, and other affective disorders. The pressing challenge therefore becomes how best to maintain mental equilibria and prevent mental and physical exhaustion.

This chapter discusses two aspects of stress management. First, it reviews evidence to support a new paradigm for how psychological homeostatic processes and metabolic functions are tightly coupled. The second part is a section on techniques for the noninvasive self-regulation of the mind–body axis. These techniques, or mind/body exercises, were discovered by yogis thousands of years ago to relieve specific common ailments. The paradigm presented here is based on recent studies that have tested ancient yogic concepts of how the autonomic nervous system (ANS) and the central nervous system (CNS) were thought to interact. Laterality, or asymmetries of function in the nervous system, provide the initial framework for new considerations of how neural structure links biology with the mind. The recent discovery of rhythmic shifts in lateralized ANS and CNS functions provides a temporal dimension to structure that may give us new perspectives on this link.

AUTONOMIC NERVOUS SYSTEM RHYTHMS AND LATERALITY

An extensively studied but not widely known example of a rhythmic shift of a lateralized autonomic function is the nasal cycle (4,5). This phenomenon is an alternating congestion and decongestion of opposite nostrils. Vasoconstriction in one nasal turbinate is paralleled by vasodilation in the other. The nasal mucosa are densely innervated with autonomic fibers. Dominant sympathetic activity on one side produces vasoconstriction in the turbinates. At the same time, the contralateral nostril exhibits dominant parasympathetic activity that causes engorgement. The nasal cycle was first documented in 1889 by Kayser, a German physician (6). He described the nasal cycle as reflecting the "alternation of vasomotor tone throughout the periphery on the two sides of the body." This observation was virtually ignored for a century. The physiology of the nasal cycle was studied and reviewed by Keuning (7). A few reports (8,9) have studied other structures in relationship to the nasal cycle.

One remarkable example of lateralized autonomic tone comes from Neligan and Strang (10). They reported observations of what they called the "harlequin color change in the newborn" who were all abnormal in some way (if only because of prematurity or infection). A few similar observations in normal babies were reported. A striking color change occurs on one half of the body and lasts anywhere from 30 s to 20 min. The baby can be in almost any position, as long as it is mostly turned on one side. The upper half of the body becomes pale and there is always a clear line of demarcation running exactly along the midline of the body. The attack could be abruptly curtailed by removing the baby from its side, but in some cases the pale and flushed sides could be reversed by turning the baby onto its opposite side. Neligan and Strang surmised "the precise distribution of the color changes suggests a temporary imbalance in the central nervous system (possibly in the hypothalamus)."

Neligan and Strang suggested that these effects may be explained in part by gravity. Heetderks (11) in 1927 observed that lateral recumbency could induce a switch of nasal dominance and also assumed that this was a gravitational effect. Heetderks concluded "that the distribution of the nasal vascular contents must be largely controlled by gravitation." In 1934, Kuno (12) described lateralized patterns of perspiration in humans and termed them the "hemihidrotic reflex." He stated that "lying on one side caused a remarkable increase in sweating universally over the upper half of the body," suggesting that gravity also played a role. Similar studies investigating posture and lateralized patterns of perspiration (13-16) demonstrate that the lateral recumbent effect of pressure can be mimicked while the subject is vertical by applying pressure to an axillary point that later increases perspiration on the contralateral side. Numerous studies of the effects of posture and pressure on the nasal cycle are reviewed by Haight and Cole (17), which showed that pressure on the axillary point, approximately equivalent to the fifth intercostal space, can induce the increased sympathetic tonus on the contralateral side of the body.

A recent study by Kennedy and co-workers (18) has provided evidence that sympathetic tonus differs greatly between the two sides of the body. They sampled antecubital venous circulation in both arms simultaneously every 7.5 min and assayed for norepinephrine (NE), dopamine (D), and epinephrine (E) levels. Figures 1 and 2 show how NE and D levels in plasma alternately rise and fall in the two arms while subjects are at rest. Figure 3 shows how NE, E, and D all covary in relatively similar fashion. Figure 4 shows how the lateralized NE levels also covary with the nasal cycle. Even though complete nasal cycle transitions were not shown in this subject during the 3 h recording period, relative fluctuations in the nasal cycle were shown to correlate significantly with the alternating levels of NE. This study demonstrates that lateralized shifts in sympathetic tonus are associated with lateralized shifts in the concentrations of neurotransmitters in peripheral circulation.

The studies of the nasal cycle reviewed by Keuning (7) showed that the average cycle is about 3-4 h and ranges from 2 to 8 h. Hasagawa and Kern (5) studied 50 human subjects and found a mean duration of 2.9 h, ranging from 1 to 6 h. All of these nasal cycle studies were done under laboratory conditions during the day, with the exception of two subjects who were studied for continuous 24 h periods by Cole and Haight (19). Laboratory conditions, which limit mobility, may skew the cycle towards longer than normal periods. The definition of a cycle and the frequency of sampling are issues that confound the discussion of cycles. There are wide variations in the reported length. One subject exhibited an alternation in dominance every 20 min for 4 consecutive cycles during a 90 min recording period (20), but on a subsequent day showed a much longer period. It is clear, however, that there is an alternating lateralization of ANS function in humans. The nasal cycle has also been demonstrated in rats and rabbits (21), in anesthetized pigs (22), and cats (23), and may occur in all mammals.

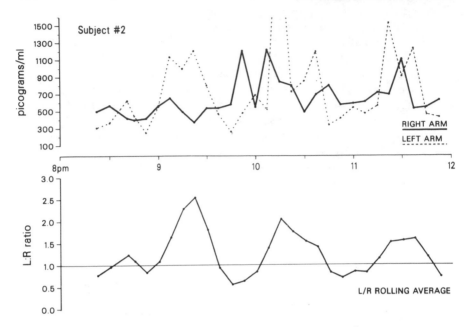

FIGURE 1 Top: Variations in plasma NE levels (pg/ml) were measured at 7.5 min intervals in both right (unbroken line) and left (hatched line) arm. Raw data are represented for subject 2 from 8:22 p.m. to 12 midnight. NE was measured by radioenzymatic assay with phenylethanolamine-N-methyltransferase and [^{3}H] SAM. The 10:08 p.m. NE value for the left arm is 2874. Bottom: The left/right ratio of the values of the two arms from above are represented as a rolling average. Values in the curve above 1.00 represent greater levels of NE in the left arm and values below 1.00 are greater levels in the right arm. Time scale is as above (reprinted from ref. 18, p. 1207, with permission from Pergamon Press).

CENTRAL NERVOUS SYSTEM RHYTHMS AND LATERALITY

Although it is generally thought that the ANS involves vegetative-visceral and homeostatic systems only, recent work shows that lateralized autonomic function is also coupled to and has a major regulatory influence on lateralized rhythms in the CNS. Werntz et al. (24,20) showed that the nasal cycle is coupled to an alternating lateralization of cerebral hemispheric activity in humans. They recorded electroencephalographic (EEG) activity continuously from corresponding sites on the two sides of the head, then rectified, integrated, and subtracted the signals. The right-left difference in signal in each of four frequency bands correlates well with the nasal cycle (Fig. 5) in 19 of 19 subjects. Relatively greater EEG amplitudes were contralateral to the dominant nostril. When the nasal cycle did not show a significant shift, no significant shift was observed in the EEG. Sapen et al. (25) showed that ANS fibers travel uncrossed between the CNS and periphery. It therefore seems likely that the hemisphere with less blood flow would be ipsilateral to the least congested nostril. Several tests have confirmed this conclusion.

In 1979, Klein and Armitage (26) observed ultradian rhythms of alternating performance efficiency with verbal and spatial skills. A group of 8 subjects performed a verbal and spatial task every 15 min for 8 h. Ultradian variations with a major peak of activity every 90–100 min were noted. Maximum performance on the verbal task was 180 degrees out of phase with performance on the other. Klein et al. (27) used lateralized cognitive tests to assess performance

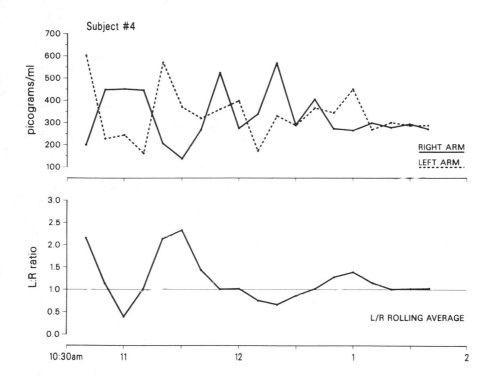

FIGURE 2 Variations in plasma DA levels (pg/ml) were measured at 7.5 min intervals in both the right (unbroken line) and left (hatched line) arms. Raw data for subject 4 is represented from 10:37 a.m. to 1:45 p.m. DA was measured by radioenzymatic assay with catechol-O-methyltransferase and [³H]SAM. Bottom: The left/right ratio of the values of the two arms from above are presented as a rolling average. Values in the curve above 1.00 represent greater levels of DA in the left arm and values below 1.00 are greater levels in the right arm (reprinted from ref. 18, p. 1208, with permission from Pergamon Press).

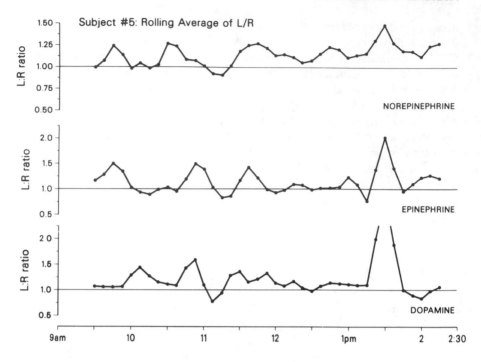

FIGURE 3 Top: The plasma variations of the left/right ratio of the two arms of subject 3 are generated by dividing the average value from the triplicate assay for NE at each time point in each arm. NE was determined by radioenzymatic assay using catechol-O-methyltransferase and [^{3}H] SAM. Time scale is 9:30 a.m. to 2:15 p.m., with plasma samples every 7.5 min. The rolling average of the left/right ratio is represented. Middle: Plasma concentrations and the rolling average of the ratios for both arms was determined as above using the same blood sample during the same assay for E. Bottom: Plasma concentrations and the rolling average of the ratios for both arms were determined as in the top section using the same blood sample during the same assay for D. Missing value at 1:30 p.m. is 2.81 (reprinted from ref. 18, p. 1209, with permission from Pergamon Press).

efficiency during different phases of the nasal cycle. They found that right nostril dominance correlates with enhanced verbal performance, or left brain activity, and left nostril dominance correlates with enhanced spatial performance. Shannahoff-Khalsa, Boyle, and Buebel (unpublished data, 1989), using cognitive tasks different from those of Klein et al. (27), have also shown that right nostril dominance corresponds to enhanced verbal skills and left nostril to spatial. Sanders, Arnold, and Shannahoff-Khalsa (unpublished data, 1988) have used the same tests as Klein et al. (27) to show again that enhanced verbal task efficiency correlates with right nostril dominance. Also in this study a mental rotation task was found to correlate with right nostril dominance. Masters (unpublished data, 1988) found a right visual field, left brain advantage when using tachistoscopic analysis for a similar mental rotation task. In 1986, Armitage (28) observed similar ultradian rhythms in EEG activity that were measured during extended task performance.

EEG experiments have also provided evidence for rhythms of alternating cerebral cortical activity during sleep in humans (28–30). LaBerge and Shannahoff-Khalsa (unpublished data, 1987) have studied the nasal cycle in relationship

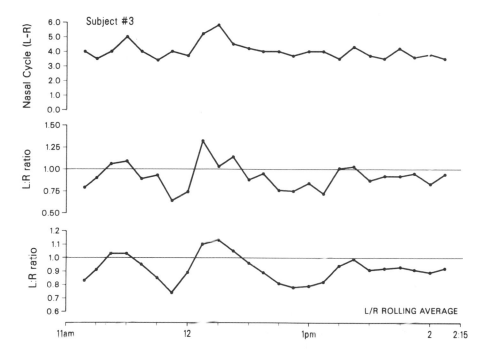

FIGURE 4 Top: The nasal cycle determination of subject 3 is plotted as the raw data of the left minus right (L–R) value versus time. The (L–R) value was measured at each time point for blood sampling (every 7.5 min). The subject fluctuates in left nostril dominance during the recording period. The nasal cycle was shifted 7 min to the left. Middle: The raw data of the plasma variations of the left/right ratio of the two arms of subject 3 are generated by dividing the average value from the triplicate assay for NE at each time point in each arm. NE was determined by radioenzymatic assay using catechol-O-methyltransferase and [^{3}H] SAM. Time scale is 11:07 a.m. to 2:07 p.m. NE values greater than 1.00 represent greater plasma levels in the left arm. Bottom: The same data as the middle section are represented here as the rolling average of the ratios, using the formula 1:2:1 (reprinted from ref. 18, p. 1210, with permission from Pergamon Press).

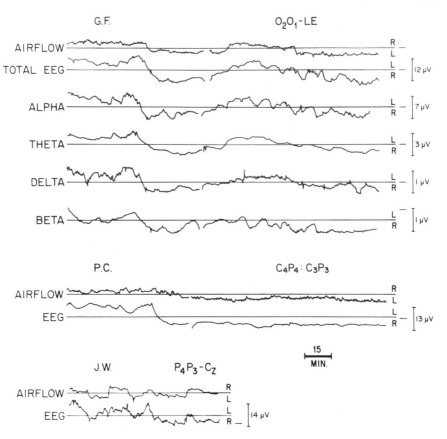

FIGURE 5 In these airflow tracings, points above the baseline indicate greater right nostril airflow and points below indicate greater left nostril airflow. Total EEG is 1–35 Hz: alpha (8–13 Hz), theta (4–8 Hz), delta (1–4 Hz), and beta (13–35 Hz) tracings were filtered through an analog filter before being integrated. This baseline is drawn to enhance visually the similarity of the basic correlation of the two phenomena. The dash to the right of the EEG tracings indicates the true zero line where the right and left EEG amplitudes are equal. The bar and its numerical equivalent next to the integrated EEG tracings represent the acutal calibrated amplitudes in microvolts. Three different subjects are exhibited here with their different profiles (reprinted from ref. 20, p. 40, with permission from Springer-Verlag).

to rapid eye movement (REM) and non-rapid eye movement (NREM) sleep. Preliminary results show that right nostril dominance is correlated with REM sleep and left nostril dominance with NREM sleep stages. Goldstein et al. in 1972 (29) and Barcaro et al. in 1986 (31) have shown that the EEG amplitudes in the two hemispheres during sleep are related to the phases of REM and NREM sleep. Goldstein et al. (29) suggest that "the difference in hemispheric amplitude relationships during NREM and REM sleep may eventually prove to be a neurophysiological concomitant of the change in brain function during these stages." Barcaro et al. (31) report that "for 9 out of 11 examined subjects, both a visual comparison with the hypnogram and a statistical analysis showed the existence of cyclic variations during the night in the delta and/or sigma correlation coefficient" of EEG. Other EEG studies in humans report similar findings (32–34), although one study failed to find a difference (35). Studies by Pivik et al. (36) and Moffitt et al. (37) correlated EEG asymmetries with sleep stages and dream recall. Others have used EEG to document alternating cerebral dominance in several nonhuman species during sleep. These include rabbits (29,38), cats (29, 39), pilot whales (40,41), dolphins (42), and fur seals (43). Other evidence in humans also suggests the existence of a natural rhythm of alternating dominance between the two cerebral hemispheres. Work by Gordon and colleagues in 1982 (44) and by Lavie et al. in 1984 (45) showed that waking from REM and NREM sleep elicits significant differences in the verbal and spatial performance ratios.

Interpretation of results from studies of hemisphere dominance during sleep and EEG studies in general has been difficult since many workers assumed that increasing EEG amplitudes correlate with decreasing mental activity. This assumption arose from work of Adrian and Matthews in 1934 (46) involving a simple arousal model in which alpha activity (8–12 Hz) was assumed to be inversely related to mental processing. This conclusion was naive, and shown by Ray and Cole in 1985 (47) to be a misinterpretation of results. They showed that alpha amplitudes depend on where mental attention is focused, that is, toward internal calculations or events (increased alpha) or toward external events and calculation based on external data (decreased alpha), not whether the eyes are opened or closed. It was presumably this confusion in the EEG literature that led Goldstein et al. (29) and others, who found greater EEG amplitudes in the left hemisphere during REM sleep, to assume that the right hemisphere is the site of REM sleep mentation. Studies of the EEG in awake subjects related to the nasal cycle, nasal cycle-cognitive studies, and studies of the nasal cycle in relation to REM and NREM sleep all suggest that the left brain is the primary site of REM sleep mentation and that the right brain is the site of NREM mentation.

BASIC REST-ACTIVITY CYCLE AND RELATED
PHYSIOLOGICAL AND PSYCHOLOGICAL RHYTHMS

Most concepts of physiological stress are concerned with the degeneration of organ function and the disruption of homeostatic systems and basal metabolic activity. But the usual concept of homeostasis implies a static state, or set point, which is then affected by shifts in environmental circumstances or stress. However, the more closely any system is studied, the more likely an underlying pattern of rhythmic activity will be discovered that more accurately describes the nature of the system, whether it be in waking states or during sleep. Although there have been numerous physiological and psychological phenomena discovered that exhibit ultradian rhythms, there has been little effort to seek relations among these supposedly independent phenomena. This lack of effort has impeded the development of an integrated view of the interactions among various systems and how they are coupled, a view that would provide a newer understanding of "homeostasis."

Kleitman may have given us one good example of a theory of interacting systems with his postulation of the basic rest–activity cycle (BRAC) (48,49). The BRAC theory had its origins in the discovery of how EEG and eye movement patterns change in concert during sleep, giving rise to the concept of REM and NREM sleeps stages. In 1957, Dement and Kleitman (50) reported cyclic variations in the EEG during sleep and their relations to eye movements, body motility, and dreaming. This study also played an important role in Kleitman's later formulation of the BRAC concept, which was supposed to explain why some psychological and physiological activities are integrated and account for the obvious patterns of intermixed locomotor activity and quiescent states during sleep. Kleitman proposed a waking correlate of the sleep pattern (61): "the BRAC is probably a fundamental variation in the functioning of the central nervous system, increasing in duration with phylogenetic progression" where "in each species of mammal studied, the BRAC also lengthens during ontogenetic development." Kleitman proposed the BRAC to be a reflection and variation of integrated events during the 24 h period. Consequently, it is easy to see how such an endogenous cycle of rest and activity could be affected by stress or overactivity.

Wada's seminal studies (52) in 1922 on hunger and its relation to activity also bear on the issues of endogenous rhythms, homeostasis, and stress. Wada proposed that food was the first form of property for primitive humans, the value of things first coming to be measured in terms of food, and primitive migration being primarily motivated by food. Wada therefore surmised that basic homeostatic mechanisms are coupled to hunger. The need to investigate the relation of the hunger rhythm with bodily movements, dreaming, motor activity, salivation, and mental activity led Wada to discover a rhythm of salivary flow that parallels the gastric hunger contraction rhythm. But, surprisingly, Wada also found that people dream more at the hunger contraction periods than during quiescence. Motor activity during waking, as judged by a hand dynamotor, showed that at hunger contraction periods the power of grip is greater than at the quiescent or after-dinner periods. Hunger contractions also correlated with scores on the Thorndike Intelligence Examination. These studies on the relation of activity to hunger predate Kleitman's concept of the BRAC. Wada recognized that "with the onset of hunger the sleeping baby awakes to feed," and in general "when the effort to satisfy hunger is thwarted, the whole organism reacts to the situation, or thwarting agent, with such hyper-tension of all organs and muscles and fibers that the excitement may lead to various types of defensive behavior." Wada therefore saw the hunger mechanism as one of the most primitive, and as certainly a central regulating aspect of physiology. This primitive rhythm and mechanism is another way of viewing the BRAC: hunt and eat, then rest. When this rhythm is disturbed, stress results. But how is this homeostatic rhythm of hunger coupled with those found in more recently discovered phenomena such as the secretion of pituitary hormones?

Richter (53) reported in 1980 that "in rats, lengths of cycles of [growth hormone] GH secretion and of cycles of feeding are 3.6–4.0 hours" and that they are phase coupled. He also suggested that "these two cyclic phenomena may be manifestations of the same timing mechanism in the brain or they could function entirely independently." Growth hormone is known to be secreted predominantly during NREM sleep in humans (54,55). Even though GH secretion does not exhibit an apparent rhythm during much of the 24 h cycle, this link with NREM is an important clue to an association between hypothalamic and cortical rhythms. Pituitary rhythms vary, however, with age, sex, and species, thus complicating any attempt to establish relations among various phenomena.

The first discovery of the pulsatile or episodic nature of pituitary hormone secretion in 1966 was the observation by Weitzman and colleagues (56) that discrete pulses of cortisol secretion reflect rhythmic secretion of adrenocorticotropic hormone (ACTH). Pituitary hormones are secreted with an ultradian rhythm (57,58), and the secretion of several of them are related to REM and NREM sleep. Luteinizing hormone (LH) secretion is coupled to REM sleep at least during puberty (59). Testosterone (T) secretion was found to be phase-linked with cortisol secretion (57), providing evidence for synchronization between the pituitary–adrenal and pituitary–gonadal axis. Testosterone is also known to be secreted in phase with penile tumescent cycles (60) during sleep, coinciding with REM sleep cycles (61). Prolactin secretion was found to increase during NREM periods (62,63). However, this finding was refuted by Van Cauter and Honinckx (57). In adult rats, the 3 h rhythms of GH and corticosterone secretion are 180 degrees out of phase, with GH being secreted during NREM sleep (64). These phase relations between GH and corticosterone secretion are similar to those found in adult humans (65,66). Plasma parathyroid hormone and calcium levels are also related to sleep stages (67), so that peaks in parathyroid hormone secretion are significantly related to NREM sleep stages 3 and 4, while elevated calcium levels are significantly related to REM sleep. Cross-correlation analysis between endorphin, an endogenous opioid, and sleep stages confirmed a relationship with REM sleep (68).

One recent study of the secretion of corticotropin-releasing hormone (CRH), the hypothalamic hormone that initiates and integrates the response to stress, revealed a diurnal rhythm in human males (69) from four samples per day. Continuous monitoring of CRH levels in the cerebrospinal fluid of adult male monkeys (70), by contrast, produced profiles characteristic of an ultradian period. Like other hypothalamic–pituitary factors, CRH may thus exhibit variations in levels of secretion that are ultradian. Even though CRH is considered a "stress" peptide, its secretion may covary with locomotor activity under normal unstressed conditions. Plasma levels of LH, for example, show a direct relationship to rhythmic motor activity or the ultradian rest-activity cycle in ovariectomized sheep (71). Rats who have lost their circadian rhythm due to lesions in the suprachiasmatic nuclei show an ultradian phase-locked relationship between locomotor activity and plasma corticosterone levels (72). Most authors do not ascribe any particular significance to the ultradian nature of pituitary hormone secretion, suggesting that the cause of this rhythmic phenomenon is unknown. However, in light of the available evidence it is reasonable to propose that such rhythms help to modulate and regulate, and reflect the coupling of the CNS with the ANS. This coupling underlies the BRAC and the accompanying coupling of psychological phenomena with rhythms of the hypothalamo-pituitary-adrenal (-gonadal) axis. It has been shown in men (but not women) that injections of luteinizing hormone releasing hormone (LHRH) prevent improvement in a spatial orientation task (right hemisphere skill), but enhance performance on a fluency task (left hemisphere skill) (73). The resulting increase in LH, which enhances left hemispheric skills, is consistent with the elevated levels of LH with REM sleep, which is a sleeping correlate of an activated left hemisphere.

In addition to the earlier work by Wada (52) on the relation of stomach contractions to dreaming and body movement, Friedman and Fisher (74) studied how "REM periods are related to a cyclic waxing and waning of instinctual drive activity mediated through the limbic system," particularly in eating behavior. They report a statistically significant waking state oral activity cycle of 80-120 min, based on subjects' use of drink, food, and tobacco. Another human study of ingestive activity shows a similar oral activity cycle (75) of about 90 min. Although both studies show considerable variability in the cycles, the range is not different from other ultradian phenomena. Ultradian rhythms of gastric pH levels in humans during night shows a range of 1.07-5.5 h, clustering around 2-3 h (76). A nocturnal study of gastric secretion in fasting subjects showed "a wide individual variation and a considerable spontaneous variation of the gastric secretion in the same individual from hour to hour and also from night to night" (77). In another study, gastric motility and pH were recorded during night sleep and showed a consistent pattern of motility decreasing and acidity increasing in deep sleep compared to levels while awake (78). Motility was markedly enhanced during REM sleep, but there was not a constant relation between the occurrence of peristaltic waves and the outbursts of rapid eye movements. Lavie et al. (79) demonstrated 100 min cycles in gastric motility during sleep, and found only minimal relations to REM periods (which may be due to the lack of adaptation nights, and a nasogastric tube sometimes with or without a balloon). They conclude that "since hunger and feeding behaviors may be weakly related to stomach contractions, it is still to be determined if appetitive behaviors have any mechanism in common with stage REM." Periodic interdigestive secretion of the pancreas, liver, and stomach was found in canines, with a peak interval of 100 min and a range of 80-130 min (80,81).

Taken together, the available evidence suggests that the ultradian rhythms of the BRAC, eating-oral-gastric rhythms, pituitary rhythms, sleep stages, and other cerebral rhythms may have central regulators in common. This conclusion can help reshape how we think about the cerebral-hypothalamic-pituitary-adrenal (-gonadal) axis with respect to stress. Rhythms also give us a new perspective on laterality.

NEURAL MATRIX FOR COUPLING MIND AND METABOLISM

Rhythmic ANS laterality and the likely regulatory role of the ANS in lateralized CNS rhythms provide compelling evidence that the ANS, via its sympathetic, parasympathetic, and enteric branches, acts as a neural matrix for coupling states of mind with metabolism. States of lateralized cerebral activation, whether during waking or sleeping, are clearly rhythmic and must have a direct relation to other important physiological and psychological phenomena and, without exception, the BRAC. Looking at these individual phenomenon without being aware of the generalized rhythms of the ANS-CNS as an integrative phenomenon evokes the tale of the blind men and the elephant. A single physical phenomenon, the nasal cycle, allows us to assess other ultradian phenomena. The nasal cycle can be measured easily and provides access to other ANS-CNS phenomena.

Besides the humoral effects of the nervous system on the immune system, the ANS serves as a neural matrix for regulation of the immune system. Bulloch (82) has shown that the ANS innervates virtually all lymphoid tissues. For example, the thymus, a dual-lobed organ, receives independent innervation from sympathetic and parasympathetic nerves for each lobe. Therefore, in light of the lateralized rhythms of the ANS, it is possible that the functions of the two lobes are rhythmic, one being active while the other is resting and regenerating. An important question is whether the two lobes are identical in their functions. Do the functions of one lobe correlate with one mode of cerebral intelligence and its related neuroendocrine state? Thymic hormones are known to have an influence on the hypothalamic–pituitary axis (83). There are also connections in the other direction. Bilateral electrolytic lesions in the anterior hypothalamus influence an animal's immune potential, causing a marked decrease in the number of nucleated spleen cells and thymocytes compared to normal or frontal cortex lesioned animals (84). Macris et al. (85) produced bilateral lesions in either the anterior or posterior basal hypothalamus of guinea pigs. Anterior lesions resulted in protection from anaphylactic shock, compared to posterior lesions or sham-operated controls. If the two thymic lobes are dissimilar, different pituitary hormones may help to facilitate one lobe of thymic function over the other.

The evidence reviewed here suggests that rhythms of lateralized lymph node and bone marrow activity may exist, and that certain splenic functions may correlate with different modes of cerebral intelligence. Therefore, the ANS is also a neural matrix for coupling mind and immunity. Various studies indicate that lateralized cerebral states may correlate with lateralized expression in the immune system. Bereavement, depression, and stress, for example, all affect immunity (86). Renoux et al. (87) showed in mice that lesions of the left frontoparietal cortex lead to depression of T-lymphocyte functions, while lesions of the right cortex augment T-cell functions. Neveu et al. (88) found the same results with T-cell functions. Neveu et al. also found that mitogenesis of B cells induced by lipopolysaccharide (LPS) was modified by cortical lesions in the same way as T cells. Left-lesioned animals showed B-cell proliferation decreased by 60% compared to controls, whereas right-lesioned animals showed B-cell mitogenesis enhanced by 120% compared to controls. The results for B cells were not found by Renoux et al., who used pokeweed as a mitogen instead of LPS.

Studies of depression in humans show greater right cerebral dysfunction by EEG (89). This result, in the light of the animal cortex lesion studies, may help explain how immunity is suppressed by abnormal right hemispheric activities in humans. Studies of hemispheric laterality and immune function have shown that left-handedness is associated with increased risk of autoimmune disease (90). Our understanding of psychoneuroimmunology may be increased by considering how the ANS acts as the neural matrix for coupling mind and immunity, especially with regard to lateralized rhythms. If we constantly shift between two separate modes of intelligence, or modes of consciousness, we may find that this rhythm is coupled to rhythms of T-cell activity and other immune factors such as lymphokine secretion. Rhythms of immune function may be an important but overlooked area of chronobiology.

Laterality also plays a role in the neuroendocrine system (for review see 91, 92), which has many significant functional asymmetries that are manifested in gonadal control, thyroid control, differential prolactin responses to right- and left-sided mastectomies in mice, differential grooming responses to right- and left-sided vagotomy in mice, and mortality rates after unilateral brain lesions in mice.

Since sudden cardiac failure is the leading cause of death in the industrialized world, it captures the attention of anyone interested in stress since the pathophysiological mechanisms remain a mystery. Strong emotions are thought to play a primary role, affecting first the CNS, which then affects the ANS to cause ventricular fibrillation. The ANS input to the heart is lateralized, with control of heart rate being more affected by the right sympathetic system and heart rhythm or arrhythomogenesis being more affected by the left (93). Laterality also exists in parasympathetically induced arrhythmias, with left vagus stimulation producing an atrioventricular (AV) block via the AV node, and right vagus stimulation producing sinus arrest via the sinoatrial node. It therefore appears that activation or interference with specific sites in either the CNS or ANS may selectively affect heart rate and rhythm (93).

The BRAC concept has led to investigations into an endogenous ultradian biorhythm manifested in heart activity. In 1974, Orr and Hoffman (94) identified a 90 min ultradian rhythm in human heart rate during both waking and sleeping. Free-running dogs were monitored via telemetry for 14–24 h in a closed environment and a 1–2 h/phase-locked rhythm of heart rate and mean arterial pressure was found (95). Another study in dogs with limited activity revealed an ultradian rhythm of mean arterial blood pressure with an average period of 158 min (96). A study in humans relating REM sleep to systolic blood pressure showed that pressure changes correlate with the cyclical changes of REM EEG patterns. Pressure increased with REM sleep (97). It therefore appears that laterality of ANS function and rhythms of cardiac function are related in a manner consistent with the relationship found in other organs. Since REM sleep seems to be the sleeping analogue of left-hemisphere dominance, we might expect to find that right nostril activity is associated with increased heart rate and blood pressure.

PENDULUM OF ANS–CNS ACTIVITY AND HOMEOSTASIS: A NEW PARADIGM FOR STRESS

Knowledge of the pendulum of alternating lateral dominance in ANS and CNS activity provides a new approach to the study of stress. The concept of a pendulum implies movement: not a single homeostatic state, but continuous alternation between two polar conditions for both mind and metabolism. The lateralized rhythm of ANS–CNS activity is an integrative temporal and structural paradigm. The pendulum effect is the key to understanding how many apparently independent physiological and psychological phenomena might be coupled. The pendulum of autonomic activity sets the frequency at which various activities are entrained. The ANS is the regulating circuitry. Stress may be defined by how long or how frequently a particular position of the pendulum is maintained. Too much left-brain activity and right sympathetic dominance may indeed be what we normally think of as stress or overactivity. It is easy to envision both acute swings and prolonged shifts toward one position of this pendulum.

The terms *ergotrophic* and *trophotropic* were coined by Hess to describe ANS functions. Ergotrophic reactions are "coupled with energy expenditure" and an "endophylactic–trophotropic" system "provides for protection and restitution" (98). Gellhorn (99) discusses these concepts at length in his discourses on ANS-somatic integration. The key concept is the antagonistic relationship of the sympathetic and parasympathetic systems in maintaining balance between these two polar states.

Left nostril/right brain dominance is unlikely to underly the fight-or-flight response, since it appears to represent the resting state of generalized increased parasympathetic tone that is antithetical to the stress response. It is also likely that peaks of immune function, regeneration, and healing occur during the increased parasympathetic state of right brain/left nostril dominance. Dramatic increases in CRH release may be coupled to right nostril/left brain dominance during the fight-or-flight response, since the apparent ultradian rhythms of CRH are likely to have their peaks during the active phase of the BRAC. Certain observations in two case studies of multiple personality disorder (MPD) are suggestive of this lateralized ANS relationship. In 1955, Ischlondsky (100) reported significant lateralized findings during a neurological examination of two different patients with similar personality traits. Each patient had:

> two diametrically-opposed personality types. One was an impulsive, irresponsible, mischievous and vindictive personality, full of rebellion against authority and of hate towards the people around her, the patient in this phase was extremely aggressive, using abusive language and scaring other patients with lurid tales of state hospitals, sex relations, etc.; in the opposed behavioral pattern to which the first personality would suddenly switch, the patient appeared dependent, submissive, shy, self-effacing, affectionate, and obedient. In a very timid way she expressed friendliness, sought affection, acceptance, and approval from the same personnel she had reviled and abused. There was no trace left of any inappropriate word or expression, no manifestation of hostility to her surroundings, and not the slightest reference

to sex. In fact, any sex thought or word would induce in her extreme fears of perdition, feelings of guilt and anxiety, depression, and shame.

In each of these two opposed mental states there was amnesia to the other, which is characteristic of MPDs: "A strong stimulus was capable of evoking the antipode of the existing mental condition." During the aggressive or active phase of the patient's behavior (100):

> examination revealed that the left and right sides of her body responded differently to sensory stimulus: while the right side was hypo-sensitive the the left side displayed hyper-sensitivity. Thus vision and hearing were unclear and far away on the right side but very clear and close on the left side. Her response to touch and pain showed a high threshold on the right, and a low threshold on the left side. Characteristically, with regard to the olfactory sense, the patient in this mental state manifested a diametrically opposed attitude: she was hyper-sensitive to smell on the right side and her *right nostril was clear*, while on the *left side* her sense of smell was absent and the *nostril congested and closed* [emphasis added]. With regard to the other neurological signs such as the size of pupils, reflexes, salivation, sweating, there was a similar difference in the response of the two sides of the body: the aggressive personality type displayed on the right side, a small pupil, a hypo-secretion of saliva, absence of sweating on sole and palm and lack of abdominal reflexes, while on the left side there was a large pupil, hypersecretion of saliva, very strong sweating on palm and sole and extremely strong abdominal reflexes.

(It is difficult to account for the observation of pupil size etc. inconsistent with nasal congestion.) Just as fast as the psyche switched to the shy, passive, and permissive personality all neurological manifestations also switched to reverse dominance: "olfactory sense proved now to be very sharp on the left side while completely absent and with nostril congested and closed on the right side." This extraordinary case study showing that lateralized ANS phenomena switch instantaneously with the psyche in two patients suggests that right nostril dominance or sympathetic dominance on the right side of the body correlates with the active phase of the BRAC and the fight-or-flight response pattern.

Other examples of laterality and the neurology of emotion and psychological profiles are reviewed by Bear (101). He states that "the patient with right-hemisphere damage may be severely impaired by unconcern, unrealistic assessment of emotional priorities, and failures in emotional communication, while left-hemisphere damage more often results in aphasia." McIntyre et al. compared left versus right temporal lobe epileptics and showed that right hemisphere foci produce an "impulsive" aggressive pattern compared with a controlled "reflective" profile of those with left hemisphere foci (102). This finding is further supported by studies in humans with one hemisphere anesthetized by barbiturates. Left hemisphere anesthesia usually produces a "depressive-catastrophic" reaction, while a "euphoric-maniacal" reaction occurs when the right hemisphere is anesthetized (103). In summary, it seems that left brain function produces an active or aggressive state if not checked by normal right brain activity and vice versa. This pendulum of cerebral activity provides a simple view of how stress may arise in the nervous system. Certainly the fight-or-flight response is an extreme swing to the left brain. Stress may alternate with a passive–depressive state, in which the right brain mode dominates and causes different physical sequelae. The patients with MPD represented completely passive, receptive victims in a state of helplessness. The neurology of this adaptive mechanism represents an interesting trait from an evolutionary perspective. This passive state has its correlate in other species that react by "playing dead" in certain situations in which escape or attack seems impossible.

STRESS, DISEASE, AND EQUILIBRIUM

The pendulum concept implies that equilibrium is defined by an equal balance of right and left neural function over time in both periphery and cortex. The midpoint in the swing corresponds to "homeostasis" in the classic sense. Is there evidence to suggest that disease can be lateralized in the periphery as a result of imbalance: can one side be more stressed than the other as reflected in dysfunction? Do some personality profiles or states of psychopathology reflect overactivation and abuse of one hemisphere?

We might think the answer to both questions is yes. But is there clinical evidence? Eccles and Eccles, in referring to lateralized autonomic tone, state that "under stress or with marked hypothalamic instability this balance may be disrupted and result in the marked autonomic asymmetry seen in migraine or Meniere's disease" (104). Such a disruption in autonomic balance may explain the asymmetrical autonomic response observed in migraine, with unilateral flushing, nasal congestion, and visual distortion. Kitrelle et al. characterize cluster headaches as recurrent, unilateral attacks of severe pain that almost always occur on the same side of the head with lacrimentation, nasal congestion, conjunctival infection, ptosis, miosis, and rhinorrhea also occurring on the same side (105).

Another curious and suggestive finding from the perspective of an ergotrophic-related state is the autonomic instability of asthmatics during sleep. Asthmatics seem to suffer more bronchoconstriction during REM sleep (106). Normal bronchodilation occurs via increased sympathetic tone, which enhances respiration, contrary to the vasoconstrictive effects of sympathetic fibers in most tissues. During REM sleep, therefore, a "weakened" or "stressed" autonomic fiber system may not "hold its own." However, even though this is not a lateralized effect of autonomic stress in the lungs, the principle of autonomic stress and lability and specific rhythmic phases holds, since REM is considered the active phase of the BRAC. Dexter and Weitzman found that REM sleep stages are also temporally related to nocturnal migraines and cluster headaches (107). In this study, sidedness was noted in only four of the seven subjects. All four experienced right-sided pain, ptosis, lacrimentation, rhinorrhea, and sometimes sweating over the right side of the face and forehead. One patient showed an alternating hemicranial headache. No report as to side was given for the other two patients. Right-sided peripheral pain with these other symptoms also suggests that the sympathetic fibers had been "weakened or strained" and hence releasing vessels caused acute dilatation. Symptoms of such headaches (and asthma) are often treated with sympathomimetics. Baust states that even though heart rate is highest during REM sleep, sympathetic tone is at its lowest, at least in the cat (108). This suggests that during REM sleep there is a propensity for failed sympathetic tone, which primarily manifests on the right side at least in this small group of subjects. This is equivalent to a lateralized stress of sympathetic function.

No simple answers can be given to the question of whether some personality profiles or states of psychopathology reflect overactivation and abuse of one hemisphere. However, the field of laterality and psychopathology has recently been well summarized by Flor-Henry (89):

> Studies strongly implicate the left frontal and/or left temporal regions in schizophrenia . . . . left hemisphere activation in acute, positive symptomology syndrome and more generally a dislocation of intrahemispheric organization, bilaterally in schizophrenia and mania . . . . Neurometabolic activity is disorganized in the frontal–temporal regions bilaterally asymmetrically (left > right) in most of the studies, with a correlation between intensity of psychopathological symptoms and degree of left hemisphere changes. . .
>
> Thalamo-striate patterns are hypometabolic on the left and hypermetabolic on the right. Correlations are established between left frontal hypometabolic activity and catatonic features, blunted affect and emotional withdrawal. Most of the first rank symptoms are associated with local circulatory changes in the left frontal or temporal region, with the notable exception of delusional mood and persecutory delusions which relate to the right posterior hemisphere. . . .
>
> Major endogenous depressions all demonstrate right hemispheric perturbation; however it is possible that the initial disturbance is left frontal. Shifts of lateral cognitive organization occur not only in schizophrenia but also in depressive psychoses. EEG changes are more bilateral in bipolar than unipolar depression and bilateral intrahemispheric disorganization is more extensive in mania (similar to schizophrenia) than in depression. The bilaterally asymmetric[al] reduction in blood flow after electroconvulsive therapy more

pronounced in the right hemisphere, again underlines the importance of right hemispheric systems in the genesis of affective psychoses, associated with reduced coherence between the left and right frontal regions

It is difficult to say whether the cause of these psychopathological conditions is the initial result of overuse or abuse, but some symptoms are suggestive. A case in point is the lateralized cognitive expression in MPD, which suggests specific adaptive mechanisms that might help such persons to cope with psychological stress and abuse.

In bilaterally structured organs, diseases such as pneumonia, kidney disease, hyper- and hypothyroid conditions, inflammation of the ovary or testicle, tumors, or skin rashes commonly have unilateral effects. The unilateral stress of ANS function deserves attention in these cases. Constellations of psychosomatic disorders may be more strongly coupled to right or left autonomic stress and dysfunction.

In a study of 980 women with unilateral breast cancer, results show a left/right ratio of 1.26. The data suggest differences in the sensitivity of left and right mammary glands to hormonal stimulation, resulting in unequal volumes of tissue at risk of carcinoma (109). When asynchronous bilateral carcinoma was documented, the disease first occurred more often in the left breast. Since this study indicates a differential sensitivity to hormonal influence, it is also possible that an autonomic correlate plays a role. In another study of breast cancer, adenocarcinoma occurred with a left/right ratio of 1.778 (110). Lateralization was also studied in 601 cases of carcinoma of the nasal cavity and paranasal sinuses in which squamous, anaplastic carcinomata, and adenocarcinoma had a pronounced left-sided predominance in the ethmoid and, to a much lesser extent, in the nose (111).

The significant differences in breast or nasal carcinoma are at best suggestive that a lateralized influence of autonomic stress plays a role. However, in a study of 151 cases of herpes zoster, with 92 cases occurring on the right and 59 on the left side of the body, stress may be an important influence (112).

Riga in 1957 (113) published observations on unilateral chronic nasal obstruction. Patients presented with a range of symptoms that he classified as:

local disorders; nasal respiratory insufficiency, hypertrophic rhinitis of the obstructed nostril and allergic disorders, and neighboring disorders; spontaneous painful sensitivity in the periphery, sinusitis, catarrh of the Eustachian tube, hypacousia and otorrhea, bronchorrhea all on the obstructed side, and distant disorders; intellectual asthenia with frequent amnesia, headaches, hyperthyroidism, cardiopulmonary asthenia with tachycardia and asthmatic disorder with sometimes hypertrophy of the left cavity of the heart and pulmonary emphysema, hepatic and gallbladder, gastritis, enterocolitis, sexual disorders, dysmenorrhea, and decrease of virility.

Eighty-nine percent of the patients with right nasal obstruction were found to be affected to some degree with this widespread and apparently unrelated array of conditions, but only 26% of the patients with left nasal obstruction were affected. This suggests that a right-sided obstruction may more seriously affect health.

NONINVASIVE ENDOGENOUS MECHANISMS FOR SELF-REGULATION

Selective Hemispheric Stimulation by Unilateral Forced Nostril Breathing

The concept for the study by Werntz et al. (20,24) on the nasal cycle and cerebral rhythm came from yogic medicine. For thousands of years yogis have been aware of this phenomenon and have experimented with how breathing is related to states of mind and metabolism. This group of early experimenters perceived the breath to be the link between the mind and body. They discovered that altering the nasal cycle by occluding the dominant nostril and force breathing through the congested side could affect mental activity, as could breathing with different rates and rhythms. This effect was documented by Werntz and colleagues (114,115). They demonstrated how unilateral forced nostril breathing could stimulate the contralateral hemisphere, producing relatively greater amplitudes in the EEG (Fig. 6). Srinivasan and Shannahoff-Khalsa (unpublished data 1987) have found similar EEG results with forced nostril breathing in a pilot study.

Work by Kristof et al. (116) suggests that the EEG activity is produced by a neural mechanism in the superior nasal meatus. This activating effect could be elicited by air insufflation into the upper nasal cavity without pulmonary exercise. Local anesthesia of the mucosal membrane suppressed the cortical effects of airflow. Servit et al. (117) showed how deep breathing through one side of the nose could activate abnormalities in patients with unilateral focal or lateralized paroxysmal abnormalities in the fronto- or occipitotemporal region.

The question of EEG amplitudes and their relation to mental activity and inactivity is important here. Yogis believe that forced nostril breathing on one side "exercises" the opposite hemisphere. The study by Klein et al. (26) showed that right nasal dominance is coupled to increased verbal performance, or left brain activity, and left nasal dominance with spatial, or right hemispheric skills. They were not able, however, to demonstrate the effects of forced nostril breathing with their subjects, possibly due to errors in experimental design. Shannahoff-Khalsa. Boyle, and Buebel (unpublished data, 1989) have shown that unilateral forced nostril breathing can alter cognitive performance in the manner predicted by yogis. Forced nostril breathing for 30 min was shown to

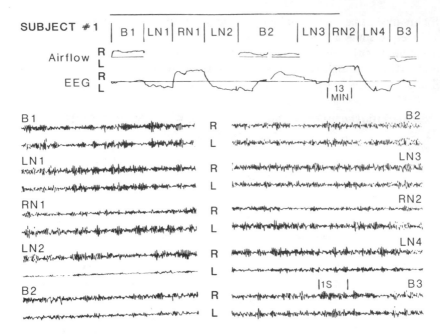

FIGURE 6 Effect of forced uni-nostril breathing on EEG asymmetry: subject 1, trial 2. Top: In the Airflow tracing the points above the baseline indicate greater right nostril airflow and points below greater left nostril airflow. Periods of forced nostril breathing are indicated. EEG tracing: points above the baseline indicate relatively greater left hemisphere EEG amplitude; points below relatively greater right hemisphere amplitude. B, baseline; LN, left nostril breathing; RN, right nostril breathing. Montage: $(O_2\text{-}P_4 ; O_1\text{-}P_3)$. Bottom: representative segments of the primary EEG that were integrated and subtracted to produce the tracings in the top section. For each pair the top tracing is from the right hemisphere and the bottom is from the left hemisphere (reprinted from ref. 115. p. 167, with permission from Springer-Verlag).

increase the task performance of the opposite hemisphere. The study by Klein et al. (26) also used shorter breathing times (15 min as well as 30 min) during their procedures. The breathing times, tests used, and the association between testing and nasal blocking seem critical. The interpretation of the expected functional relationships based on the lack of crossover by autonomic fibers coincides with the yogic interpretations.

An interesting clinical result was reported by Friedell in 1948 (118). As a physician he found that "diaphragmatic breathing with attention to both phases of respiration and the intervening pauses" coupled with "alternately closing one nostril while inhaling slowly through the other" had profound effects on patients with angina pectoris. All 11 patients studied experienced relief from symptoms with the breathing practice and were able to curtail nitroglycerin use after continued use of the technique.

It is likely that the effect of the alternate-nostril breathing exercise induces a balance in the peripheral ANS as well as in the CNS. This technique may thus help to reset the electrical patterns affecting the heart muscle, reducing the "stress" that produces chest pain due to reduced oxygen supplies. Yogi Bhajan, a master of Kundalini Yoga, suggests "angina comes when the breathing rhythm does not shift" (referring to the nasal cycle). This is supportive of the concept of stress being a prolonged swing of the pendulum of the autonomic rhythm.

Postural Effects on the ANS–CNS Rhythm

Yogis were also the first to discover how posture could alter the nasal cycle and the cerebral rhythm. Less developed practitioners lean on the "yoga danda" stick for altering the cerebral rhythm. As mentioned above (15,17), pressure on the fifth intercostal space can induce a shift in the nasal cycle. This noninvasive mechanism was used by the less adept to shift mind–body states.

Conscious Overriding of the Rhythm

An advanced yogi can consciously select which hemisphere he wants to use within the span of one breath. He can switch back and forth, fully activating one side of his brain within this very short time. The autonomic phenomenon becomes a consciously regulated activity. This level of development reflects a very advanced stage in the discipline of "self-regulation." It then becomes necessary for an individual to choose consciously which hemisphere to use. This increase in responsibility is worthwhile since emotional, mental, and psychological stress can be easily reduced as a result of the increased performance efficiency. In normal individuals, right–left cerebral balance is only a transition state that is short-lived. However, the advanced yogi can choose to operate from this state for prolonged periods. Within this state the adept practitioner begins to enjoy the fruits of the nervous system, since he or she is in conscious control.

Besides the adaptive form of this mechanism, expressed with MPD (100), Gott and co-workers (119) report a fascinating single case of a 31-year-old woman, naive to the phenomena of cerebral rhythms and nasal cycles, who has evidently trained herself without fully understanding her achievement. She was described as being able voluntarily to select and hold either of two qualitatively different state of consciousness. There is evidence of differential dominance of the left or right hemisphere in each state. "Asymmetries of EEG alpha and task performance scores indicated a state dependent shift in functional lateralization." The subject reported "that her state switch had been involuntary from early childhood. At age 16 she learned to select her state at will, thereby improving her school work and personal behavior."

HYPOTHALAMIC MODEL FOR REGULATION AND INTEGRATION OF THE ANS–CNS RHYTHM

In Swanson's recent review of the hypothalamus, he states that "it has been accepted for many years on the basis of physiological and behavioral evidence that the essential role of the hypothalamus is to integrate endocrine, autonomic, and behavioral responses that are essential for survival of the individual (homeostasis) and the species as a whole (reproduction)" (120). It may very well be that, gram for gram, the hypothalamus is the most important piece of tissue in any organism. Swanson also states that "the outstanding question has always been, what is the organization and neurotransmitter specificity of hypothalamic circuitry underlying this integration and mediating these responses?" This section will discuss a very simplistic view of how the hypothalamus may integrate and regulate the ANS–CNS rhythm, which accounts for many endocrine, autonomic, immune, and behavioral functions.

Others (57) have discussed the issues of "single" or "multiple ultradian pacemakers" with hypothalamic origins, or a "central ultradian clock" possibly outside the hypothalamus, or the "extrahypothalamic modulation" hypothesis of a hypothalamic ultradian pacemaker(s) influenced by ultradian rhythms outside the hypothalamus, or, in general, "uni-versus multioscillatory phenomena" for the various ultradian rhythms (121). There are two major points: first, are all ultradian rhythms related? And if so, are they regulated and integrated by the same pacemaker?

The model presented here suggests all ultradian rhythms are related via the proposed ANS–CNS rhythm and, second, that the hypothalamus itself is the "pacemaker." Part of the confusion over "single" vs. "multiple" ultradian pacemaker theories comes by assuming that there is no coordinated relationship between the various rhythms, and therefore, that individual pacemakers would be needed for each rhythm. This is equivalent to saying that neuroendocrine, immune, or behavioral phenomena are not coupled to autonomic phenomena. Part of this confusion may come from viewing the individual hypothalamic nuclei as independent, with no expected integrated relationship among their activities. This confusion of multi- versus single-pacemaker theories may in part stem from regulation of circadian rhythms by the suprachiasmatic nucleus (72). It is likely, however, that this nucleus also helps to couple circadian activities with the ultradian.

In the proposed model, the hypothalamus is envisioned as a single organ in which the various nuclei, like organs, are functional parts of "a" body. Everything works together and has some relationship even with distant parts. The hypothalamus works much like a clock or pacemaker in a classic sense, in which different regions, at different times, are more active.

In this model, which views the hypothalamus as a circle (Fig. 7), the two sides and their fiber systems are directly related to the ipsilateral sides of the

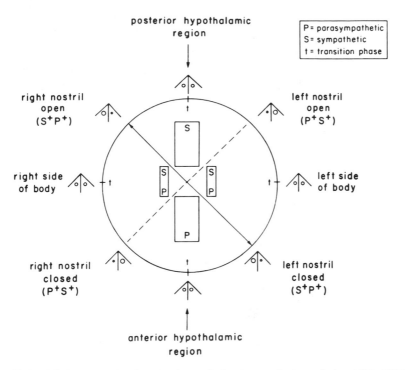

posterior hypothalamic
region

P = parasympathetic
S = sympathetic
t = transition phase

right nostril
open
(S^+P^+)

left nostril
open
(P^+S^+)

right side
of body

left side
of body

right nostril
closed
(P^+S^+)

left nostril
closed
(S^+P^+)

anterior hypothalamic
region

FIGURE 7 A model for the hypothalamic regulation of the ANS–CNS lateralized rhythm. The circle represents the hypothalamus as one organ composed of
the individual nuclei without differentiation beyond four hypothetical quadrants. A midline bisection (not drawn) of posterior to anterior regions or 12
o'clock to 6 o'clock divides the hypothalamus into right and left mirror images,
separating homologous nuclei. A perpendicular bisection separating the anterior
and posterior regions on both right and left sides (not drawn) indicates division
between parasympathetic and sympathetic regions, respectively. The hatched
line from 1:30 to 7:30 indicates a hypothetical clock time for the proposed
metabolic gradient of activity within the hypothalamus, with its expression in
the periphery where left nostril is open and right nostril is congested. The
unbroken line represents another hypothetical time in this clock, for which the
"hand" indicates the phase of the metabolic gradient of activity, here with
dominance in the right posterior quadrant producing sympathetic dominance
on the right side of the body, and right nostril open, and dominance in the left
anterior quadrant producing parasympathetic dominance and congestion in the
left nostril.

body and the cortex. This neuroanatomical relationship is supported by the work of Saper et al. (25), who show that the vast majority of autonomic fibers run ipsilaterally without the crossing-over seen in most other fiber systems running into and out of the brain. The hypothalamus is, therefore, first bisected with respect to the two sides and homologous nuclei are divided between the two halves of the circle. Second, a division is made between the rostral and caudal halves. The rostral parts are predominantly concerned with parasympathetic mechanisms, while the caudal parts are predominantly concerned with sympathetic mechanisms. Theories of this rostral–parasympathetic versus caudal–sympathetic axis are based on the work of Hess (122,98) and Ranson and Magoun (123). We now envision our circle as a clock with four quadrants. The midline posterior point is 12 o'clock, the line bisecting the posterior and anterior regions runs from 3 o'clock on the right side to 9 o'clock on the left, and so on.

This hypothalamic clock has only one hand, a rigid diameter of the circle that rotates about its midpoint. This hand specifies both the time and the nuclei that are most active. The nuclei closest to the hand determine a "metabolic gradient of activity" in the expression of their functions. This organizing principle makes the model useful for considering the possible relations of various functions and their respective nuclei. In a physical sense, the time is also told by the phase of the nasal cycle. If the hand extends from 12 to 6, equal activity is expected along this midline region where equal right and left sympathetic and parasympathetic function is expected on the two sides of the body, thus producing equal vasoconstriction–vasodilation in both nostrils. This represents a transition point in nasal dominance. A transition point also occurs when the hand is at 3 and 9 o'clock, at which the left body will have half sympathetic and half parasympathetic influence, as would be the case for the right side of the body. When the hand is at 1:30 and 7:30 the first quadrant (left side of body) shows dominant sympathetic function (open left nostril), and the third quadrant (right side of the body) shows dominant parasympathetic function (congested nostril). The opposite occurs at 4:30 and 10:30.

The proposed dynamics of the hand are as follows: the clock starts with the hand straight up (12 and 6) and then turns either clockwise to 3 and 9 o'clock or counterclockwise to 9 and 3. After it goes from 12 and 6 to 3 and 9, it resets back to 12 and 6 then reverses to 9 and 3, and again back to 12 and 6. This operation gives equal time to the functions of each quadrant and accounts, in principle, for a clocklike ANS–CNS rhythm. This clock could be the regulator and integrator for physiological and psychological phenomena. It does not presume a separation between the two, since this is a distinction that we only perceive.

Is there additional evidence to support this hypothesis? Only a few of the many pieces of supportive evidence will be included here. First, several studies show a direct neural connection between one side of the hypothalamus and an ipsilateral organ. Different studies show a direct neural link to the ovaries (124–126), testes (127), and adrenal glands (128). A study by Bakalkin et al. (129) shows an asymmetrical LHRH distribution in the rat hypothalamus: Wistar rats exhibit higher LHRH content in the right hypothalamus and albino rats exhibit higher LHRH content on the left. Bakalkin et al. state that LHRH content changes from side to side over a 24 h period and that unilateral castration or cold stress lead to a shift in LHRH distribution in the hypothalamus. When total hypothalamic dopamine and norepinephrine levels are measured in the rat over time, ultradian rhythms appear and (130) resemble those found in the periphery (18). Knobil (131) states that

> the hypothalamus of mammals contains an oscillatory or pulse generator that in the unmodulated state has a period of approximately one hour in monkeys and humans. The activation of this system initiates a cascade of neuroendocrine events that are required for normal gonadal function in both sexes. Deviation from the physiological frequency of the pulse generator leads to profound disturbances of the reproductive process.

Sometimes neuronal activity was found only on one side of the hypothalamus (Knobil, personal communication).

Another relevant finding is that the hypothalamic paraventricular nucleus seems to play a modulating role in the production of REM sleep and in the generation of its rhythm (132).

Electrical stimulation of specific regions within the hypothalamus in cats can induce bilateral and unilateral nasal constriction, retraction of the nictitating membranes, and a rise in arterial blood pressure (133). These responses occur on stimulation of regions previously described as the defense area. Many other studies support the concept of defense areas being located in the anterior regions. The work of Roszman et al. (84), for example, who placed lesions in the anterior hypothalamic region and found a decrease in the immune responses, suggests that this region is related to resting or parasympathetic functions.

The model presented here provides only a very simplified view, but may accurately describe how autonomic, neuroendocrine, immune, and behavioral activities may be regulated in concert. Knobil emphasizes the importance of not deviating from the normal pulse-generator frequency, lest profound disturbances in reproductive processes occur (131). It may be that mind–body health is determined by the metabolic gradient of activity in the various hypothalamic nuclei and that the consequent integration is a direct correlate of health. In sum, stress may directly affect this hypothalamic clock, which determines the balance of activity in the four quadrants. Different forms of stress would have an impact on the clock's timing differently. Fight-or-flight stress, catastrophic depression, and anxiety are all likely to affect different quadrants.

STRESS MANAGEMENT AND SELF-REGULATION: TECHNIQUES FROM KUNDALINI YOGA

The techniques listed in this section are thousands of years old. They were developed by groups of individuals (yogis) who learned how to master their own nervous systems. Their working knowledge of how mind and body are related had evolved to such a level of understanding that we now have a technology or user's guide for the nervous system. Although today's science has not yet proven the validity of this knowledge, the initial studies reported in this chapter involving the relationship of the nasal cycle, unilateral forced nostril breathing, and cerebral hemispheric rhythms (with some correlates, for example, cerebral REM and NREM relations) gives support for the phenomena observed in ancient times. This knowledge was taught to this author by Yogi Bhajan, a Master of Kundalini Yoga.

The credibility of these sophisticated tools comes best through their application. The stated benefits reflect claims and findings of the ancient yogic texts. The procedures presented here are presented as they were taught, without any alterations. It is advisable to not practice any of these techniques without sufficient time to relax afterwards. The breathing patterns are never to be used while or immediately before driving a car, or in combination with any controlled substances. No changes should be made in the procedures described.

Technique for Alleviating Emotional Stress and Anxiety

Sit and maintain a straight spine. Relax the arms and the hands in the lap. Focus the eyes on the tip of the nose (the end you cannot see). Open the mouth as wide as possible, slightly stressing the temporal–mandibular joint, and touch the end of the tongue tip to the upper palate where it is hard and smooth. Breathe through the nose only, while making the breath long, slow, and deep. Let the mental focus be on the sound of the breath, listen to the sound of the inhalation and exhalation. Maintain this for at least 3–5 min with a maximum of 8 min at first trial. With practice, it can be built up to a 31 min maximum.

Technique for Alleviating Fatigue and Listlessness

Sit with a straight spine. Place the palms together at the center of the chest, touching the sternum lightly, with the fingers pointing up and away at 60 degrees. Eyelids are lightly closed with the visual focus where the nose meets the eyebrows. As you inhale break the breath into four equal parts, hold a few seconds and then exhale by breaking the breath again into four equal parts, and then hold the breath out for a few seconds before inhaling again. If desired, instead of counting 1,2,3,4 to gauge the rhythm, try using the sounds Sa, Ta, Na, Ma in their place. Mentally vibrate these sounds on the inhalation

and exhalation: this adds to the effect. Their innate effect on the psyche is to help guide and correct the consciousness. On each part of the inhalation or exhalation, pull the naval point in slightly. One full cycle or breath takes 7–8 s. Continue this pattern for 3–5 min. Then inhale deeply and press the palms together with maximum force for 10 s. Relax for 15–30 s. Then repeat this entire procedure twice. When finished, if necessary, immediately lie on the back with eyes closed and relax the entire body for 2 min. Pregnant women or persons with high blood pressure can do this exercise, but must refrain from pressing the palms together at the end.

Technique for Alleviating Obsessive–Compulsive Disorders

Sit with a straight spine in a comfortable position, either with the legs crossed while sitting on the floor or in a straight-backed chair with both feet flat on the floor. Close the eyes. Use the right thumb tip to block the end of the right nostril, point the other fingers up straight, and allow the arm to relax (elbow should not be sticking up and out to the side, which creates unnecessary tension). Inhale very slowly, long and deep through the left nostril, hold in long, exhale out slowly and completely through the same nostril only (left nostril), hold out long. The mental focus should be on the sound of the breath. Continue this pattern with a maximum time of 31 min for each sitting. Begin with a comfortable rate and time, but at which the effort presents a fair challenge. Holding the breath in or out long varies from person to person. Ideal time per complete breath cycle is 1 min, and each section of the cycle lasts for 15 s. Yogic experiments claim that 90 days of 31 min per day will completely eliminate all compulsive disorders. This exercise corrects all deficits of the right hemisphere that are related to these disorders.

Technique for Expanding and Integrating the Mind

Sit with a straight spine and close the eyes; bring the mental focus to the area where the root of the nose meets the eyebrows (the third eye point). Relax the hands in the lap. Begin breathing through a curled tongue that is extended out of the mouth. The sides of the tongue are curled up and the tongue then makes a "U" shape. Break the inhale into eight equal parts. Then bring the tongue into the mouth, close it, and exhale in eight equal parts through the nose. Do not pause after completing the full inhalation or full exhalation. Continue the cycle: 8 parts in through the curled tongue and 8 parts out the nose, taking about 10 s for one complete round. If desired, try using the sounds Sa, Ta, Na Ma (twice on inhalation and twice on the exhalation) instead of counting 1,2,3,4,5,6,7,8 for each part of the breath. Mentally pair the sound of the breath with each of the different syllables in the proper sequence, or just listen to the sound of the breath itself. If you cannot curl the sides of the tongue up in this fashion, take

the breath in only through the nose in eight parts, keeping the mouth closed, and exhale out through the nose in eight parts. Curling the tongue is a genetically determined ability. If you can curl the tongue in this way it will also help to stimulate the thyroid and parathyroid glands. Start with 3-5 min, build the time up to 10-15 minutes, and then up to 31 min maximum. On completing this technique, take at least three long, slow, and deep breaths through the nose and then relax.

Technique for Stimulating the Immune System

Before doing this technique it is best to practice the technique for expanding and integrating the mind. It should be attempted just after the end, after the last three long deep breaths are taken. On the last exhalation, attempt to hold the breath out fairly completely, but relaxedly, for a minimum of 1 min. Again sit with a straight spine and keep the eyes closed. The time the breath is held out is the secret here: the longer the better. With practice, 3 min can easily be reached. The minimum time to achieve the desired effect is 1 min before the nervous system recognizes this signal. Since this is done by volition, no panic is experienced. The practitioner realizes he or she can quit at any time if desired, but only part of the brain recognizes this fact. Another part of the brain triggers an "emergency reset button" in the hypothalamus to engage all healing systems. In ancient times yogis taught this technique for treating malignant but not benign tumors. It was said to be a direct means for stimulating the immune system. This procedure can easily be practiced three times a day. This technique should not be used by pregnant women after their fourth month.

Technique for a Comprehensive, Comparative, and Intuitive Mind

This is an advanced exercise and requires substantial effort. Practice is more rigorous and is best attempted after one has developed the endurance to complete the exercise for expanding and integrating the mind for 15 min. Its format is complex and the times should be followed exactly and supervised by another to indicate time periods properly, until one has gained more experience. It has four sections, with the first three sections broken into three additional parts. The sitting posture and eye position are similar to those for the exercise for expanding and integrating the mind. Begin by using the thumb of the right hand to block the right nostril, making sure to lower the elbow to reduce strain on the arm. The breathing pattern is a series of broken breaths, and the rate is about one part per second with the fourpart breath and then less thereafter.

Section 1 (Total Time: 9 Min)

PART A. Inhale through the left nostril in 4 parts and out the left nostril in 1 part; continue this pattern for 3 min.

PART B. Inhale through the left nostril in 8 parts and out the left nostril in 1 part; continue this pattern for 3 min.

PART C. Inhale through the left nostril in 16 parts and out the left nostril in 1 part; continue this pattern for 3 min.

Section 2 (Total Time: 9 Min)

Repeat the entire procedure for section 1 completely, but start by breathing through the right nostril instead and use the left thumb to block the left nostril for this entire period.

Section 3 (Total Time: 9 Min)

With both hands relaxed in the lap, complete the breathing pattern of the three parts of section 1 without blocking either nostril. The initial phase of the nasal cycle is not a concern in this exercise or in the previous ones. One side of the nose may be more difficult to breath through.

Section 4 (Total Time: 4 Min)

Relax the hands in the lap. Curl the tongue (as in the earlier exercise) and extend it from the mouth, inhale in four parts, close the mouth and exhale in one part out the nose, four parts in through the curled tongue and one part out the nose, to continue for 4 min.

When finished completely, relax on your back for 10–30 min.

Technique for Regenerating the Central Nervous System

Sit as in the previous exercises. Keep the eyes half open and focus on the tip of the nose (the end you cannot see). The eye muscles may become sore in the beginning of practice, but this will disappear with time. Hand position is as follows: males grasp the left thumb with the right hand, closing the fingers of the right hand over the left thumb (which is now enclosed). The fingers also encompass the right thumb. Females reverse the hand posture, clasping the right thumb inside. Inhale and break the breath into 16 equal parts, then exhale and break the breath into 16 equal parts. Do not hold the breath once you have completed the inhalation or exhalation. Continue breathing in this way. Each complete breath takes about 20 s. If desired, instead of counting 1–16, mentally vibrate the sounds of Sa, Ta, Na, Ma for four cycles on the inhalation and four cycles on the exhalation. Begin with a few minutes and build up slowly to 31 min maximum time. Once you have completed the technique, take several long and deep breaths, then relax. Stop if you feel you are becoming light-headed.

This exercise was reported to help regenerate the central nervous system for those who have been damaged by drugs and alcohol. It is also said that if it is practiced for 31 min/day for 120 days, one's intuition will begin to improve remarkably.

STRESS TECHNOLOGY MEDICINE: FUTURE POSSIBILITIES

The concept of "stress technology medicine" implies a state-specific scientific approach for managing life stress. A large repertoire of yogic techniques exist for effectively coping with specific problem areas. These "mind-body exercises" were once used to help prevent stress-related illness and to regenerate the individual from the effect that stress has on the CNS. As well as the few examples given in this chapter, many others exist for common problem areas, such as addictive disorders, insomnia, eliminating and preventing heart attacks, depression, phobic disorders, immunity, or problems of the mental sphere that have yet to be recognized by modern medicine.

This technology is also useful for further development of the mind. The ancients learned ways for "guiding and correcting consciousness" and for "cleansing and restructuring" the subconscious mind (134). To many this knowledge may seem like science fiction. But 15 years ago the concepts of ANS–CNS relations giving rise to this new paradigm were also unimaginable to but a few. If concepts of another form of medicine currently have no counterpart in Western scientific concepts, it does not mean that there is nothing to be gained by applying these concepts. The world of yogic medicine has a language different than that of modern science (135). But these terms can be translated to help advance our understanding of the human nervous system and our ability to augment and facilitate its functions to improve our lives. We need a contemporary view of ancient concepts, but perhaps the experimentalists of the past have more to offer than we have ever imagined. Our future holds the possibility for developing a nearly stress-resistant and disease-resistant individual. Since this "age of stress and anxiety" is testing the glands and nerves of us all, stress technology medicine may play an important role in our health.

ACKNOWLEDGMENTS

I am grateful to Yogi Bhajan for communicating the knowledge that has made possible the scientific discoveries coauthored with my colleagues and for sharing techniques from yogic medicine. I am also grateful to Dr. Pierre Lallouette, Mrs. Sarah Grace, and Mr. John DeBeer for financial support during the preparation of the manuscript. Thanks are also given to Drs. Kenneth Klivington, Tony Hunter, David Schubert, Larry Swanson, and Theodore Melnechuk for their critical reviews of the scientific text.

REFERENCES

1. Selye H. Selye's guide to stress research. New York: Van Nostrand Reinhold, 1980: v–xiii.

2. Burchfield S R. The stress response: a new perspective. Psychosom Med 1979; 41:661–672.

3. Selye H. Stress in health and disease. Boston: Butterworths, 1976: 5–6.

4. Stoksted P. Rhinometric measurements for determination of the nasal cycle. Acta Otolaryngol (Stockh) Suppl 1953; 109:159–175.

5. Hasegawa M, Kern E B. Variations in nasal resistance in man: a rhinomanometric study of the nasal cycle in 50 human subjects. Rhinology 1978; 16: 19–29.

6. Kayser R. Uber den Weg der Athmungsluft durch die Nase. Z Ohrenheilkd 1889; 20:96–106.

7. Keuning J. On the nasal cycle. J Int Rhinol 1968; 6:99–136.

8. Beickert P. Halbseitenrhythmus der vegetativen innervation. Arch Ohr Nas Kehl Heilk 1951; 157:404–411.

9. Stoksted P. Obstructions in the nose and their influence on the pulmonary functions. Acta Otorhinolaryngol Suppl 1960; 158:110.

10. Neligan J M, Strang L B. A harlequin color change in the newborn. Lancet 1952; 1005–1007.

11. Heetderks D R. Observations on the reaction of the nasal mucous membranes. Am J Med Sci 1927; 174:231–244.

12. Kuno Y. The physiology of human perspiration. London: J & A Churchill, 1934.

13. Takagi K, Sakurai T. A sweat reflex due to pressure on the body surface. Jpn J Physiol 1950; 1:22–28.

14. Kawase T. Further studies on "pressure sweat reflex". Jpn J Physiol 1952; 3:1–9.

15. Takagi K, Kobayasi S. Skin pressure–vegetative reflex. Acta Med Biol 1955; 4:31–57.

16. Ferres M. The effect of pressure on sweating. J Physiol 1958; 143:39P–40P.

17. Haight JSJ, Cole P. Unilateral nasal resistance and asymmetrical body pressure. J Otolaryngol Suppl 1986; 16(15):1–31.

18. Kennedy B, Ziegler M G, Shannahoff-Khalsa D S. Alternating lateralization of plasma catecholamines and nasal patency in humans. Life Sci 1986; 38: 1203–1214.

19. Cole P, Haight JSJ. Posture and the nasal cycle. Ann Oto Rhino Laryngol 1986; 95:233–237.

20. Werntz D A, Bickford R G, Bloom F E, Shannahoff-Khalsa D S. Alternating cerebral hemispheric activity and lateralization of autonomic nervous function. Hum Neurobiol 1983; 2:39–43.

21. Bojsen-Moller F, Fahrenkrug J. Nasal swell-bodies and cyclic changes in the air passage of the rat and rabbit nose. J Anat 1971; 110:25–37.

22. Ashley C C, Lea T J. A method for studying the cyclic changes in nasal resistance in the anaesthetized pig. J Physiol 1978; 282:1p–2p.

23. Bamford O S, Eccles R. The central reciprocal control of nasal vasomotor oscillations. Pflugers Arch 1982;394:139–143.
24. Werntz D, Bickford R G, Bloom F E, Shannahoff-Khalsa D S. Cerebral hemispheric activity and autonomic nervous function. Soc Neurosci Abstr 1980;6:196.
25. Sapen C B, Loewry A D, Swanson L W, Cowan W M. Direct hypothalamic-autonomic connections. Brain Res 1976;117:305–312.
26. Klein R, Armitage R. Rhythms in human performance: 1-½ hour oscillations in cognitive style. Science 1979;204:1236–1237.
27. Klein R, Pilton D, Prossner S, Shannahoff-Khalsa D S. Nasal airflow asymmetries and human performance. Biol Psychol 1986;23:127–137.
28. Armitage R. Ultradian rhythms in EEG and performance: an assessment of individual differences in the basic rest activity cycle. Thesis Dissertation, 1986, Carelton University, Department of Psychology, Ottawa, Ontario, Canada.
29. Goldstein L, Stolzfus N W, Gardocki T F. Changes in interhemispheric amplitude relationships in the EEG during sleep. Physiol Behav 1972; 8: 811–815.
30. Banquet J P. Interhemispheric asymmetry during sleep. In: Koella WP, ed. Sleep 1982: 6th European congress on sleep research. Basel: Karger, 1983: 178–181.
31. Barcaro U, Denoth F, Murri L, Navona C, Stefanini A. Changes in the inter-hemispheric correlation during sleep in normal subjects. Electroencephalogr Clin Neurophysiol 1986;63:112–118.
32. Rosekind M R, Coates T J, Zarcone V P. Lateral dominance during wakefulness, NREM stage 2 sleep and REM sleep. Sleep Res 1979; 8:36.
33. Hirshkowitz M, Ware J C, Karacan I. Integrated EEG amplitude asymmetry during early and late REM and NREM periods. Sleep Res 1980;9:291.
34. Herman J H, Roffwarg H P, Hirshkowitz M. Electroencephalographic asymmetries and REM sleep dreaming. Paper presented at the Association for the Psychophysiological Study of Sleep. Hyannis, MA, 1981.
35. Antrobus J, Ehrlichman H, Wiener M. EEG asymmetry during REM and NREM: failure to replicate. Sleep Res 1978;7:24.
36. Pivik R T, Bylsma F, Busby K, Sawyer S. Interhemispheric EEG changes: relationship to sleep and dreams in gifted adolescents. Psychiatr J Univ Ottawa 1982;7:56–76.
37. Moffitt A, Hoffman R, Wells R, Armitage R, Pigeau R, Shearer J. Individual differences among pre- and post-awakening EEG correlates of dream reports following arousals from different stages of sleep. Psychiatr J Univ Ottawa 1982;7:111–125.
38. Nelson J M, Phillips R, Goldstein L. Interhemispheric EEG laterality relationships following psychoactive agents and during operant performance in rabbits. In: Harnad S, Doty R W, Goldstein L, Jaynes J, Krauthamer G, eds. Lateralization in the nervous system. New York: Academic Press, 1977: 451–470.
39. Webster W G. Hemispheric asymmetry in cats. In: Harnad S, Doty R W, Goldstein L, Jaynes J, Krauthamer G, eds. Lateralization in the nervous system. New York: Academic Press, 1977: 471–480.

40. Shurley J T, Serafetinides E A, Brooks R E, Elsner R, Kenney D W. Sleep in cetaceans. I. The pilot whale, *Globicephala scammoni* (abstr). Psychophysiology 1969; 6:230.

41. Serafetinides E A, Shurley J T, Brooks R E. Electroencephalogram of the pilot whale, *Globicephala scammoni*, in wakefulness and sleep: lateralization aspects. Int J Psychophysiol 1972; 2:129–135.

42. Mukhametov L M, Supin A Y, Polyakova I G. Interhemispheric asymmetry of the electroencephalographic sleep patterns in dolphins. Brain Res 1977; 134:581–584.

43. Mukhametov L M, Lyamin O I, Polakova I G. Interhemispheric asynchrony of the sleep EEG in northern fur seals. Experientia 1985; 41:1034–1035.

44. Gordon HW, Frooman B, Lavie P. Shift in cognitive asymmetries between wakings from REM and NREM sleep. Neuropsychologia 1982; 20:99–103.

45. Lavie P, Matanya Y, Yehuda S. Cognitive asymmetries after waking from REM and nonREM sleep in right-handed females. Int J Neurosci 1984; 23:111–116.

46. Adrian E D, Matthews B H C. Berger rhythm: potential changes from occipital lobes in man. Brain 1934; 57:355.

47. Ray W J, Cole H W. EEG alpha activity reflects attentional demands, and beta activity reflects emotional and cognitive processes. Science 1985; 228:750–752.

48. Kleitman N. Sleep and wakefulness. Chicago: University of Chicago Press, 1963.

49. Kleitman N. Basic rest activity cycle in relationship to sleep and wakefulness. In Kales A, ed. Sleep: physiology and pathology. Philadelphia: JB Lippincott, 1967.

50. Dement W C, Kleitman N. Cyclic variations in EEG during sleep and their relation to eye movements, body motility, dreaming. Electroencephalogr Clin Neurophysiol 1957; 9:673–690.

51. Kleitman N. Phylogenetic, ontogenetic and environmental determinants in the evolution of sleep-wakefulness cycles. In: Kety S S, Evarts E V, Williams H L, eds. Sleep and altered states of consciousness. Baltimore: Williams & Wilkins, 1967: 30–38.

52. Wada T. An experimental study of hunger and its relation to activity. Arch Psychol Monogr 1922; 8:1–65.

53. Richter C P. Growth hormone 3.6-h pulsatile secretion and feeding times have similar periods in rats. Am J Physiol 1980; 239:E1–E2.

54. Parker D C, Rossman L. Physiology of human growth hormone release in sleep. In: Proceedings of the fourth international congress of endocrinology. Amsterdam: Excerpta Medica (ICS 273), 1973.

55. Pawel M, Sassin J, Weitzman E. The temporal relation between HGH release and sleep stage changes at nocturnal sleep onset in man. Life Sci 1972; 11:587–593.

56. Weitzman E D, Shaumburg H, Fishbein W. Plasma 17-hydroxycorticosteroid levels during sleep in man. J Clin Endocrinol Metabol 1966; 26:121–127.

57. Van Cauter E, Honinckx E. Pulsatility of pituitary hormones. In: Schulz H, Lavie P, eds. Ultradian rhythms in physiology and behavior. Berlin: Springer-Verlag, 1985: 41–60.

58. Kripke D F. Ultradian rhythms in behavior and physiology. In: Brown FM, Graeber R C, eds. Rhythmic aspects of behavior. Hillsdale, NJ: Lawrence Erlbaum Associates, 1982: 313–343.

59. Boyar R, Finkelstein J, Roffwarg H, Kapen S, Weitzman E, Hellman L. Synchronization of augmented luteinizing hormone secretion with sleep during puberty. N Eng J Med 1972; 287:582–586.

60. Shiavi R C, Davis D M, White D, Edwards A. Luteinizing hormone and testosterone during nocturnal sleep: relation to penile tumescent cycles. Arch Sex Behav 1977; 6:97–104.

61. Karacan I, Hursch C J, Williams R L, Thornby J I. Some characteristics of nocturnal penile tumescence in young adults. Arch Gen Psychiatry 1972; 26: 351–356.

62. Parker D C, Rossman L G, Vanderlaan E F. Relation of sleep entrained human prolactin release to REM-nonREM cycles. J Clin Endocrinol Metabol 1974; 38:646–651.

63. Weitzman E D. Circadian rhythms and episodic hormone secretion in man. Annu Rev Med 1976; 27:225.

64. Kimura F, Praputpittaya C, Mitsugi N, Hashimoto R, Suzuki R. Relationship between ultradian rhythms of the sleep-wakefulness cycle and growth hormone and corticosterone secretion in rats. In: Schulz H, Lavie P, eds. Ultradian rhythms in physiology and behavior. Berlin: Springer-Verlag, 1985; 61–76.

65. Takahashi Y, Kipnis D M, Daughaday W H. Growth hormone secretion during sleep. J Clin Invest 1968; 47:2079–2091.

66. Weitzman E D, Czeisler C H, Zimmerman J C, Moore-Ede, M C. In: Martin J R, Reichlin S, Bick K L, eds. Neurosecretion and brain peptides. New York: Raven Press, 1981: 475–499.

67. Kripke D F, Lavie P, Parker D, Huey L, Deftos L J. Plasma parathyroid hormone and calcium are related to sleep stage cycles. J Clin Endocrinol Metabol 1978; 47:1021–1027.

68. Sarne Y, Lavie P, Oksenberg A, Gordon C R, Luboshitzky R. Episodic secretion of humoral endorphin in sleep. Neuroendocrinol Lett 1981; 3: 365–374.

69. Watabe T, Tanaka K, Kumagae M, et al. Diurnal rhythm of plasma immuno-reactive corticotropin-releasing factor in normal subjects. Life Sci 1987; 40: 1651–1655.

70. Kalin N H, Shelton S E, Barksdale C M, Brownfield M S. A diurnal rhythm in cerebralspinal fluid corticotropin-releasing hormone different from the rhythm of pituitary–adrenal activity. Brain Res 1987; 426:385–391.

71. Rasmussen D D, Malven P V. Relationship between rhythmic motor activity and plasma luteinizing hormone in ovariectomized sheep. Neuroendocrinology 1981; 32:364–369.

72. Watanabe K, Hiroshige T. Phase relation between episodic fluctuations of spontaneous locomotor activity and plasma corticosterone in rats with suprachiasmatic nuclei lesions. Neuroendocrinology 1981; 33:52–59.

73. Gordon H W, Corbin E D, Lee P A. Changes in specialized cognitive functions following changes in hormone levels. Cortex 1986; 22:399–415.
74. Friedman S, Fisher C. On the presence of a rhythmic, diurnal, oral instinctual drive cycle in man. Am Psychoanal Assoc J 1967; 15:317–343.
75. Oswald I, Merrington J, Lewis H. Cyclical "on demand" oral intake by adults. Nature 1970; 225:959–960.
76. Tarouini B, Lombardi P, Pernice L M, et al. Ultradian structure of gastric pH at night. Abstract presented at the 54th Annual Spring Meeting, St. Cloud State University, St. Cloud, Minnesota Academy of Science, May 2–3, 1986.
77. Levin E, Kirsner J B, Palmer W L, Butler C. The variability and periodicity of the nocturnal gastric secretion in normal individuals. Gastroenterology 1948; 10:939–951.
78. Baust W, Rohrwasser W. Das Verhalten von pH und Motilitat des Magens im naturlichen Schlaf des Menschen. Pflugers Arch 1969; 305:229–240.
79. Lavie P, Kripke D F, Hiatt J F, Harrison J. Gastric rhythms during sleep. Behav Biol 1978; 23:526–530.
80. Dimagno E P, Hendricks J C, Go V L W, Dozois R. Relationship among canine fasting pancreatic and biliary secretion, pancreatic duct pressure and duodenal phase III motor activity—Boldyreff revisited. Dig Dis Sci 1979; 24:689–693.
81. Magee D F, Naruse S. Neural control of periodic secretion of the pancreas and stomach in fasting dogs. J Physiol 1983; 344:153–160.
82. Bulloch K. Neuroanatomy of lymphoid tissue: a review. In: Guillemin R, Cohen M, Melnechuk T, eds. Neural modulation of immunity. New York: Raven Press, 1985: 111–141.
83. Hall N R, Goldstein A L. The thymus–brain connection: interactions between thymosin and the neuroendocrine system. Lymphokine Res 1983; 2:1–6.
84. Roszman T L, Cross R J, Brooks W H, Markesbery W R. Neuroimmunomodulation: effects of neural lesions on cellular immunity. In: Guillemin R, Cohen M, Melnechuk T, eds. Neural modulation of immunity. New York: Raven Press, 1985: 95–109.
85. Macris N T, Schiavi R C, Camerino M S, Stein M. Effect of hypothalamic lesions on passive anaphylaxis in guinea pigs. Am J Physiol 1970; 222: 1054–1057.
86. Stein M. Bereavement, depression, stress, and immunity. In: Guillemin R, Cohen M, Melnechuk T, eds. Neural modulation of immunity, New York: Raven Press, 1985: 29–44.
87. Renoux G, Biziere K, Renoux M, Guillaumin J M, Degenne D. A balanced brain asymmetry modulates T cell-mediated events. J Neuroimmunol 1983; 5:227–238.
88. Neveu P J, Taghzouti K, Dantzer R, Simon H, Le Moal M. Modulation of mitogen-induced lymphoproliferation by cerebral neocortex. Life Sci 1986; 38:1907–1913.

89. Flor-Henry P. Cerebral dynamics, laterality and psychopathology: a commentary. In: Takahashi R, Flor-Henry P, Gruzelier J, Niwa S, eds. Cerebral dynamics, laterality, and psychopathology. Amsterdam: Elsevier Science, 1987: 1–21.
90. Marx J L. Autoimmunity in left-handers. Science 1982; 217:141–144.
91. Gerendai I. Lateralization of neuroendocrine control. In: Geschwind N, Galaburda AM, eds. Cerebral dominance: the biological foundations. Cambridge, MA: Harvard University Press, 1984: 167–178.
92. Gerendai I. Laterality in the neuroendocrine system. Presented at the Wenner-Glen Center International Symposium on The Dual Brain, May 29–31, 1986.
93. Natelson B. Neurocardiology: an interdisciplinary area for the 80s. Arch Neurol 1985; 42:178–184.
94. Orr W C, Hoffman H J. A 90-minute cardiac biorhythm: methodology and data analysis using modified periodograms and complex demodulation. IEEE Trans Biomed Eng 1974; 21:130–141.
95. Livnat A, Zehr J E, Broten T P. Ultradian oscillations in blood pressure and heart rate in free-running dogs. Am J Physiol 1984; 246:R817–R824.
96. Blinowska K, Marsh D J. Ultra- and circadian fluctuations in arterial pressure and electromyogram in conscious dogs. Am J Physiol 249: 1985; R720–R725.
97. Snyder F, Hobson J A, Goldfrank F. Blood pressure changes during human sleep. Science 1963; 142:1313–1314.
98. Hess W R. Diencephalon, autonomic and extrapyramidal functions. New York: Grune and Stratton, 1954.
99. Gellhorn E. Principles of autonomic–somatic integrations. Minneapolis: University of Minnesota Press, 1967.
100. Ischlondsky N D. The inhibitory process in the cerebrophysiological laboratory and in the clinic. J Nerv Ment Dis 1955; 121:5–18.
101. Bear D M. Hemispheric specialization and the neurology of emotion. Arch Neurol 1983; 40:195–202.
102. McIntyre M, Pritchard P B, Lombroso C T. Left and right temporal lobe epileptics. A controlled investigation of some psychological differences. Epilepsia 1976; 17:377–386.
103. Rossi G F, Rosadini G. Experimental analysis of cerebral dominance in man. In: Darley IF, eds. Brain mechanisms underlying speech and language. New York: Grune and Stratton, 1967: 167–184.
104. Eccles R, Eccles K S J. Asymmetry in the autonomic nervous system with reference to the nasal cycle, migraine, aniscoria and Meniere's syndrome. Rhinology 1981; 19:121–125.
105. Kittrelle J P, Grouse D S, Seybold M E. Cluster headache and local anesthetic abortive agents. Arch Neurol 1985; 42:496–498.
106. Shapiro C M, Catterall J R, Montgomery I, Raab G M, Douglas N J. Do asthmatics suffer bronchoconstriction during rapid eye movement sleep? Br Med J 1986; 292:1161–1164.

107. Dexter J D, Weitzman E D. The relationship of nocturnal headaches to sleep stage patterns. Neurology 1970; 20:513–518.

108. Baust W. Autonomic function during sleep. Sleep 1974: 2nd European congress on sleep research, Rome. Basel: Karger 1974: 24–33.

109. Senie R T, Rosen P P, Lesser M L, Snyder R E, Schottenfeld, D, Duthie K. Epidemiology of breast carcinoma II: factors related to the predominance of left-sided disease. Cancer 1980; 46: 1705–1713.

110. McManus I C. Predominance of left-sided breast tumors. Lancet 1977; vol. II(8032):297–298.

111. Robin P E, Shortridge R T J. Lateralization of tumors of the nasal cavity and paranasal sinuses and its relationship to aetiology. Lancet 1979; vol. I(8118):695–696.

112. Wilson J B. Thirty one years of herpes zoster in a rural practice. Br Med J 1986; 293:1349–1351.

113. Riga I N. Neural reflex in unilateral nasal obstruction syndroma. Rev Otoneuroopthalmol 1957; 29:325–335.

114. Werntz D, Bickford R G, Bloom F E, Shannahoff-Khalsa D S. Selective cortical activation by altering autonomic function. Paper presented at the Western EEG Society Meeting, Reno, Nevada, Feb 21, 1981.

115. Werntz D A, Bickford R G, Shannahoff-Khalsa D S. Selective hemispheric stimulation by unilateral forced nostril breathing. Hum Neurobiol 1987; 6:165–171.

116. Kristof M, Servit Z, Manas K. Activating effect of nasal airflow on epileptic electrographic abnormalities in the human EEG. Evidence for the reflex origin of the phenomenon. Physiol Bohemoslov 1981; 30:73–77.

117. Servit Z, Kristof M, Strejckova A. Activating effect of nasal and oral hyperventilation on epileptic electrographic phenomena: reflex mechanisms of nasal origin. Epilepsia 1981; 22:321–329.

118. Friedell A. Automatic attentive breathing in angina pectoris. Minn Med 1948; 31:875–881.

119. Gott P S, Hughes E C, Whipple K. Voluntary control of two lateralized conscious states: validation by electrical and behavioral studies. Neuropsychologia 1984; 22:65–72.

120. Swanson L W. The hypothalamus. In: Bjorklund A, Hokfelt T, Swanson LW, eds. Handbook of chemical neuroanatomy, Vol. 5, Integrated systems of the CNS, Part 1. Amsterdam: Elsevier Science, 1987: 1–124.

121. Lavie P, Kripke D F. Ultradian circa 1-½ hour rhythms: a multioscillatory system. Life Sci 1981; 29:2445–2450.

122. Hess W R. Vegetative Funktionen und Zwischenhirn. Basel: Benno Schwabe, 1947.

123. Ranson S W, Magoun H W. The hypothalamus. Ergeb Physiol 1939; 41: 56–163.

124. Gerendai I. Unilateral complete isolation of the medial basal hypothalamus interferes with the compensatory ovarian growth following unilateral overiectomy. Neuroendocrinol Lett 1980; 2:39–43.

125. Fukuda M, Yamanouchi K, Nakano Y, Furuya H, Arai Y. Hypothalamic
      laterality in regulating gonadotropic function: unilateral hypothalamic
      lesion and ovarian compensatory hypertrophy. Neurosci Letts. 1984; 51:
      365–370.
126. Nance D M, Bhargava M, Myatt G A. Further evidence for hypothalamic
      asymmetry in endocrine control of the ovary. Brain Res Bull 1984; 13:
      651–655.
127. Mizunuma H, DePalatis L R, McCann S M. Effect of unilateral orchidec-
      tomy on plasma FSH concentration: evidence for a direct neural connec-
      tion between testes and CNS. Neuroendocrinology 1983; 37:291–296.
128. Halasz B, Szentogothai J. Histologischer Beweis einer nervosen Signaluber-
      mittlung von der Nebennierenrinde zum Hypothalamus. Z Zellforsch
      Mikrosk Anat 1959; 50:297–306.
129. Bakalkin G Y, Tsibezov V V, Sjutkin E A, Veselova S P, Novikov I D,
      Krivosheev O G. Lateralization of LH–RH in rat hypothalamus. Brain Res
      1984; 296:361–364.
130. Eriksson E, Eden S, Modigh K, Haggendal J. Ultradian rhythm in rat
      hypothalamic dopamine levels. J Neural Trans 1980; 48:305–310.
131. Knobil E. A hypothalamic pulse generator governs mammalian reproduc-
      tion. News Physiol Sci 1987; 2:42–43.
132. Piepenbrock N, Valtax J L, Malquarti V, Jouvet M. Effects of hypothala-
      mic paraventricular lesions on sleep in rats. Neurosci Letts 1985; 62:151–
      156.
133. Eccles R, Lee R L. The influence of the hypothalamus on the sympathetic
      innervation of the nasal vasculature of the cat. Acta Otolaryngol 1981;
      91:127–134.
134. Shannahoff-Khalsa D S, Bhajan Y. Sound current therapy and self-healing:
      the ancient science of nad and mantra yoga. Int J Music Dance Art Ther
      1988; 4:183–192.
135. Shannahoff-Khalsa D S. A contemporary view of life force biology: the
      merging of kundalini yoga and the neurosciences. In: Srinivasan TM, ed.
      Energy medicine around the world. Phoenix: Gabriel Press, 1988: 89–
      110.

INDEX

[Ventricular vulnerability and behavioral stress]
experimental models, 438–440
poststress state and delayed myocardial ischemia, 445–448
role of the sympathetic nervous system, 441–443

[Ventricular vulnerability and behavioral stress]
sympathetic-parasympathetic interactions and myocardial electrical stability, 443–445

Yogic medicine, *see* Self-regulation for stress management (Kundalini Yoga techniques)

ABOUT THE EDITORS

MARVIN R. BROWN is Professor of Medicine at the University of California, San Diego. The author or coauthor of over 350 scientific publications, he is a member of the American Society for Clinical Investigation, Society for Neurosciences, American Physiological Society, Endocrine Society, American Peptide Society, and American Association for the Advancement of Science. He received the B.S. degree (1969) in biology and chemistry from the University of Arizona, and M.D. degree (1973) from the University of Arizona College of Medicine, Tucson.

GEORGE F. KOOB is a member (Professor) in the Department of Neuropharmacology at the Research Institute of the Scripps Clinic, La Jolla, California, and an Adjunct Professor in the Department of Psychology at the University of California, San Diego. He is the author or coauthor of over 200 journal articles, book chapters, and books, the editor of several books, and an editorial board member of *Psychopharmacology; Pharmacology, Biochemistry and Behavior; Peptides; Behavioral Neuroscience; Behavioural Pharmacology;* and *Neuropsychopharmacology*. A member of the Society for Neuroscience, American Association for the Advancement of Science, Society of Biological Psychiatry, and Research Society on Alcoholism, among others, Dr. Koob is a Fellow of the American College of Neuropsychopharmacology. He received the B.S. degree (1969) in zoology from Pennsylvania State University, University Park, and

Ph.D. degree (1972) in behavioral physiology from the Johns Hopkins University, Baltimore, Maryland.

CATHERINE RIVIER is an Associate Research Professor at The Salk Institute, La Jolla, California. The author or coauthor of over 240 journal articles, book chapters, reviews, symposium proceedings, and abstracts, she is a member of the Endocrine Society, American Physiological Society, Society for Neuroscience, Society for the Study of Reproduction, Research Society on Alcoholism, and American Association for the Advancement of Science, among others. Dr. Rivier received a "Licence es Sciences" (1968) in animal and human physiology, animal biology, biochemistry, and microbiology, and Ph.D. degree (1972) in physiology from the University of Lausanne, Lausanne, Switzerland.